# ACROSS

# Last Minute Revision

# BIOCHEMISTRY

FIRST EDITION

*Authored by*

**Saumya Shukla** DNB Radiodiagnosis
Assistant Professor
Nizam's Institute of Medical Sciences
Hyderabad, India

**Anurag Shukla** MS MCh (Orth), UK

*Edited and Proofread by*

**Monika Shukla**

**Vibha Shukla**



JAYPEE *The Health Sciences Publisher*
New Delhi | London | Philadelphia | Panama

JAYPEE Jaypee Brothers Medical Publishers (P) Ltd

**Headquarters**

Jaypee Brothers Medical Publishers (P) Ltd
4838/24, Ansari Road, Daryaganj
New Delhi 110 002, India
Phone: +91-11-43574357
Fax: +91-11-43574314
Email: jaypee@jaypeebrothers.com

**Overseas Offices**

J.P. Medical Ltd
83, Victoria Street, London
SW1H 0HW (UK)
Phone: +44-20 3170 8910
Fax: +44 (0)20 3008 6180
Email: info@jpmedpub.com

Jaypee-Highlights Medical Publishers Inc
City of Knowledge, Bld. 237, Clayton
Panama City, Panama
Phone: +1 507-301-0496
Fax: +1 507-301-0499
Email: cservice@jphmedical.com

Jaypee Medical Inc.
The Bourse
111, South Independence Mall East
Suite 835, Philadelphia, PA 19106, USA
Phone: +1 267-519-9789
Email: joe.rusko@jaypeebrothers.com

Jaypee Brothers Medical Publishers (P) Ltd
17/1-B, Babar Road, Block-B, Shaymali
Mohammadpur, Dhaka-1207
Bangladesh
Mobile: +08801912003485
Email: jaypeedhaka@gmail.com

Jaypee Brothers Medical Publishers (P) Ltd
Bhotahity, Kathmandu, Nepal
Phone: +977-9741283608
Email: Kathmandu@jaypeebrothers.com

Website: www.jaypeebrothers.com
Website: www.jaypeedigital.com



**Inquiries for bulk sales may be solicited at:** jaypee@jaypeebrothers.com

***Last Minute Revision***

***First Edition:*** **2015**

ISBN: 978-93-5152-896-8

*Printed at* Sanat Printers

*Not only this book, my whole life is dedicated to*
*"Bhagwan Ratneshwar, my Mother and Father"*

# ACKNOWLEDGMENTS


**"To Bhagvan Ratneshwar"**

At the very outset, I fail to find adequate words, with limited vocabulary at my command, to express my emotions to 'Dear God', whose eternal blessings, divine presence, and masterly guidance helps us to fulfill all our goals.

It is very difficult to find a true Guru in this materialistic world. But I am lucky and I fail to find words to express my emotions to "Swami Swayambodhanand Sarawasati" (Swami Ji) for his colossal and beautific spiritual cosseting, without which I would never have been like this.

I will always remain obliged and grateful to my teachers Professor OP Singh, MS, FICS, MAMS; Professor VD Sharma, MS, FICS, Professor Vineet Sharma, MS, FICS, Dr Ashish Mahendra, MS, MCh, FRCS, Orthopedics Department, KGMC, Lucknow, Professor KD Khare Retired HOD, AFMC, Pune and Dr RK Singh, MS, D Orthopedic for their inspiration and encouragement, which gave succor and strength to my thoughts and mapped my way to find a modus operandi for myself.

Sometimes, it is not easy to express your emotions in words especially when you have to say thanks to your parents for their constant undemanding love, dedication, sacrifice, inspiring guidance, affectionate encouragement and never ending enthusiasm; without which this book would not have seen the light of the day.

An ostentatious use of word will not be sufficient to express my heartiest thanks to Dr SK Dikshit, Mr LN Dikshit, Dr (Mrs) Arti Shukla (MD, Obs and Gyne), Dr Smita (RIMS) and Dr Sneha Dikshit (AMU), Dr Harish Dikshit, Dr VN Shukla, Dr Shraddha Shukla, Smt Kamla Devi, Mr PS Shukla and Mr Dev S Shukla, Mr Sujit Kumar Mishra, Aditi and Kriti Tripathi and Mr Manu Shukla for their meticulous efforts during the making of this book. Their valuable and critical suggestions, constant inspiration and encouragement, instinctive corrective measures, tireless efforts, unstinted cooperation and sentimental support throughout have made this marathon task a smooth journey.

It is hard to envisage how it could have happened without the assiduously deligent and ingenious editing effort and proofreading of Dr Monika, Mrs Vibha Shukla, Mr VS Shukla. And infact this book would never have been like this without the dexterous work of Mr Sayeed and Mr Saleem.

It would be a sacrilege if I do not mention the names of my friends, whom I always find with me in every field of life.

Dr Sunil Kumar Paltan (Assistant Professor Ortho, Safai)

- Dr Gopal Singh, MS Ortho, KGMC
- Dr Sachin Awasthi, MS Ortho, KGMC
- Dr Pradeep Pandey, MS Ortho, KGMC
- Dr Saurabh Agarwal, MS Ortho, KGMC
- Dr Rudra Pratap Singh, Sr Orthopedics, GTB, Delhi
- Dr Mukul Singh, Dept Ortho, KGMC
- Dr Atul Jain, MS Orthopedics, KGMC
- Dr Harish Ghoota, MS Orthopedics, KGMC
- Dr Shaleen Verma, MS Orthopedics, KGMC
- Dr Ankur Das, MS Orthopedics, KGMC
- Dr Abhishek Manu
- Dr Nitin Joshi, MS ENT, KGMC
- Dr Sandeep Tripathi, MD Pediatrics, LHMC, New Delhi
- Dr Sandeep Rai, MS General Surgery, GSVM
- Dr Suneel Chamoli, MD Psychiatry, KGMC
- Dr Ashish Gupta, MD Radiology, KGMC
- Dr Sharad Chandra, DM Cardiology, AIIMS
- Dr Vipin Gupta, MS Gen Surgery
- Dr Anil Kumar Singh, MD, Medicine MAMC, New Delhi
- Dr Nasir Ahmed, BRDMC, Gorakhpur
- Dr Jai Jag Tambe, Sr Pediatrics, LHMC, New Delhi
- Dr Gunjan Das Agarwal, MD Radiology, KGMC
- Dr Chitwan Dubey, MS Obs and Gyne, Grants, Mumbai
- Dr Ambuj, MS General Surgery, Pune
- Dr Sandhya Mishra, DNB, Obs and Gyne, Mumbai
- Dr Chander Shekher Kumar, MS Ophthal, AIIMS
- Dr Vikas Mathur, NRSMC
- Dr Parul Kakkar, Dr Gaurav Mittal
- Dr Arijit Mitra, NRSMC
- Dr Rohit Jain, MD Patho, Ahmedabad
- Dr Gunjan Raghuvanshi, MD Patho, Agra
- Dr Vineet Kumar, MD Psychiatry, PGI Chandigarh
- Dr Nilanjana Gosh
- Dr Prajna Latika
- Dr Avneet, KGMC, Dr Gopal Singh, GSVM
- Dr Athar Mohammad, KGMC
- Mr Ananad Singh
- Mr Rajpal Singh
- Mr Rajan Singh
- Mr Inder Mohan, Mr Sumit Solanki
- Mr Pranav, Mr Ravi.

When it comes to expressing the emotions, I feel hopelessly inarticulate to Dr Abu Hatim A Rashid, MCh Pediatrics Surgery, Dr Sheeba Sarvat, Dr Shafat MD, Pediatrics, SKIMS, Srinagar (J&K), Dr Mozzam Jah, Pool Officer KGMC, Dr Arif Kamal MS Ortho, Dr Arvind Kumar, Dr Mudit Khanna and Dr Yogesh Chaudhary, for their excellent constructive evaluation, humor at the time of depression and assistance at each and every step of our work.

We are greatly indebted to many individuals who helped with the preparation of this book. In particular, we are very grateful to Dr Athar Mohammad, Dr Anurag Yadav, Dr Shobana Singh, Dr Sandeep Buratodi, Dr Mohit Dhingra, Dr Vandana Dhingra, Dr Atul Dhawan, Dr Anubhav Pandey, Dr Gaurav Anand Mishra, Dr Pallavi Chaudhary, Dr Athar (Onchology), Dr Javed, Dr Parthiv Desai, Dr Devangi Desai, Dr Arun Sharma (Jaipur), Dr Sohail Ahmad, Dr OP Gupta and Dr Sarvodaya Sinha (Grants Medical College) for their constructive suggestions.

We thank Shri Jitendar P Vij (Group chairman) M/s Jaypee Brothers Medical Publishers (P) Ltd, New Delhi, India for his thoroughly professional approach. His constant interest and input has had a significant impact on the final structure of the book. It has been a pleasure to work with an individual who constantly offered wise and superb skilled suggestions. And at last but not the least, I am thankful to Mr Kailash Singh, Mr Inder Mohan, Mr Sumit Solanki, Mr Pranav, Mr Ravi Sharma and Mr Rajkumar for their extremely diligent efforts. And infact this book would never have been like this without the dexterous work of Mr Sayeed and Mr Saleem and their team at M/s Compephere.

We are grateful to the readers of the previous edition. Suggestions from students around the country have been most helpful in the formulation of this edition. We look forward to receiving similar input in the future. We hope that anyone with an idea, suggestion, or criticism regarding this book will feel free to contact us.

Such comments are always welcome and I solicit additional corrections and criticism, which maybe addressed to us at- dr_anurag_ortho@yahoo.co.in, dr_saumyadikshit@yahoo.com, siddharth_dikshit@yahoo.com

*From the Publisher's Desk*

We request all the readers to provide us their valuable suggestions/errors (if any) *at:*

**jaypeemcqproduction@gmail.com**

so as to help us in further improvement of this book in the subsequent edition.

# CONTENTS

# Chapter -1 CARBOHYDRATE METABOLISM

## QUESTIONS

### Glycolysis

1. **Enzyme catalyzing reversible step in glycolysis is /are:**
   A. Phosphofructokinase ☐
   B. Enolase ☐
   C. Pyruvate kinase ☐
   D. Phospho-glyceromutase ☐
   E. Glyceraldehyde-3-phosphate-dehydrogenase ☐
2. **Enzyme responsible for complete oxidation of glucose to $CO_2$ to water is present in**
   A. Cytosol ☐
   B. Mitochondria ☐
   C. Lysosomes ☐
   D. Endoplasmic reticulum ☐
3. **About glycolysis true is:**
   A. Occurs in mitochondria ☐
   B. Complete breakdown of glucose ☐
   C. Conversion of glucose to 3C units ☐
   D. 3 ATP's are used in anaerobic pathway ☐
4. **Fluroide ions act by inhibiting -**
   A. Enolase ☐
   B. Hexokinase ☐
   C. Cytochrome oxidase ☐
   D. Carbonic anydrase ☐
5. **In glycolytic pathway, products formed are**
   A. Fructose-2, 6-Biphosphate ☐
   B. Fructose-1, 6-Biphosphate ☐
   C. Glyceraldehyde-3-Phosphate ☐
   D. All of the above ☐
6. **Compound that joints glycolysis with glycogenesis & glycogenolysis**
   A. Glucose 1, 6 bi phosphate ☐
   B. Glucose 1 $PO_4$ ☐
   C. Glucose 6 $PO_4$ ☐
   D. Fructose 1, 6 bi phosphate ☐
7. **Peroxidase enzyme is used in estimating**
   A. Haemoglobin ☐
   B. Ammonia ☐
   C. Creatinine ☐
   D. Glucose ☐
8. **Which of the following enzymes catalyze the irreversible steps of glycolysis?**
   A. Glucokinase, phosphofructokinase, pyruvate carboxylase ☐
   B. Hexokinase, fructose1, 6 biphosphatese, pyruvate kinase ☐
   C. Glucokinase, phosphofructokinase, pyruvate kinase ☐
   D. Enolase, fructose 1,6 biphospahatase, phosphofructokinase
9. **Key glycolytic enzymes for irreversible step (s) in glycolysis is/are:**
   A. Enolase ☐
   B. Phosphofructokinase ☐
   C. Pyruvate kinase ☐
   D. Glyceraldehyde-3-phosphate dehydrogenase ☐
   E. Hexokinase ☐
10. **In glycolysis, the first commited step is catalysed by** :
    A. 2 ,3 DPG ☐
    B. Glucokinase ☐
    C. Hexokinase ☐
    D. Phosphofructokinase. ☐
11. **The rate-limiting enzyme in Glycolysis is** :
    A. Phosphofructokinase ☐
    B. Glucose-6-dehydrogenase ☐
    C. Glucokinase ☐
    D. Pyruvate kinase ☐
12. **Glycolytic enzymes (s) inhibited by fluoride:**
    A. Hexokinase ☐
    B. Aldolase ☐
    C. Enolase ☐
    D. Pyruvate Kinase ☐
    E. Phosphofructokinase ☐
13. **Fluoride, used in the collection of blood samples for glucose estimation, inhibits the enzyme**:
    A. Glucokinase. ☐
    B. Hexokinase. ☐
    C. Enolase. ☐
    D. Glucose-6-phosphatase. ☐
14. **Fluoride inhibits which enzyme**
    A. Pyruvate kinase ☐
    B. Succinyl dehydrogenase ☐
    C. Enolase ☐
    D. Aldolase ☐
15. **Anticoagulant used to estimate glucose from a sample sent from PHC is:**
    A. EDTA ☐
    B. Calcium oxalate ☐
    C. Potassium oxalate + NaF ☐
    D. Sodium citrate ☐
16. **Which of the following anticoagutant used in estimating blood glucose prevents glycolysis -**
    A. Oxalate ☐
    B. Citrate ☐
    C. NaF ☐
    D. Heparin ☐
17. **Cancer cells derive nutrition from**
    A. Glycolysis ☐
    B. Oxidative phosphorylation ☐
    C. Increase in mitochondria ☐
    D. From a fast food joint ☐
18. **Insulin acts on which enzyme in glycoysis-**
    A. Glucokinase ☐
    B. Hexokinase ☐
    C. Glucose 6-Phosphatase ☐
    D. Adenylate kinase ☐
19. **True statements about Glucokinase is/are**:
    A. Km value is higher than normal blood sugar ☐
    B. Found in liver ☐
    C. G-6P inhibit it. ☐
    D. Has both Glucose 6 Phosphatase and Kinase activity ☐
    E. Glucose enter into cells through GLUT-2 ☐
20. **After overnight fasting, levels of Glucose transporters are reduced in**
    A. Brain cells ☐
    B. Hepatocytes ☐
    C. Adipocytes ☐
    D. RBCs ☐
21. **Within the RBC, hypoxia stimulates glycolysis by which of the following regulating pathways?**
    A. Hypoxia Stimulates pyruvate dehydrogenase by increased 2,3 DPG ☐
    B. Hypoxia inhibits hexokinase ☐
    C. Hypoxia stimulates release of all Glycolytic enzymes from Band 3 on RBC membrane ☐
    D. Activation of the regulatory enzymes by high PH ☐

**22. TCA cycle does not take place in -**
A. Hepatocyte ☐
B. Osteocyte ☐
C. Neuron ☐
D. Erythrocyte ☐

**23. Mature RBC contains all except -**
A. Enzyme of HMP shunt pathway ☐
B. Enzyme of TCA cycle ☐
C. Glycoytic enzymes ☐
D. Pyridine nubleotides ☐

**24. The end product of one stage fermentation is -**
A. Formic acid ☐
B. Pyruvate ☐
C. Lactate ☐
D. Ethanol ☐

## Shuttle Systems

**25. During gluconeogensis reducing equivalents from mitochondria to cytosol are transported by**
A. Malate ☐
B. Aspartate ☐
C. Glutamate ☐
D. Oxaloacetate ☐

**26. Malate shuttle is important in**
A. Glycogenolysis ☐
B. Glycolysis ☐
C. Gluconeogenesis ☐
D. HMP shunt ☐

## PDH Complex

**27. Congenital lactic acidosis may occur d/t defect in**
A. Pyruvate decarboxylase ☐
B. PDH complex ☐
C. Transketolase ☐
D. α-ketoglutarate dehydrogenase ☐

**28. First substrate of Kreb's cycle is:**
A. Pyruvate ☐
B. Glycine ☐
C. HCl ☐
D. Lipoprotein ☐

**29. Coenzymes for pyruvate dehydrogenase are A/E**
A. TPP ☐
B. CoA ☐
C. Lipoic acid ☐
D. FAD ☐
E. NADPH ☐

**30. Pyruvate dehydrogenase complex has all enzyme components except**
A. Decarboxylase ☐
B. Transacetylase ☐
C. Dehydrogenase ☐
D. Phosphatase ☐

**31. Pyruvate dehydrogenase contains all except -**
A. Biotin ☐
B. NAD ☐
C. FAD ☐
D. CoA ☐

**32. Pyruvate can be converted directly into all the following except :**
A. Phosphoenol pyruvate ☐
B. Alanine ☐
C. Acetyl CoA ☐
D. Lactate ☐

**33. Arsenic inhibits all except**
A. PDH ☐
B. Lipoic acid ☐
C. α-KG dehydrogenase ☐
D. Enolase ☐

**34. Thiamine deficiency causes decreased energy production because**
A. It is required for the process of transamination ☐
B. It is co-factor in oxidative reduction ☐
C. It is co-enzyme for transketolase in pentose phosphate pathway ☐
D. It is co-enzyme for pyruvate dehydrogenase. ☐

## Citric Acid Cycle

**35. Oxaloacetate + Acetyl CoA → Citrate + CoASH**
**This reaction is:**
A. Reversible ☐
B. Irreversible ☐
C. Can be reversed by catalase ☐
D. Competitive ☐

**36. In TCA cycle of tricarboxylic acid, which is first formed**
A. Isocitrate ☐
B. Citrate ☐
C. Succinate ☐
D. Fumarate ☐

**37. In TCA cycle, citrate is converted into, after losing a molecule of $H_2O$ -**
A. Isocitrate ☐
B. Cis-aconitate ☐
C. Oxaloacelate ☐
D. Glutarate ☐

**38. Which of following inhibitor in TCA cycle acts by blocking citrate -**
A. Fluroacetate ☐
B. Arsenite ☐
C. Malonate ☐
D. None of the above ☐

**39. Fluroacetate inhibits -**
A. Citrate synthetase ☐
B. Aconitase ☐
C. Succinate dehydrogenase ☐
D. Alphaketoglutarate dehydrogenase ☐

**40. Which one of the following is the correct sequential order in which the given enzymes of Kreb's cycle are formed after a molecule of acetyl CoA enters the cycle-**
A. Citrate, Oxaloacetate, Ketoglutarate ☐
B. Ketoglutarate, Oxaloacetate, Citrate ☐
C. Citrate, Ketoglutarate, Oxalocetate ☐
D. Oxaloacetate, Ketoglutarate, Citrate ☐

**41. Specific poison for succinate dehydrogenase is -**
A. Cyanide ☐
B. Malonate ☐
C. Arsenite ☐
D. Fluoride ☐
E. Malate ☐

**42. What is the substrate for the only physiologically irreversible reaction in the Kreb's Citric acid cycle-**
A. Citrate ☐
B. Alpha ketoglutarate ☐
C. Succinate ☐
D. Malate ☐

**43. Intermediate metabolite in TCA cycle are A/E:**
A. Pyruvate ☐
B. Isocitrate ☐
C. Oxaloacetate ☐
D. Malonate ☐
E. Nitric oxide ☐

**44. Which of the following substance binds to acetyl CoA and condenses OAA, inhibiting the TCA cycle:**
A. Arsenite ☐
B. Fluoroacetate ☐
C. Malonate ☐
D. Fumararte ☐

**45. Malonate competetively inhibits-**
A. Fumarate dehydrogenase ☐
B. Succinate thiokinase ☐
C. Aconitase ☐
D. Succinate dehydrogenase ☐

**46. Number of ATPs produced from adipose tissue from 1 NADH (NAD+/NADH) through respiratory**
A. 0 ATP ☐
B. 1 ATP ☐
C. 2 ATP ☐
D. 2.6 ATP ☐
E. 3 ATP ☐

**47. ATP'S are formed in the following steps of kreb's cycle:**
A. Isocitrate dehydrogenase ☐
B. Succinate dehydrogenase ☐
C. Succinate thiokinase ☐
D. Malate dehydrogenase ☐

**48. In TCA cycle, $CO_2$ is released from:**
A. Thiokinase ☐
B. Isocitrate dehydrogenase ☐
C. Citrate dehydrogenase ☐
D. Alpha ketoglutrate ☐

**49. Proper functioning of Kreb cycle does not occur with deficiency of:**
A. Thiamane ☐
B. Riboflavin ☐
C. Vitamin E ☐
D. Vit K ☐

**50. Which among the following controls is an allosteric inhibitor of TCA cycle:**
A. Pyruvate dehydrogenase ☐
B. Keto glutarate dehydrogenase ☐
C. Isocitrate dehydrogenase ☐
D. Malate dehydrogenase ☐

**51. In vivo control of citric acid cycle is effected by:**
A. Acetyl CoA ☐
B. Coenzyme A ☐
C. ATP ☐
D. Citrate ☐
E. NADH ☐

**52. Of the following groups of amino acids produce common component of the TCA cycle is:**
A. Alaine, isoleucine, leucine, lysine ☐
B. Serine, asparagines, glycine, glutamate ☐
C. Isoleucine, valine, methionine ☐
D. Prolone, leucine, tryptophan ☐

**53. Increased levels of alanine in serum after fasting suggest:**
A. Increased release of alanine from muscle ☐
B. Reduced amino acid utilization for gluconeogenesis ☐
C. Break in continuity of plasma membrane resulting in leakage of amino acids ☐
D. Decreased uptake of alanine by liver ☐

**54. During prolonged starvation, the rate of gluconeogenesis depends on**
A. Increased alanine levels in liver ☐
B. Decreased cGMP in liver ☐
C. ADP in liver ☐
D. Decreased essential fatty acids in liver ☐

**55. Transamination reaction is**
A. Net deamination with splitting of $NH_3$ ☐
B. α-ketoglutarate is $NH_2$ donor ☐
C. Transaminase enzyme & pyridoxial $PO_4$ binding is covalent ☐
D. Glutamate is formed ☐
E. Non reversible pingpong reaction ☐

**56. True about amino group of amino acid is**
A. Accepted by α-ketoglutarate ☐
B. Funneled to L- Glutamate ☐
C. Prevents oxidative breakdown ☐
D. Oxidative deamination is the 1st step to remove it ☐
E. SGPT / SGOT transfer it ☐

**57. True about glutamate dehydrogenase is A/E**
A. Liver mitochondrial enzyme ☐
B. Use both $NAD^+$ or $NADP^+$ coenzyme ☐
C. Inhibited by ADP & activated by GTP ☐
D. Reversible oxidative deamination ☐

**58. Substrate level phosphorylation is catalysed by :**
A. Succinate dehydrogenase ☐
B. Thiokinase ☐
C. Malate dehydrogenase ☐
D. Hexokinase ☐

**59. Substrate level phosphorylation is seen in the conversion of:**
A. Acetoacetate to a-keto glutarate ☐
B. Succinyl CoA to Succinate ☐
C. Fumarate to malate ☐
D. Succinate to fumarate ☐

**60. Substrate-level phosphorylation seen in reaction catalysed in:**
A. Succinate dehydrogenase ☐
B. Alfa-ketoglutarate dehydrogenase ☐
C. Succinyl CoA thiokinase ☐
D. Malate dehydrogenase ☐
E. Cis-aconitase ☐

## High Energy Compounds

**61. Which of the following is high energy phosphate bond (produce ATP on hydrolysis):**
A. F-6-phosphate ☐
B. Creatine phosphate ☐
C. Carbamoyl phosphate ☐
D. Glucose-1-phosphate ☐
E. Glucose-6-phosphate ☐

**62. High energy phosphate compounds are:**
A. ATP ☐
B. ADP ☐
C. Creatinine phosphate ☐
D. Acetyl CoA ☐
E. Glucose 1 phosphate & glucose 3 phosphate ☐

## Respiratory Chain and Oxidative Phosphorylation

**63. Among the following, the maximum redox potential is for:**
A. NADH/NAD ☐
B. Succinate/Fumarate ☐
C. Ubiquinone ☐
D. $Fe^{+3}/Fe^{+2}$ ☐

**64. In oxidative phosphorylation, the ATP production and respiratory chain are linked by :**
A. Chemical methods ☐
B. Physical methods ☐
C. Chemiosmotic methods ☐
D. Conformational changes ☐

**65. About oxidative phosphorylation true is:**
- A. Generation of ATP's ☐
- B. Generation of ADP's ☐
- C. Utilization of ATP's ☐
- D. Utilization of NADP ☐

**66. Which component transfers four protons:**
- A. NADH-Q Oxidoreductase ☐
- B. Cytochrome –C oxidase ☐
- C. Cytochrome C - Q oxidoredictase ☐
- D. Isocitrate Dehydrogenase ☐
- E. Succinate Q Reductase ☐

**67. In ETC, Oxidative phosphylartion (ATP formation) is regulated by:**
- A. NADH Co-Q reductase ☐
- B. Cytochrome C oxidase ☐
- C. Glutathione reductase ☐
- D. Isocitrate dehydrogenase ☐
- E. Co-Q-Cytochrome C reductase ☐

**68. True about ATP synthase is all except:**
- A. One rotation produce 3 ATP ☐
- B. Fo unit functions as proton channel ☐
- C. $\alpha$ and $\beta$ subunits rotate ☐
- D. Bent axle is formed by $\varepsilon$ and $\gamma$ subunits ☐

**69. Internal respiration are:**
- A. Exergonic and anabolic ☐
- B. Exergonic and catabolic ☐
- C. Endergonic and anabolic ☐
- D. Endergonic and catabolic ☐
- E. Cytochrome-C reductase involved ☐

**70. Mitochondrial membrane protein contain transporter of:**
- A. NADH ☐
- B. Acetyl COA ☐
- C. NADPH ☐
- D. ATP ☐

**71. Inernal respiration are:**
- A. Exergonic and anabolic ☐
- B. Exergonic and catabolic ☐
- C. Endergonic and anabolic ☐
- D. Endergonic and catabolic ☐
- E. Cytochrome-C reductase involved ☐

**72. Cyanide is toxic because it -**
- A. Inhibits cytochrome oxidase ☐
- B. Forms cyan meth Hb ☐
- C. Inhibits ATP carrier in mitochondria ☐
- D. Inhibits Na-K-ATP ase ☐

**73. Cytochrome oxidase in oxidative phosphorylation is inhibited by:**
- A. CO ☐
- B. $H_2S$ ☐
- C. Cyanide ☐
- D. Amobarbital ☐
- E. Rotenone ☐

**74. The electron flow in Cytochrome C oxidase can be blocked by:**
- A. Rotenone ☐
- B. Antimycin-A ☐
- C. Cyanide ☐
- D. Actinomycin ☐

**75. Cellular oxidation is inhibited by :**
- A. Cyanide ☐
- B. Carbon dioxide ☐
- C. Chocolate ☐
- D. Carbonated beverages ☐

**76. The specialized mammalian tissue/organ in which fuel oxidation serves not to produce ATP but to generate heat is:** *(AI 06)*
- A. Adrenal gland ☐
- B. Skeletal muscle ☐
- C. Brown adipose tissue ☐
- D. Heart ☐

**77. Dinitrophenol causes:**
- A. Inhibition of ATP synthase ☐
- B. Inhibition of electron transport ☐
- C. Uncoupling of oxidation and phosphorylation ☐
- D. Accumulation of ATP ☐

**78. Which of following prevent formation of ATP by blocking movement of ADP across mitochondrial membrane:**
- A. Atractyloside ☐
- B. Rotenone ☐
- C. Oligomycin ☐
- D. Ouabain ☐

**79. During phagocytosis, the metabolic process called respiratory burst involves the activation of:**
- A. Oxidase ☐
- B. Hydrolase ☐
- C. Peroxidase ☐
- D. Dehydrogenase ☐

**80. Cytosolic Cytochrome C mediates**
- A. Apoptosis ☐
- B. Electron transport ☐
- C. Krebs cycle ☐
- D. Glycolysis ☐

## Glycogen Metabolism & Storage Disease

**81. In glycogen metabolism, some metabolically important enzymes found in the liver are converted from their inactive dephosphorylated state to active phosphorylated state. Which of the following is true?**
- A. Always activated by c AMP dependent protein kinase ☐
- B. Commonly seen in fasting state than in fed state ☐
- C. Catecholamines directly cause their phosphorylation ☐
- D. ATP activates phosphorylase ☐

**82. Adrenaline acts on which enzyme in glycogenolysis-**
- A. Glucokinase ☐
- B. Hexokinase ☐
- C. Phosphorylase ☐
- D. Gluc diphosphatase ☐

**83. The major fate of glucose-6 Phosphate in tissue in a well fed state is:**
- A. Hydrolysis to glucose ☐
- B. Conversion to glycogen ☐
- C. Isomerization to fructose 6 phosphate ☐
- D. Conversion to ribulose 5 phosphate ☐

**84. In the fed state, major fate of Glucose 6-$PO_4$ in tissues is**
- A. Storage as Fructose ☐
- B. Storage as Glyceraldehyde 3-$PO_4$ ☐
- C. Enters HMP shunt via Ribulose 5-$PO_4$ ☐
- D. Storage as glycogen ☐

**85. In muscle, phosphorylase b is inactivated by:**
- A. cAMP ☐
- B. Ca ions ☐
- C. Glucose ☐
- D. ATP ☐

**86. True regarding glylcogenolysis is /are A/E**
- A. $PP_1$ is a dephosphorylating enzyme ☐
- B. Vasopressin increases it ☐
- C. Oxytocin decreases it ☐

D. $Ca^{++}$ is a synchronizer and allosteric activator ☐
E. δ subunit is catalytic ☐

**87. Phosphorylase b is maintained in an inactivated state by**
A. ATP ☐
B. c AMP ☐
C. Calcium ☐
D. Insulin ☐

**88. Which of the following is a debranching enzyme -**
A. Glycogen synthetase ☐
B. Glucose-6-phosphatase ☐
C. Amylo (1,6) glucosidase ☐
D. Amylo 1,4, - 1 , 6 transglycosylase ☐

**89. Sequence of events in glycogenolysis?** ☐
A. Phosphorylase, Glucan transferase , Debranching, Phosphorylase ☐
B. Debranching, Phosphorylase, transferase, phosphorylase ☐
C. Transferase , phosphorylase, Debranching, phosphorylase ☐
D. Any of the above. ☐

**90. In which of the following tissues, is glycogen incapable of contributing directly to blood glucose?**
A. Liver ☐
B. Muscle ☐
C. Both ☐
D. None ☐

**91. Muscle cannot make use of glycogen for energy because of deficiency of:**
A. Glucokinase ☐
B. Phosphoglucomutase ☐
C. G-6-phosphatase ☐
D. Muscle phosphorylase ☐

**92. The enzyme not present in the skeletal muscles**
A. Creatinine phosphokinase ☐
B. Hexokinase ☐
C. Phosphofructokinase ☐
D. Glucose 6 phosphatase. ☐

**93. Which of the following does not cross the cell membrane**
A. Glucose-6-phosphate ☐
B. Glucose ☐
C. Nitrous oxide ☐
D. Carbon monoxide ☐

**94. Muscles are not involved in which glycogen storage disease:**
A. I ☐
B. II ☐
C. III ☐
D. IV ☐

**95. $G_6$ phosphatase deficiency seen in:**
A. Von Gierke's disease ☐
B. Taysach's disease ☐
C. Pompe's disease ☐
D. Anderson's disease ☐
E. Fabry's disease ☐

**96. An infant has hepatorenomegaly, hypoglycemia hyperlipidemia, acidosis & normal structured glycogen deposition in liver. What is the diagnosis:**
A. Her's disease ☐
B. Von Gerke's ds ☐
C. Cori's ds ☐
D. Anderson's ds ☐
E. Pompe's ds ☐

**97. A person with von Gierke's disease has ketosis. All are true for ketosis in this patient except:**
A. Lactic acidosis ☐
B. Hypoglycemia ☐
C. Fat mobilization is less ☐
D. Hypertriglyceridemia ☐

**98. The cause of hyperuricemia and gout in glucose-6-phosphatase deficiency is :**
A. More formation of pentose ☐
B. Decreased availability of glucose to tissues ☐
C. Increased accumulation of sorbitol ☐
D. Impaired degradation of free radicals ☐

**99. Glycogen storage diseases include all the following except:**
A. Von Gierke's disease ☐
B. Fabry's disease ☐
C. Mc Ardle's disease ☐
D. Fragile syndrome ☐
E. Krabbe's disease ☐

**100. Which among the following is not a cause of fasting hypoglycemia?**
A. Glucagon excess ☐
B. Glucose 6 phospatase deficiency ☐
C. Uremia ☐
D. Glycogen synthase deficiency ☐

**101. Metabolites in HMP shunt are all except**
A. Glycerol-3 phosphate ☐
B. Sedoheptulose-7 phosphate ☐
C. Glyceraldehyde-3 phosphate ☐
D. Xylulose-5 phosphate ☐

**102. NADPH is produced by:**
A. Glycolysis ☐
B. Citric acid cycle ☐
C. Hexose monophosphate shunt ☐
D. Glycogenesis ☐

**103. Which is NOT a product of Pentose phos-phate pathway**
A. Glyceraldehyde 3-$PO_4$ ☐
B. NADPH ☐
C. Sedoheptulose $PO_4$ ☐
D. $CO_2$ ☐

**104. NADPH is generated by the action of**
A. Glucose 6 Phosphate dehydrogenase ☐
B. Glucose 1 phosphate dehydrogenase ☐
C. Glucose 1.6 diphosphate dehydrogenase ☐
D. All of the above ☐

**105. HMP shunt is of great importance in cellular metabolism because it produces -**
A. ATP ☐
B. ADP ☐
C. Acetyl CoA ☐
D. NADPH ☐

**106. Dehydrogenases of HMP shunt are specific for -**
A. FAD ☐
B. NAD ☐
C. NADPH ☐
D. FMN ☐

**107. Which one of the following enzymes use NADP as coenzyme-**
A. Glyceraldehyde-3-phosphate dehydrogenase ☐
B. Lactate dehydrogenase ☐
C. Glucose-6-phosphate dehydrogenase ☐
D. Beta hydroxy acyl CoA dehydrogenase ☐
E. Mitochondrial isocitrate dehydrogenase ☐

**108. Step in HMP pathway requiring TPP**
A. G6 PD ☐
B. 6 Phoshogluconate dehydrogenase ☐
C. Transketolase ☐
D. Transaldolase ☐

**109. The main products of HMP shunt are all except -**
A. 6-NADPH ☐
B. 2-Fructose-6-PO4 ☐
C. 1-Glyceraldehyde-3-po4 ☐
D. 1-$CO_2$ ☐

**110.Which of the following enzyme is a constituent of HMP shunt-**
- A. Glucose-6-phosphatase ☐
- B. Hexokinase ☐
- C. G-6-P dehydrogenase ☐
- D. Phosphorylase ☐

**111.Sites where HMP shunts can occur include -**
- A. Liver ☐
- B. WBC ☐
- C. Lactating mammary gland ☐
- D. Testes ☐
- E. All ☐

**112.Which of the following metabolic pathways does not generate ATP:**
- A. Glycolysis ☐
- B. TCA Cycle ☐
- C. Fatty Acid Oxidation ☐
- D. HMP Pathway ☐

**113.The most common enzyme deficiency in man is -**
- A. Glucose-6-phosphate dehydrogenase ☐
- B. Glucose-6-phosphatase ☐
- C. Hexokinase ☐
- D. Glucose-1.6-diphosphatse ☐

**114.Regarding HMP shunt all of the following are true except:**
- A. Occurs in the cytosol ☐
- B. No ATP is produced in the cycle ☐
- C. It is active in Adipose tissue, Liver and Gonads. ☐
- D. The oxidative phase generates NADPH and the Non oxidative phase generates pyruvate. ☐

**115.In G-6PD deficient patient haemolysis is due to decrease in**
- A. $H^+$ ☐
- B. TPP ☐
- C. NADH ☐
- D. NADPH ☐

## Calvin Cycle

**116.Enzymes of Calvin cycle are:**
- A. G-6-PD ☐
- B. Sedoheptulose- 1-7- bisphosphatase ☐
- C. Glyceraldehyde 3 $PO_4$ dehydrogenase ☐
- D. Phosphoribulose kinase ☐

## Gluconeogenesis

**117.Glucose can be synthesized (by gluconeogenesis ) from all except**
- A. Aminoacids eg alanine ☐
- B. Glycerol from adipose tissue ☐
- C. Acetoacetate / Fatty acids/Palmitate /GH ☐
- D. Lactate/Lactic acid/ Pyruvate ☐

**118.True about Acetyl CoA:**
- A. Precursor for synthesis of cholesterol and other steroids. ☐
- B. Form ketone bodies ☐
- C. Starting material for synthesis of fatty acid ☐
- D. Arise from glycolysis ☐

**119.Acetyl Co-A acts as a substrate for all the enzymes except** :
- A. HMG-Co A synthetase ☐
- B. Malic enzyme ☐
- C. Malonyl CoA synthetase ☐
- D. Fatty acid synthetase ☐

**120.Acetyl CoA can be converted into all of the following, Except**
- A. Glucose ☐
- B. Fatty Acids ☐
- C. Cholesterol ☐
- D. Ketone bodies ☐

**121.True about gluconeogenesis:**
- A. Prevent hypoglycemia during prolonged fasting ☐
- B. Occur in both muscle and liver ☐
- C. Fructose 2,6-biphosphate stimulate it ☐
- D. Excess of acetyl co A cause stimulation ☐
- E. Carbon skeleton of amino acid is involved in gluconeogenesis ☐

**122.Which of the following enzymes is/are involved in neoglucogenesis all except**:
- A. Phosphoglycerate kinase ☐
- B. Fructose 1, 6-biphosphatase ☐
- C. Phosphoglucomutase ☐
- D. Pyruvate carboxylase ☐
- E. Isomerase

**123.Products formed from alcohol and not intermediates of TCA cycle/glycolysis:**
- A. Acetaldehyde ☐
- B. Pyruvate ☐
- C. Lactate ☐
- D. Oxalate ☐
- E. Malate ☐

**124.In well fed state gluconeogenesis in liver is inhibited by**
- A. Protein breakdown in muscle *(AIIMS Nov 11, DNB 12)* ☐
- B. Alanine content in liver ☐
- C. ADP level ☐
- D. cGMP ☐

**125.Gluconeogenesis in Fasting state is indicated by**
- A. Citrate activation by acetyl Co-A carboxylase ☐
- B. Pyruvate Carboxylase activation by Acetyl CoA ☐
- C. Fructose 1,6 bisphosphate activates Pyruvate Kinase ☐
- D. Fructose 2, 6 bisphosphate activates PFK-1 ☐

**126.Enzyme to both common in gluconegenesis and glycolysis pathway is** :
- A. Phosphofructokinase ☐
- B. Fructose 2,6-biphosphatase ☐
- C. Hexokinase ☐
- D. Glucose 6 phosphatase ☐

**127.A genetic disorder renders fructose 1,6 – biphosphatase in liver less sensitive to regulation by fructose 2,6 – bi-phosphate. All of the following metabolic changes are observed in this disorder except**:
- A. Level of fructose 1,6-biphosphate is higher than normal ☐
- B. Level of fructose 1,6 – biphosphate is lower than normal ☐
- C. Less pyruvate is formed ☐
- D. Less ATP is generated ☐

**128.Phospho-dephosphorylation of phosphofructokinase and fructose 1, 6, biphosphatase by fructose 2, 6, Biphosphate regulation is seen in**:
- A. Brain ☐
- B. Liver ☐
- C. Adrenal Cortex ☐
- D. RBC ☐
- E. Muscle ☐

**129.Glyconeogenic capability of cell is determined by the presence of**:
- A. Pyruvate dehydrogenase ☐
- B. Glucose 6 phosphatase ☐
- C. Pyruvate carboxylase ☐
- D. Fructose 1-6 biphosphatase ☐
- E. Pyruvate carboxykinase ☐

**130.Which of the following events does not occur when concentration of glucose in the liver decreases:**

A. Inactivation of phosphofructokinase-2 (PFK-2) ☐
B. Activation of Fructose Bisphosphatase-2 (Fructose 2, 6 Bisphosphatase) ☐
C. Increased levels of Fructose 2, 6 – Bisphosphate ☐
D. Increased levels of Glucagon ☐

**131. After 50 gm of glucose is feed orally:**
A. Decrease ketone body production ☐
B. Increased lactate production upon exercise ☐
C. Decreased gluconeogenesis ☐
D. Increased gluconeogenesis ☐

## Fructose Metabolism

**132. False about hereditary fructose intolerance is:**
A. Deficiency of fructose 1- phosphate aldolase. ☐
B. Accumulation of fructose 1 - phosphate in tissues ☐
C. Hyperglycemia ☐
D. Liver & kidneys are involved. ☐

**133. Fructokinase is necessary for:**
A. Fructose-1-$PO_4$ ☐
B. Ructose 1,6 diphosphate ☐
C. Fructose 6 phosphate ☐
D. Glyceraldehyde ☐

**134. An enzyme involved in the catabolism of fructose to pyruvate in the liver is:**
A. Glyceraldehyde-3-phosphate Dehydrogenase ☐
B. Phosphoglucomutase ☐
C. Lactate-dehydrogenase ☐
D. Glucokinase ☐

## Galactose Metabolism & Intolerance

**135. A few days after birth, a child becomes lethargic, refuses feeds and vomits during breast feeding. On examination he is pot bellied. Benedict's test is positive in urine. What is the likely reducing sybstance present in urine:**
A. Glucose ☐
B. Fructose ☐
C. Sucrose ☐
D. Galactose ☐

**136. Galactosaemia commonly is due to deficiency of-**
A. Galactose-1 phosphate uridyl transferase ☐
B. Galactose-1 phosphatase ☐
C. Glucose-1 phosphatase ☐
D. Glucose-6 phosphatase ☐

**137. A newborn infant refuses breast milk since the 2nd day of birth, vomits on force-feeding but accepts glucose-water, develops diarrhea on the third day, by 5th day she is jaundiced with liver enlargement and eyes show signs of cataract. Urinary reducing sugar was positive but blood glucose estimated by glucose oxidation method was found low. The most likely cause is deficiency of :**
A. Galactose-1-phosphate uridyl transferase. ☐
B. Beta galactosidase. ☐
C. Glucose-6-phosphatase. ☐
D. Galactokinase ☐

**138. A child presents with hepatomegaly and bilateral lenticular opacities. Deficiency of which of the following enzymes will not cause such features.**
A. Galactose-1-phosphate uridyl transferase ☐
B. UDP-galactose-4-epimerase ☐
C. Galactosekinase ☐
D. Lactase ☐

**139. True regarding galactosemia:**
A. Mental retardation occurs ☐
B. Absent disaccharidase in intestine ☐
C. Defect in epimerase ☐
D. Defect in galactose 1 $PO_4$ uridyl transferase ☐

**140. Reducing sugar in urine is seen in:**
A. Fanconi anemia ☐
E. Lactose intolerance ☐
C. Galactosemia ☐
D. Phenylketonuria ☐
E. Salicylate poisoning ☐

**141. The molecule, which is the intiator of cataract formation in the eye lens and whose 1- phosphate derivative is responsible for liver failure, is:**
A. Sorbitol ☐
B. Mannitol ☐
C. Inositol ☐
D. Galacticol ☐

**142. A young man finds that every time he eats dairy products he feels very uncomfortable. His stomach becomes distended. He develops gas and diarrhea frequently. These symptoms do not appears when he eats foods other than dairy products. Which of the following is the most likely enzyme in which this young man is deficient?**
A. α-amylase ☐
B. β-galactosidase ☐
C. α-glucosidase ☐
D. Sucrase ☐

## Alcohol Metabolism

**143. In chronic alcoholism the rate limiting component for alcohol metabolism excluding enzymes is / are:**
A. NADP ☐
B. NAD ☐
C. NADPH ☐
D. FADH ☐
E. FAD ☐

**144. All are used in the diagnosis of diabetes mellitus except:**
A. FBS ☐
B. HbA1c ☐
C. D-xylose absorption test ☐
D. OGTT ☐

## Carbohydrate Classification

**145. Which of the following are enantiomers:**
A. D-Galactose & L-Glucose ☐
B. d-Galactose & 1-Glucose ☐
C. D-Mannose & L-Mannose ☐
D. d-Mannose & l-Mannose ☐
E. D-glucose and L glucose ☐

**146. Epimer combination (s) is /are**
A. D-glucose & D-fructose ☐
B. D-mannose & D-talose ☐
C. D-glucose & D-mannose ☐
D. D-glucose & D-gulose ☐
E. D- galactose & D-glucose ☐

**147. Inulin like fructans are used as prebiotics as they are non digestible. Resistance to digestion in the upper GI tract results from:**
A. Absence of digestive enzyme in the upper GIT ☐
B. Beta configuration of anomeric C2 ☐
C. Low pH of the stomach ☐
D. Presence of alpha-osidic linkages ☐

## Answers:

### Glycolysis

1. **B, D, E i.e. Enolase, Phospho-glyceromutase, Glyceraldehyde-3-phosphate-dehydrogenase**
2. **B i.e. Mitochondria** *[Ref: Harper's 28/e P-149-53; Lippincott 5/e p. 96-103; Vasudevan 6/e p. 93-97; Chatterjea 7/e P-306-10]*
3. **C i.e. Conversion of glucose to 3 C units**
4. **A i.e. Enolase** 5. **D i.e. All of the above** 6. **C i.e. Glucose 6 $PO_4$**
   *[Ref: Harper's 28/e P-149-50, 583; Lehninger 5/e p. 150-53, 582-84; Vasudevan 6/e p. 93; Chatterjea 7/e p. 306-9]*
7. **D i.e. Glucose** *[Ref: Enzymes in industry & medicine Arnold: New studies in biology; http://www.ncbe.reading.ac.uk/ncbe/protocols /pracbiotech/ pdf/glucdet.pdf]*
8. **C i.e. Glucokinase, phosphofructokinase, pyruvate kinase**
9. **B i.e. Phosphofructokinase; C i.e. Pyruvate kinase; E i.e. Hexokinase**
10. **D i.e. Phosphofructokinase** *[Ref: Harper's 29/e P-170-77; Lehinger 3/e P-541]*
11. **C i.e. Glucokinase > A i.e. Phosphofructokinase** *[Ref: Harper's 28/e p. 150, 152, 166-65; Lehninger 5th/e p.578-81]*
12. **C i.e. Enolase** 13. **C i.e. Enolase** 14. **C i.e. Enolase**
    *[Ref: Harper's 27/e P-152-53; Chatterjea 7/e P-308-10]*
15. **C i.e. Potassium oxalate + NaF** 16. **C i.e. NaF** *[Ref: Chattergea & Shinde 7/e p. 308-10; Harper's 27/e p. 152-53]*
17. **A i.e. Glycolysis** *[Ref: Harper's 27/e P-151; 26/e P-136, Lehinger 3/e P541]*
18. **A i.e. Glucokinase** *Ref: Lehninger 5/e 591, 583*
19. **A i.e. Km value is higher than normal blood sugar; B i.e. Found in liver;**
    **E i.e. Glucose enter into cells through GLUT-2** *[Ref: Lehninger 5/e p. 583-85; Chatterjea 6/e P-271; Vasudevan 3/e 73, 74]*
20. **C i.e. Adipocytes** *[Ref: Lippincott 4th/ed pg-312; Lehninger 5th/ed pg-391-93, 608, 441-42]*

21. **C i.e. Hypoxia stimulates release of all glycolytic enzymes from Band 3 on RBC membrane.**
    *[Ref: Ganong 533, 670, 720, 733, 14f; http://www.jbc.org/cgi/content/abstract/266/7/4106; http://www.pnas.org/cgi/content/full/102/7/2402]*
22. **D i.e. Erythrocytes** 23. **B i.e. Enzymes of TCA cycle**
24. **D i.e. Ethanol** *[Ref: Harper's 27/e p. 151, Lippincott's 4/e p. 96]*

### Shuttle Systems

25. **A i.e. Malate** 26. **B i.e. Glycolysis**
    *[Ref: Harper's 28/e P-155; Vasudevan 6/e p. 228; Chatterjea 7/e P-321-22]*

### PDH- Complex

27. **B i.e. PDH complex** 28. **A i.e. Pyruvate**
29. **E i.e. NADPH** 30. **D i.e. Phosphatase**
31. **A i.e. Biotin** *[Ref: Lippincott's 5/e p. 109-12]*
32. **A i.e. Phosphoenol Pyruvate** *[Ref: Harper's 28/e P-155, 165-67; Lippincott 5/e p. 105-103, 118; Shinde & Chatterjea 6/e P-305]*
33. **D i.e. Enolase**
34. **D i.e. It is coenzyme for pyruvate dehydrogenase**

### Citric Acid Cycle

35. **B i.e. Irreversible**
36. **B i.e. Citrate** 37. **B i.e. Cis aconitate**
38. **A i.e. Fluroacetate** 39. **B i.e. Aconitase**
40. **C i.e. Citrate, ketoglutarate, oxaloacetate** 41. **B i.e. Malonate**
42. **B i.e. Alphaketoglutarate** 43. **A i.e. Pyruvate, D i.e. Malonate, E i.e. Nitric oxide**
44. **B i.e. Fluoroacetate** 45. **D i.e. Succinate dehydrogenase**
46. **D i.e. 2.6 ATP** *[Ref: Lehninger 5th/e p. 630; Harper's 28/e P-143-46; Chatterjea 7/e p. 316-19; Lippincott's 5/e p. 109-13; Vasudevan 6/e p. 219]*

47. **A i.e. Isocitrate dehydrogenase; B i.e. Succinate dehydrogenase; C i.e. Succinate thiokinase; D i.e. Malate dehydrogenase**
48. **B i.e. Isocitrate dehydrogenase**
49. **A i.e. Thiamine; B i.e. Riboflavin** *[Ref: Harper's 28/e P-146]*
50. **C i.e. Isocitrate dehydrogenase** *[Ref: Debajyoti Das 101]*
51. **C i.e. ATP, E i.e. NADH**
52. **C i.e. Isoleucine, Valine, methionine**
*[Ref: Harper's 28/e P-147, 248; Lehninger 5/e p. 861]*
53. **A i.e. Increased release of alanine from muscle:** *[Ref: Harper 29/e p 192-93; Lehninger 5/e p 681, 915, 548, 598; Lippincott 5/e p 331-32]*
54. **A i.e. Increased alanine level in muscle**
55. **C i.e. Transaminase enzyme & pyridoxial $PO_4$ binding is covalent; D i.e. Glutamate is formed** *[Ref: Gray's 40/e p 974]*
56. **A, B, C, E i.e. Accepted by α-ketoglutarate; Funneled to L- Glutamate; Prevents oxidative breakdown; SGPT/SGOT transfer it**
57. **C i.e. Inhibited by ADP & activated by GTP**
58. **B i.e. Thiokinase**
59. **B i.e. Succinyl CoA to succinate**
60. **C i.e. Succinyl CoA thiokinase**

## High Energy Compounds

61. **B, C i.e. Creatine phosphate; Carbamoyl phosphate**
62. **A, C, D i.e. ATP, Creatinine phosphate, Acetyl CoA** *[Ref: Vasudevan 6/e p. 225-26; Harper 28/e p. 94; Satyanaran 3/e 222-23]*

## Respiratory Chain & Oxidative Phosphorylation

63. **D i.e. $Fe^{2+}$** *[Ref: Lippincott 5/e p. 76-77; Harper 28/e p. 99, 103-5; Chatterjea 7/e p. 133-129; Lehninger 5/e p. 708-18-515]*
64. **C i.e. Chemiosmotic methods**
65. **A i.e. Generation of ATPs**
66. **A i.e. NADH-Q Oxidoreductase; C i.e. Cytochrome C-Q oxidoreductase**
67. **A, B, E i.e. (NADH Co-Q reductase, Cytochrome C oxidase, Co-Q-Cytochrome C reductase)**
68. **C i.e. α and β subunits rotate**
69. **B i.e. Exergonic & Catabolic; E i.e. Cytochrome – C reductase involved**
*[Ref: Chatterjea 6/e P-120-130; Lehninger 3/e P- 661- 72]*
70. **A i.e. NADH, C i.e. NADPH; D i.e. ATP***[Ref: Harper's 28/e P-109-110; Lippincott 5/e p. 79-80; Lehninger 3/e P-660; Vasudevan 6/e p. 234]*
71. **B i.e. Exergonic & Catabolic; E i.e. Cytochrome C reductase involved**
72. **A i.e. Inhibits Cytochrome oxidase**
73. **A i.e. CO; B i.e. $H_2S$; C i.e. Cyanide**
74. **C i.e. Cyanide**
75. **A i.e. Cyanide**
76. **C i.e. Brown adipose tissue**
77. **C i.e. Uncoupling of oxidation & phosphorylation**
78. **A i.e. Atractyloside** *[Ref: Harper 28/e p. 108-10; Chatterjea 7/136-37; Vasudevan 6/e p. 234; Lehninger 5/e p 714; Lippincott 5/e p. 77-79]*
79. **A i.e. Oxidase** *[Ref: Robbins 7th/60; Chatterjea 6/e P-18]*
80. **A i.e. Apoptosis** *[Ref: Robbins 7/e p-29-30]*

## Glycogen Metabolism & Storage Diseases

81. **B i.e. Commonly seen in fasting state than in fed state**
82. **C i.e. Phosphorylase**
83. **B i.e. Conversion to Glycogen**
84. **D i.e. Storage as glycogen**
85. **D i.e. ATP**
86. **C and E i.e. Oxytocin decreases it and δ subunit is catalytic**
87. **D i.e. Insulin** *[Ref: Harper's 28/e p.158-62; Lippincott's 4/e p. 132-33; Chattergea & Shinde 7/e p. 327-30; Lehninger 5th/ed pg 603-04]*
88. **C i.e. Amylo 1, 6 glucosidase**
89. **A i.e. Phosphorylase, Glucan transferase, Debranching, Phosphorylase**
90. **B i.e. Muscle**
91. **C i.e. G- 6- Phosphatase**
92. **D i.e. Glucose –6 – phosphatase** *[Ref: Harper's 28/e P-146-148, 159; Lippincott 5/e p. 130; Vasudevan 6/e p. 108]*
93. **A i.e. Glucose-6-phosphate**
94. **A i.e. I**
95. **A i.e. Von gierke's disease**
96. **B i.e. Von gierke's disease**
97. **C i.e. Fat mobilization is less**
98. **A i.e More formation of pentose** *[Ref : Chatterjea 7/e P-331; 6/e p. 293]*
99. **B i.e. Fabry's disease; D i.e. Fragile syndrome; E i.e. Krabbe's disease**
100. **A i.e. Glucagon excess** *[Ref: Harper's 28/e P-160, 298; Lippincott 5/e p. 130; Lehninger 5/e p. 599; Chatterjea 7/e p. 330-31; Vasudevan 6/e p. 123, 111; Harrison 17/e p. 2459]*
101. **A i.e. Glycerol –3-phosphate**
102. **C i.e. Hexose monophosphate shunt**

103. D i.e. $CO_2$
104. A i.e. Glucose 6 phosphate dehydrgenase
105. D i.e. NADPH
106. C i.e. NADPH
107. C i.e. Glucose 6 phosphate dehydrogenase
108. C i.e. Transketolase
109. D i.e. 1 $CO_2$
110. C i.e. G-6-P- dehydrogenase
111. A i.e. Liver, C i.e. Lactating mammary gland; D i.e. Gonads
112. D i.e. HMP – Shunt *[Ref: Lippincott's 5/e p. 145-148; Harper's 28/e p. 174-78; Chattergea & Shinde 7/e p. 332-38;Lehninger 5th/e p. 630]*
113. A i.e. Glucose-6- $PO_4$ dehydrogenase *[Ref: Lippincott's 4/e p. 103]*
114. D i.e. The oxidative phase generates NADPH and non oxidative phase generates pyruvate *[Ref: Lippincott's 4/e p. 147]*
115. D i.e. NADPH *[Ref: Lippincott 5/e p. 152-54; Lehninger 5/e p. 559]*

## Calvin Cycle

116. B, D, C i.e. Sedoheptulose- 1-7- bisphosphatase; Phosphoribulose kinase; Glyceraldehyde 3 $PO_4$ dehydrogenase *[Ref: Lehninger 5/e p. 774-86]*

## Gluconeogenesis

117. C i.e. Acetoacetate / Fatty acids/Palmitate /GH
118. ALL i.e. (Precursor for synthesis of cholesterol and other steroids, Form ketone bodies, Starting material for synthesis of fatty acid, Arise from glycolysis)
119. B i.e. Malic Enzyme
120. A i.e. Glucose
*[Ref: Harper 29th/e p. 123, 164, 187-189; Chatterjae 8/e p 338, 441; Vasudevan 6/e p. 216, 450, 407; Thomas Miller (2002); Kaplan lecture notes (2007) p-201; Lippincott 4th/ed pg-- 266, 111-12, 220, 96, 119, 192, 195-96 Lehninger 5th/ed pg- 616-17, 695, 557]*
121. A i.e. Prevent hypoglycemia during prolonged fasting; D i.e. Excess of acetyl co A cause stimulation; E i.e. Carbon skeleton of amino acid is involved in gluconeogenesis *[Ref: Harper 29/e p. 187-94; Lippincott 6/e p. 331-32, 326, 329]*
122. C i.e. Phosphoglucomutase *[Ref: Harper's 29/e p. 179, 187-90; Chatterjea 8/e p. 364-69]*
123. A i.e. Acetyldehyde *[Ref: Harper's 27/e p. 225-26; Lippioncott's 4/e p. 317-18]*
124. C i.e. ADP level
125. B i.e. Pyruvate carboxylation activation
126. A i.e. Phosphofructokinase
127. A i.e. Level of Fructose 1, 6- biphosphate is higher than normal
128. B i.e. Liver
129. D i.e. Fructose 1,6 biphosphate
130. C i.e. Increased levels of Fructose 2, 6 – Bisphosphate *[Ref:Harper 29/e p. 187-93; Lippincott 5/e p. 117-122; Lehninger 5/e p. 582-87 ]*
131. C i.e. Decreased gluconeogenesis *[Ref: Lippincott 4th/ed pg-322-23,329; Teitz 6th/ed pg-376,388; Chatterjea 7th/ed pg-363-64]*

## Fructose Metabolism

132. C i.e. Hyperglycemia *[Ref: Harper's 27/e P-183; Harrison 16/e P-2321]*
133. A i.e. Fructose –1- $PO_4$ *[Ref: Harper's 27/e P-183-84]*
134. A i.e. Glyceraldehyde- 3- phosphate dehydrogenase *[Ref: Harper's 27/e P-183-184; 26/e P-169]*

## Galactose Metabolism & Intolerance

135. D i.e. Galactose
136. A i.e. Galactose–1–Phosphate uridyl transferase
137. A i.e. Galactose–1–phosphate uridyl transferase
138. D i.e. Lactase
139. A i.e Mental retardation occurs; C i.e Defect in epimerase; D i.e Defect in galactose –1 $PO_4$ uridyltransferase
140. C i.e. Galactosemia
141. D i.e. Galactitol
142. D i.e. Sucrase *[Ref: Harper's 27/e P-184-185; Chatterjea 6/e P- 312-313, 264-65, Nelson 17/e P-1268]*

## Alcohol Metabolism

143. B & C i.e. $NAD^+$ & NADPH *Ref: Lippincott 4th/ed pg- 317-18; Harper 28th/ed pg- 630-29, 218-20; Lehninger 5th/ed pg-547,664,518*
144. C i.e. D-xylose absorption test

## Carbohydrate Classification

145. **C i.e. D-Mannose & L-Mannose; D i.e. d-Mannose & l-Mannose; E i.e. D-glucose and L glucose**
146. **C, E i.e. D-glucose & D-mannose, D- galactose & D-glucose**
*[Ref: Harper 28/e p. 114-15; Lippincott 5/e p. 83-85; Lehninger 5/e p. 236-40]*
147. **B i.e. Beta configuration of anomeric C2** *[Ref: Harper 28/e p. 118-19; Lippincott 5/e p. 86-87; Lehninger 5/e p. 246-50; 'Food and Nutrition supplements: Their role in health and disease' (Springer) 1st (2001)/130; 'Colonic Microbiota, Nutrition and Health' by Gibson & Roberfroid 1st (1999)/105]*

# CARBOHYDRATE METABOLISM: REVIEW NOTES

## Glycolysis (Embden Meyerhof Pathway)

Glycolysis is the cytosolic pathway of all mammalion cells for the ***metabolism of glucose (or glycogen) to pyruvate and lactate***[Q].

- In glycolysis glucose ($C_6$) is ***converted into 3C units substances; pyruvate ($C_3$) and lactate ($C_3$)***[Q].
- All the enzymes of glycolysis are present in ***cytosol***[Q].
- This is ***not a complete breakdown***[Q] of glucose as *pyruvate further enters mitochondria* to completely degraded into $CO_2$ and $H_2O$.
- It is unique in the sense that it can function either aerobically or anaerobically.

| Aerobic Condition | Anaerobic Condition |
|---|---|
| Under aerobic condition final product is *pyruvate*[Q] | - ***Lactate***[Q] is a final product<br>- Erythrocytes, which lacks mitochondria ($O_2$ supply) completely reliant on glucose as their metabolic fuel. |

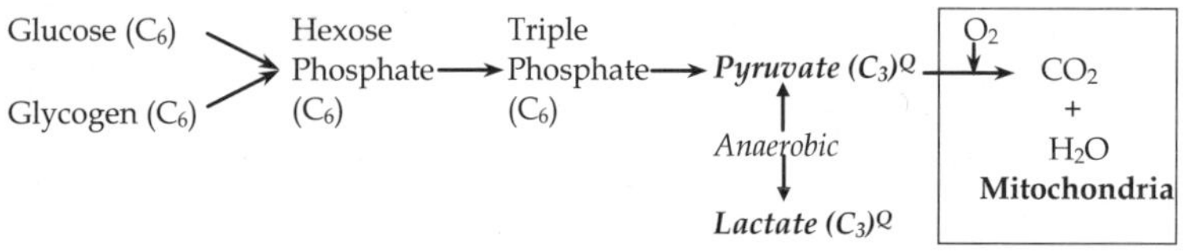


## Energy Production per Molecule of Glucose

### Common in both aerobic & anaerobic conditions

- **Steps at which energy is utilized** (ATP consumption)

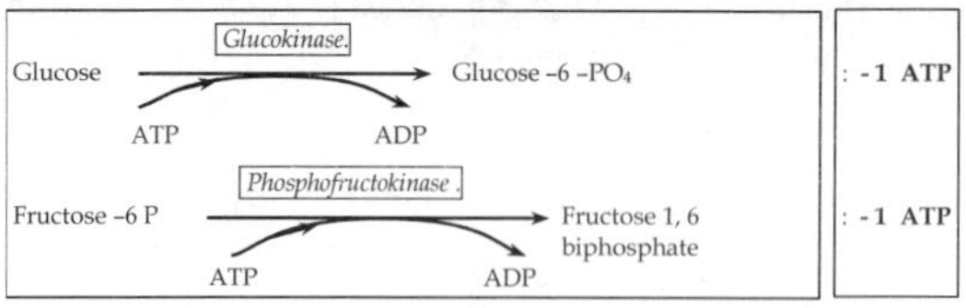


- **Steps where energy (ATP) is produced**

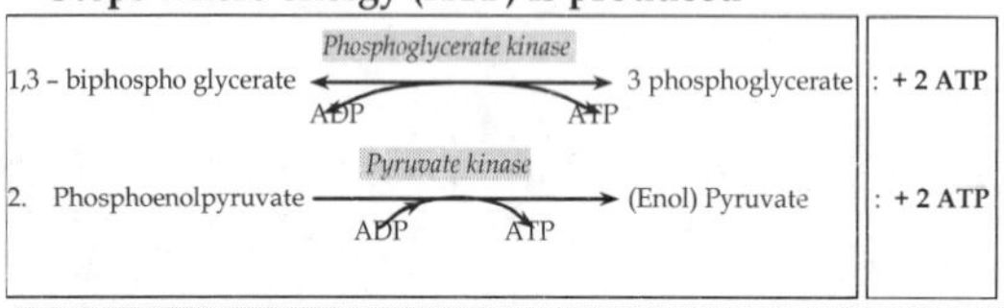


**Net ATP produced in anaerobic condition=4-2=*2ATP***[Q]

### Reaction occurring in aerobic conditions only

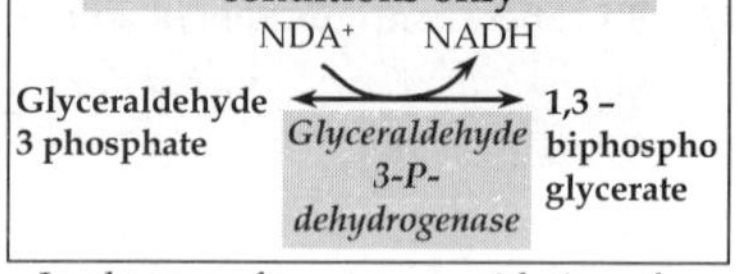


- In absence of oxygen, reoxidation of NADH at glyceraldehyde -3P - dehydrogenase stage cannot take place in electron transport chain.
- ATP gained from 1NADH according to old concept is 3ATP but according to new concept it is **1.5** or **2.5** depending on shuttle. So for 2NADH, 5 ATP will be produced (or 6 a/t old concept)
- Because **1 glucose molecule** yields **2 molecules of glyceraldehydes 3-phosphate**, the overall production of NADH per molecule of glucose is 2
- So for **2 NADH; 5ATP** will be produced (or 6 a/t old concept)
- Hence the net ATP gain in glycolysis in **Aerobic conditions** is 5 (from NADH) + 4 -2 = **7 ATP** (a/t new concept) / 6 (from NADH) + 4-2 = **8 ATP** (a/t old concept)

## Embden-Meyerhof Pathway of Glycolysis

- **Fructose – 2, 6 Biphosphate** is *not a part of glycolytic pathways but is formed during glycolysis.*
- When the body has abundant supply of glucose:
  Fructose 2,6 biphosphate is formed *from fructose -6 $PO_4$ by* the action of *phosphofructokinase -2 (PFK-2).*
- If Glucose supply is not adequate:
  Fructose 2, 6 biphosphate is converted back to Fructose - 6- $PO_4$ by PFK -2 which now acts as fructose - 2, 6 biphosphotase
- Phosphofructokinase -2 is a bifunctional enzyme.
- Fructose 2, 6 biphosphate has a ***unique role to play in the regulation of Glycolysis and Gluconeogenesis***[Q].
  - ***Positive allosteric effector of phosphofructokinase -1***[Q] (rate limiting enzyme of glycolysis)
  - ***Inhibitor of Fructose 1, 6 Biphosphatase***[Q] (enzyme of Gluconeogenesis)
- At each of 3 points where glycolytic reactions are bypassed by alternative gluconegenic reactions, simultaneous operation of both pathways would consume ATP without accomplishing any chemical or biological work, ie ATP is hydrolysed and large amount of chemical energy is dissipated as heat without any useful metabolic work being done. Therefore these uneconomical bypass processes are called **futile cycle**. However, **substrate cycle** is a better name because these provide *advantages for controlling pathways.*

That means

| | | |
|---|---|---|
| **↑ed Fructose 2, 6 - Biphosphate** | → | **↑ Glycolysis, ↓ Gluconeogenesis** |
| **↓ed Fructose 2, 6- Biphosphate** | → | **↓ Glycolysis, ↑Gluconeogenesis** |

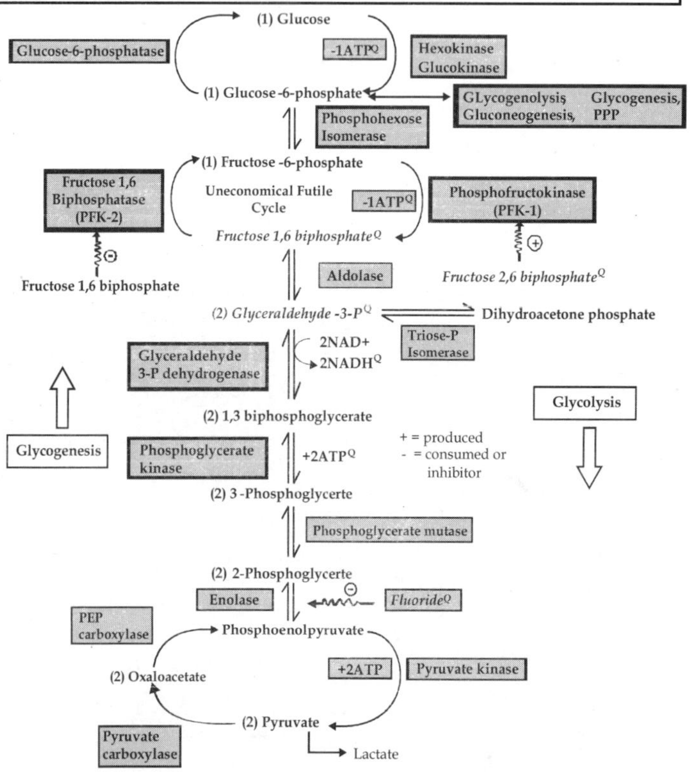


**Opposing pathways of Glycolysis & Gluconeogenesis**

## Oxidase – Peroxidase Test Strips

It is new highly specific method for estimating glucose in blood & urine. **Glucose oxidase** enzyme produce hydrogen **peroxide** & gluconic acid from glucose. And peroxidase catalyzes the reaction of $H_2O_2$ with colourlesspotassium iodide to brown iodide. This produces a colour change, the intensity of which may indicate glucose concentration in some tests (such as Boehringer, Diastix). **Horseradish peroxidase** (HRP) are used for histochemistry & ELISA because of their excellent stability, low molecular weight and its ability to produce chromogenic products (such as peroxidase labelled antibodies).

$$\textbf{Glucose} + H_2O + O_2 \xrightarrow{\text{Oxidase}^Q} \mathbf{H_2O_2} + \text{Gluconic acid } (\delta\text{-gluconolactone})$$

*Peroxidase*Q ↓ ← KI

**Brown Iodide**

## Inhibitors of Metabolic Pathway

**Kreb's cycle**

1. ***Fluoroacetate*** inhibits ***Aconitase***Q

   Citrate ⟷ (***Aconitase***) Cis-aconitate

2. ***Arsenite*** inhibits ***α- ketoglutarate dehydrogenase***Q

   α-ketoglutarate ⟷ (α-Ketoglutarate dehydrogenase) Succinyl COA

3. ***Malonate*** inhibits ***succinate dehydrogenase***Q.

   Succinate ⟷ (Succinate dehydrogenase) Fumarate

**Glycolysis**

1. ***Iodo-aetate***Q inhibits ***Glyceraldehyde 3-P-dehydrogenase***Q

   Glyceraldehyde 3 phosphate ⟷ (Glyceraldehyde 3-P-dehydrogenase) 1,3 – biphosphoglycerate

2. ***Fluoride*** inhibits ***Enolase***Q

   2 phosphoglycerate ⟷ (Enolase; **$Mg^{2+}/Mn^{2+}$**) Phospho enolpyruvate

## Enzyme (Genes) and Pathways regulated by Insulin

**Increased** Expression

**In Glycolysis**
- *Hexokinase II*Q
- *Hexokinase IV (i.e. glucokinase)*Q
- Phosphofructokinase (PFK-1)
- Pyruvate kinase

**In regulation of glycolysis/ gluconeogenesis**
- PFK-2 / FBP ase-2

**In Pentose phosphate pathway (NADPH)**
- Glucose-6-phosphate deydrogenase
- 6- phosphogluconate dehydrogenase

**In Fatty acid desaturation**
- Stearoyl CoA deydrogenase

**In Triacyl glycerol synthesis**
- Acyl-CoA- glycerol transferase

**In Fatty acid synthesis**
- Pyruvate dehydrogenase
- Acetyl CoA carboxylase
- Malic enzyme (NADPH)
- ATP citrate lyase (provides acetyl CoA)
- Fatty acid synthase complex

**Decreased** Expression

| | |
|---|---|
| PEP carboxykinase | Gluconeogenesis |
| Glucose-6-phosphatase | Glucose release to blood |

## Hexokinase and Glucokinase

- **Hexokinase**, which *catalyzes the entery of glucose into glycolytic* pathway (by converting glucose to glucose 6 $PO_4$), is a *regulatory enzyme.* Humans have 4 isoenzymes (I to IV)
- Predominant isoenzyme type of **myocyte (muscle)** is **hexokinase II > I**. It has low Km and high affinity fo glucose. It normaly acts at or near its maximal rates (because Km=0.1 is much lower than blood glucose conc. 4-5 mM) and is allosterically inhibited by their product glucose 6 – phosphate
- Predominant hexokinase isoenzyme of **liver** is **hexokinase IV (glucokinase)** which differs from hexokinase I-III of muscle in 3 respects

1. **Km** or **glucose concentration at which glucokinase is half saturated (10 mM) is higher** than usual concentration of glucose in blood. Because an efficient glucose trasporter **(GLUT-2)** rapidly equilibrates glucose concentration in cytoplasm (of liver cell) & blood, the high km of glucokinase allows its direct regulation by blood glucose level.

| Features | Hexokinase (I-III) | Glucokinase (Hexokinase IV) |
|---|---|---|
| Found in | *All tissues including fetal & adult liver* | ***Adult liver only***Q |
| **Km**<br>**Affinity** (for glucose) | ***Low (0.1 mm)***Q<br>**High** | ***High (10 mM)***Q<br>**Low** |
| Stability | More | Less (labile) |
| phosphorylate | Any hexose (non specific) | Glucose (specific) |
| **Allosteric inhibition** | ***Glucose – 6- PO₄***Q | ***Fructose-6-phasphate***Q |

**High blood glucose** level (After carbohydrate rich meal)

Excess glucose transported into hepatocytes & converted to glucose – 6 $PO_4$ by glucokinase. Because it is only half saturated at 10 mM glucose, its activity continues to rise as glucose concentration rises to >10 mM

So its ***main function is to clear glucose from blood at levels > 100 mg/dl***[Q].

**Low blood glucose** level (after fasting)

Glucose concentration in hepatocyte is low due to its *low affinity* (high km) and the glucose generated by gluconeogenesis leaves the cell before being trapped by phosphorylation.

So it ***makes glucose available to tissue at lower blood glucose levels***[Q].

| Glucose feeding | No change | Increased |
|---|---|---|
| **Fasting /DM** | Not much change | Decreased |
| GH, Glucocortico-steroids | Inhibit | Inhibit |
| Insulin | Induce | Induce |
| Function | Make glucose available to tissues for oxidation at lower blood glucose level | Clear glucose from blood after meals (leves > 100 mg/dl) |

2. ***Glucokinase is not inhibited by glucose-6 – $PO_4$***[Q] and it can therefore continue to operate when the accumulation of glucose – 6- $PO_4$ completely inhibits hexokinase I- III.
3. Glucokinase is inhibited by reversible binding of **regulatory protein** specific to liver (and more tightly in presence of **allosteric effector fructose -6- phosphate)**. Glucose competes with fructose 6-$PO_4$ for binding & cause dissociation of regulatory protein from hexokinase (in nucleus), relieving the inhibition. Whereas during fast, (glucose <5 mM), fructose 6-$PO_4$ triggers inhibition of glucokinase by regulatory protein, so liver does not complete with other organs for scarce glucose

★ Glucose enter into cells by *GLUT – 2* in the liver *under control of insulin*. GLUT –2 has higher km value for glucose hence transport glucose only when blood sugar is high.

★ **GLUT-4** Work *in muscle* cells and *adipocytes*.

## Glucose Transporters

**Insulin dependent (sensitive)**
Facilitated transport

| | |
|---|---|
| - *Adipose tissue*[Q]<br>- **Skeletal Muscle**<br>- **Heart** | **GLUT-4** |

↓
**Decrease in fasting**

**Insulin insensitive (not dependent)**

**Active transport**

- Intestine epithelium
- Renal tubules
- Choroid plexus

**Facilitated transport**

| | |
|---|---|
| RBC<br>Liver<br>Brain | GLUT-1<br>GLUT 2<br>GLUT 3 |
| Intestine, Testis, Kidney, Sperm | GLUT 5 |
| Leukocyte, Spleen | GLUT6 |
| Lens<br>Cornea | |

## Shuttle System

Mitochondrial (inner) membrane is impermeable to NADH. The NADH generated in **glycolysis** are transported from cytoplasm to mitochondria for oxidation by shuttles (mainly matale)

**Malate shuttle**

- This is more common and universal shuttle used mainly in liver, kidney & heart
- *Oxidation of reduced* **NADH + $H^+$** in mitochondria *yields* ***3 ATP***[Q] ***(old)/ 2.5 ATP (new)***
- When body utilized malate shuttle, net ATP production by glycolysis – TCA cycle per glucose molecule oxidized will be *38* ***ATP***[Q]**/32 ATP** (new).
- The complexity of this system is d/t impermeability of mitochondrial membrane to O.AA, which must react with glutamate & transaminate to aspartate and α - ketoglutarate before transport through mitochondrial membrane & reconstitution to O.A.A in cytosol.

**Glycerophosphate shuttle**

- This is present in some tissue (*e.g. brain, white skeletal muscle*) and absent in others (e.g. Heart muscle)
- ***FAD***[Q] dependent so *only* ***2 ATP***[Q] *(old)*/**1.5 ATP** (new) are produced.
- When body utilizes this system, net ATP production is ***36 ATP***[Q] (old)/**30 ATP** (new.)

**Malate Shuttle**

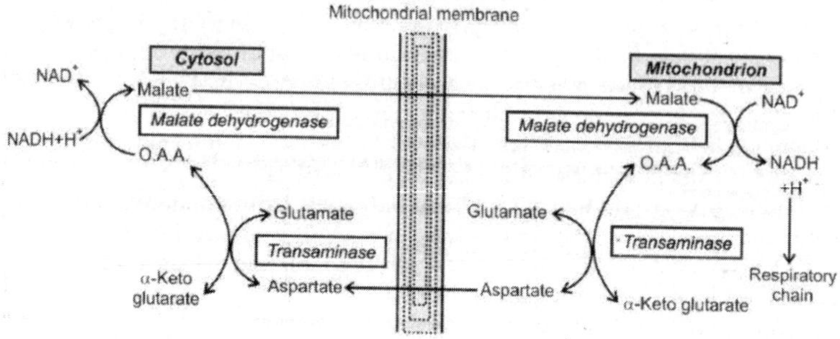

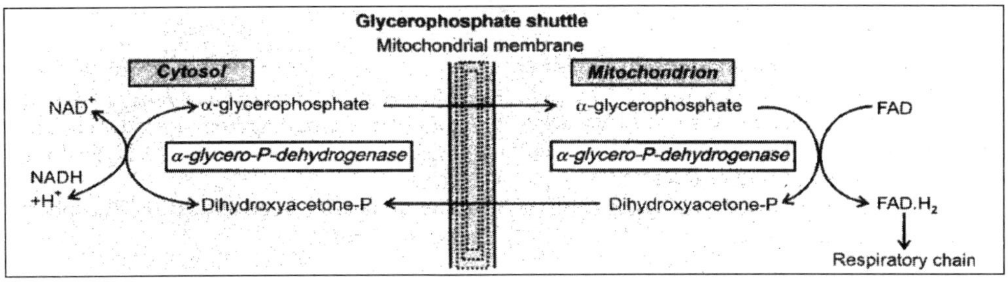


## Pyruvate Dehydrogenase (PDH) Complex

It is not the part of TCA cycle, but is the *major source of acetyl CoA – a 2 carbon substrate for cycle.* The **irreversibility** of PDH reaction precludes the formation of pyruvate from acetyl CoA, and explains why glucose cannot be formed from acetyl CoA by gluconeogenesis. PDH complex is a multimolecular aggregate of 3 enzymes components and 2 regulatory enzymes.

| **Component enzyme** | Coenzyme |
|---|---|
| $E_1$ = **Pyruvate dehydrogenase (decarboxylase)** | ***Thiamine pyrophosphate (TPP)***Q |
| $E_2$ = **Dihydrolipoyl trans acetylase** | ***Lipoic acid & CoA***Q |
| $E_3$ = **Dihydrolipoyl dehydrogenase** | ***FAD, & NAD+***Q |

| **Regulatory enzyme** | Activator of enzyme | Action |
|---|---|---|
| **PDH kinase** (c-AMP- independent) | ATP, Acetyl CoA, NADH | Phosphorylates & inhibits (turn.off) E1 |
| **PDH phosphatase** | $Ca^{++}$ | Dephosphorylates or activates (turn on) $E_1$ |

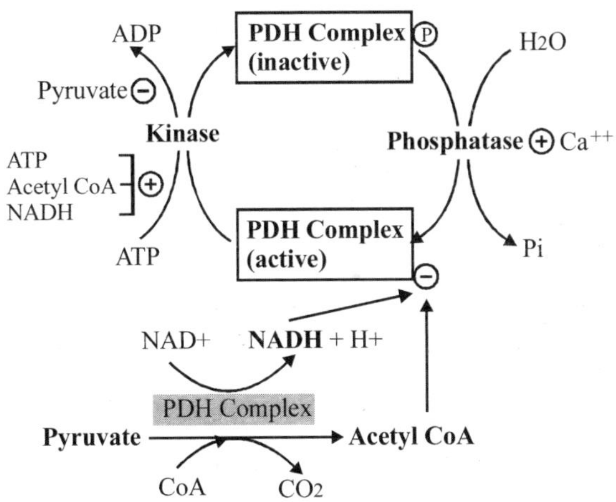


★ Pyruvate is a potent inhibitor of *PDH kinase* therefore it activates E1.

★ Acety CoA & NADH formed in this reaction allosterically inhibit active form of $E_1$

★ **So energy produced in complete aerobic oxidation of 1 glucose molecule is 30-32 ATP** (new concept)

| **Aerobic glycolysis** | **PDH complex reaction** | **Cirtic Acid Cycle** |
|---|---|---|
| **5-7 *ATP***Q | 2NADPH or **5 ATP** | **10 ATP** x 2 i.e. **20 ATP** |

★ Each glucose molecule gives rise to 2 pyruvate molecules & so 2 TCA cycles occur.

- *X-linked dominant deficiency in E1 component of PDH complex*, although rare, is the most common cause of ***congenital lacticacidosis***Q. This enzyme deficiency results in inability to convert pyruvate to acetal CoA, causing pyruvate to be converted to lactic acid via lactate dehydrogenase. This mainly affects *brain which relies on TCA cycle for most its energy* & is particularly sensitive to acidosis.
- **Leigh syndrome** *(subacute necrotizing encephalomyelopathy)* occurs d/t defects in mitochondrial ATP production as a result of mutation of *PHD complex, electron transport chain or ATP synthase*. It can affect both nuclear & mitochondrial DNA.

## Fate of Pyruvate

- *7 reversible reactions* of glycolysis are used in synthesis of glucose from lactate to pyruvate (i.e. gluconeogenesis). But the *3 irreversible reactions* must be circumvented by 4 alternate reactions that enegetically favour the synthesis of glucose. And these reactions are unique to gluconeogenesis. **The first road block in synthesis of glucose from pyruvate (gluconeogenesis) *is irreversible conversion of PEP to pyruvate by pyruvate kinase in glycolysis*** [Q]. In gluconeogenesis, pyruvate is first carboxylated by pyruvate carboxylase to OAA, which is then converted to PEP by PEP – carboxykinase.
- Conversion of phosphoenol pyruvate(PEP) to pyruvate is one of the three irreversible step (barrier) in simple reversible glycolysis. So this conversion is achieved by 2 enzymes.

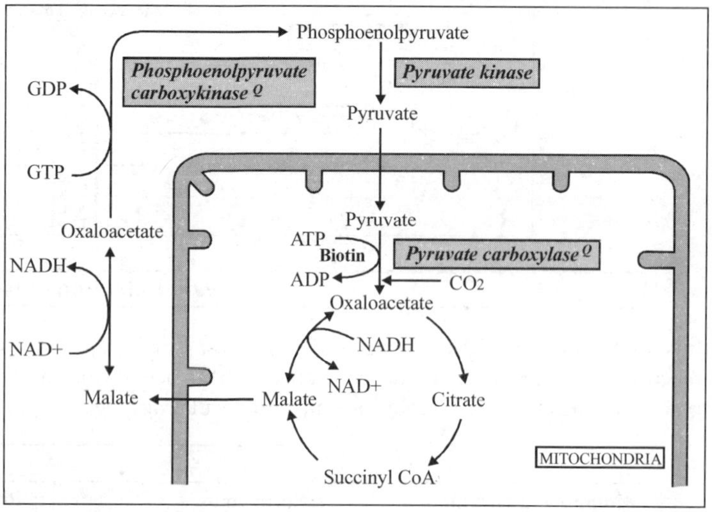


- **Pyruvate carboxylase:** Pyruvate has to be first converted to oxaloacetate in mitochondria.
- **Phosphoenol pyruvate carboxykinase:** OAA is then converted to phosphoenolpyruvate in cytosol

### Fate of Pyruvate (End product of glycolysis)

- **Oxidative decarboxylation** by *pyruvate dehydrogenase complex*, in tissues with *high oxidative capacity* such as cardiac muscle, irreversibly converts pyruvate to **acetyl CoA** (a **major fuel of TCA cycle and a building block** *for fatty acid synthesis*)
- **Carboxylation** by *biotin dependent pyruvate carboxylase* converts pyruvate to ***oxaloacetate*** **(OAA)**. This replenishes the citric acid cycle intermediates and provides substrate for gluconeogenesis.
- **Anaerobic glycolysis** occurs in tissue which are poorly vascularized/or lack mitochondria such as *exercising muscle, cornea & lens of eye, kidney medulla, testes, leucocytes & RBC.* **Lactate** formed by action of *lactate dehydrogenase* is the final product.
- **Transamination** by *alanine amino transferase (ALT/SGPT)* converts pyruvate to ***alanine*** [Q]

## Arsenic (As) poisoning

**Arsenite (trivalent As) inhibits (dehydrogenases)** enzymes **that require lipoic acid co-enzyme** (primary mechanism)

- ***$E_2$ of pyruvate dehydrogenase (PDH) complex*** [Q]
- ***α-ketoglutarate dehydrogenase*** [Q]
- ***Branched chain α- ketoacid dehydrogenase*** [Q]

**Arsenate (Pentavalent As)** *competing with inorganic phosphate as a substrate* (also occurs)

- Arsenate competing as a substrate for **glyceraldehydes -3- phosphate dehydrogenase**, forms a complex that spontaneously hydrolyzes to form 3-phosphoglycerate. By bypassing the synthesis of 1, 3-BPG and phosphate transfer from it, the cell is usually deprived of energy usually obtained from glycolysis. So it inhibits net ATP & NADH production without inhibiting the pathway itself.
- As also replaces phosphate on F1 domain of ATP synthase resulting in formation of ADP- arsenate that is rapidly hydrolyzed.

## Citric Acid Cycle/Krebb's Cycle

Citric acid cycle is a series of reaction in ***mitochondria***[Q] that *oxidize acetyl CO-A* and reduce coenzyme that upon reoxidation are linked to the formation of ATP.

Mn = **"C, Cis, I, O, α, S², F, M, O"**

- In bracket carbon content of each compound is written
- Release of $CO_2$ l/t decrease in one carbon atom
- Two irreversible steps of TCA are
  - *Oxaloacetate → citrate*
  - *α-ketoglutarate → succinyl CoA*
- ⊖—— indicates inhibitors of TCA

★ New concept
**1NADH = 2.5 ATP**
**1 FADH₂ = 1.5 ATP**

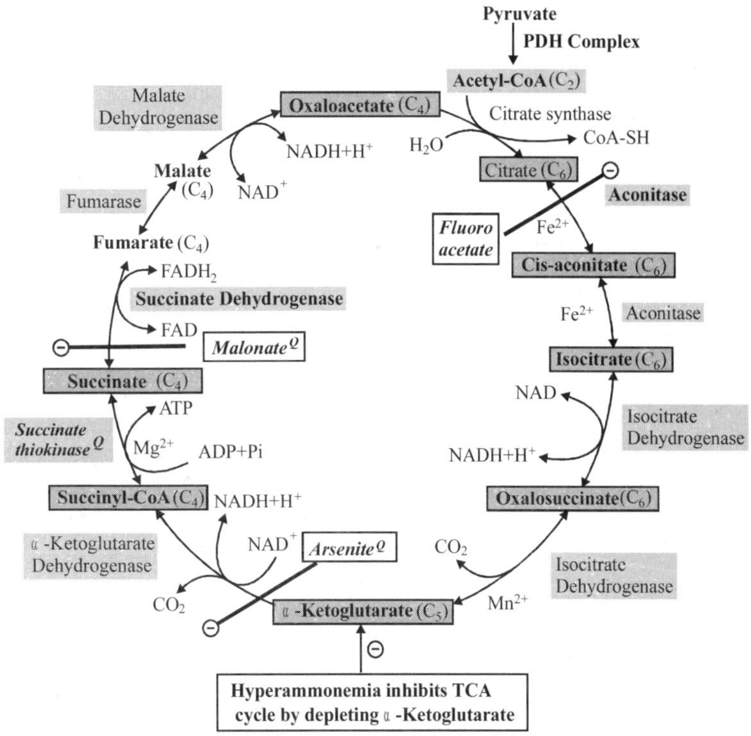


[see coloured Plate 20]

### Inhibitors of TCA (Citric Acid /Kreb's) Cycle

- **Aconitase** which isomerizes citrate to isocitrate, is *non competitively inhibited* by a ***rat poison fluoroacetate***[Q]. **Fluoroacetate (with acetyl CoA)** is converted to **fluoroacetyl CoA**, which ***condenses with oxaloacetate to form***[Q] **fluoro-citrate** – a potent *non competitive inhibitor of aconitase* – resulting in **citrate accumulation**.
- **Alpha ketoglutarate dehydrogenase** enzyme (which converts *α-ketoglutarate to succinyl CoA by oxidative decarboxylation) is non-competitively inhibited* by **arsenite (trivalent arsenic)** causing the substrate alpha ketoglutarate to accumulate. Arsenite forms a stable complex *with thiol group of lipoic acid* making it unavailable to serve as a coenzyme.
- *Oxidation of succinate to fumarate* by **succinate dehydrogenase** is competitively inhibited by **malonate**. Succinate dehydrogenase is the only enzyme of TCA cycle that is embedded in inner mitochondrial membrane and so also functions as **complex II of electron transport chain.**
- **Hyperammonemia** (↑$NH_3$) usually due to urea cycle defect inhibits TCA cycle by ***depleting α-ketoglutarate***[Q].

| Inhibitor of TCA cycle | Enzyme | Inhibition Type |
|---|---|---|
| **Fluoroacetate** (Rat poison) | *Aconitase*[Q] | **Non-competitive** |
| **Arsenite (Trivalent Arsenic)** | **Alpha-ketoglutarate dehydrogenase** | Non-competitive |
| **Malonate** | *Succinate dehydrogenase*[Q] | Competitive |
| **Ammonia Intoxication** | ***By depleting Alpha-ketoglutarate***[Q] | |

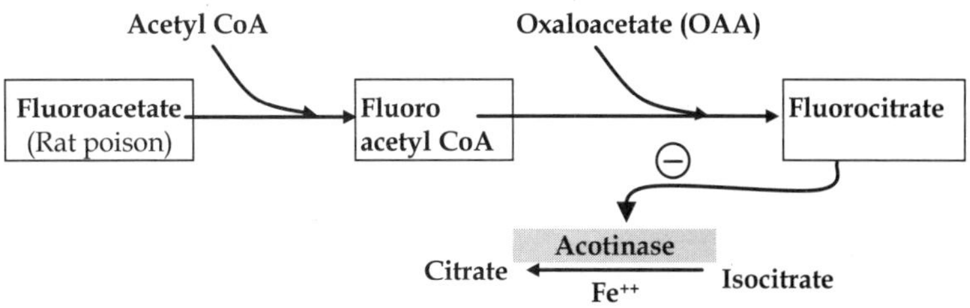


### 4-B Complex Vitamins are Essential in the TCA (Citric Acid) Cycle

**Riboflavin[Q] ($B_2$)**
In the *form of **FAD***, a cofactor in
- *α- ketoglutarate dehydrogenase complex*
- *succinate dehydrogenase.*

**Niacin**
In the form of ***NAD***, the electron acceptor *coenzyme for three dehydrogenase*
- *Isocitrate dehydrogenase*
- *α- ketoglutarate dehydrogenase*
- *Malate dehydrogenase*

***Thiamine*[Q] ($B_1$)**
As thiamine diphosphate (TDP/TPP), *coenzyme for decarboxylation in **α-ketoglutarate dehydrogenase** reaction.*

**Pentothenic acid**
As part of **coenzyme A**, the cofactor attached to active carboxylic acid residue such as *acetyl CoA & succinyl CoA.*

## Energy Production in TCA Cycle

### NADH Production

- ***3 molecules of NADH***[Q] are produced in one turn of cycle in the following reaction
  - Isocitrate ⟷ Oxalosuccinate (*Isocitrate dehydrogenase*[Q])
  - α- ketoglutarate ⟶ Succinyl CoA (*α- ketoglutarate dehydrogenase*[Q])
  - Malate ⟷ OAA (*Malate Dehydrogenase*[Q])
- Each NADH gives **3 ATP** (old concept) / **2.5 ATP** (new concept). So NADH oxidation in one TCA cycle provides ***9ATP***[Q] (old) / **7.5 ATP** (new).

### $FADH_2$ Production

***1 molecule of*** $FADH_2$[Q] is produced in the following reaction

- Succinate ⟷ Fumarate (*succinate dehydrogenase*[Q])

Each $FADH_2$ gives *2ATP*[Q] (old concept) / **1.5 ATP** (new concept)

### ATP / GTP synthesis

***1 GTP/ATP***[Q] is produced by *substrate level phosphorylation* [ It is production of ATP 'at the substrate level' without ***the participation of electron transport chain.***]Q

Succinyl CoA ⟷ Succinate (***Succinate thiokinase***[Q])

★ ***Over all 12 ATP***[Q] (old) / **10 ATP** (new) are formed **per turn of the citric acid cycle.**

| Substrate | ATP Production | |
|---|---|---|
| | New value | Old value |
| **NADH** | **2.5** | 3 |
| **FADH** | **1.5** | 2 |
| **Glucose** | **32** | 38 |
| **Acetyl CoA** | **10** | 12 |
| **Palmitate** | **106** | 129 |

## Regulation of Citric Acid Cycle by

### Availability of ADP[Q]

- ↑ADP → Stimulates TCA cycle
- ↑ATP/ ↓ADP→ cycle depressed

### Supply of $NAD^{+}$[Q]

- ↑$NAD^+$ → Stimulates cycle
- ↑NADH →Inhibits cycle

### Regulation of selective enzyme activity

- Citrate synthase
- ***Isocitrate dehydrogenase***[Q]
- α- ketoglutarate dehydrogenase complex

- In addition to above

*Succinate dehydrogenase* is inhibited by OAA, and availabily of OAA depends on *malate dehydrogenase* which is controlled by NADH / $NAD^+$ ratio.

## Involvement of the Citric Acid Cycle in Transamination and Gluconeogensis

**Valine, Isoleucine** and **Methionine**[Q] produce ***succinyl COA*** which is an important component of TCA cycle.
[Mn: **Successful VIM**]

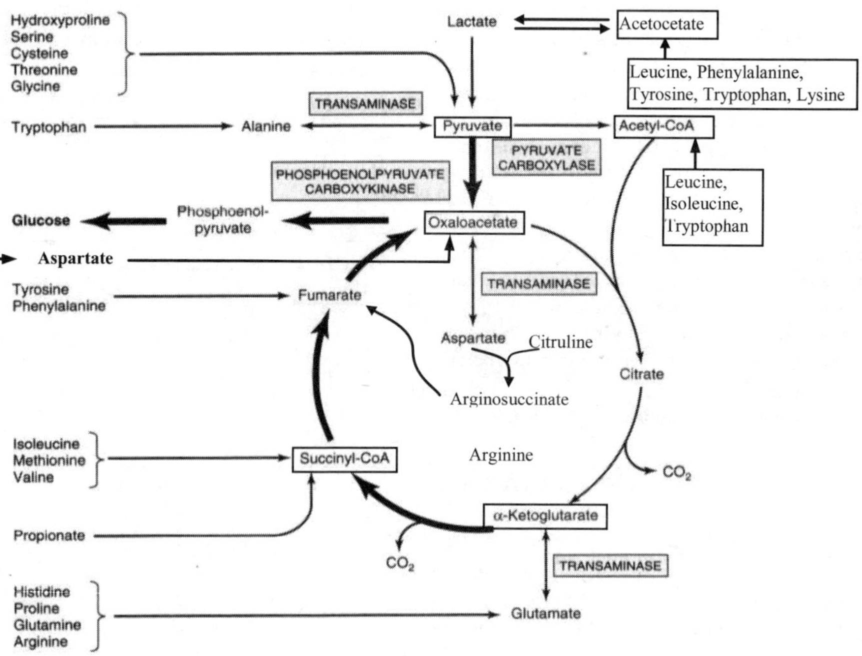


★ The bold arrows indicate the main pathway of gluconeogenesis

## Glucose – Alanine Cycle

- **Alanine transportes toxic ammonia (amino group) from skeleton muscles to liver** via a pathway called glucose – alanine cycle.
- It is important to remember that **resting muscles use fatty acids** as its major fuel source. Whereas **exercising muscles initially use glycogen stores** (by anaerobic glycolysis & convert it to lactate / pyruvate) **and then use free fatty acids** provided by mobilization of TAG from adipose tissue (when glycogen reserves are depleted) so these aminoacids are not directly utilized as fuel source by muscles.
- During first few days of fasting, there is ***rapid breakdown of muscle protein, providing aminoacids (alanine & glutamine mainly) that are used by liver for gluconeognesis***Q. *Because muscles do not have glucagon receptors, muscle proteolysis is initiated by fall in insulin and is sustained by the rise in glucocorticoids.* Alanine & glutamine are produced by catabolism of branched chain aminoacids. By ***several weeks of fasting, rate of muscle proteolysis decreases paralleling a decline in the need for glucose as a fuel for the brain which has started using ketone bodies as a source of energy***Q.
- In tissues that degrade aminoacid for fuel (mainly skeletal muscle), amino group is collected in form of L-glutamate (d/t transamination)
- This **glutamate** (containing toxic α-amino group) can be transported to liver by converting it to glutamine or it can transfer its α-amino group to **pyruvate**, a easily available product of muscle glycolysis by the action of **alanine aminotransferase (ALT/SGPT)**. The **alanine** so formed passes into blood to liver.
- In liver cell cytosol **alanine aminotransferase (ALT/SGPT)** transfers amino group from alanine to α-ketoglutarate forming pyruvate (which enters gluconeogenesis) and glutamate (under go oxidative deamination)
- Vigrously contracting muscles operate anerobically producing pyruvate & lactate (from glycolysis) and $NH_3$ (from aa break down). **Alanine-glucose cycle** in concert with Cori cycle send these products to liver where pyruvate & lactate are incorporated into glucose (by gluconeogenesis and returned back to muscle) and $NH_3$ is converted to urea for excretion. So the **energetic burden of gluconeogenesis is imposed on liver and all available ATP in muscle is devoted to muscle contraction.**
- In the fasting state, the **output of alanine from skeleton muscle is in far excess of its concentration in the muscle proteins that are being catabolized**. Because it is **also formed by transamination of pyruvate produced by glycolysis of muscle glycogen**. Alanine is exported to the liver, where it is transaminated ***back to pyruvate, which serves as a substrate for gluconeogenesis***Q. **The use of alanine to transport ammonia from skeleton muscles to liver is an example of intrinsic economy** of living organisms. Thus glucose – alanine cycle **provides an indirect way of utilizing muscle glycogen to maintain blood glucose in fasting state**. The ATP required for hepatic synthesis of glucose from pyruvate is derived from the oxidation of fatty acids.

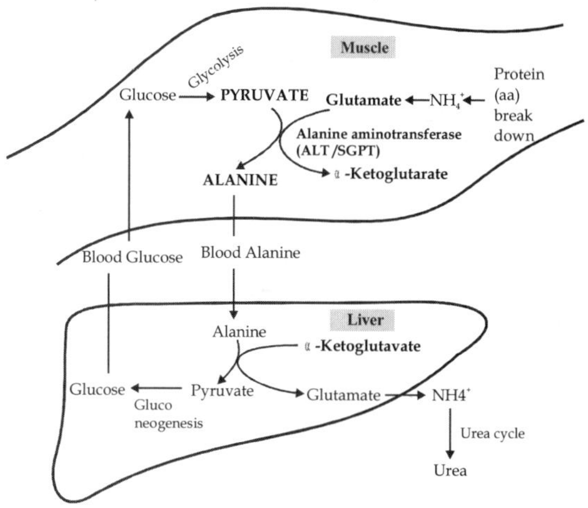


**Alanine - Glucose Cycle**

**Glucose - Alanine cycle:** Skeletal muscle transport $NH_3$ to liver in form of alanine, resulting in reciprocal transfer of glucose to muscle, This cycle is called Glucose - Alanine cycle.

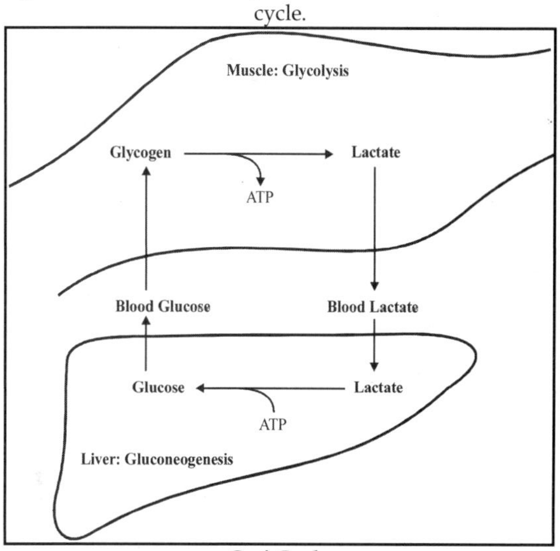


**Cori Cycle**

## Reversible Oxidative Deamination: (L) Glutamate Dehydrogenase (GDH)

- **Transamination** (1st step in catabolism of aa) *transfers amino group of many α-amino acids to α-keto glutarate*, thus converting it to **L-glutamate**. The reaction predominatly occurs in **cytosol of hepatocytes (liver cells)**.
- L glutamate is transported from cytosol to mitochondria of hepatocyte. ***Only (predominantly) mitochondrial matrix contain glutamate dehydrogenase which oxidatively deaminates glutamate to α-ketoglutarate (α-keto acid) and free amonia***Q (α-amino group is liberated as $NH_3$). A/t vasudevan this reaction occurs in only liver; a/t Lippincott 252 this occurs in liver & kidney.
- GDH, a **Zn containing** *metalloenzyme* of **m**itochondrial **m**atrix, is a tetramer (i.e. has 4 polypeptide chain each containing 1 Zn molecule). It is the ***only enzyme that can use either NAD+ or NADP+ as coenzyme***Q (or acceptor of reducing equivalent). $NAD^+$ is used in oxidative deamination and NADPH is used in reductive amination (i.e. reverse reaction).
- ***Oxidative deamination is a freely reversible reaction***Q. The direction depends on relative concentration of substrate, product (glutamate, α-ketoglutarate, $NH_3$) and ratio of oxidized to reduced coenzyme. So in well fed state glutamate levels are high resulting in oxidative deamination, whereas in starvation it synthesize amino acids by reductive amination.

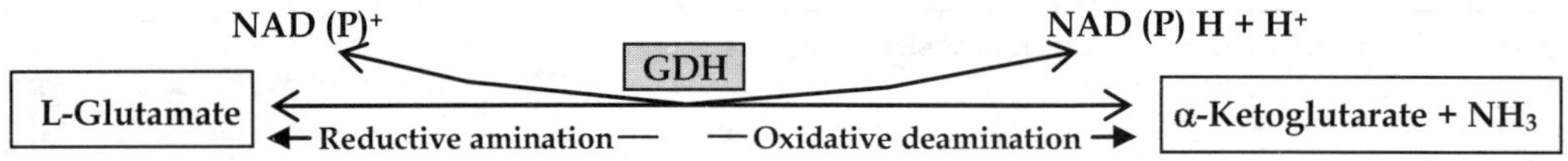


- **Liver GDH** is ***allosterically activated by ADP and inhbited by ATP, GTP and NADH***[Q]. Thus when energy levels are low in cell, amino acids are catabolized by GDH for energy production. Mutations that alter GTP binding site cause permanent activation of GDH, & result in hyper insulinism-hyper-ammonia syndrome characterized by ↑NH3 and ↓glucose in blood.
- **Trans deamination** is sequential action of *transamination f/b oxidative deamination*, and provide a pathway where by the amino groups of most amino acids can be released as NH3. *Transamination takes place in cytoplasm of all cells of body (mainly liver, kidney, muscle, heart etc)* and form glutamate. Toxic glutamate is transported to liver as non-toxic glutamine (most tissue) and alanine (from muscles), and finally oxidatively deaminated in mitochondria of liver (mainly).
- Minor pathways of deamination are L/D/Mono-amino oxidase; dehydrase, desulfhydrase and histidase (non oxidative) etc.

## Substrate & Oxidative Phosphorylation

There are *two types of phosphorylation of ADP to ATP*

### Substrate level phosphorylation

- Is production of ATP 'at the substrate' without the participation of electron transport chain
- Formation of ATP does not require ATP
- Respiratory chain does not participate
- It is not affected by dinitrophenole

- In TCA cycle

Succinyl CoA —*Succinate thiokinase*[Q]→ Succinate

- In Glycolysis

1, 3- biphos-Phoglycerate —*Phosphoglycerate Kinase*[Q]→ 3 phospho glycerate

Phosphoenol Pyruvate —*Pyruvate Kinase*[Q]→ (Enol) pyruvate

### Oxidative Phosphorylation at Respiratory Chain Level

| Generation of High Energy Phosphate In Catabolism of Glucose | | | Number of (P) Formed per Mole of Glucose |
|---|---|---|---|
| **Pathway** | **Reaction Catalyzed by** | **Method of ~ Production** | |
| **Glycolysis** | Glyceraldehyde-3-phosphate dehydrogenase | Respiratory chain oxidation of 2 NADH | 6* |
| | Phosphoglycerate kinase | Phosphorylation at substrate level | 2 |
| | Pyruvate kinase | Phosphorylation at substrate level | 2 |
| | | | 10 |
| Allow for consumption of ATP by reactions catalyzed by hexokinase and phosphofructokinase | | | -2 |
| | | Net | 8 |
| | Pyruvate dehydrogease | Respiratory chain oxidation of 2 NADH | 6 |
| | Isocitrate dehydrogenase | Respiratory chain oxidation of 2 NADH | 6 |
| | α-ketoglutarate dehydrogenase | Respiratory chain oxidation of 2 NADH | 6 |
| **Citric acid cycle** | Succinate thiokinase | Phosphorylation at substrate level | 2 |
| | Succinate dehydrogenase | Respiratory chain oxidation of 2 $FADH_2$ | 4 |
| | Malate dehydrogenase | Respiratory chain oxidation of 2 NADH | 6 |
| | | Net | 30 |
| Total per mole of glucose under **aerobic conditions** | | | 38 |
| Total per mole of glucose under **anaerobic conditions** | | | 2 |

★ It is assumed that NADH formed in glycolysis is transported into mitochondria via the malate shuttle. If the glycerophosphate shuttle is used, only 2 ~ (P) would be formed per mole of NADH, the total net production being 26 instead of 38. The calculation ignores the small loss of ATP due to a transported of $H^+$ into the mitochondrion with pyruvate and a similar transport of H+ in the operation of the malate shuttle, totaling about 1 mol of ATP. Note that there is a substantial benefit under anaerobic conditions if glycogen is the starting point, since the net production of high-energy phosphate in glycosis is increased from 2 to 3, as ATP is no longer required by the hexokinase reaction.

## High Energy Compounds

These compounds release **at least 7 Kcal /mol (i.e. > 7 K cal/mol or > 25 KJ/mol)** on hydrolysis; they have large Δ G° (free energy of hydrolysis) from *7-15 Kcal/mol*. The high energy bond is indicated by a *squiggle bond (~)*. These include

| High Energy Compounds | Δ G° (Kcal/mol) | Energy release (KJ/mol) |
|---|---|---|
| • **Phosphate Compounds** | | |
| 1. Pyrophosphates: Nucleotides like **ATP, GTP, UTP, UDP-glucose** | | |
| - ATP → ADP + Pi | **7.3** | 30.5 |
| - ATP → AMP + PPi | 10.7 | 45.6 |
| 2. Phosphagens: like **Creatine phosphate (CP) or phosphocreatine** | 10.5 | 43.1 |
| 3. Acyl phosphates: like **1, 3-Biphosphoglycerate (BPG)** | 10.1 | 49.4 |
| 4. Enol phosphates like **phosphoenol pyruvate (PEP)** | 14.8 | 61.9 |
| 5. **Carbamoyl phosphate** | 12.3 | 51.4 |
| 6. **Amino acyl adenylate (amino acyl AMP/cycline AMP)** | 12.0 | 50.0 |
| 7. **Acetyl phosphate** | 10.3 | |
| 8. **Arginine phosphate** | 10.0 | |
| 9. **Inorganic pyrophosphate** | 8.0 | |
| • **Sulfur Compounds** | | |
| 10. Sulfonium compounds like **S- adenosyl methionine (SAM)** | 8.0 | |
| 11. Thioester **CoA derivatives like Acetyl CoA, Succinyl CoA, Fatty acyl CoA, HMG CoA** | 7.7 | |
| 12. **Adenosine phosphosulfate** (active sulfate) | | |

## Low Energy Compounds

These liberate **< 7 Kcal/mol** on hydrolysis at pH7 (i.e. lower than energy liberated by hydrolysis of ATP to ADP + Pi)

These include

| Low Energy Compounds | Δ G° (Kcal/mol) |
|---|---|
| 1. **ADP** – AMP + Pi | 6.5 |
| 2. **Glucose 1 phosphate** | 5.0 |
| 3. **Fructose 6 phosphate** | 4.0 |
| 4. **Glucose 6 phosphate** | 3.5 |
| 5. **Glycerol 3 phosphate** | 2.2 |

★ All values of Δ G° and energy released are negative (-)

## Redox Potential (Eo) & Electron Transport Chain (ETC)

- Mitociondrial ETC consists of a series of sequentially acting electron carriers, accepting & donating either 1 or 2 electrons. Free energy is released as electrons are transferred from an **electron donor (reducing agent / reductant)** to an **electron acceptor (oxidizing agent / oxidant)**. 3 types of electron transfer occur and term reducing equivalent is used to designate a *single electron equivalent* in any form.
  - Direct transfer of **electrons (e-) to cytochromes** for reduction of **Fe3+ to $Fe^{2+}$**
  - Transfer as a **hydrogen atom, ($H^+ + e^- = \bullet H$)** to **FMN, FAD** and **coenzyme Q (Ubiquinone)**
  - Transfer as **hydride ion (:$H^-$)** bearing 2 electrons to **$NAD^+$**
- Oxidation (loss of $e^-$) of one substance is always accompanied by reduction (gain of $e^-$) of another substance. For example oxidation of NADH to $NAD^+$ is accompanied by (a/b) reduction of FMN to $FMNH_2$. So oxidation – reduction reactions are sum of 2 separate half reactions one an oxidation & other a reduction reaction. Thus $NAD^+$ /$NADH_2$ form a **redox pair** and FMN /$FMNH_2$ forms other.
- **Standard recuction potential / Redox potential (E°)** in *volts*, is a *quantitative measurement of the tendency of a redox pair (couple) to donate or accept electron under standard potential.* The pairs are ordered from most negative to most positive E° i.e. is in increasing order of E°. **More negative** the E°, the greater is the tendency of reductant member of that pair to **lose electron. More positive** the greater is the tendency of oxidant member of that pair to **accept electron.** *So electron flow spontaneously from lower to higher (i.e. more negative to more positive) redox potential.*
- The change in free energy (Δ G°) is directly related to Δ E° (i.e. E° of electron accepting pair – E° of electron donating pair). The standard free energy required for phosphorylation of ADP to ATP is + **7.3 Kcal/mol.**

$$\Delta G = nF \Delta E°$$

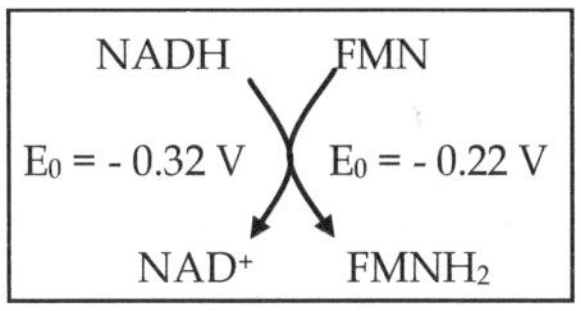


F = Faraday constant (23.1 K Cal/Volt-mol)

n = Numbers of e- transferred (1 for cytochrome, 2 for NADH, $FADH_2$ and CoenzymeQ)

Transport of a pair of e- from NADH (complex I) to $O_2$ via ETC produces 52.58 Kcal and so produce 3 ATPs from 3 ADP & 3 Pi (3 x 7.3 = 21.9 K Cal/ mol) per O atom reduced. Hence **P:O ratio** is **3:1** for NADH (and 2:1 for $FADH_2$ because complex I is bypassed). The remaining energy is used in anciliary reactions or released as heat. But now recent studies have shown that 2.5 ATP is produced per **0.5** mol (1/2 $O_2$) = per atom of O from NADH (P:O ratio = **2.5:1**). And $FADH_2$ generate 1.5 ATP (P:O ratio = 1.5:1)

| Redox Pair | | Redox potential (E° volts) |
|---|---|---|
| Ferredoxin ($Fe^{+3}$ / $Fe^{+2}$) | | - 0.432 |
| $2H^+/H_2$ (at pH7) | | - 0.414 |
| **α-Ketoglutarate /Isocitrate** | | - 0.38 |
| Acetoacetate / β Hydroxy butyrate | | - 0.35 |
| **NADP+ / NADPH** | | - 0.324 |
| **NAD+ / NADH** | | - 0.320 |
| Lipoate (ox / red) | | - 0.29 |
| Glutathione (ox / red) | | - 0.23 |
| **FAD / $FADH_2$** | | - 0.22 |
| Pyruvate / Lactate | | - 0.19 |
| **Oxaloacetate / Malate** | | - 0.17 |
| $2H^+$ / $H_2$ (at PH0) | | 0 |
| **Fumarate / Succinate** | | + 0.03 |
| **Ubiquinone / Ubiquinol** | | + 0.045 |
| **$Fe^{3+}$ / $Fe^{2+}$ in Cytochromes** | b | + 0.077 |
| | $C_1$ | + 0.22 |
| | C | + 0.254 |
| | a | + 0.29 |
| | $a_3$ | + 0.35 |
| **$Fe^{+3}$ / $Fe^+$** | | + 0.771 |
| **$O_2$ / $H_2O$** | | 1+ 0.82 |

## Electron Transport Chain (ETC)/Respiratory Chain

- Energy rich molecules like glucose are ultimately metabolized to $CO_2$ and water. The metabolic intermediates of these oxidation reactions donate electrons to NAD /FAD to form energy rich coenzymes **NADH/FADH$_2$.**
- These energy rich reduced coenzymes, in turn, donate electrons to *a specialized series of electron carriers / donors arranged a/t redox potential (E°)* – collectively called ETC.
- ETC is present in **inner mitochondrial membrane** & is the final common pathway in aerobic cells by which electrons obtained from different fuels of body flow to oxygen. This requirement of $O_2$ makes the ETC the **respiratory chain**, which accounts for the greatest portion of body's use for oxygen.
- Electrons flow through the ETC through a redox span of **1.1 volts** from $NAD^+$ / NADH to $O_2$ / $H_2O$
- The components of respiratory chain contain 4 large protein complexes (initial 2 are flavoproteins & last 2 are cytochromes) and 2 mobile electron carriers – coenzyme Q & cytochrome C.
- The chain reaction of e- transport starts with formation of NADH (by various **substrate dehydrogenases** removing hydrogen atom as in TCA cycle – isocitrate / α-ketoglutarate / malate - dehydrogenase). Transfer of hydride ion (:$H^-$, bearing 2 electrons) and a free proton ($H^+$) to $NAD^+$ l/t formation of NADH (having 2 $e^-$) plus a free proton ($H^+$). ETC consists of
-

| **Component** of ETC | **Prosthetic Group/Electron flow** | **Features** |
|---|---|---|
| **Complex I: NADH dehydrogenase/ NADH-Ubiquinone (CoQ) oxidoreductase / NADH-CoQ reductase** | **FMN**, non heme iron sulfur proteins **(FeS)**<br>NADH→FMN<br>↓<br>Fes<br>↓<br>CoQ | - It is a large L shaped 42 subunit protein which accepts 2$e^-$ & 1 $H^+$ from NADH and transfer it to CoQ<br>- **12 Kcal/mol** of released energy is utilized to pump **4 protons ($H^+$)** out of mitochondria into inter membranous space. |
| **Complex II: Succinate dehydrogenase /Succinate -Q- Reductase** | **FAD, FeS**<br>Succinate→FAD<br>↓<br>Fes<br>↓<br>CoQ | - It is a small 4 subunit protein which accepts e- from succinate & transfer it to CoQ.<br>- It is **not a proton pump** as energy liberated is not enough to pump protons.<br>- It also contain **heme b** that is not in direct path of $e^-$ transfer but serve to **reduce** the frequency with which **$e^-$ leak out of system**, moving from succinate to molecular $O_2$ to produce reactive oxygen species |
| **Coenzyme Q (CoQ)/Ubiquinone/Q** | - This **only nonprotein** member of ETC is a *lipid soluble benzoquinone with long hydrophobic isoprenoid tail (side chain).*<br>- It is called ubiquinone as it is *ubiquitous (present everywhere) quinone derivative. Menaquinone (of bacteria) & plastoquinine (of chloroplast)* have analogous roles<br>- It can accept 1 or 2 electrons to become semiquinone or ubiquinol respectively. So it can act at the junction of 2e- donor & 1e- acceptor (Q cycle).<br>- Because it is small & hydrophobic, Q is a **mobile carrier** freely diffusible within the lipid bilayer of inner mitochondrial membrane and can shuttle b/w other less mobile e- carriers.<br>- It has a central role in coupling e- flow to proton (H+) movment as it carries both e- & H+.<br>- **For transferring to complex III it accepts hydrogen atom (e- & H+) from.**<br>1. $FMNH_2$ produced in **complex I** (from FMN)<br>2. $FADH_2$ produced in **complex II**<br>3. $FADH_2$ produced in β-oxidation by **acyl CoA dehydrogenase** (through **ETF-ubiquinone- oxidoreductase**) and by **glycerol 3 phosphate dehydrogenase**. These bypass complex II & I. | |

## Oxidative Phosphorylation

- As electrons ($e^-$) are transported down the ETC, they *lose* much of *their free energy.* Some part of this energy is **captured & stored as ATP** (from ADP + Pi) in a process called **oxidative phosphorylation.** The remainder (not trapped as ATP) energy is used for ancilliary reactions like *$Ca^{+2}$ transport into mitochondria & to generate heat.*
- Electron transfer down the ETC is energetically favoured because NADH is a strong electron ($e^-$) donor and $O_2$ an avid acceptor.
- **Mitchelle- chemiosmotic hypothesis** of proton pump & ATP synthase
  - It states that ETC is responsible for ATP production b/o electro-pH gradient produced d/t associated proton pumping (i.e. proton pump is a link b/w ETC and oxidative phosphorylation).
  - As we know, electron transport through **complex I, III and IV** also transports (pumps) **4, 4 and 2 protons (H+)** respectively across inner mitochondrial membrane from matrix to inter membrane space.
  - This associated proton transport creates **an electrical gradient** (*outside is positive* relative to inside) of 0.15-0.20V; and a **pH gradient** (*outside pH is lower* than inside d/t more H+ ion concentration) of 0.75 -1.4. This generates a proton motive force (PMF) of 0.224V corresponding to a free energy change of 5.2 Kcal/mol of protons.
  - The energy generated by proton gradient is enough to synthesize ATP by **ATP synthase (complex V)**. So the proton gradient is a link that couples oxidation (ETC) to phosphorylation (ATP synthesis)
  - **Complex V: ATP synthase** (also k/a **$F_1/F_0$ ATPase** because it can also catalyze hydrolysis of ATP to ADP + Pi) has $F_0$ and $F_1$ subunits. **$F_o$ unit** spans inner mitochondrial membrane and serves as **proton channel**, whereas **F1 unit phosphorylates ADP to ATP**.
  - Protons that have been pumped out to inter membrane space, creating electrical and pH gradient, they **reenter** the **mitochondrial matrix by passing through a proton channel in $F_o$ domain of ATP synthase (complex V).**
  - This re-entery of protons *rotates $F_0$ unit thus producing conformational changes in extra membranous $F_1$ domain*, and at the same time, dissipating the pH and electrical gradients. The conformational changes of $F_1$ unit allow phosphorylation of ADP + Pi to ATP, and release ATP.
- **Paul Boyer's Binding Change mechanism** of **rotational catalysis**
  - It states that ATP synthesis by proton gradient is comparable to a *'water driven hammer minting coin'*. $F_0$ is wheel, flow of

| | | |
|---|---|---|
| **Complex III: Cytochrome $bC_1$ complex /Ubiquinone cytochrome C oxido-reductase / Cytochrome reductase** | Fe-S, **Heme** group (a porphyrin ring & iron, which is reversibly converted from $Fe^{3+}$ to $Fe^{2+}$ form)<br>Q → Cyt b<br>↓<br>Cyt $C_1$<br>↓<br>CytC | - It transfers electron from CoQ to cytochrome C. - 10 Kcal/mol of released energy is utilized to **pump 4 protons**[Q] out of mitochondria into inter membranous space.<br>- **Q cycle** couples e- & H+ transport in complex III & involves **cytochrome $b_1$, $b_H$ (b562, b566), cytochrome $C_1$ and Rieske Fe - S** (an unusual iron sulfur protein in which one of the iron atom is linked to 2 histidine -SH rather than 2 cysteine- SH groups), oxidation of $QH_2$ (ubiquinol) to Q (ubiquinone) is coupled to reduction of 2 molecules of cytochrome via cytochrome C |
| **Cytochrome c** | - Soluble carrier protein of intermembrane space<br>- After its single heme group accepts an electron from complex III, cytochrome c moves to complex IV to donate electron to a binuclear copper centre | |
| **Comple IV Cytochrome c oxidase / cytochrome oxidase** | 2 Heme groups (of cyt a, $a_3$), **2 copper ions** of $Cu_A$, $Cu_B$<br>**Cyt C → CuA**<br>↓<br>**Cyta**<br>↓<br>**Cyt a3**<br>↓<br>**CuB**<br>↓<br>$O_2$ | - It transfer electrons from cytochrome C to the final acceptor $O_2$ converting (reducing) it to water ($H_2O$).<br>- $O_2$ remains tightly bound to complex IV ($a_3$) until it is fully reduced to $H_2O$, this minimizes the release of ROS.<br>- It pumps **2 proton (H+)** out into inter membrane space for every pair of electron passing down the chain by complex IV |

proton is water fall, and structural changes in $F_1$ l/t ATP coin being minted for each turn of wheel.

- 3 Beta (catalytic sites) sub units of F1 has 3 conformational states

1. **L state** binds to substrate & product with with loose affinity
2. **T state** binds substrate tightly & catalyzes ATP synthesis
3. **O state** is open and does not bind to substrate or product; i.e. release product (ATP)

- For complete rotation of $F_1$ unit through 3 states **10 protons** are translocated. As the ATP is released, the original conformation of enzyme ($F_1$) is assumed

- So the energy is actually required for producing conformational change (not for ATP synthesis). And the energy surplus produced by proton gradient is stored as chemical energy ATP.

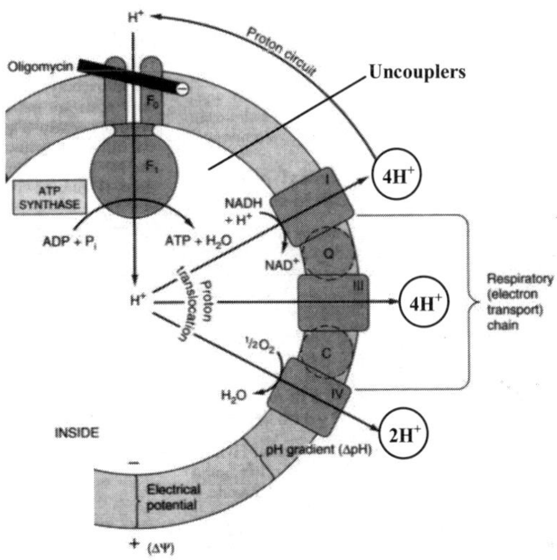


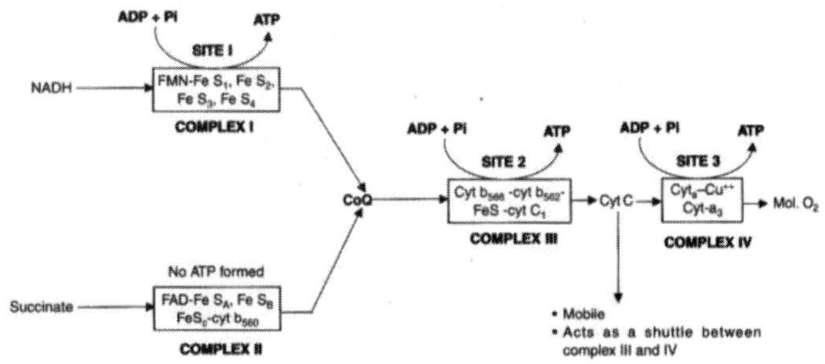


Four complexes of Electron Transport Chain

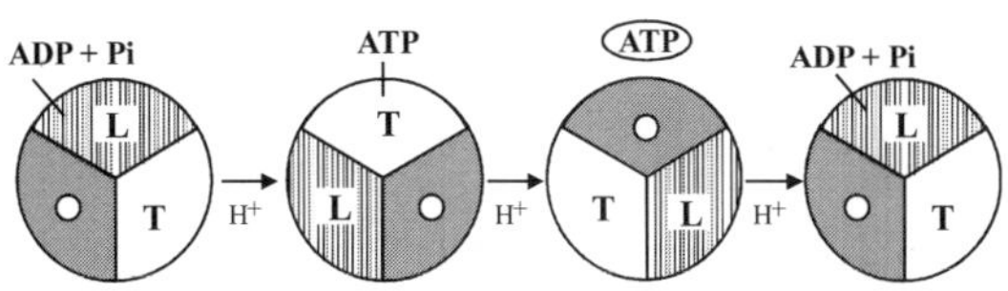


Paul Boyer's Binding Change Model of Rotational Catalysis

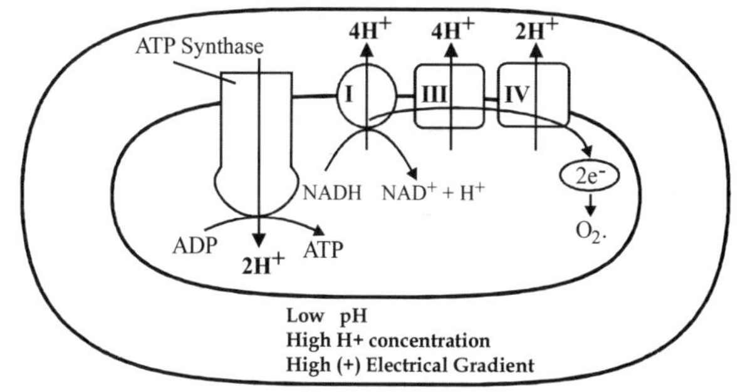


Mitchell Chemi-Osmotic Hypothesis

## Mitchell's Chemi-Osmotic Theory

**Mitchell's chemiosmotic theory**[Q] postulates that energy from oxidation of respiratory chain components is coupled to the translocation of hydrogen ions (proton, $H^+$) from the inside to outside of inner mitochondria membrane Respiratory chain ***complexes I, III & IV***[Q] acts as a **proton pump**. Inner mitochondrial membrane is impermeable to ions in general but particularly to protons which accumulates outside the membrane creating **a electro- chemical potential difference** ($\Delta\mu H^+$)
The $\Delta\mu H^+$ is used to drive a membrane located **ATP synthase** which functions as a *rotary motor to form ATP.*

| $F_0$ Subunit complex | $F_1$ Subunit complex |
|---|---|
| - A *membrane protein* complex which forms ***proton channel***[Q]<br>- It is a *disk of "C" protein* subunit<br>- Attached to it is ***"bent axle"*** formed by ***Y- subunit*** & ***ε- subunit***[Q]<br>- Protons passing through the disk of "C" units cause it & attached Y- unit to rotate<br>- Uncoupling agent dinitrophenol allow leakage of $H^+$ across the membrane, thus collapsing the electrochemical proton gradient. *Oligomycin specifically blocks conduction of $H^+$ through $F_0$ subunit* | - Composed of 9 polypeptide chains (3α, 3β, 1γ, 1 σ & 1ε) project into *matrix* and contain *phosphorylation mechanism*<br>- ***3 α & 3- β subunits, which are fixed to the membrane and do not rotate***[Q]<br>- The Y- subunit fits inside $F_1$ sub complex<br>- *ADP & Pi are taken up sequentially by the β subunits to form ATP,* which is expelled as the rotating Y subunite squeeze each β subunit in turn. Thus ***3 ATP molecules are generated per rotation***[Q]. |

★ **Ionophores** are lipophilic molecules that complex specific cations & facilitate their transport eg *valinomycin ($K^+$), dinitrophenol.*

★ **Familial infantile mitochondrial myopathy & renal dysfunctions** involves severe diminution or absence of most oxido reductases of the respiratory chain. **MELAS** (**m**itochondiral **e**ncephalopathy **l**actic **a**cidosis & **s**troke) is caused by mutation in mitochondrial DNA & is d/t NADH: ubiquinone oxidoreductase (complex I) or cytochrome oxidase deficiency. It may be involved in *Alzheimer is disease* & *diabetes mellitus.*

## Transporter System in Inner Mitochondrial Membrane

Although the outer membrane is freely permeable to most ion & small molecules, the inner mitochondrial membrane is **impermeable to most small ions** like $H^+$, $Na^+$, $K^+$; and **small molecules** such as ADP, ATP, Pyruvate and other metabolites important to mitochondrial function. The relative impermeability of inner mitochondrial membrane necessitates exchange transporters

**Inner mitochondrial membrane is freely permeable to unchanged small molecules such as,**

- $O_2$ - $H_2O$
- $CO_2$ - $NH_3$
- Monocarboxylic acids such as 3-OH-butyric acid, acetoacetic & acetic

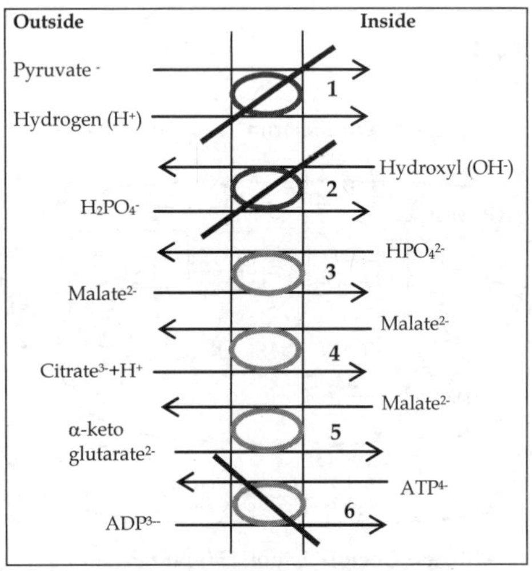


★ **N- ethyl- Maleimide, hydroxycinnamate** and **atractyloside** inhibit *pyruvate symport, phosphate transporter and adenine nucleotide transporter*

★ Transporters are named on the name of product they take inside mitochondria

| Transporters | Exchange / Transport |
|---|---|
| **1. Pyruvate symport** | Transport pyruvate & hydrogen ions in same direction (inwards) |
| **2. Phosphate transporter** | Exchange phosphate for hydroxyl ions |
| **3. Dicarboxylate transporter** | Exchange dicarboxylate (malate 2-) ions for phosphate |
| **4. Tricarboxylate transporter** | Exchange tricarboxylate (citrate) for malate |
| **5. α-ketoglutarate transporter** | Exchange alpha ketoglutrate for malate |
| **6. Adenine Nucleotide transporter** | Exchange ADP for ATP |
| **7. Glutamate-Aspartate transporter** | Glutamate is converted to aspartate and aspartate is exchanged for $H^+$ ion |

**Transporters are required for**

- *Long chain fatty acids* require carnitine system
- *Pyruvate*
- Dicarboxylate & tricarboxylate anions and aminoacids
- ***ADP enter & ATP exit***[Q]
- *NADH* is transported by **malate and glycerophosphate shuttle**
- ***NADPH***[Q]
- Mitochondria accumulate cations such as $K^+$, $Na^+$, $Ca^{2+}$ and $Mg^{2+}$ and *Pi.*
- **Creatine phosphate shuttle** bring outside the ATP generated in mitochondria
- Alpha-ketoglutarate transporter and glutamate / aspartate transporter are used in **malate shuttle** for transfer of reducing equivalents from cytosol into mitochondria.
- Transporter for glutamine, ornithine, neutral amino acids and carnitite (**carnitine acyl carnitine translocase**).

# Poisons Inhibiting the Respiratory Chain

## Inhibitors of Electron Transport Chain (ETC)

- ETC inhibitors, **prevent the passage (transport) of electrons** by binding to a specific component of chain, thus blocking the **oxidation-reduction reaction**. So all electron carriers located before the block are fully reduced, whereas those located *after the block are oxidized.*
- Inhibition of ETC *blocks ATP synthesis* as both processes are tightly coupled. And *reactive oxygen species (ROS)* like superoxide ($O_2^{-}\bullet$), hydroxyl radicals ($OH^\bullet$) and hydrogen peroxide ($H_2O_2$) are produced d/t incomplete reduction of $O_2$ to $H_2O$. ROS can damage DNA, proteins & cause lipid peroxidation.

| Site of action | Inhibitor (Poison) | Mechanism |
|---|---|---|
| **Complex I: NADH-CoQ reductase (or NADH dehydrogenase complex)** | - **Amobarbital** (amytal) & **seco barbitals** = Barbiturates<br>- **Rotenone** (fish poison & insecticide)<br>- Myxothiozole | Blocks e- transfer through complex I (i.e. from Fe S to CoQ / *ubi quinone*) |
| | - **Piericidin A** (antibiotic) | Blocks e- transfer by ***competing with CoQ*** |
| | - Chlorpromazine (tranquilizer)<br>- Guanethidine (a hypotensive alkyl guanide) | |
| **Complex II: Succinate - CoQ Reductase (Succinate dehydrogenase)** | - ***Malonate***[Q] | Competitive inhibitor of complex II inhibiting e- transfer from succinate to FAD |
| | - Carboxin<br>- TTFA | Inhibit e- transfer from Fe S to CoQ (through complex II) |
| **Complex III: CoQ - Cyt C reductase (Cytochrome reductase)** | - **Antimycin A**<br>- **BAL** (British anti lewisite or **Dimercaprol**), antidote of war gas<br>- Napthoquinone<br>- Phenformin (hypoglycemic drug) | Inhibits transfer of e- from cyt b to $C_1$. |
| **Complex IV: Cytochrome oxidase (Cyt c oxidase)** | - **Carbon monoxide (CO)**[Q] | Capture $O_2$ binding site |
| | - **Cyanide (CN-)**<br>- **Hydrogen sulfide ($H_2S$)**<br>- **Azide ($N_3^-$)** | Inhibit terminal $e^-$ transfer from $a_3$ to molecular $O_2$ (arrest respiration) |

★ DCMU (Dichlorophenyl dimethyl urea) competes with Q B for binding site in PS II

## *Inhibitors of Oxidative Phosphorylation (ATP synthesis)*

| **- Oligomycin** (antibiotic)<br>**- Venturicidin** | **- Atractyloside** (glycoside)<br>**- Bongregate** (pseudomonads toxin) | **Ionophores** |
|---|---|---|
| - **Binds** to **Fo domain of ATP synthase, closing the proton (H+) channel, blocking reentry of protons** through ATP synthase into mitochondrial matrix<br>- This l/t *accumulation of H+ at higher concentration in inter membrane space.* Because the pH & electrical gradient cannot be dissipated, e- transport stops b/o difficulty of pumping any more protons against steep proton gradient.<br>- Inhibition of phosphorylation inhibits e- transport<br>- So Oligomycin completely blocks oxidation & phosphoryla-tion by blocking the flow of protons through ATP synthase and prevents stimulation of $O_2$ uptake by ADP & phosphorylation of ADP to ATP | - **Blocks adenine nucleotide transporter (translocases)** responsible for ***movement of ADP into & ATP out of the mitochondria***[Q] ***across the inner mitochondrial membrane***[Q]<br>- It ***Inhibits ATP-ADP exchange***[Q].<br>- Adequate supply of ADP is blocked thus preventing phosphorylation and ATP formation. | - Ionophores are lipid soluble compounds that increase the permeability if lipid bilayer to certain ions.<br>- These are of 2 types<br>1. **Valinomycin** (mobile ion carrier)<br>2. **Gramicidin** (channel formers)<br>- Valinomycin allow K+ to permeate mitochondria and dissipate proton ($H^+$) gradient. |

**Oligomycin & venturicidin** inhibits $F_o$ & $CF_o$ ; **DCCD** (dicyclohexyl carbodimide) blocks proton flow through $F_o$ & $CF_o$; and **aurovertin** inhibits F1 domain of **ATP synthase (complex V)**

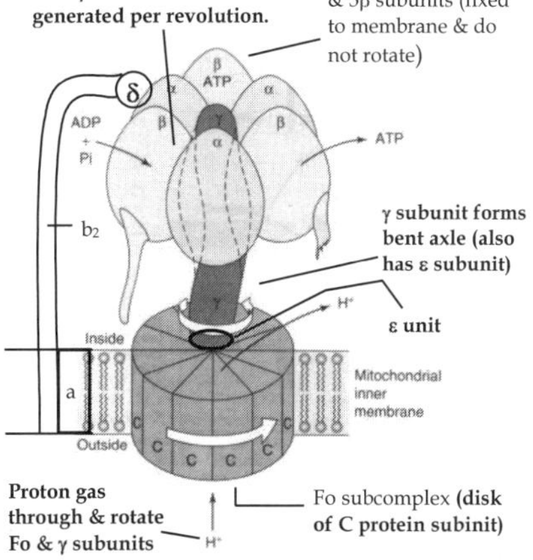


## Uncouplers of Oxidative Phosphorylation

- Uncouplers *uncouple oxidation (electron transport chain) from phosphorylation.* This dissociation of oxidation from phosphorylation will allow oxidation to proceed, but the energy instead of being trapped into ATP by phosphorylation is dissipaled as heat.
- Uncouplers create a **proton leak removing proton gradient** i.e. allowing protons to re-enter mitochondrial matrix without capturing any energy as ATP. The energy is released as heat and the process is called **non-shivering thermogenesis.**
- Uncouplers are (mostly) *toxic in vivo*, causing respiration to become uncontrolled, since the *rate is no longer limited by concentration of ADP or Pi*. These allow mitochondria to use $O_2$ regardless of whether or not there is any ADP or Pi available.
- Uncouplers (eg DNP) are amphipathic & *increase permeability of lipoid inner mitochondrial membrane to protons, thus reducing electro- chemical potential & short circuiting ATP- synthase.* In this way oxidation can proceed without phosphorylation (i.e., without ATP synthesis). So energy is lost as heat (**chemiosmotic theory**). So these are toxic in vivo. Examples are

| Natural/Physiological Uncouplers | Synthetic Uncouplers |
|---|---|
| - **Uncoupling proteins (UCP)** occur in *inner mitochondrial membrane (of mammals* including humans) *adipocytes.* **Thermogenin (UCP-1)** is responsible for non shivering thermogenesis (heat production) in **brown fat** to maintain body heat, in response to cold in *neonates* and during arousal in *hibernating animals*. UCP-1 is activated by *fatty acids* and brown fat (unlike white fat) uses almost 90% of its respiratory enrgy for thermogenesis. UCP-2 and 3 are also found in humans but their importance remains unclear.<br>- **Long chain fatty acids (FA)** in brown fat<br>- Essential fatty acid (EFA) deficiency<br>- Excess of **thyroxine hormone**<br>- Unconjugated *hyperbilirubinaemia* | - **2, 4 Dinitrophenol★** (2,4-DNP)<br>- **2, 4 Dinitrocresol★** (2,4-DNC)<br>- **CCCP★** (Chloro carbonyl cyanide phenyl hydrazone; the most active uncoupler)<br>- **FCCP★** (tri fluora carbonyl cyanide phenyl hydrazone)<br>- **Dicoumarol** (vitamin K analogue, anti coagulant)<br>- **Aspirin** & other salicylates in high doses; this is the reason of fever d/t toxic overdose<br>- ***Valinomycin*** (produced by streptomyces; **a $K^+$ ionophore,** transport $K^+$ from cytosol to matrix & $H^+$ viceversa thus decreasing proton gradient)<br>- **Calcium** ($Ca^{++}$ transport into mitochondria is coupled with uptakes of Pi and oxidative phosphorylation. But the energy produced is spent to pump the $Ca^{++}$ into mitochondria. So $e^-$ transport proceeds but no energy is stored as ATP)<br>★ Are hydrophobic proton carriers |

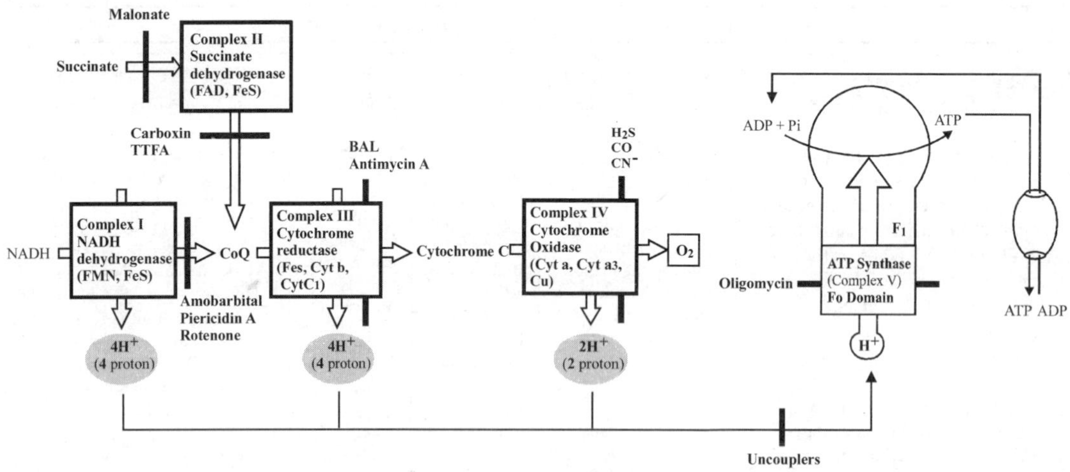


## Mechanism of Apoptosis

**Extrinsic (death- receptor- initiated) pathway**

- **Death receptors** are members of **TNF** (tumor necrosis factor esp *TNF1*) family that contain a **cytoplasmic death domain** involved in protein- protein interaction. The pathway is initiated by engagement of cell surface death receptor.
- When **Fas** binds to its ligand FasL (a death receptor) their cytoplasmic death domain binds with **FADD (Fas associated death domain)**, which in turn binds an inactive form of ***caspase – 8 (& in humans caspase- 10)***.
- Multiple procaspase 8 molecules cleave one another to generate active caspase –8. This pathway can be inhibited by **FLIP**.

**Intrinsic (mitochondrial) pathway**

- Growth factors & survival signals stimulate antiapoptotic. **Bcl – 2 protein** (named after B cell lymphoma & is homologous to C. elegans protein C ed 9)
- **Antiapoptotic Bcl- 2** & **Bcl- x** proteins normally reside in mitochondria & cytoplasm
- When cells are deprived of survival signals or subjected to stress Bcl – 2 / Bcl-x are lost from mitochondrial membranes & replaced by **pro-apoptotic Bak, Bax**, and **Bim**. So the permeability of mitochondrial membrane increases and **cytochrome C** & **AIF** leaks out.
- Cytochrome C binds to **Apaf-1 (apoptosis activating factor 1**, homologous to Ced 4 of c. elegans) and complex activates **caspase – 9**
- **Apoptosis inducing factor (AIF)** enter cytosol & bind to various inhibitors of apoptosis.

## Glycogen Phosphorylase and Glycogenolysis

- Mobilization of stored glycogen is caused **by glycogen phosphorylase**, which degrades *glycogen to glucose 1 phosphate*. It is often referred to simply as **phosphorylase** – so honoured because it was the first phosphorylase to be discovered. It was the first enzyme shown to be allosterically regulated & controlled by reversible phosphorylation and for which detailed 3 dimensional structures of active & inactive forms were revealed by x-ray crystallography.
- Phosphorylase exists in 2 inter convertible forms: **phosphorylase a** which is catalytically active, and **phosphorylase b** which is less active (or inactive). This conversion from inactive to active phosphorylase is done by active phosphorylase kinase b or **phosphorylase kinase a,** an enzyme responsible for transferring a phosphoryl group to ser residues in each of the 2 identical subunits of glycogen phosphorylase.
- **Epinephrine & nor epinephrine (in muscle** during activity) or **glucagon** (in **liver** when blood glucose level is too low) *increase concentration* of **C-AMP,** which inturn activates **C- AMP dependent protein kinase (protein kinase A, or PKA).** PKA then **phosphorylates & activates phosphorylase b kinase (to phosphorylase kinase a)**, which catalyzes phosphorylation and activation of serine residues of **glycogen phosphorylae** , and thus stimulating glycogen breakdown. In muscle this provides fuel for glycolysis to sustain muscle contraction whereas in liver it counters the low blood glucose levels.
- Both phosphorylase and phosphorylase kinase (a) are

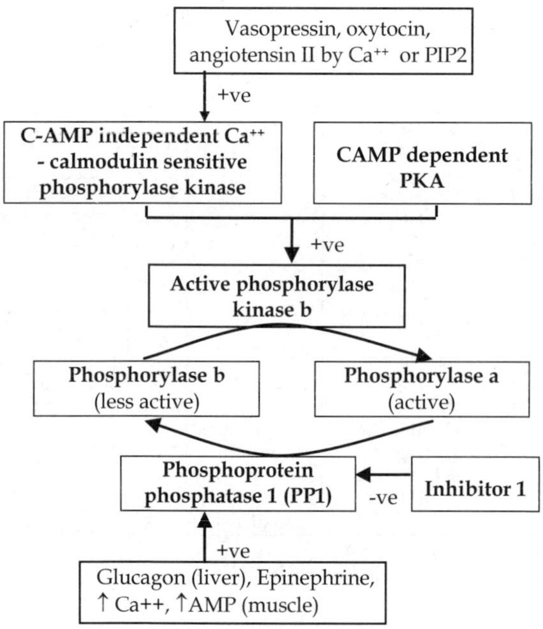

dephosphorylated and inactivated by **phosphorylase α phosphatase or phosphoprotein phosphatase 1** (PP1). In resting muscles. Protein **inhibitor 1**, when activated after phosphorylation by cAMP dependent protein kinase,inhibit PP1. In liver insulin increases activity of **phosphodiesterase** (which hydrolyze C-AMP) and indirectly stimulate PP1 resulting in decreased glycogenolysis.

- In liver, cAMP independent glycogenolysis occurs in response to $\alpha_1$ *adrenergic stimulation by epinephrine or norepinephrine*. This involves stimulation of **$Ca^{++}$ / calmodulin sensitive phosphorylase kinase** by Ca++. It is also activated by ***vasopressin, oxytocin, & angiotensin II***Q acting either through $Ca^{++}$ or PIP2
- ***$Ca^{++}$ ion is responsible for intiation & synchronization of both muscle contraction and glycogenolysis (or activation of phosphorylase)***Q. Muscle phosphorylase kinase (c̲ activates phosphorylase) is a tetramer of α, β, γ, and δ subunits.
  - **α, and β,** subunits contain serine residue that are activated by cAMP dependent protein kinase.
  - **δ** subunit is identical to Ca++ binding protein calmodulin & binds 4 $Ca^{++}$
  - **γ catalytic subunit** is activated (by δ- calcium binding) even while the enzyme is in dephosphorylated state b; the fully activated & phsphorylated a form occurs in high concentrations of calcium.
- **Allosteric control** of phosphorylase occurs through

**In muscle**

- **Activation**
  - $Ca^{++}$ (through δ subunit of phosphorylase kinase)
  - **C- AMP**
  - 5′ AMP
- **Inhibition**
  - ***ATP***Q
  - Glucose 6 phosphate

**In Liver**

- **Activation**
  - CAMP
- **Inhibition**
  - ***ATP***Q
  - Glucose 6 phosphate
  - ***Free glucose***Q

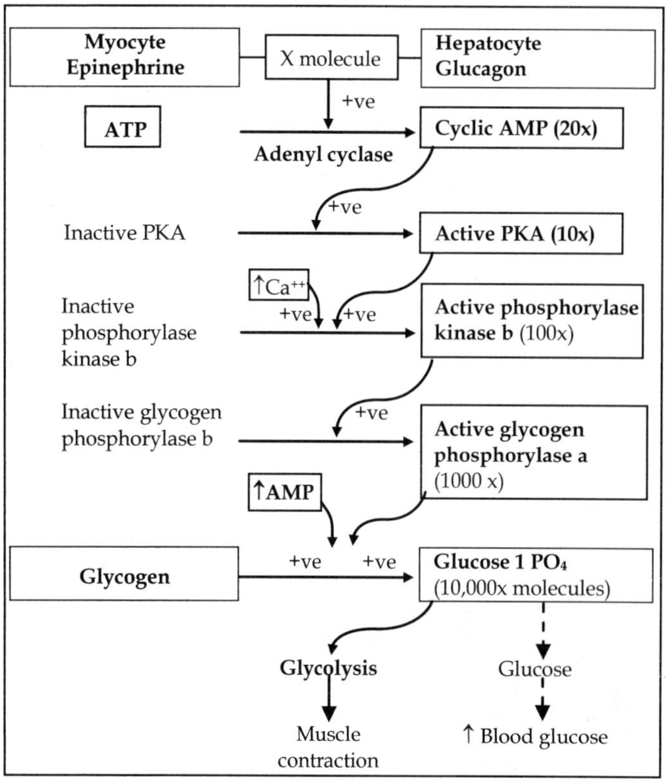


| Factors maintaining active phosphorylase | Allosteric Inhibitors of glycogen phosphorylase (inactivating it) | Factors maintaining inactive phosphorylase |
|---|---|---|
| - ***C- AMP dependent protein kinase***Q<br>- ***Adenyl cyclase, Cyclic AMP and hormones***Q increasing C-AMP.such as **epinephrine (in muscle)**, norepinephrine, **glucagon** (in liver) & thyroid hormone<br>- Calmodulin component of phosphorylase kinase<br>- ***Calcium***Q<br>- ***5AMP*** (allosteric activator in muscle only)<br>- ***Inhibitor-1*** (inhibits PP-1) | - ***ATP & Glucose 6 phosphate (in muscles & liver both)***Q<br>- ***Glucose (in liver but not in muscles)*** Q | - ***Protein phosphatase 1***Q (PP-1)<br>- ***Glucose 6 phosphate***Q<br>- ***Insulin***Q<br>- Phosphodiesterase (hydrolyze cAMP) |

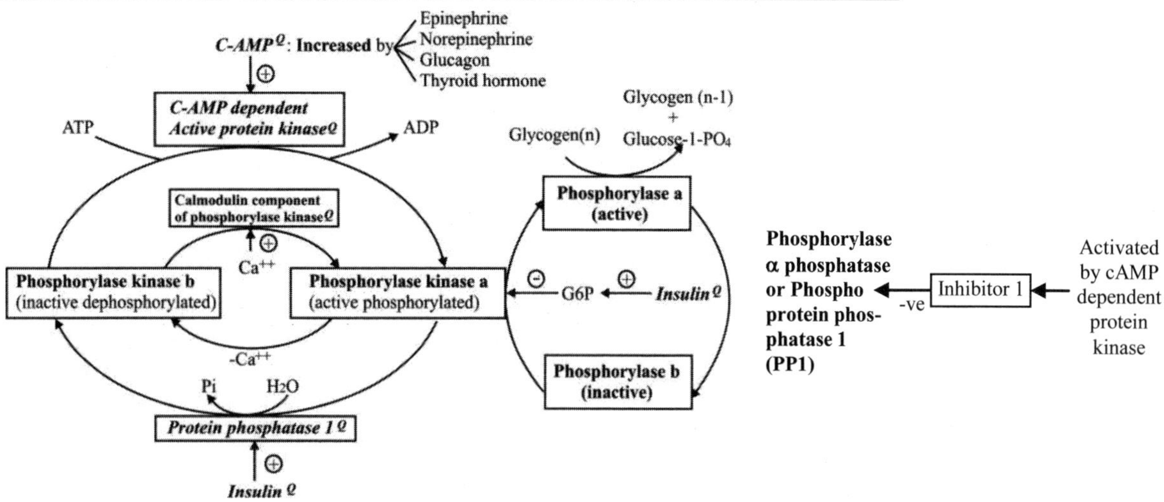

## Glycogenesis and Glycogenolysis

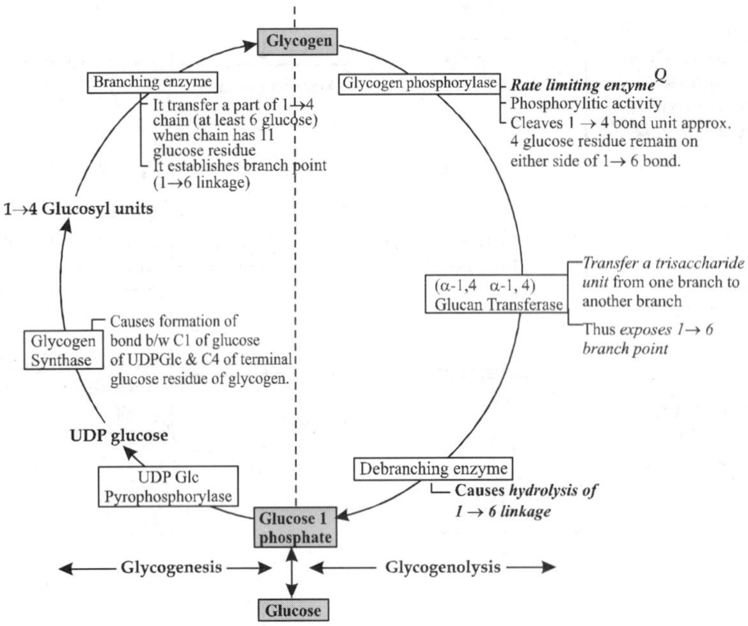


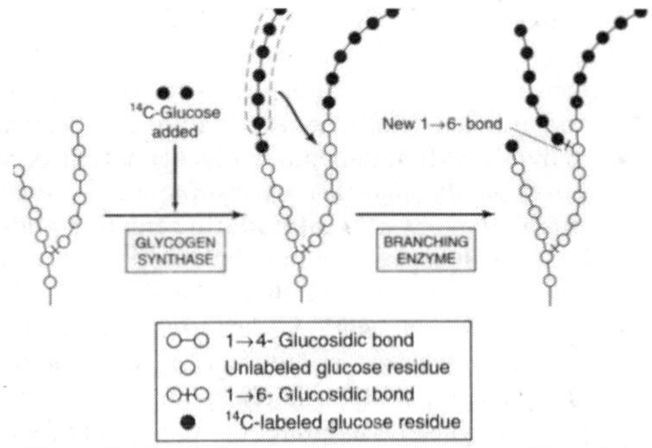


The biosynthesis of glycogen. The mechanism of branching as revealed by adding 14C-labeled glucose to the diet in the living animal and examining the liver glycogen at further intervals

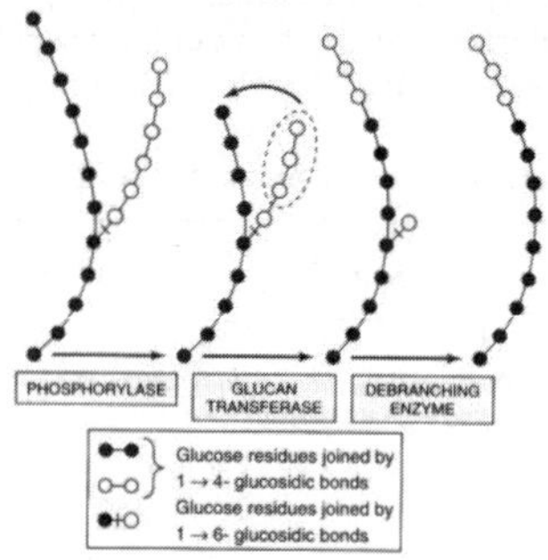


Steps in glycogenolysis

In well fed state (also called *absorptive stage*) ***insulin suppresses glucose -6- phosphatase activity and causes glucose 6 – phosphate to enter glycogenesis***[Q] (to form glycogen).

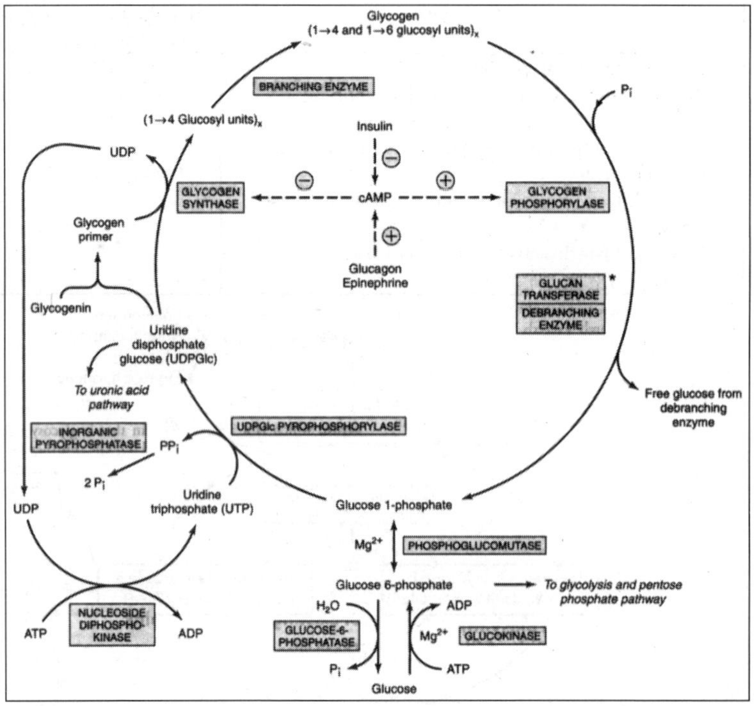


Pathway of glycogenesis and of glycogenolysis in the liver. Two high-energy phosphates are used in the incorporation of 1 mol of glucose into glycogen. (+), stimulation; (-), inhibition. ***Insulin decreases the level of cAMP only after it has been raised by glucagons or epinephrine – i.e. it antagonizes their action***[Q]. Glucagon is active in heart muscle but not in skeletal muscle. At asterisk: Glucan transferase and debranching enzyme appear to be two separate activities of the same enzyme.

## Glycogen Storage Diseases (Glycogenosis)

| Type | Name | Deficient Enzyme | Organ involved primarily | Clinical Features |
|---|---|---|---|---|
| O | - | Glycogen synthase | Liver | Hypoglycemia (low blood glucose), hyper ketonemia (high ketone bodies), early death. |
| Ia | Von Gierke's disease | *Glucose 6 phosphatase*Q | *Liver*Q | - Glycogen (**normal structured** but metabolically unavailable) accumulation in liver & renal tubule cells l/t hepatorenomegaly and failure (of both)<br>- **Hypoglycemia, hyper lipemia, hypercholesterolemia, hyper triglyceridemia** *(d/t increased fat mobilization)*Q, **hyper ketonemia (ketosis), lactic acidemia (lactic acidosis) and hyper uricemia** |
| Ib | - | Endoplasmic reticulum glucose -6- Phosphate transporter (microsomal -6- P translocase) | *Liver* | - **High susceptibility to recurrent bacterial infections** d/t neutropenia and impaired neutrophil function<br>- Rest as Type Ia |
| Ic | - | Microsomal Pi transporter | *Liver* | As type Ia |
| II | Pompe's | Lysosomal glucosidase ($\alpha 1 \rightarrow 4$ & $\alpha 1 \rightarrow 6$) or **Acid maltase** | Skeletal & Cardiac muscle | - Fatal accumulation of glycogen in lysosome<br>- **Infantile-juvenile** form: muscle hypotonia & death from **heart failure by age 2.**<br>- **Juvenile-adult form** : myopathy & muscular dystrophy |
| IIIa | Forbe's or Cori's, Limit dextrinosis | Liver & muscle debranching enzyme | Liver, Skeletal & Cardiac muscle | - *Hepatomegaly in infants*, myopathy (muscle weakness), fasting hypoglycemia<br>- Accumulation of characteristic branched polysaccharide (**limit dextrin**) |
| IIIb | Limit dextrinosis | **Liver debranching enzyme** (muscle enzyme normal) | Liver | As type IIIa but *no muscle involvement (weakness)* |
| IV | Andersen's, Amylopectinosis | Branching enzyme | Liver, Skeletal muscle | - Hepato-spleenomegaly, myoglobin in urine, death d/t cardiac or liver failure before age 5<br>- Accumulation of polysachride with few branch points. |
| V | Mc Ardle's | Muscle (Myo) phosphorylase | Skeletal muscle | - Exercise induced cramps & pain d/t poor exercise tolerance; blood lactate is very low after exercise<br>- Muscle glycogen content is abnormally high (2.5-4%); myoglobin in urine. |
| VI | Her's | Liver phosphorylase | Liver | Hepatomegaly (d/t accumulation of glycogen), mild hypoglycemia & generally good prognosis. |
| VII | Tarui's | Muscle & erythrocyte phosphofructo kinase (PFK)-1 | Muscle, RBC | As type V with **hemolytic anemia** |
| VIII | | Liver phosphorylase kinase | Liver | As type VI |
| IX | | Liver & muscle phosphorylase-kinase | Liver, muscle | As type VI with accumulation of glycogen in muscle. |
| VIb | | Leukocyte & Liver phosphorylase kinase | Leukocytes & Liver | As type VI |
| X | | C-AMP dependent protein kinase | Liver | Hepatomegaly; accumulation of glycogen in liver |
| XI | Fanconi-Bickel | Glucose transporter (GLUT-2) | Liver | Failure to thrive, hypatomegaly, renal failure and rickets. |

★ Fabry's disease and krabbe's disease are sphingolipidoses. **Fragile X- syndrome** is caused by *abnormal expansion of trinucleotide repeats* (CGG/ CCG expansion lead to fragile site on chromosomes)

| Disease | Deficiency/Absent Enzyme |
|---|---|
| Fabry's disease | deficiency of α- ***Galactosidase***Q |
| Farber's disease | deficiency of ceramidase |
| Forbe's disease | ***Absence of debranching enzyme***Q. |

## Von Gierke's Disease (Type Ia Glycogen storage Disease)

| | |
|---|---|
| Inheritance | **AR**Q |
| **Chromosome** | 17 |
| **Enzyme defect** | *Glucose 6 phosphatase*Q |
| **Organs affected** | **Liver** (primary), kidney, intestinal mucosa |
| **Glycogen Stored** | ***Normal in structure but metabolically not available***Q |
| Appearance | *Doll like face* with fatty cheeks, thin extremities and protuberant abdomen (d/t **hepato-reno megaly)** |

Glucose 6 phosphatase (present in liver but not in muscle) *converts glucose 6-PO4 (obtained from glycogenolysis) to glucose*. So deficiency l/t **hypoglycemia**.

**Metabolic Abnormalities & Clinical Presentation**

- **Fasting hypoglycemia** d/t unavailability of glycogen
- **Hyper lipemia (hyper lipidemia), acidaemia & ketosis** occurs as a result of utilizing fat as energy source (i.e. **increased fat mobilization**).
- Excess acetyl CoA obtained from β- oxidation is diverted for **increased cholesterol, fatty acid** and **ketone body synthesis** resulting in xanthomas, fatty infiltration of liver, hepatorenomegaly (protuberant abdomen) & doll like face with fatty cheeks
- Persistent hypoglycemia has 2 effects
  - *Inhibits insulin secretion* which *inturn inhibits protein synthesis* l/t *stunted growth (dwarfism) and thin extremities*
  - *Stimulates secretion of catecholamines* which cause muscle glycogen to break down producing *lactic acidosis*
- Hyperuricemia an gout (d/t more pentose ***formation and decreased excretion)***Q. It has 2 reasons

1. Increased production:
   - ***Accumulated G-6- Phosphate enters the HMP shunt and l/t increased production of pentoses***Q
   - Pentose acts as substrate for *PRPP synthetase* (Phospho Ribosyl pyro phosphate synthetase) and result in *increased production of purines*
   - Purines are catebolized to uric acid.
2. Decreased renal excretion of uric acid is caused by *increased lactic acid level which competes with uric acid for excretion.*

## 6- Phosphogluconate Pathway / Hexose Mono Phosphate (HMP) Shunt / Pentose Phosphate Pathway (PPP)/Warburg-Dickens-Lipman-Pathway

- It is an *alternate pathway for complete oxidation of glucose*, which is not ***meant for production of energy (ATP)***Q. Like glycolysis, enzymes of PPP are ***cytosolic***Q. But unlike glycolysis
  - the **irreversible oxidative portion of PPP** occurs in specialize tissue like ***liver, lactating mammary glands & adipose tissue***Q which are active in fatty acid synthesis, in ***adrenal cortex***Q which is active in NADPH dependent synthesis of steroids and in ***erythrocytes***Q which require NADPH to require glutathione reduced. It also occurs in ***lens, cornea, testes and ovary but not in non lactating mammary gland and unimportant in skeletal muscle***Q. Whereas glycolysis occurs in all tissues.
  - It is *multicyclic process*, 3 molecules of glucose 6 phosphate gives rise to 3 molecules of CO2 and 3 molecules of 5 carbon sugar, which rearranges to give 2 molecules of glucose 6- phosphate and 1 molecule of glyceraldehyde 3- phosphate. ***$CO_2$ is produced in HMP shunt which is never produced in E.M. pathway***Q.

| 6 Carbon Glucose –6 P (3 molecules) | → | 5 Carbon Sugar (3 molecules) +3$CO_2$ |
|---|---|---|
| | | ↓ Rearrange |
| | | 6 carbon Glucose– 6–P (2 molecules) + 3 carbon Glyceraldehyde–3–P (1 molecule) |

  - ***Oxidation is achieved by dehydrogenation using $NADP^+$ not $NAD^+$ as hydrogen acceptor***Q.
- HMP shunt can be divided into 2 phases: (1) **oxidative non reversible phase** that l/t formation of ribulose 5-$PO_4$, $CO_2$ and 2 molecules of NADPH for each molecule of glucose – 6 – $PO_4$ oxidized. (2) **non-oxidative reversible phase** that occurs in all cells synthesizing nucleotides & nucleic acids; and mainly *involve* ***two transketolase (transfer 2 carbon units) and one transaldolase (which transfer 3 carbon units)*** *reactions.*
- ***Glucose 6 $PO_4$ dehydrogenase is the rate limiting enzyme and uses $NADP^+$ as a coenzyme***Q. **Transketolase** ***requires thiamine pyrophosphate (TPP)***Q. Other enzymes requiring TPP are ***pyruvate de carboxylase***Q of pyruvate dehydrogenase complex, ***α –ketoglutarate dehydrogenase***Q of TCA cycle, & ***branched chain α -keto acid deydrogenase***Q of branched chain aminoacid metabolism.
- ***No ATP is directly produced or consumed in HMP shunt***Q. Its ***major function is to provide NADPH***Q (required for fatty acid & steroid synthesis) ***and pentose sugar***Q (for nucleic acid & nucleotide synthesis). Summary of PPP is

| 3 glucose – 6- $PO_4$ + NADP+ | → | 2 glucose – 6- $PO_4$ + 1 glyceraldehyde-3- $PO_4$ + 3$CO_2$ + 6NADPH + 6$H^+$ |
|---|---|---|

★ **Insulin** & **thyroid hormone** enhance the activity of HMP shunt

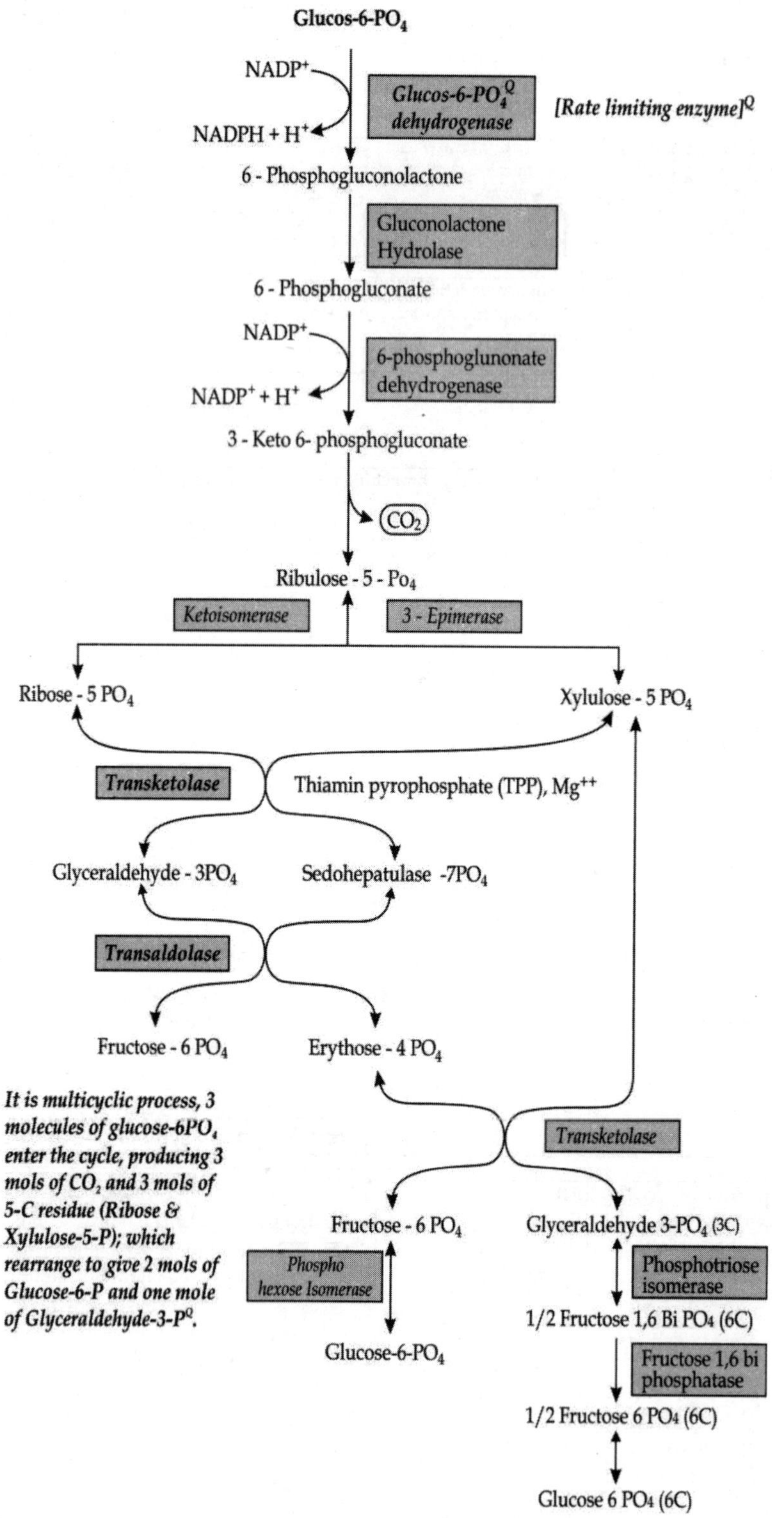


✱ ***It is multicyclic process, 3 molecules of glucose-6$PO_4$ enter the cycle, producing 3 mols of $CO_2$ and 3 mols of 5-C residue (Ribose & Xylulose-5-P); which rearrange to give 2 mols of Glucose-6-P and one mole of Glyceraldehyde-3-P***Q.

[see coloured plate 21]

## Glucose-6-$PO_4$ Dehydrogenase (G6PD) Deficiency

- It is a ***X-linked recessive disorder***[Q] that causes episodic hemolytic anemia because of ***decreased ability of RBCs to deal with oxidative stresses, due to impaired generation of NADPH***[Q].
- ***G6PD is the first and rate limiting enzyme of the HMP shunt which is responsible for the production of NADPH in the cells***[Q].

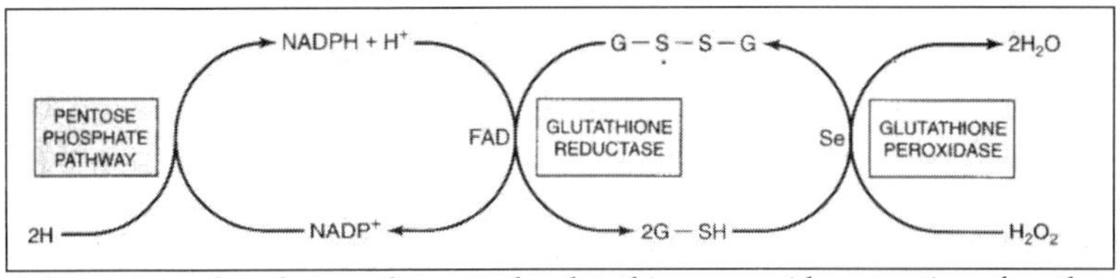


Role of the pentose phosphate pathway in the glutathione peroxidase reaction of erythrocytes. (G-S-S-G, oxidized glutathione; G-SH, reduced glutathione; Se, selenium cofactor)

- NADPH acts as a ***cofactor for glutathione reductase***[Q] that generates reduced form of glutathione.
- Reduced glutathione is a potent antioxidant and removes $H_2O_2$ by enzyme ***glutathione peroxidase***
- In the absence of reduced glutathione, $H_2O_2$ accumulates and decrease the life span of RBC by causing oxidative damage to cell membrane leading to hemolysis.
- **Favism** by eating **Fava beans** (eg as an ingredient of falafel- a Mediterranean food) *l/t hemolytic anemia, jaundice, even kidney failure & death may occur in peoples with G6PD deficiency.*

## Carbon ($CO_2$) Assimilation /Fixation = Calvin Photosynthetic Carbon Reduction Cycle

- Plants synthesize carbohydrate from $CO_2$ and water by process of photo synthesis in plastids (chloroplast). It occurs in 3 stages – fixation of $CO_2$ into 3 phosphoglycerate, conversion of 3 phosphoglycerate to glyceraldehydes 3 phosphate and regeneration of ribulose 1, 5 biphosphate from triose (glyceraldehydes 3) phosphate.
- Overall 3 molecules of ribulose 1, 5 biphosphate fixes 3 molecules of $CO_2$ to form 6 molecules of glyceraldehyde 3 phosphate (18 carbons) in equilibrium with dihydroxy acetone phosphate. The formation of glyceraldehyde from 3 phosphoglycerate *is reversal of corresponding glycolysis steps, with one exception that cofactor is* NADPH rather than NADH.
- In 3rd stage 5 of 6 molecules of triose (glyceraldehyde 3) $PO_4$ (=15C) are used to regenerate 3 molecules of starting material ribulose 1, 5 biphosphate (15 carbons) involving many of the same reactions used in oxidative **pentose phosphate pathway** (but in reverse direction). This **reductive pentose phosphate pathway** also uses few extra enzymes like sedoheptulose, 1, 7 biphosphatase etc that make the reductive cycle irreversible.
- **Fructose 6 phosphate** is a key intermediate in stage 3 and can lead either to regeneration of ribulose 1, 5 biphosphate or to synthesis of starch.
- **6 NADPH and 9 ATPs** are required for synthesis of each triose phosphate (glyceraldehyde 3 $PO_4$) from $CO_2$ & $H_2O$. so summary of calvin cycle is

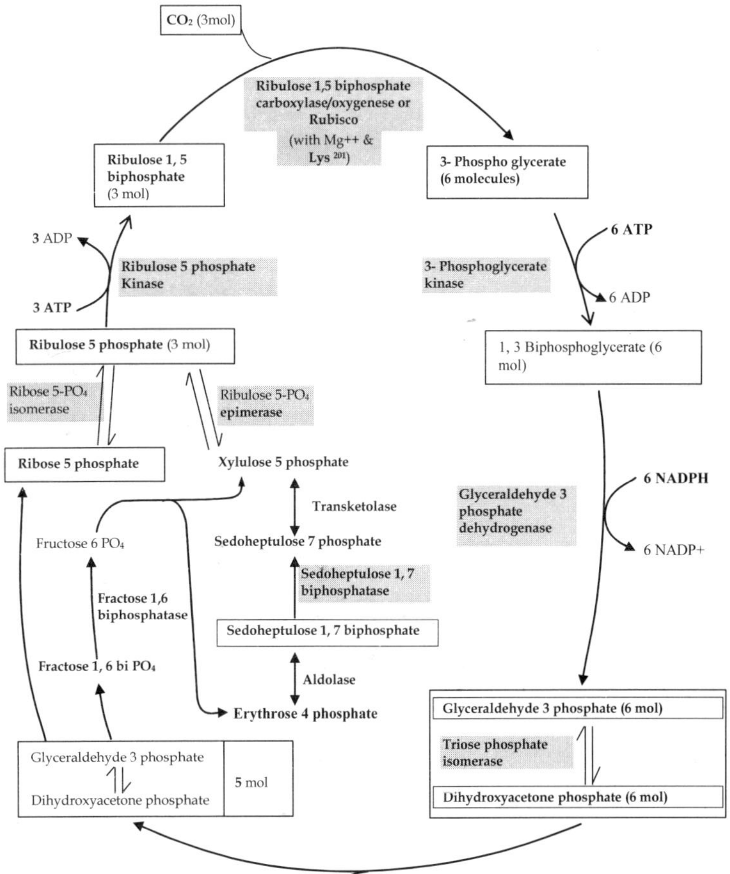


**Glyceraldehyde 3 phosphate** (1 molecule) used immediately for ATP production by glycolysis or converted to **fructose 6 phosphate** ultimately forming starch (in chloroplast) or sucrose (in cytoplasm) to be stored for later use

$$3CO_2 + 5H_2O + \mathbf{6NADPH + 9\ ATP \rightarrow Glyceraldehyde\ 3\ phosphate\ (G3P)} + 6NADP^+ + 9\ ADP + 2H^+ + 8Pi$$

## Gluconeogenesis

It is the formation of glucose or glycogen from noncarbohydrate sources. **Substrate for gluconeogenesis** (as per priorities) are

1. **Glucogenic aminoacids** grouped by site of entry in TCA cycle

**Amino acid that form pyruvate**
Mn – **"Sir Try All 39 Glass Cyst"**

| | |
|---|---|
| Sir | **Ser**ine |
| Try all | **Try**ptophan |
| 3 | **Thre**onine |
| 9 | ***Alanine***[Q] |
| Glass | **Gly**cine |
| Cyst | **Cyst**eine |

- Form **Oxaloacetate**
  Mn – **"As Per"**
  - **Aspar**agine
  - **Aspar**tate
- Form **Fumarate**

| | |
|---|---|
| P | Phenyl alanine |
| T | Tyrosine |

Form **Sucinyl CoA**
Mn –**"3 Will meet1 Lucy"**

| | |
|---|---|
| 3 | - **Thre**onine |
| Will | - **Val**ine |
| Meet | - **Met**hionine |
| 1-Lucy | - iso-**Leu**cine |

Form **α-Ketoglutarate**
Mn **"His Glues Are Prolific"**

| | |
|---|---|
| His | **His**tidine |
| Glues | **Glu**tamate |
| | **Glu**tamine |
| Are | **Ar**ginine |
| Prolific | **Pro**line |

2. ***Lactate***[Q] 3. ***Pyruvate***[Q] 4. ***Glycerol***[Q] (obtained from lipolysis of fat) [Mn "**G < P < L**"]
5. ***Propionic acid***[Q] (important in ruminants)

## Ketogenic A.A

Those A.A that are converted to *acetoacetate*; or one of its precursors (acetyl CoA or acetoacetyl CoA)

- ***Leucine***[Q]
- ***Lysine***[Q]

A.A that are **both Glucogenic & Ketogenic**

| | | |
|---|---|---|
| T | - | Tyrosine |
| | | Tryptophan |
| I | - | Isoleucine |
| P | - | Phenylalanine |

**Carbohydrate (pyruvate), oxidation of fatty acids (beta- oxidation)** and ethanol, **ketogenic amino acids, ketone bodies (ketolysis), HMG CoA**, thioesterification of acetate and Clevage of citrate **form Acetyl CoA**, which is used in

**TCA (Citric acid cycle /Oxidative phosphorylation)**
↓
**Energy (10 –ATP) + $CO_2$**
- Combines with oxaloacetate to form citric acid, which initiates **TCA cycle** to generate ATP via oxidative phosphorylation
- Each molecule of acetyl CoA produce **10 ATP** (new concept)

★ All pathways of fat, protein & carbohydrate catabolism l/t production of acetyl CoA which is oxidized in TCA to yield ATP

**Acetylation reaction**
↓
- **Detoxification** of xenobiotics & drugs like isoniazid, sulfonamides, & PAS
- **Acetyl choline synthesis**
- **Melatonin synthesis**

★ **Pantothenic acid** is coenzyme for acetylation reaction.

**Cholesterol synthesis**
↓
- **Steroidogenesis**
- **Steroid hormone, vitamin $D_3$ formation**

★ **Acetyl CoA & Malonyl CoA** are used in **lipogenesis**

**- Fatty acid synthesis**
**- Lipogenesis**
↓
- **Synthesis & elongation of fatty acids (lipogenesis)**
- Synthesis of ether lipids eg *plasmalogense & platelet activating factor (PAF)*

**Ketogenesis**
↓
**Ketone body formation**
↓
**Energy**

## Fate of

### Acetyl CoA

- In **Citric Acid Cycle**
  Acetyl CoA + O.A.A —*Citrate Synthase*→ Citric Acid
- In **Cholesterol Synthesis**
  Acetyl CoA —*Thiolase*→ Aceto Acetyl CoA —*HMG CoA Synthase*→ HMG CoA
- In Fatty Acid Synthesis
  Acetyl CoA —*Acetyl CoA Carboxylase*→ Malonyl CoA

  Fatty Acid Synthase Enzyme
  **Acetyl Transacylase** | **Malonyl Transacylase**
  ↓
  Acetyl-Malonyl Enzyme
- In **β oxidation**
  3 Keto acyl CoA —*Thiolase*→ Acyl CoA + Acetyl CoA

### Pyruvate

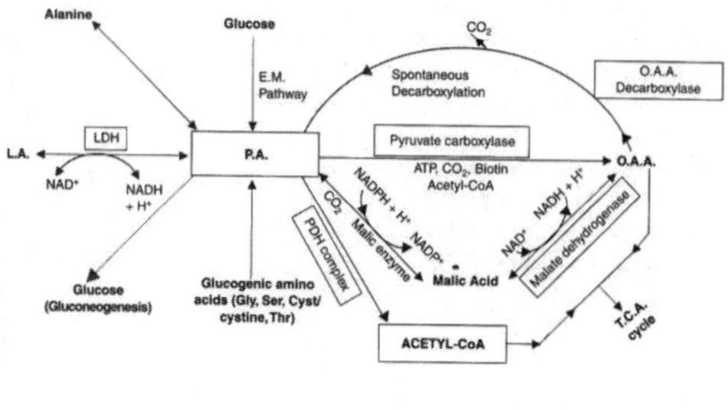


★ **Acetyl CoA carboxylase is also known as Malonyl CoA Synthetase**

## Gluconeogenesis

- The **carbon skeletons for gluconeogenesis** are derived primarily from ***glucogenic aminoacids & lactate from muscle and glycerol from adipose tissue***Q. **Although the lactate produced in muscle** (by anaerobic glycolysis during intense exercise) **is *used by liver for gluconeogenesis (through Cori cycle); the muscles do not participate in gluconeogenesis*Q. *Liver and kidney are the major gluconeogenic tissues*Q.**
- ***Gluconeogenesis prevent hypoglycemia during short and long term (= prolonged) fasting***Q i.e. begins 4-6 hours after the last meal becomes fully active as stores of liver glycogen are depleted and peaks at 5-7 days of fasting .
- ***Gluconeogenesis is stimulated by excess of acetyl CoA and decrease in fructose 2, 6 biphosphate concentration***Q.
  1. **Although acetyl CoA cannot be used as a substrate for gluconeogenesis,** it is an **allosteric activator** of pyruvate **carboxylase** and an **allosteric inhibitor of pyruvate dehydrogenase.** So acetyl CoA (produced by β oxidation) pushes pyruvate to gluconeogenesis
  2. **Gluconeogenesis is favoured by activation of fructose 1,6 biphosphatase ( F 16 BPase d/t decreased availability of its inhibitor F,1, 6 biphosphate)** and by **induction of PEPCK** by glucagon.
- It is **synthesis of glucose or glycogen from** non carbohydrate precursors (substrates) such as **glucogenic aminoacids** (forming **pyruvate**, oxaloacetate, alpha KG, succinyl CoA, fumarate), **lactate, glycerol and propionate. Liver and kidneys** are major gluconeogenic tissues; the kidney contributing upto 40% of total glucose synthesis in fasting state and more in starvation. Gluconeogenic key enzymes are expressed in **small intestine** but their role in fasting state is unclear.
- A supply of **glucose** is necessary for **nervous system (brain) & erythrocytes (RBC)**. Glucose is important in *maintaining the level of intermediates of citric acid cycle* even when fatty acids are the main source of acetyl CoA. Gluconeogenesis also *clears lactate produced by muscles & erythrocytes, and glycerol produced by adipose tissue.* Failure of gluconeogenesis is fatal b/o hypoglycemic brain dysfunction and excessive gluconeogenesis in critically ill (injured / infected) patients also has poor outcome.
- It *involves glycolysis*, the *citric acid cycle* plus some special reactions.
- *Main Pathway* of gluconeogenesis *is **a reversal of glycolytic pathway*** but **thermodynamic 'barriers'** prevent a simple reversal of glycolysis. There are *four such energy barriers which are irreversible.* Three non equilibrium reactions in glycolysis and one in glycogen metabolism prevent simple reversal of glycolysis for glucose /glycogen synthesis (gluconeogenesis) and they are
- **Propionate** is a major source of glucose in **ruminants**. It **non ruminant** (eg **humans**) propionate arises from ***beta-oxidation of odd chain fatty acids (eg ruminant lipids), oxidation of isoleucine & side chain of cholesterol***Q, and is a minor substrate for gluconeogenesis.

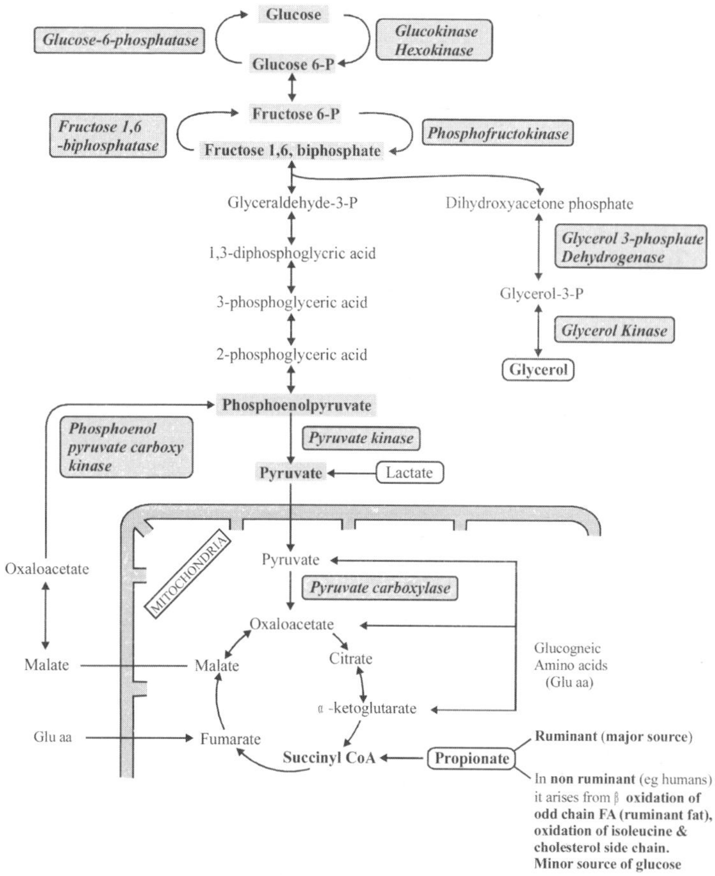


**Major pathways of gluconeogenesis and glycolysis in liver**

[see coloured Plate 22]

| Irreversible Thermodynamic Barrier Reactions | Enzyme in Glycolysis, Glycogen metabolism (4th) | Reversed in Gluconeogenesis by key Enzymes |
|---|---|---|
| Phosphoenol pyruvate (PEP) → Pyruvate | *Pyruvate Kinase*Q | *Pyruvate carboxylase & PEP carboxy kinase*Q |
| Fructose 6 phosphate → Fructose 1, 6 biphosphate | Phospho fructokinase (PFK)1 | Fructose 1, 6 biphosphatase |
| Glucose → Glucose 6 phosphate | *Gluco/Hexo-Kinase*Q | *Glucose 6 phosphatase*Q |
| Glycogen → Glucose 1 phosphate | Glycogen phosphorylase, Glucan transferase, Debranching enzyme | UDP Glc phosphorylase, Glycogen synthase, Branching enzyme |

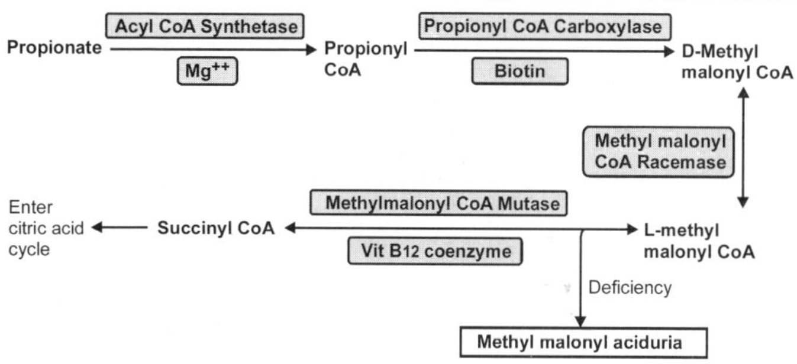

# Regulation of Gluconeogenesis & Glycolysis

## Regulatory & Adaptive Enzymes a/w Carbohydrate Metabolism

- Since glycolysis and gluconeogenesis share the same pathwy but in opposite directions, they must be regulated reciprocally. **Availability of glucogenic precursors (substrates)** is the most important factor, along with **circulating level of glucagon**, in movement to movement **regulation of gluconeogenesis**.
- In carbohydrate metabolism enzyme activity is **regulated by 3 mechanisms**

| Enzyme | Enzyme Activity in | | Transcription Regulator | | Allosteric Regulation | |
|---|---|---|---|---|---|---|
| | High Energy state (Carbohydrate Feeding) | Low Energy state (Fasting/ Diabetes) | Inducer | Repressor | Activator | Inhibitor |
| **Glycogenolysis, Glycolysis, & Pyruvate oxidation** | Increase 1-6 except 2 | Decrease 1-6 except 2 | | | | |
| **1. Glycogen synthase** | ↑ | ↓ | | | Insulin, glucose 6-phosphate | Glucagon |
| **2. Hexokinase** | - | - | | | | Glucose 6 phosphate |
| **3. Glucokinase** | ↑ | ↓ | **Insulin** | Glucagon | | |
| **4. Phosphofructo-kinase (PFK)1** | ↑ | ↓ | **Insulin** | Glucagon | **AMP,** fructose 6-P, fructose 2 , 6 biphosphate, Pi | Citrate, ATP, glucagon |
| **5. Pyruvate kinase** | ↑ | ↓ | **Insulin, fructose** | Glucagon | Fructos 1, 6 biphosphate, insulin | ATP, alanine, glucagon, nor epinephrine |
| **6. Pyruvate dehydrogenase** | ↑ | ↓ | | | CoA, NAD+, insulin, ADP, pyruvate | ***Acetyl CoA***[Q], NADH, ATP (fatty acid ketone -bodies) |
| **Gluconeogenesis**<br>**7. Pyruvate carboxylase** | | | **Glucacortico-steroids,** | Insulin | **Acetyl CoA**[Q] | **ADP**[Q] |
| **8. PEP carboxykinase** | | | **glucagon ,** | | Glucagon? | - |
| **9. Glucose 6-phosphatase** | | | **epinephrine** | | - | - |

### Slow Adaptive changes in enzyme activity (Induction & Repression) from alteration in rate of Enzyme Synthesis or Degradation or both.

- Induction & repression of key enzymes (*catalyzing physiologically irreversible non equilibrium reactions*) is **slow & requires several hours.**
- Activity of enzymes catalyzing reactions in opposite direction varies **reciprocally** so the effects are reinforced.
- For example **insulin** secreted in response to excess of blood glucose enhance synthesis of *key enzymes of glycolysis and antagonize* the effect of epinephrine, glucocorticoids and glucagon stimulated cAMP thereby suppressing synthesis of *key enzymes of gluconeogenesis*.

**Excess of glucose (Carbohydrate Feeding)**

→ **Increased Insulin** → **Increased activity of enzymes involved in glucose utilization (glycolysis &** lipogenesis)

→ **Decreased Glucocorticoids, Glucagon, Epinephrine** → **Decreased** activity (synthesis) of key enzymes of **gluconeogenesis**

### Covalent Modification by Reversible Phosphorylation

- It is **rapid**
- In response to **fasting** (decrease in blood glucose), **glucagon & epinephrine,** inhibit glycolysis and stimulate gluconeogenesis in liver by **increasing cAMP concentration. c-AMP dependent protein kinase activity** leads to phosphorylation & inactivation of **pyruvate kinase**

**Fasting / Diabetes**

→ **Decreased insulin & glycolysis enzymes**

→ **Increased glucocorticoids, glucagon (cAMP), epinephrine** and enzymes of **gluconeo-genesis**

### Allosteric Modification

It is **instantaneous** and examples of allosteric regulation include

**A. Allosteric activation of hepatic pyruvate carboxylase by acetyl CoA increases gluconeogenesis** and **reciprocal inhibition of pyruvate dehydrogenase** by acetyl CoA sparing pyruvate from oxidation (in TCA).

- **Gluconeogenesis in fasting state** is ***indicated by increased activity (activation) of pyruvate carboxylase by Acetyl CoA***[Q]. As a result of increased lipolysis (in fasting state & diabetes), the liver is flooded with fatty acids. The rate of formation of acetyl CoA by beta- oxidation of these fatty acids exceeds the capacity of liver to oxidize it to $CO_2$ & $H_2O$. As a result, **acetyl CoA accumulates and cause allosteric activation of hepatic pyruvate carboxylase.** At the same time acetyl CoA **inhibits pyruvate dehydrogenase** (by activating PDH kinase). Thus acetyl CoA can divert pyruvate towards gluconeogenesis and away from TCA.

**Beta- oxidation of FA (fasting)**

↓

**Acetyl CoA**

→ **Allosteric activation of pyruvate carboxylase (in liver)**

→ **Reciprocal inhibition of PDH**

**Metabolic Fate of Pyruvate**

↓ Pyruvate is converted to oxaloacetate (entering gluconeogenesis)

↓ Inhibits conversion of pyruvate to acetyl CoA. Thus pyruvate is diverted away from TCA

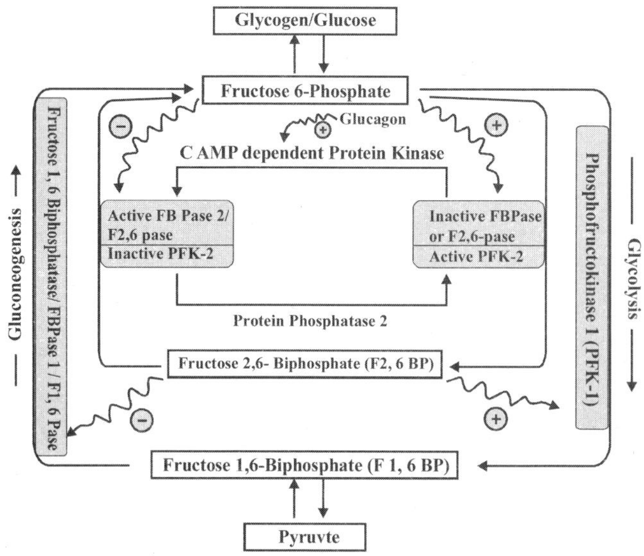


**B. Allosteric regulation by Energy levels within cells**

- **5′AMP acts as an indicator of energy status of cells.** A small decrease in ATP (d/t its use in energy requiring proesses) causes a several fold increase in AMP so that AMP acts as a **metabolic amplifier (sensitive signal) of change in energy status of cell.**
- Energy rich state of cell (ie high ATP & low AMP levels) stimulate gluconeogenesis (an energy requiring pathway). Whereas energy poor state (elevated levels of AMP) increase glycolysis (for energy / ATP formation)

**PFK-1 and Fructose 1, 6 Biphosphatase are reciprocally regulated (allosterically) by AMP**

- **Fructose 1, 6 biphosphatase is allosterically inhibited by AMP** (decreasing gluconeogenesis) and simultaneously AMP **activates phosphofructokinase (phosphofructokinase 1)** increasing glycolysis & **phosphorylase** increasing glycogenolysis.
- **PFK1 occupies a key position in regulating glycolysis** in response to energy status of cell. It is activated by 5′ AMP and is inhibited by citrate & normal ATP concentrations. As a consequence of inhibition of PFK-1, glucose 6 phosphate accumulates, which in turn inhibits uptake of glucose in extrahepatic tissue by inhibition of hexokinase.

**C. PFK-1 & FBP ase1are reciprocally regulated (allosterically) by Fructose 2, 6 Biphosphate**

- **Fructose 2, 6 Biphosphate** is most potent positive allosteric **activator of phosphor fructokinase 1** (increasing glycolysis) and **inhibitor of fructose 1, 6 biphosphatase /FBPase 1 /or F 1, 6 pase** (decreasing gluconeogenesis). Thus it *(F2, 6 BP) plays a unique role in regulation of glycolysis & gluconeogenesis in liver*[Q].
- **PFK1 is virtually inactive in the absence of F2, 6 biphosphate (d/t inhibition caused by ATP, citrate glucagon).** F2, 6 biphoshate increases PFK1's affinity for its substrate fructose 6 phosphate and reduces its affinity for allosteric inhibitors ATP & citrate; thereby increasing glycolysis. F2, 6 BP has opposite effect on FBPase1 : it inhibits FBpase 1 (or fructose 1, 6 biphosphatase) by reducing its affinity or increasing km for its substrate fructose 1, 6 biphosphate

**Fructose 2, 6 Biphosphate (F2, 6 BP)**

- **Allostric activation of PFK-1 by increasing** its **affinity for** its substrate **fructose 6 phosphate** & reducing affinity for its allosteric inhibitors ATP & citrate
  ↓
  **Increase glycolysis**
- **Allosteric inhibition** of **FBPase 1 (Fructose 1, 6 biphosphatase or F1, 6 pase) by reducing its affinity or increasing Km for** its substate **fructose 1, 6 biphosphate**
  ↓
  **Decrease gluconeogenesis**

- **In well fed state with abundant supply of glucose (& so fructose 6 phosphate)**
  ↓
  **Allosteric Stimulation of PFK-2 and inhibition of FBPase 2 by fructose 6 phosphate**
- **Fasting state**
  ↓
  **Glucagon enhances FBPase 2 and inhibits PFK-2 activity**

- Therefore **decreased sensitivity of FBpase 1 to regulation (inhibition) by fructose 2, 6 biphosphate increases gluconeogenesis;** ***thereby decreasing levels of fructose 1, 6 biphosphate, pyruvate and ATP***[Q].
- Cellular **levels of allosteric regulator fructose 2, 6 biphosphate (F2, 6BP) depends on the relative rates of its formation (by phosphofructokinase 2 or PFK2) and breakdown (by fructose 2, 6 biphosphatase or FBPase 2).** PFK-2 and FBPase 2 are 2 separate enzymatic activities of a **single bifunctional protein (enzyme)**. This bifunctional enzyme is **under allosteric control of fructose 6 phosphate which stimulates kinase (PFK-2) and inhibits phosphatase** (FBpase 2). The balance of these activities are **regulated by glucagon & insulin; as glucagon enhances FBPase 2 activity & inhibits PFK-2 activity** (via cAMP dependent protein kinase) whereas insulin has opposite effect.

**Feed – Fast Cycle**

**After Feeding**

- Liver is a glucose producing rather than a glucose using tissue. However after a meal containing carbohydrate, the liver becomes a net consumer of glucose, retaining ~ *60 of every 100 gm of glucose* presented by portal system.

**After Fasting (starvation)**

- ↑ glycogen degradation (glycogenolysis)
- ↑ gluconeogenesis
- ↑ fatty acid oxidation
- ↑synthesis of ketone bodies (ketogenesis)
- ↑ degradation of TAG

- Hepatic metabolism of glucose is increased by
  - ↑ phosphorylation of glucose
  - ↑ glycogen synthesis
  - ↑ activity of HMP
  - ↑ glycolysis
  - ↓ gluconeogenesis
- Fat metabolism: ↑ Fatty acid & TAG synthesis
- Aminoacid metabolism: ↑protein synthesis and ↑ amino acid degradation
  But the liver has limited capacity to degrade branched chain aminoacids leucine, isoleucine and valine; they pass through the liver essentially unchanged and are preferentially metabolized in muscle.

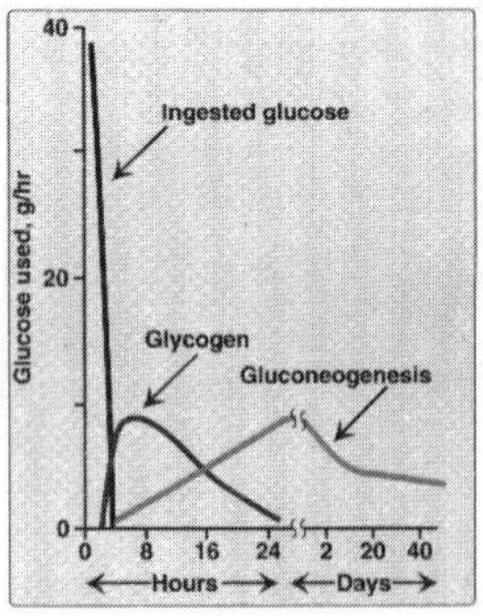


**Sources of blood glucose after ingestion of 100g of glucose**

## Fructose Metabolism

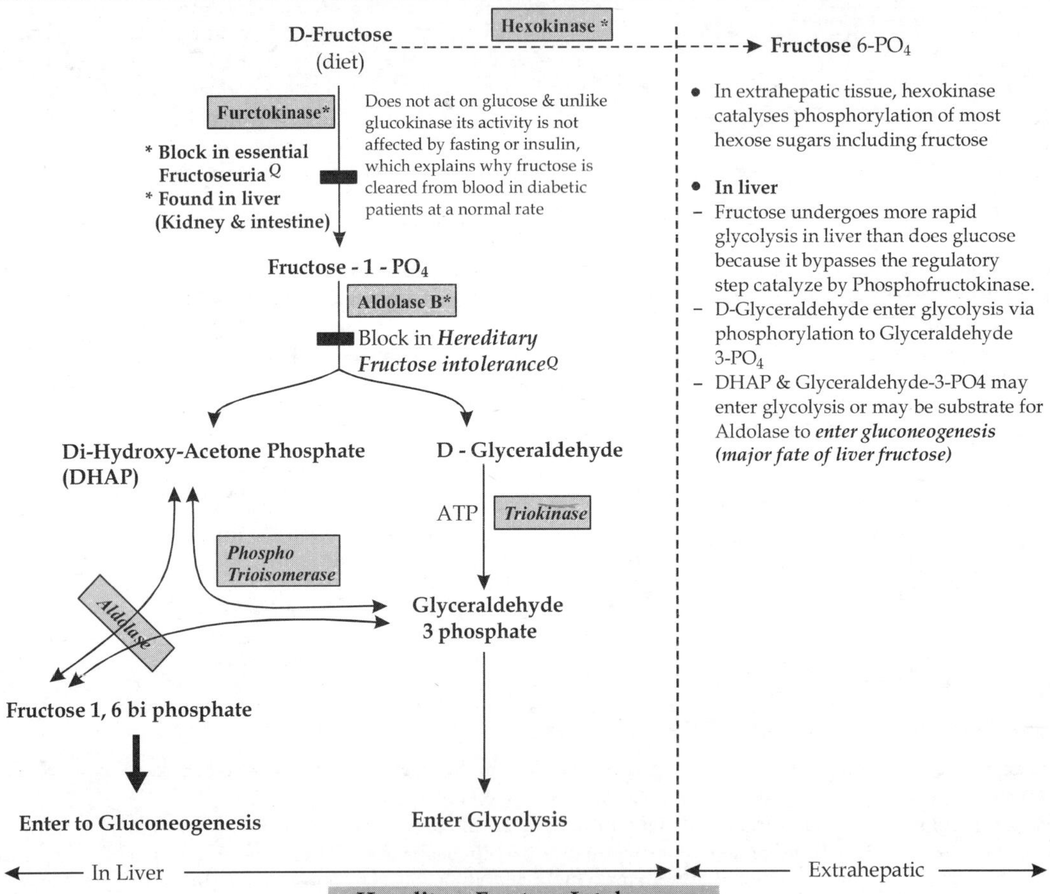


- In extrahepatic tissue, hexokinase catalyses phosphorylation of most hexose sugars including fructose
- **In liver**
  - Fructose undergoes more rapid glycolysis in liver than does glucose because it bypasses the regulatory step catalyze by Phosphofructokinase.
  - D-Glyceraldehyde enter glycolysis via phosphorylation to Glyceraldehyde 3-$PO_4$
  - DHAP & Glyceraldehyde-3-PO4 may enter glycolysis or may be substrate for Aldolase to ***enter gluconeogenesis (major fate of liver fructose)***

### Hereditary Fructose Intolerance

| Hereditary fructose intolerance is due to ***deficiency of fructose 1, 6- biphosphate aldolase B in the liver, kidney and intestine***[Q]. | |
|---|---|
| **Mechanism** | **Clinical Presentation** |
| • Aldolase B catalyzes fructose 1-$PO_4$ to DHAP and D-glyceraldehyde.<br>• Its deficiency causes ***excessive rise of fructose -1- $PO_4$ and fructose in blood***[Q]<br>↓<br>***Hypoglycemia***[Q] | • This is severe disease of infants that appears with the ingestion of fructose containing food<br>• Administration of fructose or sucrose leads to ***Hypoglycemia***[Q] accompanied by nausea, vomiting, convulsion & profuse sweating.<br>• Continued intake leads to<br>- ***Hepatomegaly***[Q]<br>- ***Jaundice***[Q]<br>- ***Proximal renal tubular dysfunction***[Q]<br>- ***Intellectual impairment***[Q] |
| **Treatment:** Complete elimination of all sources of sucrose, fructose and sorbitol from the diet. | |

## Glactosemia

An inherited ***Autosomal recessive***[Q] disorder, in which there is inability to convert galactose to glucose in normal manner. This may occur *due to deficiency* of following enzymes:

| **Galactose 1-$PO_4$ uridyl transferase** (classical & most common) | **UDP galactose -4 epimerase** (Rare) | **Galactokinase** (Minor) |
|---|---|---|
| - Manifests with in a few days after birth ***(after ingestion of milk)***[Q]<br>- Failure to thrive<br>- ***Hepto splenomegaly***[Q]<br>- Jaundice, Ascites<br>- ***Hypoglycemia***[Q]<br>- ***Mental retardation***[Q]<br>- ***Cataract***[Q], ***(oil drop cataract)***[Q] | Feature of uridyl trans ferase deficiency +<br>- Nerve deafness<br>- Hypotonia<br>- ↑in cellular UDP Galactose | *Cataract*[Q]<br>Affected infant is other wise asymptomatic. |

- Infants are subject to ***bacterial sepsis (especially with E.coli)***[Q] this may be *leading cause of death*.
- **Biochemical & urinary finding**
  - Increase blood galactose level
  - ***Decreased blood glucose***[Q]
  - ***Galactosuria (reducing sugar galactose** in urine gives **positive Benedict's test)***[Q]
  - Albuminuria
  - Amiaciduria: Glycine, Alanine, Serine
- **Treatment:** ***Galactose free diet***[Q].

### Galactose Metabolism

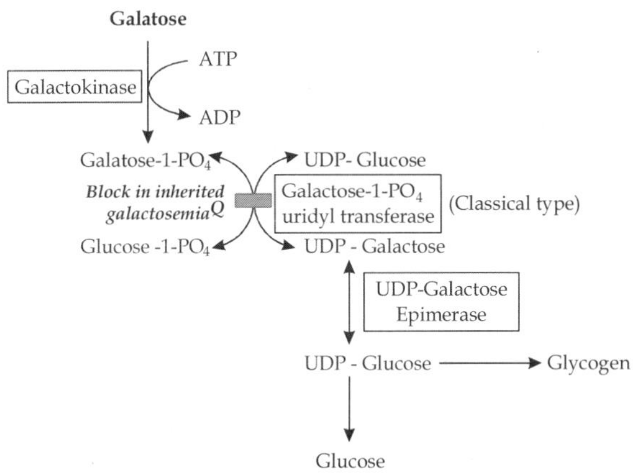


### Cataract

| **In Galactosemia is due to accumulation of galactitol**[Q]**.** | **In Diabetes is due to accumulation of sorbitol**[Q] **in lens.** |
|---|---|
| • The increased galactose conc. in blood and eye is reduced to *Galactitol* by *aldolase reductase,*<br>• Galactitol can not escape from lens cells and accumulates to form cataract. | ↑Concentration of glucose in blood & eye is *reduced to sorbitol* by aldolase reductase. |

## Ethanol (Alcohol) Metabolism

***Major path in liver involves 2 oxidation reactions by alcohol & aldehyde dehydrogenase & NAD+***[Q]

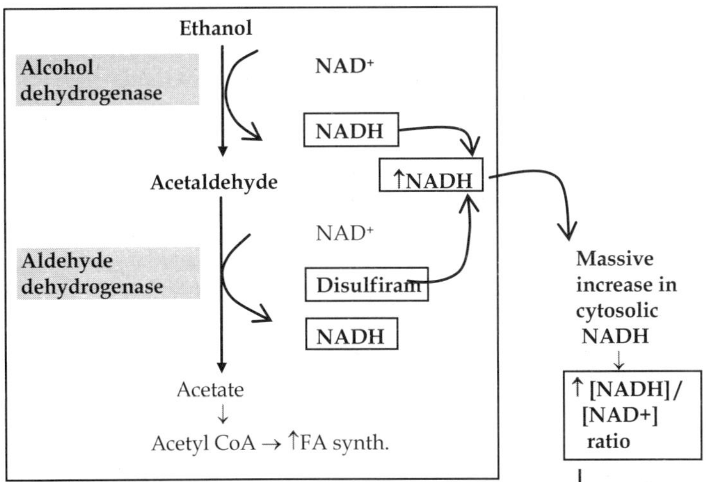


- Minor path takes place via cytochrome P450 dependent **microsomal ethanol oxidizing system (MEOS)** involving *NADPH*[Q] & $O_2$
- This system increases in activity in chronic alcoholism & may account for increased metabolic clearance

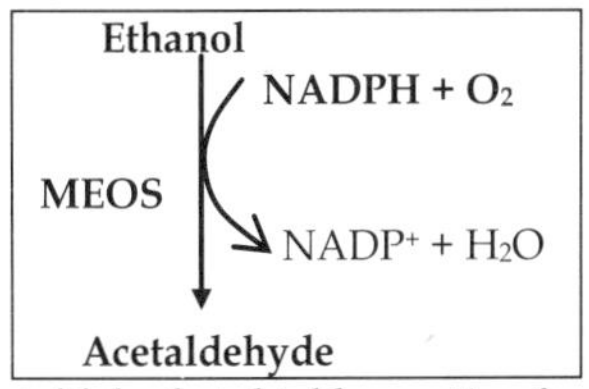


★ **Acetaldehyde** is highly reactive & can *form adducts* with protein nucleic acids & other molecules

★ *Ethanol interpolates* into biological membranes, expanding them and increasing their fluidity. It alters membrane active transport, AP, & neurotransmitter release esp affecting brain.

↑ [NADH]/[NAD+] ratio:

- Favours reduction of pyruvate to lactate and oxaloacetate to malate
  - **↑lactate / pyruvate ratio**
    - **Hyperlacticacidemia**
    - ↓ excretion of uric acid
    - Aggravate **gout**
  - **↓gluconeogenesis** (because both pyruvate & oxaloacetate are intermediates)
    ↓
    **Precipitate hypoglycemia** in individuals who have depleted their stores of liver glycogen or are using insulin.
- - **Inhibits fatty acid oxidation**
  - **↑esterification of FA** to form triacyl glycerol resulting in fatty liver
- Inhibits glycerophosphate dehydrogenase l/t elevated glycerophosphate

# Classification of Carbohydrate Structure

## Aldose and Ketose

- Monosacchrides are classified a/t the number of carbon atoms they contain eg triose for 3C, tetrose for 4C etc. Most oxidized functional group of **aldoses** is aldehyde and **ketoses** is ketone. In other words, if the carbonyl group is at an end ($C_1$) of carbon chain (in an aldehyde group) the monosacchride is aldose and if the carbonyl group is at any other position (eg $C_2$ in a ketone group) the monosaccharide is a ketose. Most aldoses have –ose (except few like glyceraldehyde) and ketoses have – ulose (except few like fructose) suffix.

## Epimers

- Carbohydrate isomers that differ in configuration around only one carbon atom (with the exception of carbonyl carbon) are called **epimers**. For example
- **Erythrose and threose** are $C_2$ epimers
- **Ribose** is epimer of **arabinose** (at $C_2$) and **xylose** (at $C_3$) but arabinose and xylose are not epimers as they differ in $C_2$ & $C_3$ positions.
- **Lyxose** is epimer of **Xylose** (at $C_2$) and **arabinose** (at $C_3$) but arabinose and Xylose are not epimers as they differ in $C_2$ & $C_3$ positions.
- **Glucose** is epimer of **mannose** (at $C_2$) and **galactose** (at $C_4$) but mannose & galactose are not epimers.
- **Allose** is epimer of **altrose** ($C_2$), **glucose** ($C_3$) and **gulose** ($C_4$) but altrose, glucose & gulose are not epimers
- **Talose** is epimer of **galactose** ($C_2$), **idose** ($C_3$) and **mannose** ($C_4$) but galactose, idose & mannose are not epimers.

| $^1$CHO | CHO | CHO | CHO | CHO | CHO | CHO | CHO |
|---|---|---|---|---|---|---|---|
| H - $^2$C - OH | OH - C - H | H - C - OH | HO - C - H | H - C - OH | HO - C - H | H - C - OH | HO - C - H |
| H - $^3$C - OH | H - C - OH | HO- C - H | HO - C -H | H - C - OH | H - C - OH | HO- C - H | HO- C - H |
| H - $^4$C - OH | H - C - OH | H - C - OH | H - C - OH | HO- C - H | HO- C - H | HO - C - H | HO - C - H |
| H - $^5$C - OH | H - C - OH | H - C - OH | H - C - OH | H - C - OH | H - C - OH | H - C - OH | H - C - OH |
| $^6CH_2OH$ | $CH_2OH$ | $CH_2OH$ | $CH_2OH$ | $CH_2OH$ | $CH_2OH$ | $CH_2OH$ | $CH_2OH$ |
| D-Allose | D-Altrose | D-Glucose | D-Mannose | D-Gulose | D-I dose | D-Galactose | D-Talose |

## Enantiomers (Optical/Stereo-Isomers)

- **Enantiomers (optical isomers or stereoisomers)** are pairs of structures that are **mirror images of each other but not identical**, similar to left and right hand which are the same but opposite. These are non super imposable and are designated as **D and L-sugar**. Each enantiomer often *shows different chemical reactions* with other enantiomers. Because of presence of many enantiomers in living beings, there is usually a marked difference in effects of two stereoisomers. For example only one of drug stereoisomer produces desired effect while the other does not.
- Isomers that are mirror images of each other are called **enantiomers (optical isomers)** and the 2 membes are designated as 'D' or 'L' sugars. In **L** form the OH group on the **asymmetric (chiral) carbon** *(i.e. a carbon linked to 4 different atoms or groups)* farthest from carbonyl carbon is on **left**, whereas in **D isoform** it is on the **right. Racemase** enzymes inter convert D & L enantiomers. In general, a molecule with n chiral centers have $2^n$ **stereoisomers** (enantiomers). Glyceraldehyde (triose) has 1 chiral carbon so $2^1 = 2$ stereoisomers, whereas hexoses have 4 chiral carbons so $2^4 = 16$ stereoisomers.
- The *presence of asymmetric carbon atoms provides optical activity to compound.* A beam of polarized light, when passed through a solution of optical isomer, is rotated either to **right, dextro rotatory (+)** or to **left, (levorotatory (-)**. *Stereochemistry (D/L forms) is independent of the direction of rotation of polarized light*, so D (+), D (-), L (+) or L (-) forms exist. Glucose being dextrorotatory is also called dextrose and naturally occurring fructose is D (-).

## Isomers

**Isomers** are compounds that *have same chemical formula but have different structures*. For example glucose, fructose, galactose, mannose, idose, talose, gulose, allose, and altrose all are isomers with same chemical formula $C_6H_{12}O_6$.

| Carbon | Generic | Aldoses | Ketoses |
|---|---|---|---|
| 3 | **Trioses** ($C_3H_6O_3$) | **Glycerose** (glyceraldehyde) | **Dihydroxy-acetone** |
| 4 | **Tetroses** ($C_4H_8O_4$) | **Erythrose,** Threose | **Erythrulose** |
| 5 | **Pentoses** ($C_5H_{10}O_5$) | **Ribose, Xylose** Arabinose, Lyxose | **Ribulose Xylulose** |
| 6 | **Hexoses** ($C_6H_{12}O_6$) | **Glucose, Gulose, Galactose, Mannose,** Allose, Altrose, Idose, Talose | **Fructose,** Psicose, Sorbose, Tagatose |
| 7 | **Heptoses** ($C_7H_{14}O_7$) | - | **Sedoheptulose** |
| 9 | **Nonoses** ($C_9H_{18}O_9$) | **Neuraminic Acid** | |

## Pyran/Furan; Haworth Projection; Chair Conformation

- The ring structure of monosaccharides are either similar to **pyran** (a *6 membered ring consisting of 5 carbon & 1 oxygen*) or **furan** (a 5 membered ring consisting of 4 carbon & 1 oxygen) and are called **pyranose** or **furanose.**
- Cyclic structures are drawn in **Haworth projection** in which *bonds nearest to the viewer* (viewing from side & above the plane of ring) *are bold and thickened* and OH groups are above or below the plane of ring. However, the 6 membered pyranose ring is *actually in form of (two) chair conformation* and is not planar as Haworth perspective suggested. Two **conformations** (like chair) are **interconvertible *without the breakage of covalent bond whereas 2 configurations (like Alpha & Beta) can be inter converted only by breaking a covalent bond.***
- If the hydroxyl group of anomeric carbon of ring sugar is not linked to other compound by a glycosidic bond, the ring can open and the sugar is called **reducing sugar**. Because it acts as a reducing agent with **chromogenic Benedict's** or **Fehling's solutions.** So the reagent gets reduced and sugar becomes oxidized. Only state of oxygen in aldehyde group decide if sugar is reducing or non reducing.

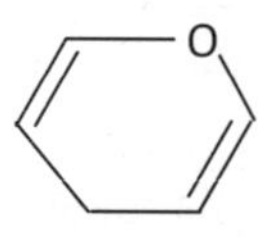


**Pyran**

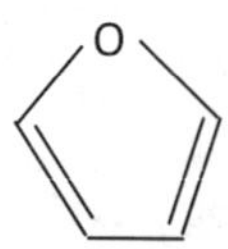


**Furan**

### Fischer Projection Formula; Diastereomers (Anomers)

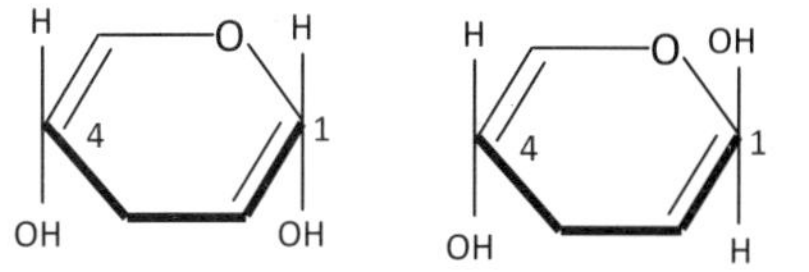

α-D-Gluco β-D- Gluco pyrnose

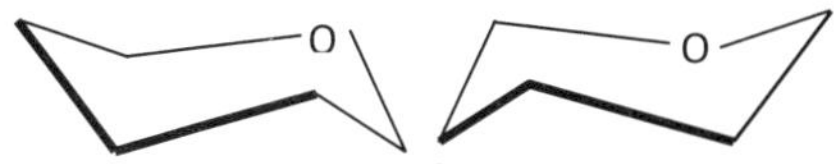

2 Chair conformations

- **In Fischer projection formula** to represent 3 dimensional sugar structure on paper, horizontal bonds project out of plane of paper *towards* the reader, whereas vertical bonds project behind the plane of paper, away from reader.
- $\geq$ 99% of sugars with 5 or more carbons exist in **cyclic (ring) form** (i.e. $\leq$ 1% is in **open chain** or **acyclic form**) in which the aldehyde group (of aldose) or Keto group (of ketose) has reacted with the alcohol (OH) group on the same sugar to form **hemiacetals** or **hemiketals**. This cyclization makes the carbonyl carbon ($C_1$ of aldose & $C_2$ of ketose) asymmetric (now called **anomeric carbon**) generating **alpha and beta anomers**. Because these are not mirror images of each other they are also called **diastereomers**, and can be spontaneously inter converted by **mutarotation process**. The **alpha anomer** has **same side** and **beta anomer** has **opposite side orientation of hydroxyl (OH) group at anomeric & farthest chiral centers**, in Fischer projection. Biological enzymes use alpha or Beta forms preferentially like glycogen is synthesized from alpha where as cellulose from Beta – D glucopyranonose.

### Inulin like Fructan Prebiotics (ILF)

- **Prebiotics** are *nondigestible food ingredients* that should *pass harmlessly through upper gastrointestinal tract* to be a *substrate for advantageous probiotic agents (colonic bacteria) in the large bowel*. These beneficially affect the host by *selectively stimulating the growth or activity of health promoting colonic bacteria like lactobacilli & bifidobacteria*.
- Inulin is a polysaccharide of fructose (& so a **fructosan**) found in roots & tubers of dandelions, dahlias and artichokes. It is easily soluble in water and is used to **determine GFR**. But it is not hydrolyzed by intestinal enzymes and acid. So **non digestible oligosaccharide (NDO)- inulin like fructans** are most widely used & studies prebiotics.
- Inulin like fructans are **non digestible** in upper digestive tract b/o their **β-configuration of anomeric $C_2$**. Their **Beta glycosidic bonds (linkages)** resist the hydrolysis by enzymes & acid. As human digestive enzymes **α–amylase (in saliva)** and **disaccharidases** (like isomaltase, maltase, sucrase, lactase synthesized by small intestinal mainly jejunal mucosal cells) can break **α (1 → 4) and α (1 → 6) glycosidic bonds** respectively; trehalase breaks α (1 → 1) bond.
- Humans lack β- (1 → 4) endoglucosidase and therefore are unable to digest cellulose containing *β (1 → 4) glycosidic bonds between glucose residue* and chitin (exoskeleton of arthropods) containing *β (1 → 4) glycosidic linkage b/w N-acetyl glucosamine residue.*
- ILF pass through small bowel without degradation and with out inhibiting (even actually promoting) the absorption of nutrients & minerals like $Fe^{+2}$, $Ca^{+2}$ and $Mg^{+2}$ (i.e. harmless passage through upper digestive tract).
- ILF reach colon in intact form and become substrates for *beneficial health promoting probiotic bacteria like bifidobacteria and lactobacilli.*

# Chapter -2 FAT METABOLISM

## QUESTIONS

### Lipids of Physiological Significance

1. **All are true except**
   A. Linoleic acid is found in soyabean oil ☐
   B. Linolenic & linoleic acids are cis derivatives containing double bonds. ☐
   C. Arachidonic acid contain five double bonds. ☐
   D. Monoenoic acids contain one double bond at 9th position. ☐
2. **Which among the following is a cardioprotective fatty acid?**
   A. Palmitic acid ☐
   B. Stearic acid ☐
   C. Oleic acid ☐
   D. Omega-3 fatty acids ☐
3. **True statement about fatty acid:**
   A. Polyunsaturated FA is essential for membrane structure ☐
   B. Biologically arachidonic acid is essential to life ☐
   C. Hydrogenated vegetable oils contains Trans fatty acid ☐
   D. Most of the naturally occurring unsaturated FA exists as trans-isomer ☐
4. **False about trans fatty acid**
   A. Increase risk of cardiovascular disease ☐
   B. Fried foods have high content of TFA ☐
   C. Hydrogenation increases TFA ☐
   D. Hydrogenation decreases TFA ☐
   E. It ↑ LDL & ↓ HDL ☐
5. **The most essential fatty acid is**
   A. Linoleic acid ☐
   B. Linolenic acid ☐
   C. Arachidonic acid ☐
   D. Palmitic acid ☐
6. **Essential fatty acid is/are:**
   A. Palmitic acid ☐
   B. Linoleic acid ☐
   C. Linolenic acid ☐
   D. Free fatty acid ☐
   E. Oleic acid ☐
7. **Maximum source of linoleic acid is**
   A. Coconut oil ☐
   B. Sunflower oil ☐
   C. Palm oil ☐
   D. Vanaspati ☐
8. **Which of these fatty acids is found exclusively in breast milk:**
   A. Linolaete ☐
   B. Linolenic ☐
   C. Palmitic ☐
   D. Docosahexanoic acid ☐
9. **The following fatty acid does not belong to W6 series**
   A. Linoleic acid ☐
   B. Arachidonc acid ☐
   C. Gamma linolenic acid ☐
   D. Alpha linolenic acid ☐
10. **Gangliosides consists of:**
    A. Long chain fatty acid (LCFA) ☐
    B. Alcohol- sphingosine ☐
    C. Phosphate ☐
    D. Sailic acid ☐
    E. Glycerol ☐
11. **Which of the following is correct in regards of function of phospholipid:**
    A. Cell-cell interaction ☐
    B. Signal transduction ☐
    C. Surfactant ☐
    D. Acute inflammatory mediator ☐
    E. Activates membrane enzyme ☐
12. **Glycosphingolipidis made up of:**
    A. Glucose ☐
    B. Glycerol ☐
    C. Sphingosine ☐
    D. Fatty acids ☐
    E. Thromboxane A2 ☐
13. **Alcoholic group is found in:**
    A. Ganglioside ☐
    B. Sphingomyelin ☐
    C. Cerebroside ☐
    D. Terpen ☐
14. **Not a predisposing factor for atherosclerotic plaque formation?**
    A. Apo E deficiency ☐
    B. Alpha 2 – macroglobulin ☐
    C. Oxidised LDL ☐
    D. Increased homocyctiene ☐

### Acylglycerol & Sphingolipid Metabolism

15. **Molecular change in Lysosomal storage disorder is:**
    A. Defective fusion of lysosomes and phagosomes ☐
    B. Increased synthesis of some substrates ☐
    C. Mutation of genes encoding lysosomal hydrolases ☐
    D. Membrane defect of lysosomes ☐
16. **Which of the following is/are not sphingolipidosis:**
    A. Tay sach's disease ☐
    B. Sandhoff's disease ☐
    C. Krabbe's disease ☐
    D. Wolman disease ☐
    E. Fabry's disease ☐
17. **True about gaucher disease:**
    A. Due to deficiency of enzyme sphingomyelinase ☐
    B. Due to deficiency of enzyme Beta-Gluco-cerebrosidase ☐
    C. Deposition of glucosylceramide ☐
    D. Foam cell depositon ☐
    E. PAS staining positive ☐
18. **Sphingomyelinase Deficiency is seen in:**
    A. Niemann-Pick disease ☐
    B. Farber's disease ☐
    C. Tay Sach's disease ☐
    D. Krabbe's disease ☐
19. **Gaucher's disease is due to deficiency of enzyme** :
    A. Sphingomyelinase ☐
    B. β-Glucosidase ☐
    C. Hexosaminidase-A ☐
    D. β-Galactosidase ☐
20. **Splenomegaly seen in A/E:**
    A. Neimann pick's disease ☐
    B. Krabbe's disease ☐
    C. GM2 gangliosidosis ☐
    D. Gaucher's disease ☐
    E. Sialodosis ☐

21. **In Gaucher's diseases, there is deficiency of-**
A. Glucocerebrosidase ☐
B. Glucokinase ☐
C. Sphingomyelinase ☐
D. G-6PD ☐

22. **Accumulation of sphingomyelin in phagocytic cells is feature of**
A. Gauchers disease ☐
B. Niemann pick ds ☐
C. Tay sachs disease ☐
D. Downs syndrome ☐

23. **Enzyme deficiency seen in genetic disease like:**
A. Tay sach's disease ☐
B. Gaucher's disease ☐
C. Cystic Fibrosis ☐
D. Wilson's disease ☐
E. Familial hypercholesterolemia ☐

## Lipid Transport

24. **Which of the following lipoproteins does not move towards charged end in electrophoresis**
A. VLDL ☐
B. LDL ☐
C. HDL ☐
D. Chylomicrons ☐

25. **The human plasma lipoprotein containing the highest percentage of triacylglycerol by weight is:**
A. VLDL ☐
B. Chylomicrons ☐
C. HDL ☐
D. LDL ☐

26. **Triglycerides are maximum in:**
A. Chylomicrons ☐
B. VLDL ☐
C. LDL ☐
D. HDL ☐

27. **Dietary triglycerides are transported by**
A. Chylomicrons ☐
B. VLDL ☐
C. LDL ☐
D. HDL ☐

28. **Maximum content of triglycerides are found in**
A. HDL ☐
B. LDL ☐
C. Chylomicrons ☐
D. VLDL ☐

29. **The most important carrier of cholesterol in plasma is:**
A. Chylomicrons ☐
B. HDL ☐
C. VLDL ☐
D. LDL ☐

30. **Highest amount of cholesterol is present in:**
A. HDL ☐
B. LDL ☐
C. VLDL ☐
D. IDL ☐
E. Chylomicrons ☐

31. **Cholesterol is transported to extrahepatic tissues by:**
A. IDL ☐
B. VLDL ☐
C. HDL ☐
D. LDL ☐
E. Chylomicrons ☐

32. **Main transporter of cholesterol to peripheral tissue is:**
A. HDL ☐
B. LDL ☐
C. IDL ☐
D. VLDL ☐
E. Chylomicron ☐

33. **Apoprotein A is found in :**
A. Chylomicrons ☐
B. VLDL ☐
C. HDL ☐
D. LDL ☐

34. **Which of the following has highest electrophoretic mobility and least lipid content:**
A. Chylomicrons ☐
B. HDL ☐
C. LDL ☐
D. VLDL ☐
E. IDL ☐

35. **One of the following is having least density:**
A. Chylomicron ☐
B. HDL ☐
C. LDL ☐
D. VLDL ☐

36. **Good cholesterol found in:**
A. HDL ☐
B. LDL ☐
C. VLDL ☐
D. IDL ☐
E. PDL ☐

37. **Apo $B_{48}$ and apo $B_{100}$ are expressed as two different apoproteins because of difference in :**
A. RNA editing ☐
B. RNA splicing ☐
C. Chromosomal loci ☐
D. Apo B gene ☐

38. **Which helps in the transport of chylomicrons from intestine to liver :**
A. Apoprotein B ☐
B. Apoprotein A ☐
C. Apoprotein C ☐
D. Apoprotein E ☐

39. **Endogenous triglycerides in plasma are maximally carried in :**
A. VLDL ☐
B. Chylomicrons ☐
C. LDL ☐
D. HDL ☐

40. **Which of the following is an activator of LCAT-**
A. Apo B 100 ☐
B. Apo B 48 ☐
C. Apo E ☐
D. Apo AI ☐

41. **All of the following statements about apoproteins are true Except:**
A. Apoprotein A-I activates LCAT ☐
B. Apoprotein C-I activates lipoprotein lipase ☐
C. Apoprotein C-II inhibits lipoprotein lipase ☐
D. Apoprotein C- II activates lipoprotein lipase ☐

42. **Best marker of dyslipidemia**
A. TG & cholesterol ☐
B. LDL / HDL ratio ☐
C. Cholesterol ☐
D. APO AI ☐

43. **Most important in causing coronary artery disease (CAD) is**
A. HDL ☐
B. LDL ☐

C. VLDL
D. Triglycerides

**44. Dietery cholesterol is delivered transported to extra hepatic tissue by :**
A. VLDL
B. LDL
C. Chylomicrons
D. IDL

**45. All of the following statements about LDL are true except:**
A. It delivers cholesterol to cells
B. It contains only one Apoprotein
C. It is a marker for cardiovascular disease
D. It contains Apo-$B_4$

**46. All the statements regarding LDL receptors are true except:**
A. Present only in the extra-hepatic tissues
B. Clathrin-coated pits contain the receptor on cell membrane
C. It is taken into the cells by endocytosis
D. Increased cellular cholesterol down-regulates the synthesis of LDL receptors

**47. Cholesterol present in LDL :**
A. Represents primarily cholesterol that is being removed from peripheral cells.
B. Binds to a receptor and diffuses across the cell membrance.
C. On accumulation in the cell inhibits replenishment of LDL receptors.
D. When enters a cell, suppresses activity of acyl-CoA: cholesterol acytranferase ACAT.

**48. All of the following statements are true regarding lipoproteins except:**
A. VLDL transports endogenous lipids
B. LDL transports lipids to the tissues.
C. Increased blood cholesterol is associated with increased LDL receptors
D. Increased HDL is associated with decreased risk of coronary disease

**49. Which receptors are present in liver for uptake of LDL:**
A. Apo E
B. Apo A and Apo E
C. Apo E and Apo B100
D. Apo B100

**50. All of the following statements about Lipoprotein Lipase are true, Except**
A. Found in adipose tissue
B. Found in myocytes
C. Deficiency leads to hypertriacylglycerolemia
D. Does not require CII as cofactor

**51. Lipoprotein with seavenging action is:**
A. HDL
B. LDL
C. VLDL
D. None

**52. A young male patient presents with LDL 600mg/dl, triglycerides 140 mg/dl. What would be the most likely finding on physical examination**
A. Tendon xanthoma
B. Planar xanthoma
C. Lipemia retinalis
D. Tuberoeruptive xanthoma

**53. A patient was diagnosed with isolated increase in LDL. His father and brother had the same disease with increased cholesterol. The likely diagnosis is:**
A. Familial type III hyperlipoproteinemia
B. Abetaliporoteinemia
C. Familial lipoprotein lipase deficiency (type 1)
D. LDL receptor mutation

**54. Which of the following is increased in lipoprotein lipase deficiency:**
A. VLDL
B. LDL
C. HDL
D. Chylomicrons

**55. In Familial hypercholesterolemia there is deficiency of :**
A. LDL receptor
B. Apo protein A
C. Apo protein C
D. Lipoprotein lipase.

**56. Familial hypercholesterolemia is:**
A. Deficient LDL receptors
B. Deficient HDL receptors
C. HMG CoA reductase deficiency
D. Deficient VLDL receptors

**57. Which of the following types of hypertriglyceridemia is associated with an increase in chylomicron and VLDL remnants?**
A. Type I
B. Type IIa
C. Type III
D. Type IV

**58. In Abetaltipoproteinemia result in absence of:**
A. Chylomicron
B. LDL
C. VLDL
D. HDL
E. TG

**59. A person on a fat free carbohydrate rich diet continues to grow obese. Which of the following lipoproteins is likely to be elevated in his blood?**
A. Chylomicrons
B. VLDL
C. LDL
D. HDL

**60. Increased level of lipoprotein(a) predisposes to:**
A. Liver cirrhosis
B. Atherosclerosis
C. Nephrotic syndrome
D. Pancreatitis

## Cholesterol Synthesis & Excretion

**61. In cholesterol synthesis, which is rate limiting amino acid:**
A. HMG CoA reductase
B. HMG CoA synthetase
C. 7 alpha hydroxylase
D. Phosphofructokinase

**62. Which of the following enzymes is common to the synthesis of cholesterol and ketone bodies:**
A. HMG -Co-A Reductase
B. HMG-Co-A Lyase
C. HMG-Co-A Synthase
D. Thiokinase

**63. Cholesterol structurally belongs to molecule:**
A. Steroid
B. Carbohydrate
C. Urea
D. Peptide

**64. Fatty acids of cholesterol are mainly:**
A. Oleic acid

B. Linoleic acid ☐
C. Linolenic acid ☐
D. Palmitic acid ☐
E. Stearic acid ☐

**65. For reduction of cholesterol, the best management includes:**
A. Cholesterol restricted diet ☐
B. High fiber diet ☐
C. Diet with high unsaturated FA and low saturated FA ☐
D. Diet with low unsaturated FA and high saturated FA ☐
E. Cholesterol restricted diet, high fiber and diet with low saturated FA to unsaturated FA ratio ☐

**66. Hypolipidemic agents act on:**
A. HMG CoA synthetase ☐
B. HMG CoA oxygenase ☐
C. HMG CoA reductase ☐
D. HMG CoA hydratase ☐
E. HMG CoA mutase ☐

**67. Bile acids are derived from :**
A. Fatty acids ☐
B. Cholesterol ☐
C. Bilirubin ☐
D. Proteins ☐

**68. Bile acids synthesized in liver (Primary bile acids):**
A. Lithocolic acid ☐
B. Cholic acid ☐
C. Chenodeoxycholic acid ☐
D. Deoxycholic acid ☐
E. Taurocholic acid ☐

## Fatty Acid Synthesis And Metabolism

**69. Which biochemical reaction does *not* occur in the mitochondria:**
A. Kreb's cycle ☐
B. Urea cycle ☐
C. Gluconeogenesis ☐
D. Fatty acid synthesis ☐

**70. Mitochondria is involved in all of the following, except:**
A. ATP production ☐
B. Apoptosis ☐
C. Tricarboxylic acid cycle ☐
D. Fatty acid biosynthesis ☐

**71. NADPH is required for :**
A. Gluconeogenesis ☐
B. Glycolysis ☐
C. Fatty acids synthesis ☐
D. Glycogenolysis ☐

**72. NADPH is used in:**
A. Fatty acid synthesis ☐
B. Ketone synthesis ☐
C. Gluconeogenesis ☐
D. Glycolysis ☐

**73. In synthesis of fatty acids energy is supplied by:**
A. NAD ☐
B. FAD ☐
C. GTP ☐
D. NADPH ☐

**74. The most important source of reducing equivalents for fatty acid synthesis in the liver is:**
A. Glycolysis ☐
B. TCA cycle ☐
C. Uronic acid pathway ☐
D. HMP pathway ☐

**75. The first step in fatty acid synthesis involves:**
A. Acetyl CoA carboxylase ☐
B. β-Hydroxyl CoA dehydrogenase ☐
C. Acetyl dehydrogenase ☐
D. Pyruvate kinase ☐

**76. Acetyl CoA is necessary for:**
A. Aminoacid synthesis ☐
B. Fatty acid synthesis ☐
C. Glucose storage ☐
D. All ☐

**77. In fatty acid synthesis CO2 loss occurs in which step**
A. Hydration ☐
B. Dehydration ☐
C. Condensation reaction ☐
D. Reduction ☐

**78. Saturated acyl enzyme formation causes:**
A. Freeing of PAN-SH site ☐
B. Freeing of Cyst – SH site ☐
C. Both ☐
D. None ☐

**79. Carbon atoms added in FA synthesis**
A. 2 in Ist cycle & 4 in IInd cycle ☐
B. 4 in Ist cycle & 2 in IInd cycle ☐
C. 2 in Ist cycle & 2 in IInd cycle ☐
D. 4 in Ist cycle & 4 in IInd cycle ☐

**80. All participate in Fatty acid synthesis except**
A. Hydratase ☐
B. Reductase ☐
C. Transacylase ☐
D. Dehydrogenase ☐

**81. PAN-SH site of fatty acid synthase complex accepts:**
A. Acetyl CoA ☐
B. Malonyl CoA ☐
C. Propionyl CoA ☐
D. All ☐

**82. True about mitochondrial chain elongation of fatty acid is/are**
A. Operates under anaerobic conditions ☐
B. Operates aerobically ☐
C. Common pathway ☐
D. Not a common pathway ☐
E. Pyridoxal-Phosphate & NADPH is required ☐

**83. In which organelle (s) of hepatocyte, the elongation of long chain fatty acid takes place:**
A. Endoplasmic reticulum (ER) ☐
B. Golgi body ☐
C. Mitochondria ☐
D. Lysosomes ☐
E. Ribosome ☐

## Triacylglycerol and Phosphoglycerol Synthesis

**84. Regarding synthesis of triacyl glycerol in adipose tissue, all of the following are true except:**
A. Synthesis from Dihydroxyacetone phosphate ☐
B. Enzyme Glycerol kinase plays an important role ☐
C. Enzyme Glycerol 3 phosphate dehydrogenase plays an important role ☐
D. Phosphatidate is hydrolyzed ☐

## β - Oxidation Of Fatty Acids

**85. The substance essential for transfer of fatty acids across mitochondrial membrane:**
A. Ceratine ☐
B. Ceratinine ☐
C. Carnitine ☐
D. Coenyzme A ☐

**86. All are true about β-oxidation except:**
- A. Activation of FA is a must ☐
- B. Carnitine palmitoyl transferase I is present in outer mitochondrial membrane ☐
- C. Carnitine palmitoyl trasferase II is present in mitochondrial matrix ☐
- D. FA activation requires 2ATP. ☐

**87. β-oxidation of odd-chain fatty acids produces:**
- A. Succinyl CoA. ☐
- B. Propionyl CoA ☐
- C. Acetyl CoA ☐
- D. Malonyl CoA ☐

**88. How many ATP's are formed in case of stearic acid by β-oxidation-**
- A. 7 ☐
- B. 18 ☐
- C. 56 ☐
- D. 147 ☐

**89. β-oxidation of palmitic acid yields**
- A. 3 acetyl CoA ☐
- B. 129 ATP net ☐
- C. 131 ATP net ☐
- D. 16 Acetyl CoA ☐
- E. 96 ATP from citric acid cycle ☐

**90. Beta-Oxidation is peroxisome is differentiated from that occurring in mitochondria by:**
- A. Acetyl CoA ☐
- B. $H_2O_2$ formed ☐
- C. Different enzymes are found in different sites ☐
- D. NADH is required ☐

**91. Refsum's disease is due to deficiency of which of the following enzyme?**
- A. Malonate dehydrogease ☐
- B. Thiophorase ☐
- C. Succinate thiokinase ☐
- D. Phytanic alpha oxidase ☐

## Eicosanoids

**92. Which of the following is a suicide enzyme?**
- A. Lipoxygenase ☐
- B. Cyclooxygenase ☐
- C. 5′ nucleotidase ☐
- D. Thromboxane synthase ☐

## Ketogenesis (Ketone Body Formation)

**93. The immediate precursor in the formation of acetoacetate from acetyl Co A in the liver is:**
- A. Mevalonate ☐
- B. HMG CoA ☐
- C. Acetoacetyl CoA ☐
- D. 3-hydroxy-butyryl ☐

**94. Which organ does not utilise ketone bodies:**
- A. Liver ☐
- B. Brain ☐
- C. Skeletal muscles ☐
- D. Cardiac muscles ☐

**95. Ketone bodies cannot be utilized by:**
- A. Heart ☐
- B. Brain ☐
- C. Skeletal muscles ☐
- D. RBC s ☐

**96. In a well fed state, acetyl CoA obtained from diet is least used in the synthesis of :**
- A. Palmity CoA ☐
- B. Citrate ☐
- C. Acetoacetate ☐
- D. Oxalosuccinate ☐

**97. In a well fed state, the activity of CPT-I in outer mitochondrial membrane is inhibited by:**
- A. Glucose ☐
- B. Pyruvate ☐
- C. Acetyl CoA ☐
- D. Malonyl CoA ☐

**98. All of the following statements are correct about metabolism in brain except :**
- A. Fatty acids are utilised in starvation ☐
- B. 60% of total energy is utilized during resting stage ☐
- C. Ketone bodies are used in starvation ☐
- D. Has no stored energy ☐

**99. If starvation exceeds 7 days, the major nutritional supply of the brain comes from**
- A. Fatty acids ☐
- B. Ketone bodies ☐
- C. Protein breakdown ☐
- D. Carbohydrate breakdown ☐

**100. Energy source used by brain in later days of Starvation is**
- A. Glucose ☐
- B. Ketone bodies ☐
- C. Glycogen ☐
- D. Fatty acids ☐

**101. In a patient with starvation for 72 hrs which of the following would be seen:**
- A. Increased glycogenolysis ☐
- B. Increased ketosis due to break down of fats ☐
- C. Degradation of proteins ☐
- D. Increased gluconeogenesis ☐

**102. All of the following are increased in starvation except:**
- A. Lipolysis ☐
- B. Ketogenesis ☐
- C. Gluconeogenesis ☐
- D. Glycogenesis ☐
- E. Glycogenolysis ☐

**103. All of the following metabolic changes occur during prolonged fasting when compared with fasting for 12-24 hours, except:**
- A. Brain use of ketone bodies increases ☐
- B. Liver gluoneogenesis increases ☐
- C. Muscle protein degradation decreases ☐
- D. Brain use of glucose decreases ☐

**104. Which of the following metabolic events will not occur following 12-24 hour of fasting**
- A. Increase in free fatty acids ☐
- B. Increase in ketone bodies ☐
- C. Decrease in Glycogen ☐
- D. Decrease in Serum Proteins ☐

**105. In starvation, bran utilizes glucose peferentially but not in liver because:**
- A. Low km value of hexokinase ☐
- B. Low km glucokinase ☐
- C. High km glucokinase ☐
- D. High blood flow ☐

**106. Ketone body formation without glycosuria seen in:**
- A. DM ☐
- B. DI ☐
- C. Prolonged starvation ☐
- D. Obesity ☐

**107. Which substrate is/are used to provide energy for body:**

A. Ketone bodies ☐
B. Glucose ☐
C. Free fatty acids ☐
D. Creatine phosphate ☐
E. Collagen ☐

**108. In starvation, nitrogen is carried from muscle to liver and kidney by:**

A. Alanine ☐
B. Aspartic acid and Serine ☐
C. Glycine ☐
D. Asparagines ☐

**109. In a seriously ill patient, addition of amino acids in the diet results in a positive nitrogen balance. The mechanism for this is:**

A. Increased absorption of amino acids from the intestine ☐
B. Enhanced rates of gluconeogenesis ☐
C. Increased secretion of insulin ☐
D. Increased Growth hormone secretion ☐

**110. Starvation and diabetes mellitus can lead on to ketoacidosis which of the following features is in favour of ketoacidosis due to diabetes mellitus.**

A. Increase in glucagon/insulin ratio, increased CAMP and increased blood glucose ☐
B. Decreased insulin, increased free fatty acid which is equivalent to blood glucose ☐
C. Decreased insulin, increased free fatty acid which is not equivalent to blood glucose ☐
D. Elevated insulin and free fatty acid, equivalent to blood glucose ☐

**111. Rothera's test for detection of:**

A. Proteins ☐
B. Glucose ☐
C. Fatty acid ☐
D. Ketones ☐

**112. A destitute woman is admitted to the hospital with altered sensorium and dehydration; urine analysis shows mild proteinuria and no sugar; what other test would be desirable:**

A. Fouchet ☐
B. Rothera ☐
C. Hays ☐
D. Benedicts ☐

## Answers:

### Lipids of Physiological Significance

1. **C i.e. Arachidonic acid contain five double bonds** *[Ref: Harpers 28/e P-121-23; Lippincott's 5/e p. 181-82]*
2. **D i.e. Omega-3 fatty acids**
3. **C, B, > A i.e. (Hydrogenated vegetable oils contains Trans fatty acid; Biologically arachidonic acid is essential to life > Polyunsaturated FA is essential for membrane structure)**
4. **D i.e. Hydrogenation decreases TFA**
5. **A i.e. Linoleic acid**
6. **B i.e. Linoleic acid; C i.e. Linolenic acid**
7. **B i.e. Sunflower Oil**
8. **D i.e. Docosahexanoic Acid** *[Ref: Lippincott's 6/e p. 182; Park 16/e p.407; Lehninger 5th/e p. 345, 815-16; Harper 28/e p.122; Vasudevan 6/e p.437]*
9. **D i.e. Alpha linolenic acid** *[Ref: Harper's 27/e P-123; 26/e P- 113, 191]*
10. **A, B, D i.e. Long chain fatty acid (LCFA), Alcohol- sphingosine, Sailic acid**
11. **A i.e. Cell-cell interaction, B i.e. Signal transduction; C i.e. Surfactant; D i.e. Acute inflammatory mediator, E i.e. Activates membrane enzymes** *[Ref: Lehninger 5/e p. 256, 350-55; 829; Chatterjea 7/e p. 45, 58- 61; Vasudevan 6/e p. 81-82; Lippincott 5/e p. 201-2, 209-10, 217]*
12. **A, C, D i.e. Glucose, Sphingosine, Fatty acids**
13. **A i.e. Ganglioside, B i.e. Sphingomyelin, C i.e. Cerabrosides***[Ref: Lippincott's 5/e P-211; Harper's 28/e P-208-9]*
14. **B i.e. Alpha 2 – macroglobulin** *[Ref. Harper 28/e p. 216, 232; 575; Vasudevan 6/e p. 292-300, 335]*

### Acylglycerol & Sphingolipid Metabolism

15. **C i.e. Mutation of genes encoding lysosomal hydrolases** *[Ref: Harrison 17/e p- 2452-53; Harper's 27/e P-541]*
16. **D i.e. Wolman disease** *[Ref: Harper 29/e p. 235, 233; Lippincott's 6/e p. 212, 210; Vasudevan 7/e p. 193, 91-93; Chatterjea 8/e p. 11, 50, 63, 424]*
17. **B, C, E i.e. Due to deficiency of enzyme Beta-Gluco-cerebrosidase, Deposition of glucosylceramide, PAS staining positive** *[Ref: Harper 28/e p 210; Harrison17/e p- 2452-54; Robbins 7/e p 163-164; Vasudevan 6/e p.168-69; Chatterjea 7/e p 58-59; Lippincott 5/e p 212; Lehninger 5/ 356]*
18. **A i.e. Niemann-Pick disease**
19. **B i.e. β-glucosidase**
20. **B i.e. Krabbe's disease**
*[Ref: Harrison 17/e P 2452-57; Lippincott's 5/e P-208-217; Harper's 28/e P-210, Chatterjea 7/e p. 60, Harrison 16/e p. 2316- 17]*
21. **A i.e. Glucocerbrosidase**
22. **B i.e. Niemann pick ds**
23. **A i.e. Tay- sach's disease; B i.e. Gaucher's disease** *[Ref: Harper's 27/e P-215; Lippincott's 3/e P-210]*

### Lipid Transport

24. **D i.e. Chylomicrons** *[Ref: Lippincott 5/e p-227-28; Chatterjea 7/e p 419-18; Harper 28/e p 213]*
25. **B i.e. Chylomicrins** *[Ref: Lippincott's 5/e P-227-28]*
26. **A i.e. Chylomicron**
27. **A i.e. Chylomicrons**
28. **C i.e. Chylomicrons**
29. **D i.e. LDL**
30. **B i.e. LDL**
31. **D i.e. LDL**
32. **B i.e. LDL** *[Ref: Harper's 27/e P-218; 26/e P-206, Shinde & Chatterjea: Biochemistry 6/e P- 386]*
33. **C i.e. HDL**
34. **B i.e. HDL**
35. **A i.e. Chylomicron** *[Ref: Harper's 28/e P-213-14; Lehninger 5/e p. 836-37]*
36. **A i.e. HDL** *[Ref: Harper's 27/e p. 238; Lippincott's 4/e p 242- 43]*
37. **A i.e. RNA editing** *[Ref: Harper's 27/e P-218]*
38. **A i.e. Apoprotein B**
39. **A i.e. VLDL**
40. **D i.e. Apo AI**
41. **C i.e. Apoprotein C II inhibits lipoprotein lipase**
*[Ref: Harper's 28/e p. 212-15; Chattergea 7/e p. 419-21; Devlin 5/e p. 712; Lippincott's 100, 177, 189, 227 – 34]*
42. **B i.e. LDL / HDL ratio**
43. **B i.e. LDL**
44. **B i.e. LDL**
45. **D i.e. It contains Apo-$B_4$**
*[Ref: Harper 28th/ed pg-216; Lehninger 5th/ed pg- 843; Journal of American college of nutrition, Vol 27, No-1, 1-5 (2008) Chattarjea 7th/ed pg. – 374-75; Lippincott 4th/ed pg-234-31]*
46. **A i.e. Present only in the extra-hepatic tissues:** *[Ref: Harper29/e p 242, 255-57; Lehninger 5/e p 837-41; Lippincott 5/e p 233-31]*
47. **C i.e. On accumulation in the cell inhibits replenishment of LDL receptors.**
48. **C i.e. Increased blood cholesterol is associated with increased LDL receptors**
49. **C i.e. Apo E and Apo B100**

50. **D i.e. Does not require CII as cofactor**
*[Ref: Lippincott 4th/ed pg-228-29; Lehninger 5th/ed pg- 837-39; 346, 649; Harper 28th/ed pg-134- 35, 215-16, 232]*
51. **A i.e. HDL** *[Harper's 27/e P-221-223; 26/e P-209, 210; Chatterjea 6/e P- 386]*
52. **A i.e. Tendon Xanthoma**
53. **D i.e. LDL receptor mutation**
54. **D i.e. Chylomicrons**
55. **A i.e. LDL receptor**
56. **A i.e. Deficient LDL receptor**
57. **C i.e. III**
*[Ref: Harper's 29/e p. 232; Harrison 18/e p. 3148-49; Lippincott's 4/e p. 178, 229- 232, 380; Chattergea 7/e p. 424 – 27]*
58. **A i.e. Chylomicron, B i.e. LDL, C i.e. VLDL, E i.e. TG** *[Ref. Harrison 16/e P-2288; Harper's 27/e P-239]*
59. **B i.e. VLDL** *[Ref: Harper's 27/e P-219-220; 26/e P-211-12]*
60. **B i.e. Atherosclerosis** *[Ref: Harper 27/e p. 239; Lippincott's 4/e p. 237; Robbins 7/e p. 521]*

## Cholesterol Synthesis & Excretion

61. **A i.e. HMG COA reductase**
62. **C i.e. HMG-Co-A Synthase**
63. **A i.e. Steroid**
64. **D i.e. Palmitic acid; E i.e. Stearic acid**
*[Ref: Lehninger 5/e p 355-60, 831-35; Vasudevan 6/e p 147-52; Chaterjea 8/e p 431-35; Lippincott 5/e p 196-98; Harper 29/e p 210-13, 251-55]*
65. **E i.e. Cholesterol restricted diet, high fiber diet with low saturated FA to unsaturated FA ratio.**
66. **C i.e. HMG COA reductase**
67. **B i.e. Cholesterol** *[Ref: Harper's 27/e P-230,236;26/e P-218; Chatterjea 6/e P-374; KDT 5/e P-577]*
68. **B i.e Cholic acid; C i.e. Chemodeoxycholic acid. E i.e. Taurocholic acid**

## Fatty Acid Synthesis

69. **D i.e. Fatty acid synthesis** *[Ref: Harper's 29/e P-217-24; Lippincott 5/e p. 184-186, 194; Chatterjea 8/e p. 414-419]*
70. **D i.e. Fatty acid biosynthesis.**
71. **C i.e. Fatty acid synthesis**
72. **A i.e. Fatty acid synthesis**
73. **D i.e. NADPH**
74. **D i.e. HMP pathway**
75. **A i.e. Acetyle CoA Carboxylase;**
76. **B i.e. Fatty acid synthesis**
77. **C i.e. Condensation reaction**
78. **A i.e. Freeing of PAN-SH site**
79. **B i.e. 4 in Ist cycle & 2 in IInd cycle**
80. **D i.e. Dehydrogenase**
81. **B i.e. Malonyl CoA**
82. **A i.e. Operates under anaerobic conditions; D i.e. Not a common pathway; E i.e. Pyridoxal-Phosphate & NADPH is required**
83. **A & C i.e. ER and Mitochondria** *[Ref: Lippincott 4th/ed pg- 187; Harper 28th/ed pg- 196, 199; Lehninger- 812-15]*

## Triacylglycerol and Phosphoglycerol Synthesis

84. **B i.e. Enzyme glycerol Kinase Plays an important role** *[Ref: Lippincott/s 4/e p. 181-88, 174- 76 , Harper 27/e p. 226, 209-11]*

## β - Oxidation of Fatty Acids

85. **C i.e. Carnitine** *[Ref: Harper's 28/e P-184-86; Lippincott 4/e p. 191]*
86. **C i.e. Carnitine palmitoyl trasferase II is present in mitochondrial matrix**
87. **B i.e. Propionyl CoA** *[Ref: Harper's 27/e P-188-89; 26/e P- 182, 181; Shinde & Chatterjea P-348, 347]*
88. **D i.e. 147** *[Ref: Lehninger 5th/e p. 65-57; Harper 28/e p. 191; 27/e p. 189]*
89. **B i.e. 129 ATP net; E i.e. 96 ATP from citric acid cycle**
90. **B i.e. $H_2O_2$ formed**
91. **D i.e. Phytanic alpha oxidase** *[Ref: Harper 28th/ed p. 191, 493; Lippincott 4th/ed pg--195; Lehninger 5th/ed pg- 665; Nelson 17/ed pg-2077]*

## Eicosanoids

92. **B i.e. Cyclooxygenase** *[Ref: Harper 29/e p. 224-226]*

## Ketogenesis (Ketone Body Formation)

93. **B i.e. HMG CoA**
94. **A i.e. Liver**
95. **D i.e. RBCs**
96. **C i.e. Acetoacetate** *[Ref: Harper 29/e p 210-14; Lippincott 5/e p 195-97]*
97. **D i.e. Malonyl CoA** *[Ref: Harper 29/e p 212-14, 247-48; Lippincott 5/e p 330-31, 193-98]*

98. **A i.e. Usilize fatty acids in Starvation;** 99. **B i.e. Ketone bodies;** 100. **B i.e. Ketone bodies**

101. **D i.e. Increased Gluconeogenesis** *[Ref: Ganong 22/e P- 299-301, 342-43, 349- 50; Lehininger 2/e P- 842- 45; Chatterjea 6/e P- 362-65, 465; NMS 3/e P-517; Lippincott's 3/e P-294]*

102. **D i.e. Glycogenesis** 103. **B i.e. Liver gluoneogenesis increases** 104. **D i.e. Decrease in serum Proteins** *[Ref: Lippincott 5/e p 321-33; Mark's (2012) p 35-36; Vasudevan 6/e p 107-108; Chattarjea 8/e p 535-35; Ganong 22/e p 350]*

105. **A i.e. Low Km value of hexokinase C i.e. High Km value of glucokinase**

106. **C i.e. Prolonged Starvation** *[Ref: Lippincott's 3/e P-89, 293; Lahninger 2/e P- 840 – 49]*

107. **A i.e. Ketone bodies; B i.e. Glucose; C i.e. Free fatty acids; D i.e. Creatine phosphate**

108. **A i.e. Alanine** *[Ref: Lippincott 3/e P 294; Lahninger 2/e P 843]*

109. **C i.e. Increased secretion of insulin** *[Ref: Ganong 22/e p. 345-46]*

110. **A i.e. Increase in glucagons / insulin ratio, increased C- AMP & increased blood sugar.** *[Ref: Lehnenger 2/e P- 847- 49; Lippincott 2/e P 297; Ganong 22/e P- 350, 336- 49]*

111. **D i.e. Ketones** *[Ref. Vasudevan 6/e p. 372, 319, 305, 64, 251-50, 288, 279; Lehninger 5/e p. 241; Satyanarayana 3rd/295; 'Practical Biochemistry for Students' by Malhotra 4th/e 43-47, 'Laboratory Manual of Biochemistry' by Chary & Sharma (2004) / 21]*

112. **B i.e. Rotheras** *[Ref: Chatterjea 6/e P-652-60]*

# FAT METABOLISM: REVIEW NOTES

## Fatty Acids

F.A. are aliphatic carboxylic acids. The chain may be saturated (containing *no double bonds* & end in –'**Anoic**') or unsaturated (containing one or more double bond & end in – '**Enoic**'). Carbon atoms are numbered from carboxyl carbon (carbon No 1). The carbon atoms adjacent to carboxyl carbon (Nos. 2, 3 & 4) are also k/a $\alpha$, $\beta$ & $\gamma$ respectively, and the *terminal methyl carbon* is K/a $\omega$ *or n- carbon*. $\Delta$ indicates number & position of double bonds eg $\Delta^9$ = a double bond between carbons 9 & 10; $\omega 9$ = a double bond on the 9th carbon counting from $\omega$ carbon. So

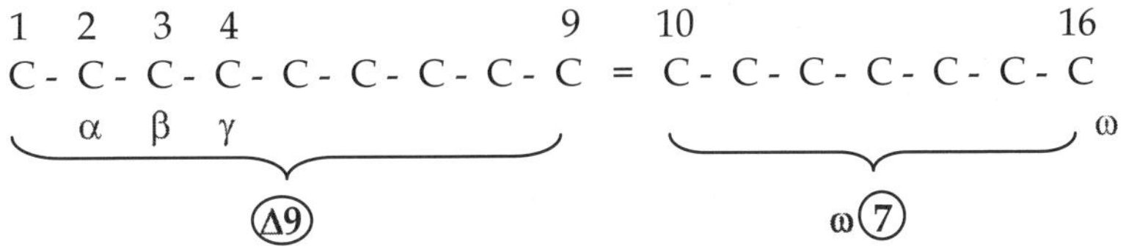


this is 16 carbon atom monoenoic acid (unsaturated fatty acid with one double bond) that is $\Delta^9$ *and* $\omega^7$

### Saturated Fatty Acids (SFA)

- Saturated fatty acids (having no double bond) are major component of meat product (beef fat) making it white, greasy & *solid at room temperature*. Other main sources are *dairy product* and some vegetable oils such as coconut & palm oils (used in latin American & Asian food).
- Consumption of saturated fat is a/w **increased incidence of coronary heart disease (by increasing total plasma cholesterol & LDL cholesterol), and increased risk of prostate & colon cancer**. So limiting intake of saturated fats is strongly advised.
- SFA with 14 (Myristic) & 16 (palmitic) carbon chain lengths are most potent in increasing serum cholesterol. Whereas, stearic acid (18 carbon) found in chocolate etc has little effect on blood cholesterol.

| Name | Number of (Atoms) |
|---|---|
| Acetic | 2 |
| Propionic | 3 |
| Butyric | 4 |
| Valeric | 5 |
| Caproic | 6 |
| Capric | 10 |
| Lauric | 12 |
| Myristic | 14 |
| **Palmitic** | **16** |
| **Stearic** | **18** |
| Lignoceric | **24** |

### Unsaturated Fatty Acids (UFA)

- Contain one (**monounsaturated**) or more double bond (**polyunsaturated**). Are named *monoenoic, dienoic trienoic, tetra enoic, pentaenoic & hexaenoic* according to numbers of double bond 1,2 3, 4, 5, & 6 respectively
- **Monounsaturated fatty acids (MUFA)** like **olive oil rich in oleic acid** (when substituted for saturated FA in diet) **lower both total plasma cholesterol & LDL cholesterol, but maintain or increase HDL cholesterol; thus decreasing incidence of coronary heart disease.**
- Effect of polyunsaturated fatty acid (PUFA) on cardiovascular disease is influenced by location of double bond ($\omega_3$ = at 3rd bond position / $\omega_6$ = at 6th bond position starting from methyl end).
- Consumption of $\omega_6$ or n-6 PUFA (mainly **linoleic acid**, 18:2 (9, 12)) when substituted for SFA, **lower plasma cholesterol & LDL cholesterol**, but **HDL** which protects against coronary heart disease is **also lowered**. So the powerful benefits of lowering LDL are only partially offset because of decreased HDL. *Nuts, avocados, olives, soyabean* and various vegetable oils including *sesame, cottonseed, corn oil, sunflower oil, canola oil, safflower oil* etc are common sources of $\omega_6$ PUFA.
- Dietary **$\omega_3$ PUFA** *suppress cardiac arrhythmias, reduce serum triacyl glycerols, decrease tendency of thrombosis, lower BP and substantially reduce risk of cardiovascular mortality* (i.e. are **cardioprotective**) but they have *little effect on LDL or HDL cholesterol level*. The $\omega_3$ PUFA mainly Alpha-linolenic acid, 18:3 (9, 12, 15) are found in plants (its acceptable range is 0.6 – 1.2% of total calories). Flax seed oil, canola oil, soyabean oil are rich in ω-3 PUFA. **Fish oil (salmon fat)** containing long chain ω-3- **DHA** (docosahexaenoic acid) and **EPA** (eicosapentaenoic acid) are ω-3 PUFAs. Two fatty fish meals per week are recommended.
- **Mediterraneen diet rich in MUFA (olive oil) and ω-3 fatty acids (from fish oils & some nuts)** but low in saturated fats is a/w ↓ LDL & total cholesterol but little change in HDL: hence decreased risk of coronary heart disease. Plasma triacyl glycerols are unchanged.
- Arachidonic acid a precursor of prostaglandins & leukotrienes is ω-6 PUFA.

| No. of Carbon atoms | No. of double bonds | Position of double bonds | Family | Common Name | Systemic Name | Occurrence |
|---|---|---|---|---|---|---|
| 16 | 1 | $\Delta^9$ | $\omega^7$ | **Palmitoleic** | Cis- 9- Hexadece- noic | In nearly all fats |
| 18 | 1 | $\Delta^9$ | $\omega^9$ | **Oleic** | Cis- 9- octadecenoic | Possibly the most common fatty acid in natural fats (olive oil) |
| 18 | 1 | $\Delta^9$ | $\omega^9$ | **Elaidic** | Trans-9- actadecenoic | Hydrogenated and ruminant fats |
| 18 | 2 | 9, 12 | $\omega^6$ | **Linoleic** | all –cis- 9,12- octadeca dienoic | Corn, peanut, cottonseed, soyabean, and many plant oils |
| 18 | 3 | 9, 12, 6 | $\omega^6$ | **γ - Linolenic** | all – cis- 6, 9, 12- octadeca trienoic | Some plants, eg. oil of evening primrose, borage oil; minot fatty acid in animals |
| 18 | 3 | 9, 12, 15 | $\omega^3$ | **α - Linolenic** | all –cis- 9,12, 15 octa-decatrienoic | Frequently found with linoleic acid but particularly in **linseed** oil |
| 20 | 4 | 5, 8, 11, 14 | $\omega^6$ | **Arachidonic** | all –cis-5,8, 11, 14- Eicosatetraenoic | Found in animals fats and in peanut oil; important component of phospholipids in animals |
| 20 | 5 | 5, 8, 11, 14, 17 | $\omega^3$ | **Timnodonic** | all –cis- 5, 8, 11, 14, 17- Ecosapentaenoic | Important component of fish oils eg. **cod liver, mackerel, menhaden, salmon oils.** |
| 22 | 6 | 4, 7, 10, 13, 16, 19 | $\omega^3$ | **Cervonic** | all –cis- 4, 7, 10, 13, 16, 19- Docosahexaenoic | Fish oils, phospholipids in brain. |
| 24 | 1 | 15 | | **Neurvonic acid** | | |

| Fatty acid type | Metabolic Effect | | Clinical Effect |
|---|---|---|---|
| | LDL | HDL | |
| **Trans fatty acid** | ↑ | ↓ | **Increased** incidence of **coronary heart disease** |
| **Saturated fatty acid** | ↑ | Little effect | **Increased** incidence of **coronary heart disease**<br>Increased risk of **prostate & colon cancer** |
| **Monounsaturated fatty acid (MUFA)** | ↓ | ↓ | **Decreased** incidence of coronary heart disease |
| **ω-6 polyunsaturated fatty acid (PUFA)** | ↓ | ↓ | **Decreased** incidence of coronary heart disease |
| **ω-3 Polyunsaturated fatty acid (PUFA)** | Little effect | Little effect | **Decreased** incidence of **coronary heart disease**<br>Decreased risk of **sudden cardiac death**<br>**Decreased** tendency for **thrombosis**, reduce **BP** & serum **triacylglycerols** and suppress **cardiac arrhythmias** |

## Trans Fatty Acids (TFA)

### Procedure & Purpose

- Lipid rich food, when exposed too long to oxygen (air), may *spoil and become rancid d/t oxidative cleavage of double bond in unsaturated fatty acids,* which produces aldehyde and carboxylic acids of shorter chain length & therefore *higher volatility.*
- To improve/increase the shelf life and volatility (stability at high temperature in deep frying), commercial vegetable oils are subjected to **partial hydrogenation / hardening.**
- Hardening *converts many cis double bonds in FA to single bonds and increase the melting temperature* of oils, so that they are more nearly *solid at room temperature.* **Margarine** is produced from liquid vegetable oils by partial hydrogenation.
- But the undesirable effect of partial hydrogenation procedure is production of trans fatty acids i.e *some cis* ***double bonds are converted to trans double bonds***Q. So trans

### Biological Significance

- Trans fatty acids do not occur naturally in plants, but occur in small amount in animals (**ruminant fat** arising from action of microorganisms in the rumen)
- Many fast foods are **deep fried in partially hydrogenated vegetable oils** & therefore contain high levels of trans fatty acids. So TFA is a major component of many commercial baked goods, like cookies, cakes and most deep fried foods. A clue to presence of TFA is "**partially hydrogenated**" word used in the list of ingredients.
- Dietary intake of trans fats **raise the level of triacyl glycerol & LDL (bad) cholesterol,** increase the body's inflammatory response

fatty acids are chemically unsaturated fatty acids but behave like saturated fatty acid (i.e. they are atherogenic).

- Soft margarine, low in trans fatty acid (or containing not at all) is produced by refined technology

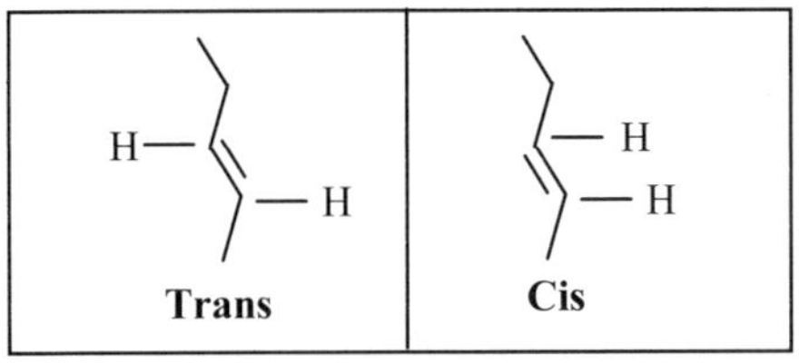


Fatty Acid

(another risk factor for heart disease) and **decrease the level of HDL (good) cholesterol** and so a/w higher incidence of cardiovascular disease, and avoiding these fats in diet substantially reduces the risk of coronary heart disease.

- Consumption of trans fatty acid is a/w ***increased risk of cardiovascular disease, diabetes mellitus***[Q] (d/t increased insulin resistance) and adversely affect endothelial function.

## Essential Fatty Acid

- ***Dietary essential fatty acids in humans are linoleic acid and α- linolenic acid***[Q], because we lack enzymes needed to synthesize them. Plants provide these EFA. **Linoleic acid is the precursor of ω-6-arachidonic acid** and so prostaglandins. **So the arachidonic acid becomes EFA if linoleic acid is deficient in diet**. α-linolenic acid is precursor of ω-3-fatty acids required for growth and development.
- Those fatty acids that ***cannot be synthesized by human bodies***[Q] and must be provided in diet. The most important essential fatty acid is → ***Linoleic acid***[Q] (because it serves as a basis for the production of other EFA)

| EFA | Dietary Source |
|---|---|
| **Linoleic acid**[Q] | Safflower oil |
| **Linolenic acid**[Q] | *Soyabean oil*[Q] |
| **Arachidonic acid** | *Meat, egg, milk*[Q] |
| **Eicosapentaenoic acid** | *Fish oil*[Q] |
| ***Docosahexanoic Acid***[Q] | ***Breast milk*** |

**Dietary sources of linoleic acid**

| | |
|---|---|
| *Safflower oil*[Q] | *73%*[Q] *(max)*[Q] |
| *Corn oil*[Q] | 57% |
| *Sunflower oil*[Q] | 56% |
| *Soyabean oil*[Q] | 51% |

- Humans require but do not have the enzymatic capacity to synthesize omega-3 PUFA α linolenic acid (ALA; 18:3 ($\Delta^{9,12,15}$), and must therefore obtain it in diet. However from ALA; humans can synthesize 2 other omega PUFAs: eicosapentaenoic acid (EPA; 20 : 5 ($\Delta^{5,8,11,14,17}$) and docosahexaenoic acid (DHA; 22:6 ($\Delta^{4,7,10,13,16,19}$). An imbalance between dietary ratio of omega 6 & omega 3 (optimal is between 1:1 and 4: 1) PUFAs is associated with increased risk of cardiovascular disease.
- Mammalian hepatocytes can introduce ***double bonds at $\Delta^9$ position of FA but not between C-10 and methyl terminal end. So mammas can not synthesize linoleate, 18:2 ($\Delta^{9,12}$) or α- linolenate 18:3 ($\Delta^{9,12,15}$)***[Q].

  However, plants can synthesize both; the desaturases that introduce double bonds at $\Delta^{12}$ and $\Delta^{15}$ positions are located in ER and chloroplast. So these are **essential fatty acids** for mammals; they must be obtained from dietary plant material. ***Once ingested linoleate may be converted to other PUFAs, particularly γ-linolenate***[Q], eicosatrienoate and eicosatetraenoate (arachidonate), all of which can be **made only from linoleate**

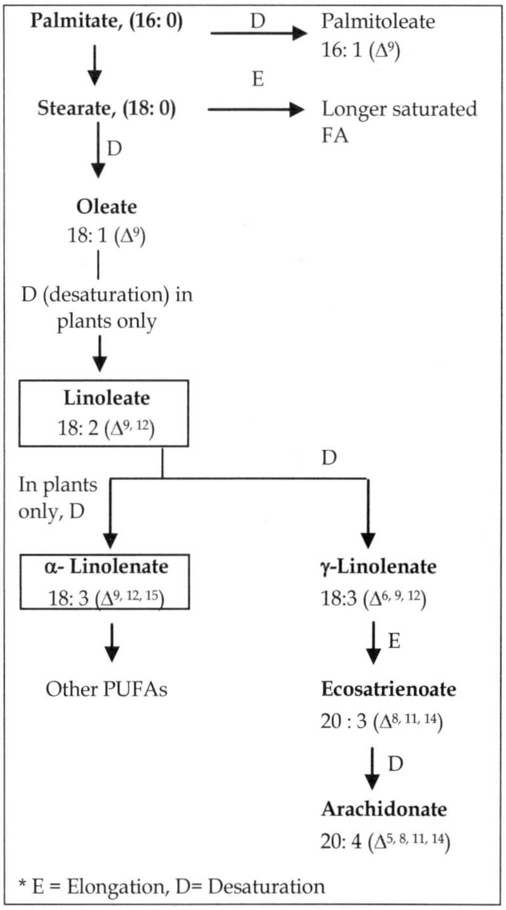


## (Polar) Membrane Lipids

- Lipids are heterogenous group of compounds that are relatively *insoluble in water and soluble in nonpolar solvents like ether and chloroform.*
- All major lipids have either **glycerol or sphingosine back bone**, to which *1 or more long chain alkyl groups and a polar head group* are attached. In glycerophospholipid, galacto (sulfo) lipid and triacyl glycerol, the alkyl groups are *fatty acids in ester linkage* whereas, sphingo (both phospho & glyco) lipids contain single fatty acid in amide linkage to sphingosine backbone.

## Phospholipids (PL)

- Phospholipids contain **phosphoric acid residue** in addition to *fatty acid and alcohol*
- So PLs are **phosphatidic acid** derivatives in which the *phosphate is esterified with the OH group of suitable alcohol (glycerol or sphingosine).*
- Both types of PLs are found in membranes & play a role in generation of lipid signaling molecules.

## Glycolipids (GL)

Glycolipids contain both *carbohydrate* and *lipid*. The carbohydrate portion is antigen determinant and so the glycolipids are antigenic. Two types include

### Glycero-phospholipids (Phospho-glycerides)

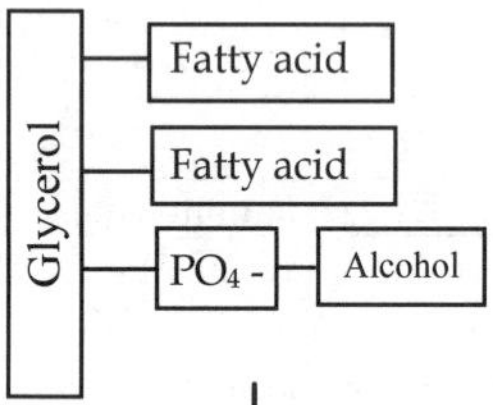


### Sphingo-phospholipids (Phospho-sphingolipids)

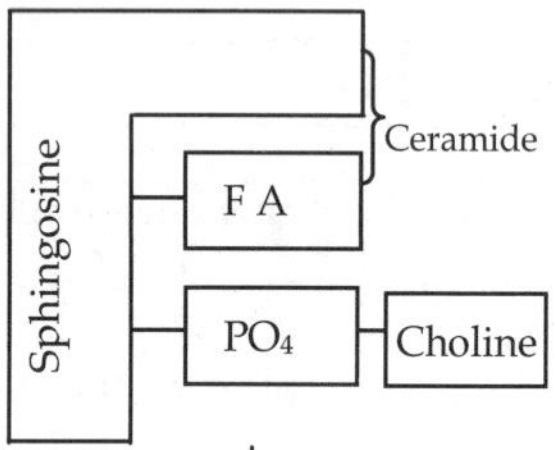


### Glyco-sphingolipids

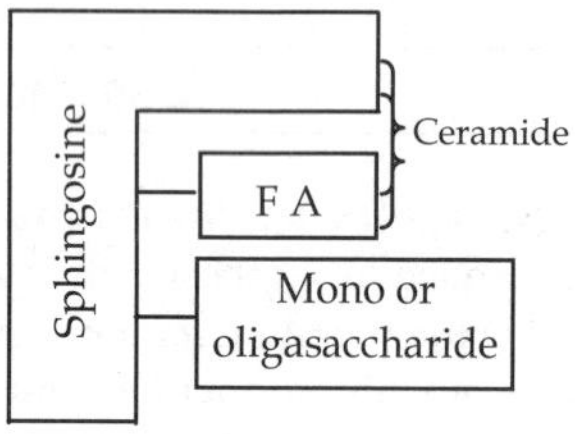


### Galactolipids (sulfolipids)

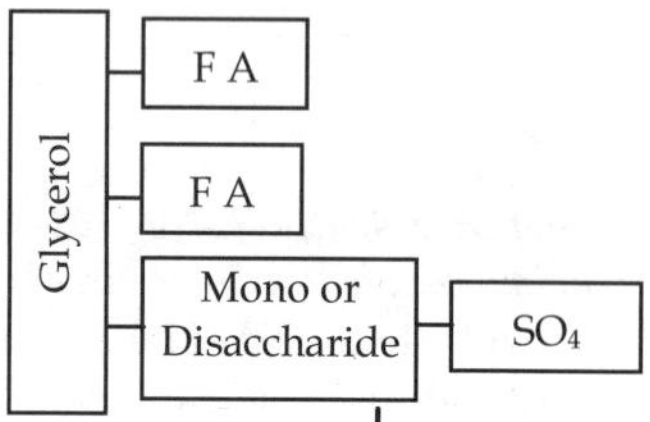


- Phosphoglyceride contain *glycerol backbone linked to 2 fatty acid, a phosphate group and an alcohol* (like serine/ ethanolamine/ choline/ inositol/ glycerol)
- **Phosphatidic acid** is the *simplest (parent)* phosphoglyceride (PG) and is the precursor of other members of this group. All PGs contain (or are derivative of) *phosphatidic acid* (diacyl glycerol with a $PO_4$ group on 3rd carbon).
- PGs are formed from **phosphatidic acid (PA)** and an alcohol

| Glycerophospho-lipid | Components<br>Head group | Common | Net charge (at pH7) |
|---|---|---|---|
| **Phosphatidic acid (PA)** | (Parent compound) | | -1 |
| Phosphotidyl choline (**Lecithin**)<br>Phosphatidyl ethanolamine (**cephalin**) | Choline<br><br>Ethanolamine | **PA** | 0<br><br>0 |
| Phosphatidyl serine<br>Phosphatidyl glycerol | Serine<br>Glycerol | | -1<br>-1 |
| Phosphatidyl inosital 4- 5, biphosphate | Myo Inositol 4, 5-biphosphate | | -4 |
| **Cardiolipin** | Diphosphatidyl glycerol | | -2 |

- Saturated ($C_{16}$ or $C_{18}$) fatty acid at $C_1$ and unsaturated fatty acid ($C_{18}$ or $C_{20}$) is attached in ester linkage to $C_2$ (2nd carbon) of glycerol.
- A highly charged or polar head group is attached through a phosphodiester linkage to third carbon. In this head group $PO_4^{-3}$ *bears a negative charge at neutral pH. The polar alcohol may be negatively charged (phosphotidylinositol 4, 5, biphosphate), neutral (phosphotidyl serine) or positively charged*

- All **sphingo-lipids** (ie **sphingosine containing lipids)** are formed from ceramide. **Ceramide** is synthesized from **serine aa in ER** and works as 2nd messenger in cell cycle/ differentiation/ senescence and apoptosis. 3 types of sphingolipids are: **phosphosphingolipids (eg sphingomyelin), glycosphingolipids (eg cerebrosides, globosides** and **gangliosides)** and **sulfatides (or sulfo-glyco sphingolipids).**
- Sphingolipids are composed of 1 mol of long chain **amino alcohol sphingosine (4- sphingenine) backbone** linked to 1 mol of **long chain fatty acid** through an amide linkage (at $C_2$) (i.e. = **ceramide**) and a polar head ($PO_4$ in phosphospingolipids & mono/oligo-saccharide in glycosphingolipid) group joined by **phosphodiester bond** in phosphosphingolipids and by **O-glycosidic bond** in glycosphingolipids.
- C- 2 bears fatty acid (saturated or monounsaturated with 16, 18, 22 or 24 carbon) in amide linkage.
- **Ceramide** is structurally similar to diacyl glycerol & is parent compound.

### Sphingomyelin (sphingophospho-lipid)

- It consists of **ceramide** (i.e. **sphingosine amino alcohol** backbone attached at $C_2$ to **long chain FA** through an amide linkage) and a polar head group. **Phosphoryl choline** or

### Glycosphingolipids

- It consists of **ceramide (sphingosine + fatty acid) and antigenic carbohydrate (mono/oligosaccharide)**
- Like phospholipids, these are essentially present in all membranes but are particularly abundant in **nerve tissue**. They are located in **outer leaflet of plasma membrane**, where they interact with extracellular environment and play role in regulation of cellular inter action, growth and development. So when the cell division/growth is dysregulated,

- In **galactolipids**, 1 or 2 galactose residues are connected by glycosidic linkage to C-3 of 1, 2 diacyl glycerol
- Galactolipids found predominantly in plants are localized in *internal (thylakoid) membrane of chloroplasts.* They make 70-80% of total membrane lipids of vascular plants and are *most abundant membrane lipid in biosphere.*
- This phosphate free lipid is evolved to conserve PO4, a limiting plant nutrient in soil, for more critical roles
- **Sulfolipids** in plant membrane bear negative

*(phosphotidyl choline or phosphotidylethanolamine).*

- Phosphoacylglycerol containing choline (i.e. **phosphotidyl choline / Lecithins)** ***are the most abundant phospholipids of cell membrane***[Q] & represent a large proportion of body's *store of choline.* Choline is important in nervous transmission as acetylcholine and as store of labile methyl groups.
- **Dipalmitoyl lecithin** is very active surface active agent and a major constituent of the ***surfactant***[Q].
- **Phosphatidyl ethanolamine (cephalin) & phosphatidylserine** (found in most tissue) differ from phosphatidyl choline only in that *ethanolamine or serine, respectively, replaces choline.*
- **Phosphatidylinosilot** is a ***precursor of second messengers (i.e. help in signal transduction)***[Q].
- **Lysophospholipids** are intermediates in the metabolism of phosphoglycerols.
- In **cardiolipin** 2 phosphatidic acids (PA) share a single glycerol (i.e. 2PA esterified through their $PO_4$ groups to glycerol) hence the name is **diphosphatidyl glycerol**. It is found exclusively in **inner mitochondrial membrane**, where it maintain ETC. It is antigenic and is recognized by antibodies raised against *Treponema pallidum (syhillis bacteria).*
- Some PGs have **ether linked fatty acids (Ether lipids)** like

1. **Plasmalogens** which constitute 10% of PL of brain & heart muscles. These resemble *phosphotidyl ethanolamine (abundant in nerve tissue) &/ or phosphotidylcholine* (abundant in heart muscle) but possess an ether link on Sn -1 instead of ester link (i.e. ester linked fatty acid at carbon 1 is replaced by **ether linked unsaturated alkyl group**).
2. **Platelet activating factor (PAF)**, an unusual ether phosphoglyceride **has saturated alkyl group in ether link** to carbon 1 and an acetyl residue (rather than FA) at carbon 2 of glycerol backbone. PAF is synthesized by variety of cells. It **binds to surface receptors** triggering potent ***acute inflammatory & thrombotic events***[Q]. PAF is one of the most potent bioactive molecule it ***activates inflammatory cells & mediates hypersensitivity, anaphylactic & acute inflammatory reactions***[Q]. It causes ***platelet aggregation & degranulation***[Q] and activate neutrophils & alveolar macrophages ***to generate superoxide radicals***[Q] (killing bacteria).

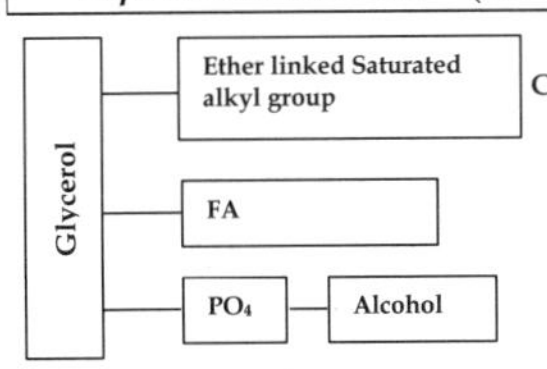


Plasmalogens

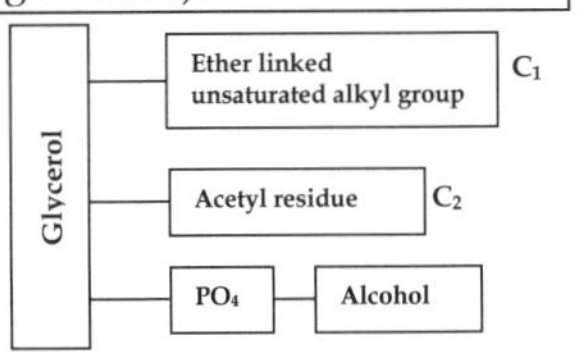


Platelett activating factor

★ All cells except mature RBCs can synthesize phospholipids, whereas triacyl glycerol synthesis occurs only in liver, lactating mammary glands, adipose tissue and intestinal mucosal gland.

★ Lung maturity of fetus is gauged by determining the **dipalmitoyl lecithin (DPPC) to sphingomyelin (L/S ratio)** in amniotic fluid. A $\geq$ 2 ratio indicate maturity and major shift from sphingomyelin to DPPC synthesis that occur in pneumocyte at 32 weeks gestation.

★ A ceramide (containing 30 carbon FA) is major component of skin & regulates it's *water permeability.*

**phosphoethanolamine** (as polar head groups) are attached to carbon 1 of sphingosine through *phosphodiester bond.*

- It is found in as an constituent of **myelin** in nervous tissue.

there is dramatic change in glycosphingolipid composition of plasmamembrane

- Glycosphingolipids have been identified as a source of *blood group antigens, embryonic antigens, tumor antigens.*
- They serve as cell surface receptors for *cholera & tetanus toxins* and for certain microbes & viruses.
- Genetic disorder a/w inability to degrade glycosphingolipids l/t lysosomal accumulation of these compounds.
- These can be of two types

charged sulfonate head group

- In this sulfonated lipid, glucose residue is joined to diacylglycerol in glycosidic linkage.

**Neutral (Uncharged) glycosphingolipids = Neutral glycolipids**

- It consists of **ceramide linked to 1 or more sugar residues** at carbon 1

1. **Cerebroside** (i.e. **ceramide mono saccharide)**/are the simplest neutral glycosphingolipids and they contain either a galactose (**galactocerebroside**) or glucose (**glucocerebroside**). Galactocerebroside are found in plasma membranes of neural tissue and gluco cerebroside, which occur in *plasmamembrane of non neural tissue* serves primarily as an *intermediate in the synthesis & degradation of more complex glycosphingolipids.*

▪ As the name suggest, cerebrosides are found mainly *in brain & peripheral nervous tissue.* Different galacto /gluco- cerebrosides may differ in type of FA attached to sphingosine.

2. **Globoside (ceramide oligosaccharide)** are produced by *attaching additional mono saccharide (including N-acetyl galactosamine) to glucocerebrosides.* **Globosides** contain 2 or more sugars, usually D- glucose, D-galactose or N-acetyl D galactosamine

**Cerebroside (gluco/galacto)** =
Ceramide+Glucose/Galactose
(Cer - Glc / Gal)
**Globoside (Lactosylceramide)** =
Cer - Glc - Gal
**Globoside (Forsman antigen)** =
Cer - Glc - 2 Gal - 2 Gal Nac

**Neutral Storage Lipid (triacyl glycerol)**

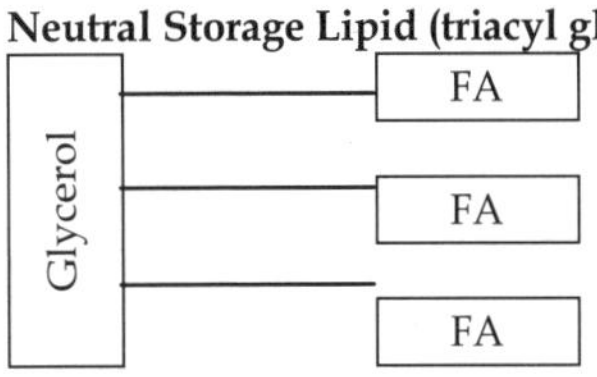


**Acidic (Negatively charged) glycosphingolipids**

- It consists of **ceramide** l/t **N-acetyl neuraminic acid = NANA/sialic acid (in gangliosides)** or a **sulfate group** on a galactose (in **sulfatides**)
- Negative charge at physiological pH is provided by *NANA/sulfate group*

1. **Gangliosides** are derivatives of *ceramide oligosaccharide* (glucosyl ceramide) that contain oligosaccharide as their polar head group & **$\geq$1N acetyl neuraminic acid (Neu 5 Ac = NANA)** a sialic acid at termini. These are found in ganglionic cells of CNS, particularly at the nerve endings. They have receptor & other functions. Notation G (for ganglioside). Subscriptio M, D, T, or Q indicate whether there is 1 (mono) 2 (di), 3 (tri) or 4 (quatro) molecules of NANA in ganglioside. Additional number designate monomeric sequence of carbohydrate attached to ceramide. *$GM_3$* is the simplest ganglioside G represent ganglioside; M is a monosialo containing; & 3 is a number assigned on the basis of chromatographic migration. *$Gm_1$*,is receptor in intestine for cholera toxin.
2. **Sulfatides** are sulfoglycosphingolipids i.e. cerebrosides that contain **sulfated galactosyl residue.** These sulfogalactosyl ceramide are found predominantly in **nerve tissue (myelin)** & *kidney.*

## Ceramide

- **Phospatidylcholine** → **Sphingomyelin**
- On combination with **Monosaccharide Sugar residue**
  - **UDP-galactose** → **Galactocerebroside**
  - **UDP-glucose** → **Glucocerebroside**
- **Oligosaccharide (≥2 UDP sugar residue)** → **Globoside** → (+ **NANA**) → **Ganglioside**

## Risk of Atherosclerosis & Coronary Heart Disease (CHD)

- **LDL cholesterol** (especially **oxidized LDL**) uptake by macrophage is responsible for formation **of foam cells** – the hallmark of atherosclerotic plaque. A positive correlation exists b/w plasma LDL cholesterol concentration & atherosclerosis. LDL is degraded in liver (70%) and extrahepatic tissues (30%), both expressing **LDL (apo-B-100, E) receptor**.
- **LDL (apo-B-100, E) receptor** is **defective** in familial hypercholesterolemia, increasing blood LDl cholesterol levels and causing **premature atherosclerosis**.
- **Apoprotein A-I** is a measure of HDL (good) cholesterol & **apo-B** measures LDL (bad) cholesterol. Hence **ratio of Apo B/AI** is the most reliable index of atherosclerosis (cardiovascular disease). Ratio of 0.4 is very good and ratio of 1.4 has highest risk of heart accidents.
- **Lipoprotein (a)**, which inhibits fibrinolysis, consists of 1 mol of LDL attached to 1 mol of apo (a). It increases risk of coronary heart disease (& atherosclerosis) if levels are > 30 mg/dl.
- High plasma **homocysteine** levels (> 15 μmol/L), increased **hs-CRP** (i.e. high sensitivity C-reactive protein), high levels of serum triglyceride & **long chain saturated fatty acids** (e.g. stearic acid), hypertension, diabetes mellitus and smoking are risk factors for atherosclerosis and coronary heart disease.
- **Atherosclerosis** & **coronary heart disease** occurs in familial **lipoprotein (a)/Lp(a) excess**, familial hypercholesterolemia type II a (**defective LDL receptor apo B-100**), familial type III hyperlipoproteinemia/ broad beta / remnant removal disease/ familial dysbeta lipoproteinemia (**abnormal apo E**). Coronary heart disease also occurs in familial hyper triacylglycerolemia type IV and **hepatic lipase deficiency**.

## Lysosomal Storage Disease

Lysosomal storage disorder is *accumulation of specific macromolecule within cells* that are normally metabolized by cells. This is because of deficiency of one or other lysosomal enzyme.

### Mucopolysaccharidoses (MPS)

| Type | Syndrome | Enzymatic Defect | Accumulated / Urinary metabolite |
|---|---|---|---|
| I | **Hurler** or **Scheie** | ***α- L- Iduronidase*[Q]** | - ***Dermatan sulfate*[Q]**<br>- ***Hepran sulfate*[Q]** |
| II | **Hunter** | *Iduronate sulfatase* | ***Heparan sulfate*[Q]** |
| III A | **Sanfilippo A** | *Heparan sulfate N-sulfatase (sulfamidase)* | |
| III B | **Sanfilippo B** | *α-N- Acetyl glucosaminidase* | |
| III C | **Sanfilippo C** | *Acetyl CoA*<br>*- α-glucosaminidase*<br>*- N-acetyl transferase* | |
| III D | **Sanfilippo D** | *N- Acetylglucosamine 6 sulfatase* | |
| IV A | **Moriquio- A** | *N-acetyl Galactosamine – 6- sulfatase* | - Keratan sulfate<br>- Chondroitin –6 sulfate |
| IV B | **Morquio -B** | *β- Galactosidase* | - Keratan sulfate |
| VI | **Maroteauxlamy** | *N- acetyl galactosamine 4- sulfatase (aryl sulfatase β* | Dermatan sulfate |
| VII | **Sly** | *β- Glucronidase* | - Dermatan sulfate<br>- Heparan sulfate<br>- Chondroitin 4/6- sulfate |

Clinical features of MPS: Coarse facies. Valvular heart disease, mental retardation, **hepatosplenomegaly**, skeletal deformity, joint stiffness, corneal clouding, & vacuolated / granulated lymphocytes.

### Neutral glycosphingolipidoses

| Disorder | Fabry disease | Gaucher disease | Nieman-Pick disease A&B |
|---|---|---|---|
| Deficient enzyme | ***α- Galactosidase A*[Q]** | ***Acid-β- glucosidase/gluco cerebrosidase*[Q]** | ***Sphingomyelinase*[Q]** |
| Stored material | *Globotriacyl ceramide* | ***Glucosyl ceramide*** | ***Sphingomyelin*[Q]** |
| Clinical features | - ***Cutaneous angiokeratoma (i.e. reddish purple skin rash)*[Q]**, corneal dystrophy<br>- ***Painful acroparesthesis i.e. burning pain in lower extremity)*[Q]**<br>- Hypohydrosis, kidney & heart failure.<br>- X- linked disorder, onset in childhood,<br>- No hepatospleenomegaly, skeletal disease and hematological involvement | - No CNS and opthalmological involvement in type 1 (adult) form<br>- ***PAS staining positive Gaucher cells*[Q]** in bone marrow, cytopenia<br>- Lipid as bilayered stacks in elongated distended lysosomes on EM | - Pulmonary infiltrates & lung failure<br>- **Foam cells in bone marrow[Q]**<br>- Pleomorphic inclusion of lipid in lysosomes concentric parallel lamella (on electron microscopy = EM<br>- Mental retardation, seizures, **hepato spleenomegaly**, macular degeneration<br>- Osteoporosis in type B only |

### Leukodystrophies

| Disorder | Enzyme defect | Accumulated lipid | Clinical Features |
|---|---|---|---|
| **Krabbe's disease (globoid cell** | *Galactosyl ceramidase/ β* | *Galactosylceramide Galactosyl* | - *Globoid bodies* (glycolipid- laden |

**Mucolipidoses (MLS)**

| | Disorder | Enzyme defect | Accumulated | Clinical features |
|---|---|---|---|---|
| I | **Sialidosis** | *Sialidase (neuraminidase)* | Glycoprotein fragments Sialyloligosaccharides | MPS II phenotype – coarse facies, pebbly skin lesions, joint stiffness |
| II | **I- Cell disease** | UDP- N- acetyl glucosamine: glucoprotein- N- acetylglucosamininylphospho transferase (Acid hydrolases thus lack phosphomannosyl residues) | Glycoprotein fragments Glycolipids | Coarse facies, gingival hypoplasia, absence of mucopolysacchariduria |
| III | **Phosphotransferase** | As with ML-II but deficiency is incomplete | Glycoprotein fragments Glycolipids | Coarse facies, stiffness of hands & shoulder |

**Glycoproteinoses**

| | | |
|---|---|---|
| **Fucosidosis** | $\alpha$ -Fucosidase | Glycopeptides, oligosaccharides |
| **Mannosidosis α, β** | Mannosidase α/β | Oligosaccharides |
| **Aspartylglucosaminuria** | Aspartylglucosaminidase | Aspartyl glucosamine, glycopeptides |
| **Schindler's disease** | α-N-galatosaminidase | |

★ Clinical features – Coarse facies, enlarged tongue, angiokeratomas

| | | | |
|---|---|---|---|
| **leukodystrophy)** | *galactosidase*[Q] | *sphingosine* | macrophages) in white matter<br>- Mental & motor retardation<br>- Blindness & deafness |
| **Metachromatic leukodystrophy** | *Arylsulfatase A*[Q] | *Cerebroside sulfate* | - Mental Retardation<br>- Progressive paralysis<br>- Dementia in adult form<br>- Nerve stain yellowish brown with cresyl violet (metachromasia) |
| **Multiple sulfatase deficiency** (Active site cysteine to Cα formyl glycine converting enzyme) | **Aryl sulfatases A, B & C and steroid sulfatase** | Sulfogalactosyl ceramide (sulfatide), steroid sulfates, proteoglycans mucopoly saccharides | - Absent activity of all cellular sulfatases<br>- MR, HS omegaly, retinal degeneration, & skeleletal involvement |

**$GM_2$ gangliosidoses**

| | | | |
|---|---|---|---|
| **Tay Sach's disease** | *β- Hexosaminidase A*[Q] (HAD- A) | *$GM_2$ gangliosides* | - Mental retardation, seizures, macrocephaly, ***hyperacusis and cherry red spot in both***[Q].<br>- Hepatosplenomegaly & skeletal involvement only in sandhoff ds. |
| **Sandhoff's disease** | β- Hexosaminidase A and B [HAD- A,B] | $GM_2$ gangliosides | |

**Disorder of neutral lipids**

| | | | |
|---|---|---|---|
| **Wolman disease** | Acid lysosomal lipase | Cholesterol esters, triglycerides | *Adrenal calcification*, hepatospleenomegaly, mild, mental retardation |
| **Cholestery ester storage disease** | Acid lysosomal lipase | Cholesteryl ester | Hepatomegaly, cirrhosis |
| **Farber disease** | **Acid ceramidase** | Ceramide | Macular degeneration, arthropathy, subcutaneous nodules |

## Sphingolipidoses

- **Sphingolipidoses** (a part of **lysosomal lipid storage diseases)** are a group of **autosomal recessive (except for Fabry disease which is X-linked) inherited** diseases that are caused by a **genetic defect in the degradation (catabolism) of sphingo (or glycosphingo) lipids containing sphingosine.**
- Common features of all sphingolipidoses include
  1. **Rate of synthesis of stored sphingolipid is normal but a specific lysosomal hydrolytic enzyme for degradation is deficient** resulting in accumulation of usually only a single sphingolipid containing ceramide (the substrate for enzyme). It can also result from defects in **lysosomal activator proteins (eg saposins)** that facilitate access of lysosomal hydrolases to short carbohydrate chains as degradation proceeds.
  2. Enzymatic activity is **affected in all tissues similarly.** Accumulation of sphingolipids in neurons cause **neurodegeneration and shortening of lifespan.**
  3. The **incidence is low in most populations except for Gaucher, Tay Sachs and Niemann- Pick disease** (which show high incidence in few ethinic groups). All are **AR except Fabry's disease** which has **x-linked** inheritance.
  4. Can be diagnosed by measuring **enzyme activity** (in cultured fibroblasts or peripheral leukocytes) or by **DNA analysis**. Prenatal diagnosis uses cultured amniocytes or chorionic villi. **Histological examination** can be also useful eg **shell like inclusion bodies in Tay Sachs** and **wrinkled (crumpled) tissue paper appearance of cytoplasm in Gaucher disease.**
  5. Treatment is **not effective** for many diseases. Although **recombinant human enzyme replacement therapy** and **bone marrow transplantation** can successfully treat Fabry's and Gaucher's disease. **Substrate deprivation therapy** (to stop synthesis), **chemical chaperone therapy** and gene therapy (under investigation) are other alternatives.
- Sphingolipidoses include (1) **Neutral glycosphingo lipidoses** (eg **Fabry's, Gaucher's and Niemann Pick disease A and B);** (2) **Generalized GM1 gangliosidoses**; (3) **GM2 gangliosidoses (eg Tay Sachs & Sandhoff's diseases);** (4) **Leukodystrophies (eg Krabbe globoid cell leukodystrophy**, **metachromatic leukodystrophy** and multiple sulfatase deficiency) (5) **Lactosyl ceramidoses** and; (6) **Farber's disease.**
- **Wolman's disease and cholesteryl ester storage diseases are** not sphingolipidoses as these are a/w **accumulation of triglycerides & cholesterol esters (not sphingolipid/ ceramide).**
- **Multiple sclerosis** is a demyelinating disorder (not sphingolipidoses) in which the lipid composition of white matter resembles that of gray matter because of **loss of both phospholipids** (esp **ethanolamine plasmalogen**) **and of sphingolipids from white matter.** The CSF shows raised phospholipid levels.

## Lysosomal Storage Diseases without

**AR inheritance**

- MPS II – Hunter
- Fabry's disease
- ★ Both are *X-linked*

**Neurological involvement**

- MPS IV A, Morquio
- MPS VI B, Morquio
- MPS VI, Maroteaux- lamy
- Cholesterylester storage disease
- Gaucher's disease type I

**Hepatospleenomegaly**

- ***Tay- sach's disease***Q
- ***Fabry's disease***Q
- Mucolipidos is III; pseudo- Hurler polydystrophy
- ***Krabbe's disease***Q
- Metachromatic leukodystrophy
- ★ Cholestery ester storage disease (only hepatomegaly)

**Skeletal involvement**

- Tay- sach's disease
- Fabry disease
- Niemann- Pick disease, neuropathic type A
- Krabbe's disease
- Metachromatic leukodystrophy
- Wolman's disease
- Cholesteryl ester storage disease
- Farber disease

**Opthalmologic involvement**

- MPS III (Sanfilippo) A, B, C, D
- Gaucher's disease type I
- Fucosidosis
- β- Mannosidosis
- aspartyl glucosaminuria
- Krabbe's disease
- Wolman disease
- Cholesteryl ester storage disease

**Hematological involvement**

- $GM_2$ gangliosidoses (i.e. Tay Sach's & Sandhoff's disease)
- Fabry's disease
- Krabbe's disease
- Metachromatic leukodystrophy
- Disorders of neutral lipids (i.e. Wolman, Faber & cholesteryl ester storage disease)

★ Neurological involvement means mental retardation for all lysosomal storage diseases (LSD) except **Fabry disease** where it is in form of ***painful acroparesthesias (i.e. burning pain in lower extremities)***Q. And in *$GM_2$ gangliosidoses (Tay sach's & Sandhoff's disease), Niemann- Pick disease, β -Mannosidosis* and sialidosis (myoclonus), MR is associated with seizures.

★ In *all MPS and ML* opthalmological involvement, is in form of **corneal clouding** *except in MPS II, Hunter disease*, which causes *retinal degeneration*. And ML III, pseudo- Hurler polydystrophy also show mild retinopathy and hyperopic astigmatism along with corneal clouding. Retinal degeneration is also present in *multiple sulfatase deficiency*; and *macular degeneration* in *Farber disease* & Niemann – Pick disease A & B. Optic atrophy is seen in metachromatic leukodystrophy; corneal dystrophy & vascular lesions in Fabry disease. Cherry red spot is found in ***$GM_2$ gangliosidoses (Tay sach's & Sandhoff's disease), Sialidoses and, GM1 gangliosidoses***Q.

## Classification and Separation of Lipoproteins (Based on)

**Electrophoretic mobility (Frederickson's Method)**

- Lipoproteins are separated on their *charge/ size ratio*. Mostly on paper /agarose electrophoretic media.
- **Increasing order of electrophoretic mobility** towards charged (anode) end is

| Lipoprotein | Migrate into |
|---|---|
| **Chylomicron** | ***Do not migrate & remain at origin***Q |
| **LDL** (β-lipoprotein) | β- globulin region |
| **VLDL** (pre-β-lipoprotein) | Pre β-globulin region |
| **HDL** (α-lipoprotein) | $\alpha_1$ globulin region |

**Density (SP unit) based ultracentrifugation (Gofman-Method)**

- Increase in lipid /protein ratio decreases the density of lipoprotein and increase the floatation property of lipoprotein.
- Svedberg units of floatation (SF unit) is the rate at which lipoprotein floats through NaCl and is = $10^{-13}$ cm/S/dyne/g at 26°c
- In ultracentrifugation separation technique, only *the order of LDL & VLDL* is reversed (as compared to electrophoresis).

| | |
|---|---|
| **Chylomicron** | **Floats** d/t lowest density |
| **VLDL** | |
| **LDL** | |
| **HDL** | Settles below d/t highest density |

**Apolipoproteins (Alaupovic Method)**

| Lipoprotein Family | Apolipo protein | Density class |
|---|---|---|
| A | A-I & AII | HDL |
| B | Apo B ($B_{48}$ & $B_{100}$) | LDL & VLDL |
| C | Apo CI, CII, CIII | LDL, VLDL & HDL |
| D | Apo-D | $HDL_3$ |
| E | Apo E (arginine rich) | LDL, VLDL & HDL |

| | Chylomicron | VLDL | LDL | HDL |
|---|---|---|---|---|
| Triacylglycerol | 90% | 60% | 8% | 5% |
| Protein | 2% | 5% | 20% | 40% |
| Phospholipids | 3% | 15% | 22% | 30% |
| Cholesteral & Cesters | 5% | 20% | 50% | 25% |

Liporoteins is composed of

Neutral Lipid are
(Hydrophobic)
- Triacylglycerol
- Cholesterol and chlolesterol esters

Surrounding shell
(Hydrophillic)
- Proteins (Apolipoproteins)
- Phospholipids
- (Unesterified cholesterol)

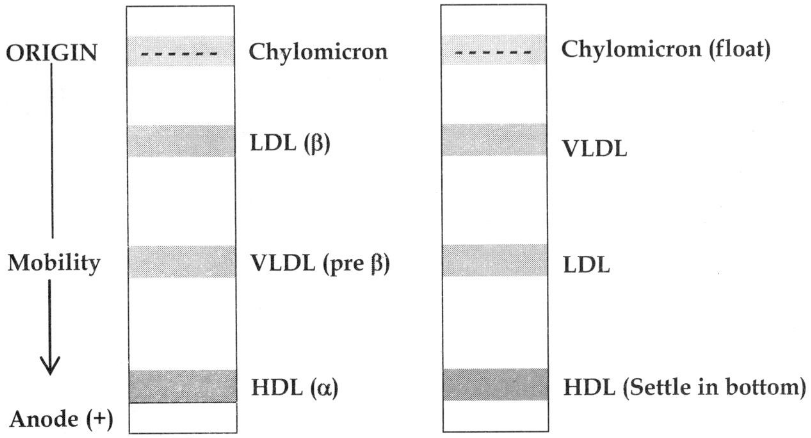


**Electrophoretic separation** **Ultracentrifugation (Density based)**

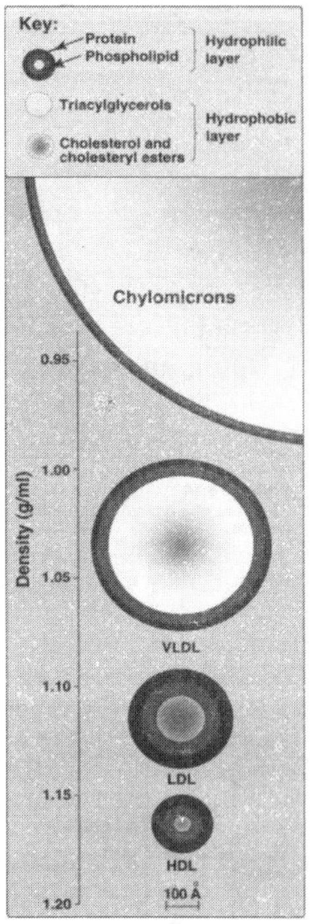


Approximate size and density of serum lipoproteins. Each family of lipoproteins exhibits a range of sizes and densities; this figure shows typical values
[Note: The width of the rings approximates the amount of each component]

## Features of Lipoproteins

The density of lipoprotein decreases as the proportion of lipid to protein increases.

| Lipoprotein | Source | Diameter (nm) | Density (g/mL) | Composition: Protein (%) | Composition: Lipid (%) | Main Lipid Composition | Apolipoprotiens |
|---|---|---|---|---|---|---|---|
| Chylomicrons | Intestine | 90-1000 | <0.95 | 1-2 | 98-99 | Triacylglycerol | A-I, A-II, A-IV[1], B-48, C-I, C-II, C-III, E |
| Chylomicron remnants | Chylomicrons | 45-150 | <1.006 | 6-8 | 92-94 | Triacylglycerol, phospholipids, cholesterol | B-48, E |
| VLDL | Liver (intestine) | 30-90 | 0.95-1.006 | 7-10 | 90-93 | Triacylglycerol | B-100, C-I, C-II, C-III |
| IDL | VLDL | 25-35 | 1.006-1.019 | 11 | 89 | Triacylglycerol, cholesterol | B-100, E |
| LDL | VLDL | 20-25 | 10.19-1.063 | 21 | 79 | Cholesterol | B-100 |
| HDL | Liver, intestine, VLDL, chylomicrons | | | | | Phospholipids, cholesterol | A-I, A-II, A-IV, C-I, C-II, C-III, D[2], E |
| $HDL_1$ | | 20-25 | 1.019-1.063 | 32 | 68 | | |
| $HDL_2$ | | 10-20 | 1.063-1.125 | 33 | 67 | | |
| $HDL_3$ | | 5-10 | 1.125-1.210 | 57 | 43 | | |
| Preβ-HDL[3] | | <5 | >1.210 | | | | A-1 |
| Albumin/free fatty acids | Adipose tissue | | > 1.281 | 99 | 1 | Free Fatty acids | |

**Abbreviations :** HDL, high-density lipoproteins; IDL, intermediate-density lipoproteins; LDL, low-density lipoproteins; VLDL, very low density lipoproteins.
1 Secreted with chylomicrons but transfers to HDL
2 Associated with HDL2 and HDL3 subfractions
3 Part of a minor fraction known as very high density lipoproteins (VHDL).

- **Diameter and Lipid Content**: *decreases* from upward to downward i.e
  - *Chylomicron* has highest diameter and highest lipid content
  - *HDL* has lowest diameter & has least lipid content.
- **Density and protein content:** Increases on going downward i.e.
  - HDL has highest density & has max. protein content.
  - ***Chylomicron has least density***[Q].

- Maximum content of **TG,s** is seen in → ***chylomicron***Q
- Maximum content of ***exogenous TG's*** → chylomicrons
- Maximum content of ***endogenous*** **TG's** is in → ***VLDL***Q
- Maximum **cholesterol** is in → ***LDL***Q.

**HDL**

- HDL are ***synthesized in the liver***Q.
- This is ***highest density***Q lipoprotein (because least lipid content)
- It has highest electrophoretic mobility
- Apoprotein associated with HDL are ***APO A, APOC II, & APOE***Q.

| Chylomicrons | VLDL | LDL | HLD |
|---|---|---|---|
| • Lipoprotein particles with<br>- ***Lowest density***Q<br>- ***Largest size***Q<br>- Maximum amount of lipid<br>• Are assembled ***in intestinal mucosal cells***Q.<br>• Carry exogenous ***dietary TG's to peripheral tissues***Q. | • Are ***produced in the liver***Q.<br>• Are *composed predominantly of TG (also cholesterol ester & cholesterol)*<br>• Carry ***endogenous TG from liver to peripheral tissue***Q. | • ***Contain high concentration of cholestrol & cholesterol esters (bad cholesterol)***Q<br>• ***Provide cholesterol to the peripheral tissue***Q.<br>• LDL is ***causative for coronary disease***Q. | • Synthesized *in liver* & are released into blood by exocytosis.<br>• *Remove free cholesterol from extrahepatic tissue &* esterify it.<br>• *Esterified cholesterol is carried to liver* where HDL is degraded & *cholesterol is removed.*<br>• ***Protective in coronary disease (scavenging action)***Q |

## Chylomicrons & VLDL

Triglycerides (TG) are manly found in – ***chylomicrons & VLDL***Q.

| **Endogenous** ***(from Liver)***Q | **Exogenous** ***(from diet)***Q |
|---|---|
| Maximum in ***VLDL***Q | Max content ***in chylomicron***Q. |

**Chylmicrons**: are found *in chyle* formed only by the lymphatic system *draining the intestine*. They are responsible for transport of all dietary lipids into circulation.

**VLDL**: transport *TG from the liver to extrahepatic tissue.*

★ ***The only apolipoprotein, that remains associated with chylomicrons along its entire journey (from intestine to liver) is apo-B48).***Q

**Intestine Fat**
*(Dietary triglycerides)*Q
↓
Carried by
**Chylomicron** (nascent)
***(B-48)***Q
← Apo C II, E (HDL provides)
↓
**Chylomicron** ***($B_{48}$, C, E)***
↓ (Lipoprotein lipase) — Apo C → HDL; FA → Extrahepatic tissue
↓
**Chylomicron remnant**
**($B_{48}$, E)**

- 90% of TG is lost
- Cholesterol & cholesterol esters retained
- They are taken up by liver by apo E specific receptor mediated endocytosis. Receptor can be :
  LDL (apo B-100, E)
  LRP (LDL receptor related protein)

↓
**Liver**

- Cholesterol ester & remaining Triglycerides are hydrolyzed and metabolized by hepatic lipase

**Lvier Fatty acid**
*(Endogenous triglycerides)*Q
↓
Carried by
**VLDL** (nascent)
***(B-100)***Q
← Apo C II, E (HDL provides)
↓
**VLDL** ***($B_{100}$, C, E)***
↓ (Lipoprotein lipase) — Apo C → HDL; FA → Most of it Supplied to Extrahepatic tissue
↓
**VLDL remnant (IDL)**
**($B_{100}$, E)**

- precursor of IDL
- It can be :
  - **Converted to LDL (Mainly)**
  - **Taken up by liver via LDL (apo B-100, E) receptors** → **Liver**

**Lipoprotein lipase**

- located on wall of blood cappilaries
- Anchored to endothelium by heparan sulphate
- found in adipose tissue, lactating mammary gland, heart, aorta, lung, diaphragm, kidney, spleen.
- ***Activators : Phospholipid & apo C-II***Q
- ***Inhibitors : apo AII & apo C-III***Q
- It is not active in adult liver and not present in blood.
- Released on heparin administration.
- Insulin enhances its synthesis in adipocytes
- Function : It hydrolizes triglycerides (to FA & glycerols) of chylomicron and VLDL resulting in loss of 90% TG & loss of apo-C.

★ Only one molecule of B100 is present in each of these lipoprotein particles & this is conserved during transformation. So each LDL particle is derived from a single precursor VLDL particle.

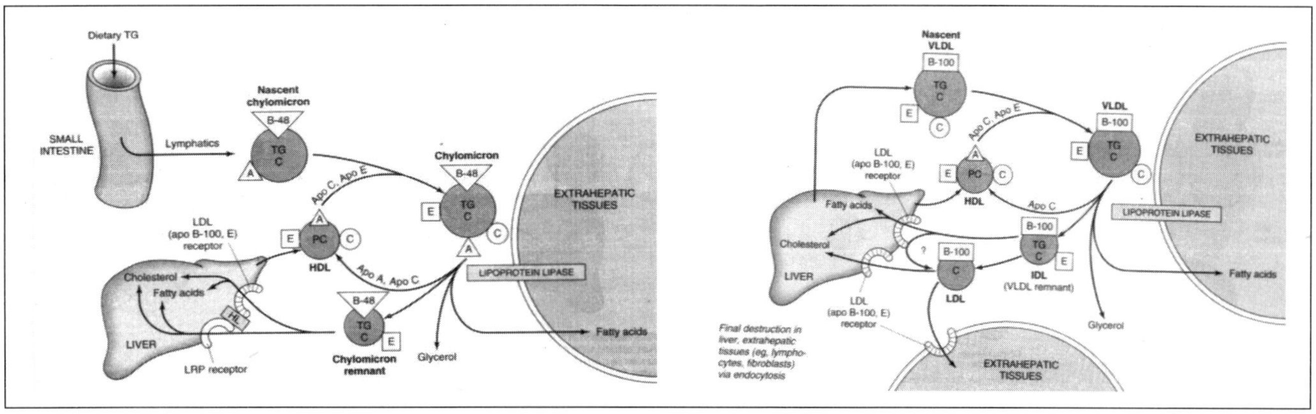


## Apolipoprotein

- Lipoproteins are composed of **neutral (non-polar) lipid core** (containing *triacyl glycerol and cholesteryl ester*) surrounded by a *single surface layer shell* of **amphipathic** (polar) *apolipoproteins, phospholipids and nonesterified (free) cholesterol.* These amphipathic compounds are oriented so that their *polar groups are exposed on the surface*, thus making the particle soluble in aqueous solution. The triacyl glycerol & cholesterol of lipo proteins are either *exogenous* (obtained from diet) or *endogenous* (de novo synthesized). The protein part of lipoprotein is k/a **apoprotein** or **apolipoprotein** which constitutes nearly 70% of some HDL and as little as 1% of chylomicron. Some apolipoproteins are integral & cannot be removed, whereas others are free to transfer to other lipoproteins. Actual apolipoprotein & lipid content of each lipoprotein class is variable because of constant interchange of these between them.
- ***Apo AI & apo AII***[Q] are major apoproteins of **HDL ($\alpha$ -lipoprotein)**. The main apoprotein of **LDL ( $\beta$ – lipoprotein)** and **VLDL (pre $\beta$ -lipoprotein)** is ***B-100***[Q]. **Chylomicron** mainly contains ***B- 48***[Q]. B-100 is one of the longest single polypeptide chain & is synthesized in liver, whereas, B-48 is 48% of B-100 d/t introduction of stop signal by RNA editing enzyme. It is formed by same mRNA but in intestine.
- Apo B-48 and Apo B-100 are synthesized from same Apo B gene and same ApoB- m-RNA. **Apo B 100 is a 100 KDa protein synthesized in liver by full length translation** of corresponding mRNA of Apo B gene. Apo – B-100 forms part of *LDL, IDL and VLDL*. **Apo B-48** is a 48 KDa protein (48% shorter form of Apo B-100) **synthesized in intestine by partial translation of same mRNA of Apo B gene**. Apo B 48 forms part of **chylomicron & chylomicron remnant**. This difference between the sizes of Apo B100 and Apo B48 occurs because **post transcriptional processing (editing)** of Apo B mRNA , **deaminates the cytidine (C) to uracil (U) in intestine** at 2153 position. After **cytidine deamination** the **CAA codon** (which codes **glutamine in liver**) becomes **UAA (nonsense or stop codon)** in intestine. This results in shorter apo B-48 protein being made in intestine (and incorporated into chylomicron) than is made in the liver full length Apo B-100, incorporated in to VLDL.
- **Apoprotein C –I, C- II and C- III** are smaller polypeptides freely transferable between chylomicrons, VLDL and HDL. **Apoprotein E** is found in chylomicron, chylomicron remnant, HDL and IDL.
- Functions of apoproteins are

**Enzyme cofactors / inhibitors**

| Enzyme | Apoprotein function |
|---|---|
| **Lipoprotein lipase** | - *Apo-CII (main) & CI are co factors*[Q]<br>- *Apo AII & apo C III are inhibitors*[Q] |
| **Lecithin: cholesterol acyl transferase (LCAT)** | Apoprotein **AI is cofactor** |
| **Cholesteryl** ester transfer protein | Apo – **CI** is inhibitor |

**As ligand** on lipoprotein particle for interaction with liprotein receptors in tissue eg.

| LDL receptor | *B-100 & E*[Q] |
|---|---|
| **LDL receptor related protein (LRP) or remnant receptor** | APo-E |
| HDL receptor | Apo AI |

**Form part of structure**

- Apoprotein **B** is structural protein for *chylomicron, VLDL, IDL & LDL*
- Apoprotein **AI** is structural protein for *HDL.*

★ LCAT is also a part of HDL

## Low Density Lipoprotein (LDL)

- It is derived **from VLDL** (after going through **IDL stage**) by *loss of triacyl glycerol*.
- Each LDL paricle ***contain a single apo B-100 molecule***[Q] and is derived from single VLDL precursor
- It has ***highest cholesterol and cholesteryl ester content***[Q]. It transports 70% of total cholesterol
- The *primary function of LDL particle is to provide cholesterol to peripheral tissues* (or return it to liver).
- Cholesterol in LDl is called **bad cholesterol** because it is transported to arteries, where it is oxidized by free radicles and retained in arterial proteoglycans starting the formation of ***atherosclerotic plaques. So it increases risk of coronary artery disease***[Q], stroke and peripheral vascular disease.
- While there is growing consensus that ***levels of apolipoprotein (apo) B and the ratio of apo B/apo- AI*** are more accurate predictors of CVD risk but it will take time before apoprotein terminology is recognized by general public & recommended by National cholesterol Education program. Till then it may be more efficacious to continue adhering to already familiar & proven measurements of ***LDL-cholesterol/HDL- cholesterol ratio.***

- It is measured indirectly by using *Friedewald equation* i.e.
  1. LDL cholesterol (in mg/dl) = Total cholesterol – HDL cholesterol – (0.20 x Triglycerides)
  2. LDL cholesterol (in mmol/l) = Total cholesterol – HDL cholesterol – (0.45 x Triglycerides)
- American Heart Association guide lines (2003) for fasting LDL cholesterol levels & risk of CAD

| LDL Fasting Level | | CAD Risk |
|---|---|---|
| Mg/dL | Mmol/L | |
| <100 | < 2.6 | Optimal LDL, corresponding to reduced but not zero risk |
| 100-129 | 2.6-3.3 | Near optimal LDL |
| 130-159 | 3.3-4.1 | Borderline High LDL |
| 160-189 | 4.1-4.9 | High LDL level |
| >190 | >4.9 | Very high LDL, corresponding to highest risk of heart disease |

## LDL (apo B 100, and apo E) Receptors

- **Liver** and many **extrahepatic tissues** express the ***negatively charged glycoprotein LDL (apo B-100, E) receptors***[Q] on the *cell membrane in depressed coated pits* that are coated on cytosolic side with a protein called **clathrin** (which stabilizes the shape of pit)
- It is so designated because it is ***specific for apo B-100 but not B-48***[Q], which lacks the carboxy terminal domain of B-100 containing the LDL receptor ligand, and it ***also takes up lipoproteins rich in apo E***[Q].
- So these receptors can take up LDL, VLDL remnant (i.e. IDL), and chylomicron remnant. The LDL is metabolized via LDL receptor. Approximately 30% of LDL is degraded in extrahepatic tissue and 70% in liver.
- The glycoprotein LDL receptor spans the membrane, the B100 binding region being at the exposed amino terminal end. After binding , ***LDL is take up intact with receptor by endocytosis***[Q]. The vesicle containing LDL loses its clathrin coat & fuses wit similar vesicles, forming larger vesicles called **endosomes**. The pH of endosomes fall d/t proton pumping activity of **endosomal ATPase** which allows separation of LDL from its receptor. The receptor migrates to one side of endosome, whereas LDL stays free within the lumen of vesicle. This structure is called **CURL – Compartment for uncoupling of Receptor & Ligand**. This leads to

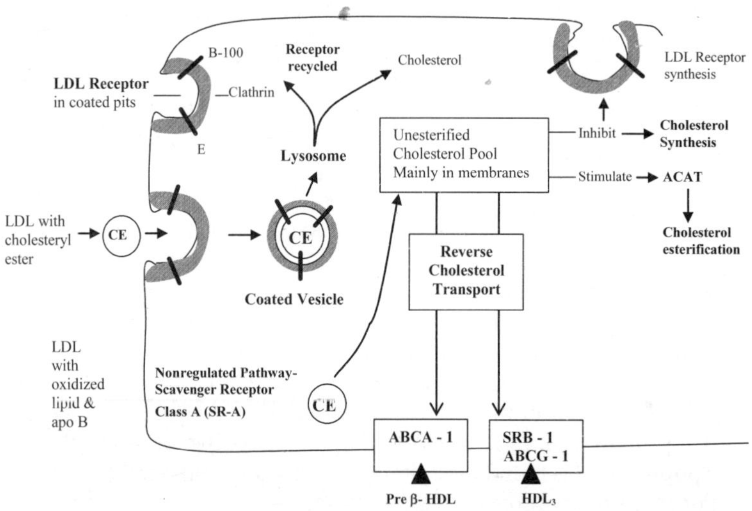


**Hydrolysis of apoprotein and cholesteryl esters** (present in LDL) in **lysosome** and ***translocation of cholesterol into the cells***[Q]

This influx of cholesterol inhibits cholesterol synthesis and uptake by

- *Inhibiting transcription of genes encoding HMG CoA synthase, HMG CoA reductase* & other enzymes involved in cholesterol synthesis
- ***Inhibiting synthesis (replenishment/recruitment or transcription) of new LDL receptors***[Q] via SREBP (sterol regulatory element binding protein) pathway, thus decreasing their number in plasma membrane

Because cholesterol is esterified by **ACAT** (***acetyl CoA-cholesterol acyl transferase), cholesterol influx stimulates ACATactivity promoting cholesterol esterification***[Q]

**LDL receptors** are **recycled** back to the cell surface

- ***LDL receptor is defective***[Q] in *familial hyper cholesterolemia*, a genetic condition which increases blood LDL cholesterol levels and ***cause premature atherosclerosis and coronary artery disease (CAD)***[Q].

## Lipoprotein Lipase (LL)

- It is an *extracellular enzyme* that is located on capillary walls, anchored to *endothelium by negatively charged proteioglycan chains of heparan sulfate.*
- It is *not normally found in blood;* however following *heparin injection,* LL is released from its heparan sulfate binding sites into circulation.
- Lipoprotein lipase is found in capillaries of most tissues but ***predominantly in adipose tissue, cardiac & skeletal muscles, lactating mammary glands***Q, and also in spleen, lung, renal medulla, aorta and diaphragm. ***Adult liver does not have this enzyme***Q (Lippincot) / It is not active in liver - *Harper*
- Hepatic lipase , bound to sinusoidal surface of liver cells, does not significantly attack chylomicrons or VLDL triacylglycerol, but rather is involved in chylomicron remnant and HDL metabolism. It is also released by heparin.
- ***Triacyl glycerols (TAG) of chylomicron and VLDL are hydrolyzed by lipoprotein lipase***Q, progressively through diacyl glycerol to mono acyl glycerol and finally to free fatty acids and glycerol. ***Both phospholipids & apo CII are required as cofactors for LL activity, while apo A II and apo CIII act as inhibitors***Q.
- The formed fatty acids are stored (by adipocyte) & used for energy (by cardiac & skeletal muscles, and renal cortex). And if not immediately taken up by cells , some of it are transported back to circulation attached to albumin until their uptake does occur.
- Lipoprotein lipase synthesis and transfer to luminal surface of capillary is stimulated by insulin (fed state). The ***highest concentration of LL is in cardiac muscles***Q, reflecting that *fatty acids provide much of the energy for cardiac functions.*

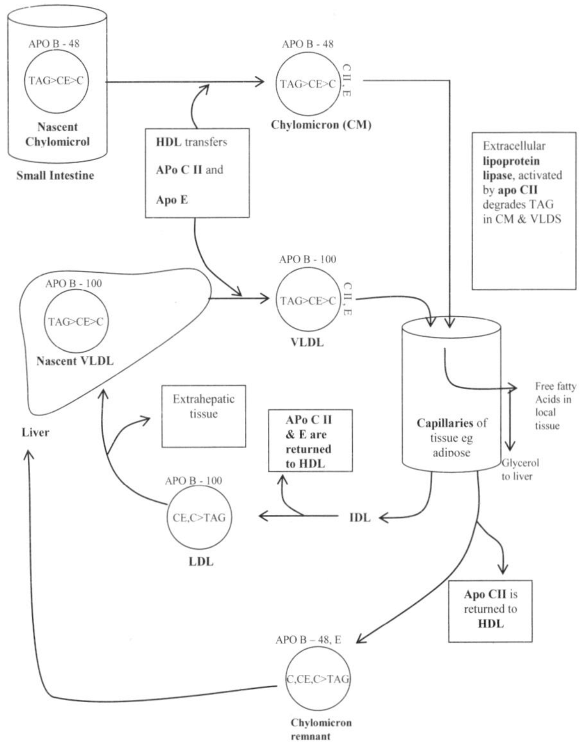


- ***Heart lipoprotein lipase has a low Km and adipose enzyme has a large Km***Q (about 10 times more than heart LL) for triacyl glycerol. This allows heart continuing access to circulating fuel, even when plasma lipoprotein concentrations are low whereas, *adipocytes* can remove fatty acids from circulating lipoproteins and store them as TAG only when lipoprotein concentrations are elevated. This also ***enables the delivery of fatty acids to be redirected from adipose tissue to heart in starved state***Q (when plasma TAG is low). A similar redirection occurs in **lactating mammary glands** for milk synthesis.

## Frederickson Classification of Hyperlipoproteinemias

| Type | Name | Basic defect | Elevated lipoprotein | Electrophoretic classification | Triglycerides | VLDL (pre β) | LDL (β) | HDL (α) | Cholesterol | Refrigeration test | Clinical feature |
|---|---|---|---|---|---|---|---|---|---|---|---|
| I | **Familial lipoprotein lipase deficiency /chylomicronemia syndrome** | - *LPL deficiency*Q<br>- Abnormal LPL<br>- *Apo C-II deficiency*Q causing inactive LPL | *Chylomicrons*Q | Hyper chylomicronaemia | ↑ | ↑ | ↓ | ↓ | Normal | Creamy layer, infranate clear or slightly turbid (Lactescent) | - Erruptive xanthomas<br>- Pancreatitis<br>- Autosomal recessive<br>- ***No atherosclerosis***Q |
| **IIa** | **Familial hyper cholesterolemia/defective apo B /sitosterolemia** | - *Defective LDL receptor*Q<br>- Mutation is apo-B 100, PCSK-9, ABCG8,<br>- ABCG S & ARH | ***↑LDL & hypercholesterolemia***Q | Hyper β-lipoproteinemia (heavy βband) | Normal (-) or ↑ | ↑ (may be) | ↑ - | - | ↑ - | Clear (yello orange tint) | - Tendon tuberous xanthomas<br>- Coronary & peripheral atherosclerosis<br>- ***Autosomal dominant***Q<br>- No pancreatitis |

| | | | | | | | | | | | |
|---|---|---|---|---|---|---|---|---|---|---|---|
| IIb | **Familial combined hyperlipidemia** | Unknown | *LDL & VLDL*[Q] | Heavy β and pre β band | N | ↑ | ↑ | - | N or ↑ | Clear to slightly turbid | - Coronary & peripheral atherosclerosis<br>- No pancreatitis & no xanthoma |
| III | **Familial dysbetalipoproteinemia/Broad β disease / Remnant removal disease** | - ***Abnormality in apo E***[Q] | ***Chylomicron & VLDL remnants of density <1.019*** *(β – VLDL)*[Q] | **Broad β** lipoproteinaemia (**Broad floating β band**) | ↑ | ↑ | ↓ | - | ↑[Q] | Turbid to opaque with thin clear layer | - Palmar tuberoeruptive Xanthomas<br>- Coronary & peripheral atherosclerosis<br>- Autosomal dominant<br>- No pancreatitis |
| IV | **Familial hyper triacylglycerolemia** | - Over production of VLDL often with glucose intolerance & hyperinsulinemia<br>- Un known /Apo A-V | *VLDL*[Q] with cholesterol rise and HDL & LDL tend to be subnormal | Hyper pre β lipoproteinaemia | ↑ | ↑ | ↓ | ↓ | ↑ | Turbid to opaque | - Autosomal dominant<br>- Commonly associated with coronary heart disease, type II diabetes mellitus, obesity, alcoholism & administration of progestational hormones<br>- No pancreatitis & no xanthoma |
| V | **Familial hyper triacylglycerolemia** | - Apo A – V / unknown | *Chylomicron & VlDL*[Q] | Heavy (hyper) chylomicron & pre β bands | ↑ | ↑ | ↓ | ↓ | ↑ | Creamy layer infranate turbid to opaque (Lactescent) | - Autosomal dominant<br>- Eruptive xanthomas<br>- pancreatitis |

★ *Normal TG's in 2 & ↑ed s. cholesterol in 2,3*[Q]

| | Abetalipoproteinemia | Dysbetalipoproteinemia |
|---|---|---|
| **Pathogenesis** | Caused by *mutation* in the gene encoding *microsomal triglyceride transfer protein (MTP)*, this prevent loading of apo – B with lipid & there is ***defective synthesis or secretion of Apo- B***[Q] | Is due to ***defective form of apoprotein E***[Q].<br>[Apo- E plays a crucial role in the catabolism of chylomicron and VLDL.] |
| **Lipoprteins level** | Absent / ↓***Chylomicron***[Q]<br>Absent / ↓ ***VLDL***[Q]<br>Absent / ↓***LDL***[Q] | ↑***Chylomicron remnant***[Q]<br>↑***VLDL remnant***[Q]<br>LDL normal |
| **Plasma lipid abnormalities** | ***Low cholesterol***[Q] (d/t decreased LDL)<br>***Low TG,s***[Q] (d/t decreased chylomicron & VLDL) | **Increased TG's (mainly)**[Q]<br>***Increased VLDL cholesterol***[Q] |
| **Clinical features** | - ***Malabsorption of fat***[Q]<br>- Early childhood diarrhea & failure to thrive.<br>- ***Neuropathy***[Q]<br>- ***Spinocerebellar degeneration (Ataxia)***[Q]<br>- ***Retinitis pigmentosa***[Q]<br>- ***Acanthocytosis***[Q] | - ***Tuberous xanthoma***[Q]<br>- Deposition of cholesterol in palmar creases ***(striae palmaris)***[Q]<br>- ***Risk for atherosclerosis***[Q] & its complication is increased |
| **Treatment** | - Vitamin E<br>- Low fat, High caloric diet | • Drugs:- HMG COA reductase inhibitor<br>- Febrates, Niacin<br>- Estrogen replacement therapy (In postmenopausal women)<br>• Low – cholesterol, low fat diet |

## Cholesterol: Structure, Esterification & Transport

- **Sterols** are structural lipids present in the membranes of most eukaryotic cells. It has **steroid nucleus**, consisting of 4 fused rings, 3 with 6 carbons and 1 with 5 carbons. The steroid nucleus is almost planar and is relatively rigid; the fused ring do not allow rotation about C-C bonds.
- **Cholesterol**, the **major sterol of animal tissues**, is amphipathic, with a polar head (OH group at C3) and a non polar hydrocarbon body (steroid nucleus & hydrocarbon side chain at C-17) about as long as a 16 carbon fatty acid in its extended form.
- Plants have **stigmasterol** & fungi have **ergosterol.** Bacteria cannot synthesize sterols. The sterols of all eukaryotes are synthesized from 5 carbon **isoprene subunits**, as are **fat soluble vitamins**, **quinones** and **dolichols**
- **Cholesterol** is the *most important steroid (sterol)* and precursor of all other steroids in body eg: - Corticosteroids, Sex hormones, ***Bile acid***[Q], ***Vitamin D***[Q].
- Cholesterol occurs in body as **free form** (that exchanges readily between tissues & liproproteins) and **ester form.** Of the cholesterol absorbed, 80-90% in the lymph is **esterified with long chain fatty acids** (to form cholesterol ester). Esterified form is transported as lipoproteins & is not readily exchangeable and used for storage also. ***Highest proportion of circulating cholesterol is found in LDL (beta lipoproteins) which takes cholesterol to tissue & also in HDL which carry it from tissues to liver for degradation (scavanger)***[Q].
- **Esterfication of cholesterol**: Cholesterol may be combined with long chain FA such as Linoleic acid (50%), Oleic acid (18%), Palmitic acid (11%), Arachidonic acid (5%), and other fatty acid (16%).

| In tissue | In Plasma |
|---|---|
| By transfer of acyl group from acyl COA to cholesterol *by enzyme ACAT* (acyl: cholesterol acyl transferase) | By transfer of acyl group (mostly unsaturated) from lecithin to cholesterol *by enzyme. LCAT* (Lecithin: cholestero acyl transferase)<br>Lecithin + Cholesterol —LCAT→ Lysolecithin + cholesterol ester |

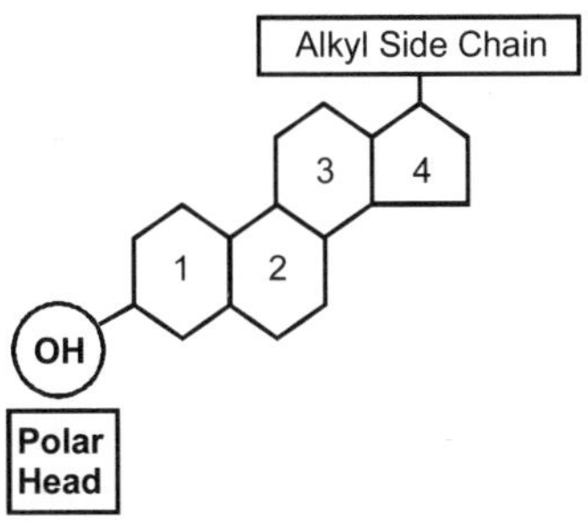


**Cholesterol with Steroid Nucleus**

## Cholesterol Synthesis

- Sir **John Cornforth** & **Vladimir Prelog** described synthetic pathway and received Nobel Prize (1975).
- Cholesterol is synthesized in **liver, adrenal cortex, testes, ovaries & intestine. Although all nucleated cells** can synthesize cholesterol, including arterial walls. Enzymes for cholesterol synthesis are partly located in **endoplasmic reticulum (ER)** and partly in **cytoplasm**.
- ***Acetyl CoA is the starting material & source of all carbon atoms in cholesterol***[Q]. The synthesis can be divided into 5 steps.

### 1. Synthesis of Mevalonate

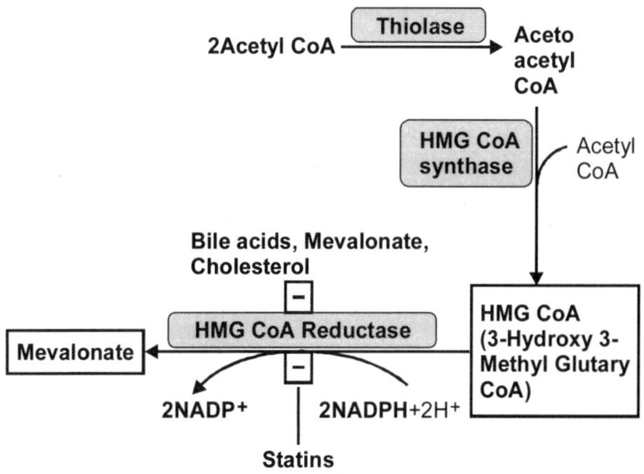


**Cholesterol synthesis** is controlled by ***regulation of HMG COA reductase, which is a rate limiting enzyme***[Q].

**HMG COA Reductase activity**

| Increased by | Decreased by |
|---|---|
| • Insulin<br>• Thyroid | • Mevalonate (immediate product)<br>• Cholesterol (ultimate product)<br>• Glucagon<br>• Glucocorticoid<br>• Drugs: - ***Hypolipidemic drugs***[Q]<br>- Atorvastatin<br>- Simvastatin<br>- Lovastatin<br>- Other statins |

### 2. Formation of Isoprenoid units by loss of $CO_2$

Mevalonate is phosphorylated sequentially using ATP by **3 kinases (mevalonate, 5 phospho mevalonate & 5 diphosphomevalonate kinase)** and then decarboxylated by 3, 5 diphospho mevalonate decarboxylase to form **5 carbon atom active isoprenoid unit (ie isopentenyl diphosphate)**.

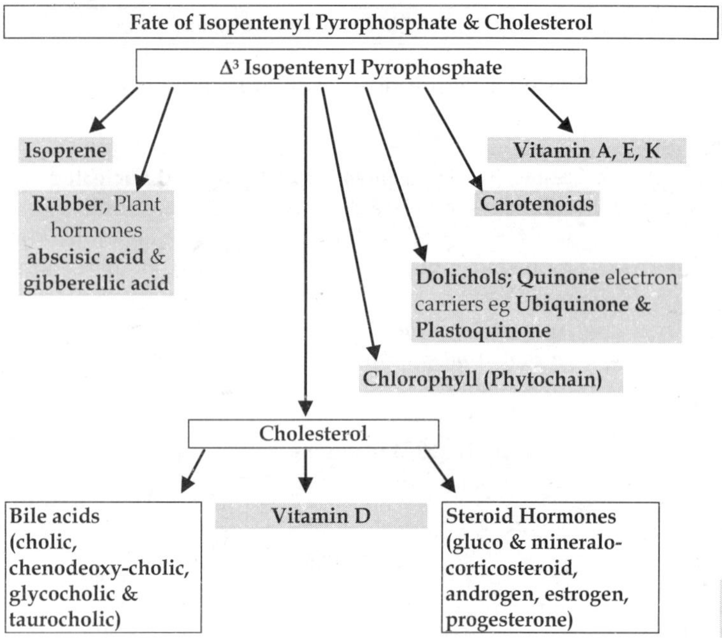


### 3. Condensation of 6 Isprenoid units form Squaline

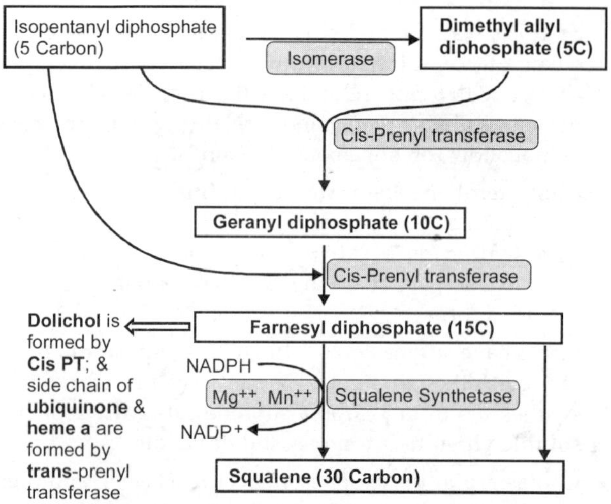


### 4. Formation of parental steroid, Lanosterol by Cylization of Squalene

**Endoplasmic reticulum enzyme, squalene epoxidase** converts squalene to squalene 2,3 epoxide by transferring methyl group on C14 to C13 and on C8 to C14. **Ring closure (cyclization)** is catabolize by **oxidosqualene-lanosterol cyclase** to form lanosterol.

### 5. Formation Cholesterol (in ER membrane)

Methyl groups on $C_{14}$ & $C_4$ are removed to form **14 desmethyl lanosterol** & then **zymosterol**; The double bond, between $C_8$-$C_9$ is remove to $C_5$-$C_6$ in 2 steps forming $\Delta^{7,24}$ Cholestadienol and then **desmosterol (24-dehydrocholesterol)**. The double bond of side chain is reduced to finally produce cholesterol by **$\Delta^{24}$ reductase** (enzyme inhibited by **triparanol**).

**Other Rate limiting Enzymes of Different Pathways**

| Pathways | Rate limiting Enzymes |
|---|---|
| **Glycolysis** | *Phospho fructokinase (PFK)-1* [Q] |
| **Glycogenesis** | *Glycogen synthase*[Q] |
| **Glycogenolysis** | *Glycogen phosphorylase*[Q] |
| **Gluconeogenesis** | *Phosphoenol pyruvate (PEP) carboxykinase*[Q]; *F1, 6 biphosphalase* |
| **Citric acid (TCA) cycle** | Alpha- ketoglutarate dehydrogenase |
| **HMP shunt (PPP pathway)** | *Glucose 6 phosphate dehydrogenase*[Q] |
| **Fatty acid synthesis** | *Acetyl CoA carboxylase*[Q] |
| **Cholesterol synthesis** | *HMG-CoA reductase*[Q] |
| **Ketone body formation** | *HMG CoA synthesase*[Q] |
| **Bile acid synthesis** | *7-alpha hydroxylase*[Q] (regulated by **farnesoid x-receptor or FXR)** |
| **Lipolysis** of adipose tissue | *Hormone sensitive triacylglycerol lipase*[Q] |
| Purine synthesis | PP ribose – P-glutamyl amidotransferase |
| **Uric acid synthesis** | **Xanthine oxidase**[Q] |
| **Urea cycle** | **CPS I (mitochondria)** |
| **Pyrimidine synthesis** | CPS (carbamoyl phosphate synthetase II) |
| Purine salvage pathway | **HGPRT ase; APRT ase (adenine phosphoribosyl** transferase) |
| **Heme synthesis** | ALA synthase |
| Catecholamine | DOPA decarboxylase |
| GTP formation | IMP dehydrogenase |
| Tetrahydro biopterin formation | GTP cyclohydrolase I |

## Measures to Lower Blood Cholesterol (CH)

**Dietary alteration**

- Diet *lower in cholesterol & saturated fatty acid*[Q]
- *Increase dietery fiber*[Q] intke
- Substitution of PUFA and monosaturated FA for saturated

**Hypolipidemic drugs**

| Drugs | Mechanism of action | Effect on lipid |
|---|---|---|
| • **HMG- COA Reductase inhibitor**<br>- Lovastatin<br>- Simvastatin<br>- Atorvastatin | *↓CH synthesis by inhibition of HMG -COA reductase*[Q] | • *↑LDL receptors*[Q]<br>• ↓LDL<br>• ↓TG's<br>• ↑HDL |

FA. i.e. ***saturated/unsaturated FA ratio is low***[Q].

- Lipid lowering effect of PUFA (Poly Unsaturated FA):
  - ↑cholesterol excretion from intestine
  - ↑cholesterol oxidation (catabolism to bile acid)
  - LDL receptor upregulation.

| | | |
|---|---|---|
| • **Bile acid sequestrant**<br>- Cholestyramine<br>- Cholestipol | • *↓Bile acid absorption, ↑ hepatic conversion of CH to bile acid*[Q]<br>• ↑LDL receptor on hepatocytes | ↓ LDL<br>↑ HDL |
| • Fibric acid derivatives<br>- Gemfibrozil | • *↑Activity of lipoprotein lipase*[Q]<br>• ↓ release of FA from adipose tissue | ↓ TG<br>↓ LDL<br>↑ HDL |
| • **Nicotinic acid** | • *↓Lipolysis in adipocytes*[Q]<br>• ↓ Production of VLDL | ↓ LDL<br>↓ TG's<br>↑ HDL |

## Bile Acids

| Primary bile acids | Secondary bile acids |
|---|---|
| Synthesized *in liver from cholesterol*<br>- ***Cholic and chenodeoxycholic acid***[Q]<br>- ***Glycine & Taurine conjugate***[Q] of cholic & chemodeoxycholic acid | Produced *in intestine from primary bile* acid by bacterial action<br>- Deoxycholic acid<br>- Lithocholic acid & their glycine and taurine conjugate. |

## Formation of Bile Acids

**Cholesterol**

↓ ***7-α-hydroxylase***[Q] - ***Rate limiting step***[Q]; NADPH + H⁺, $O_2$, C-vitamin, Cytochrome P-450 — Mn: **"NOCC"**

**7-α-OH cholesterol**

↓ ***7-α-hydroxylase***[Q] - ***Rate limiting step***[Q]; NADPH + H⁺, $O_2$, CoA-SH — Mn: **"NOCC"** → Propionyl CoA [NOCC]

**In Liver**

**Primary bile acids & their Glycine and Taurine Conjugate**

- **Cholyl CoA** → Glycine | Taurine → ***Glycocholic acid***[Q], ***Taurocholic acid***[Q]
- **Chenodeoxy cholyl CoA** → ***Glyco and Taurochenodeoxy cholic acid***[Q]

In intestine (Bacteria): Decojugation + 7-α-dehydroxylation

**Secondary bile acids**

- ***Deoxycholic acid***[Q]
- **Lithocholic acid**[Q]

## De Novo Fatty Acid Synthesis

- Fatty acid synthesis requires

**Multienzyme complex**

- 7 enzyme multicomplex ***Fatty acid synthase***[Q]
- **Acetyl Co enzyme A carboxylase (rate limiting enzyme)**

**Coenzymes & Cofactors**

Mn- **"Be Human"**

| | |
|---|---|
| - *Biotin*[Q] | Be |
| - $HCO_3^-$ (Source of $CO_2$) | Hu |
| - *Mn*$^{2+}$[Q] | M |
| - ATP | A |
| - *NADPH*[Q] | N |

**Building Block**

***Acetyl CoA***[Q]

**Site**

***Cytosol***[Q]

- This takes place in cytosol. ***Acetyl Co enzyme A***[Q] is *primer (starting material)* for formation of *palmitic acid (palmitate $C_{16}$ fatty acid)*. ***Propionyl CoA*** acts as primer for synthesis of *long chain* fatty acid having an *odd number* of carbon atoms.

## Fatty Acid Synthase Complex

- It is a polypeptide containing *7 enzyme activities* – Harper
- It is a multienzyme complex, made up of an ellipsoid dimer of identical polypeptide monomeric units arranged in head to tail fashion. Each monomeric unit contains *six enzymes & an ACP molecule (Acyl carrier protein) – Chaterjae.*
- It is functional only when the two monomeric units are in association with each other. Order of enzyme from end to end in each monomeric unit is.

Mnemonic – **"KAS TAAM – HER KAR ACP"** i.e.

**K**eto **A**cyl **S**ynthase, **T**rans **A**cylase < **A**cetal / **M**alonyl **H**ydratase, **E**nol, **R**eductase, **K**eto **A**cyl **R**eductase, **ACP** – Thioesterase

- Active sites of enzyme

| At **Ketoacyl Synthase** end | At **ACP end** |
|---|---|
| *Cysteine – SH (Cys – SH)*<br>This site of monomer *I* accepts *Acetyl – CoA* | *Pantothenyl – SH (Pan- SH)*<br>This site of monomer *II* accepts *malonyl -CoA* |

Mnemonic- "**Ist AC of IInd PM**" i.e. Monomer **I** accepts **A**cetyl CoA & has **C**ys – SH active site; Monomer **II** has **P**an-SH active site & accepts **M**alonyl CoA.

- ***Ist** and **rate limiting step** is **formation of malonyl from acetyl CoA**[Q]* in presence of ***acetyl CoA carboxylase**[Q]* by fixation of $CO_2$ (so called *$CO_2$ fixation reaction.*)

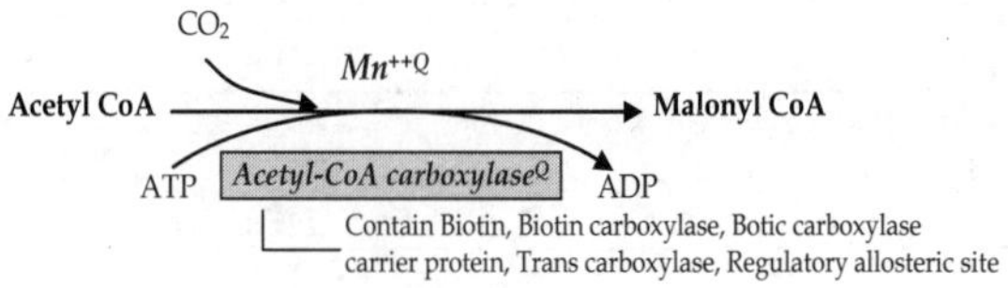


* This is a ***rate limiting irreversible reaction**[Q]*
* **Citrate** is an *activator* and **palmityl CoA** is *inhibitor* of enzyme

## Fatty Acid Synthesis

Once malonyl CoA is synthesized rest of fatty acid synthesis reaction takesplace with FA synthase complex. Now *Acetyl CoA binds to cys -SH end of KAS (unit I) and malonyl CoA binds to Pan-SH end of ACP (unit II)* The *coenzyme A is removed* from both of these and *Acetyl (acyl) - malonyl enzyme* is formed This whole reaction is catalyzed by enzyme transacylase.

↓

Now, the acetate attacks malonate ( that means acetyl group from Cys-SH site is shifted to malonyl group of Pan-SH site) to form 'aceto - acyl- ACP'. As Aceto acetate is attached to pan - SH of monomer II, Cys - SH of monomer I becomes free.

This is a ***condensation reaction*** catalyzed by *condensing enzyme - ketoacyl synthase.* There is ***loss of one molecule of $CO_2$***

↓

Now aceto- acetate (or 3- ketoacyl group) undergoes ***reduction, dehydration and reduction*** again, catalyzed by ketocyl reductase, Hydratase an enoyl recuctase respectively, to ultimately form *saturated acyl - S- enzyme.* All the above three reactions occur *on Pan-SH of monomer II.*

↓

Once *saturated acyl - S - enzyme* is formed; it is now *transferred to the 'cys -SH'* of monomer I, ***freeing the Pan - SH site**[Q]*. (which will accept another malonyl group in each cycle, adding two carbon atoms per cycle)

↓

This cycle starts with **2 carbon** atom- acetyl CoA & **3 carbon** atom - malonyl CoA l/t formation of **5 carbon** atom compound acyl - malonyl enzyme. With a release of $CO_2$ (i.e. **1 Carbon atom**) ultimately a **4 carbon** atom compound, saturated acyl enzyme is formed. With repetition of each cycle 3 carbon atoms are added (in form of malonyl CoA) and 1 carbon atom is released (in form of $CO_2$); thus resulting in ***addition of 2 carbon atom in each cycle**[Q]*. So after 7 cycles ***(1 first + 6 repetitions = 4+ 6x2 = 16C)**[Q]*

Palmitic acid (16 - C compound) is formed.

↓

Palmitic acid is liberated from the enzyme complex by the seventh enzyme- *thioesterase (deacylase)*

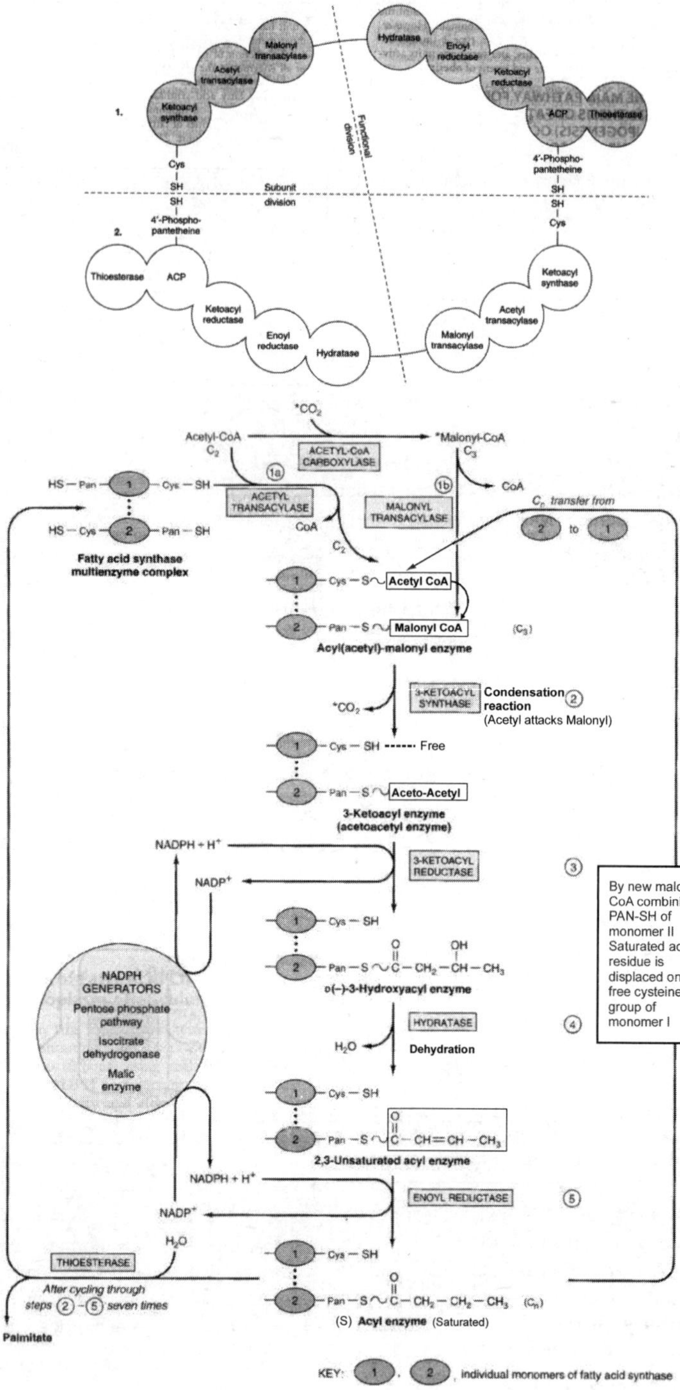


Biosynthesis of long-chain fatty acids. Details of how addition of a malonyl residue causes the acyl chain to grow by two carbon atoms. (Cys, cysteine residue; Pan, 4'-phosphopantetheine). The blocks in dark blue contain initially a C2 unit derived from acetyl-CoA (as illustrated) and subsequently the Co unit formed in reaction 5.

## Fatty Acid Chain Elongation

| Mitochondrial System | Microsomal System |
|---|---|
| 1. ***Not a common pathway***[Q] | 1. ***Usual common pathway for chian elongation***[Q] |
| 2. Operates in ***mitochondria***[Q] | 2. Operates in "microsomal" system. Chain elongation of FA takes place in ***endoplasmic reticulum (ER)***[Q] |
| 3. Palmityl-CoA is usually the starting material and converted to stearyl-CoA. Other long-chain FA may be elongated. | 3. Acyl group that may acts as "Primer" molecule; May be saturated FA series from C10 to C16 and some unsaturated C18 FA. End-product is next higher homologue of the 'Primer' acyl-CoA molecule. |
| 4. ***Operates under "anaerobic" conditions. It is favoured by a high NADH/NAD⁺ ratio in cells***[Q]. Also in presence of excessive ethanol oxidation in liver. | 4. ***Requires presence of $O_2$***[Q] |
| 5. Acetyl-CoA (two carbon unit) is directly incorporated into the palmityl CoA molecule | 5. Acetyl moiety (two carbon) is added through Malonyl CoA and not directly by incorporating C-2 units. |
| 6. NADPH is required which is provided by HMP shunt. | 6. NADPH is required as a reductant provided by HMP shunt. |
| 7. ***Pyridoxal-P is required as a coenzyme***[Q] of the "condensing enzyme" in the first reaction to incorporate C-2 unit. | 7. ***Pyridoxal-P is not required***[Q] |

**Animal Cell**

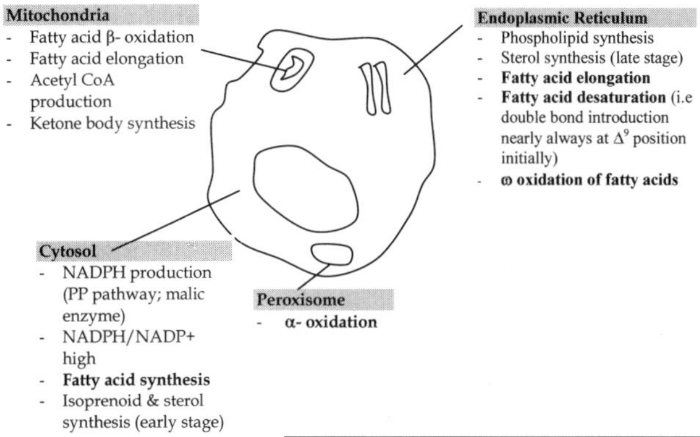


**Plant Cell**

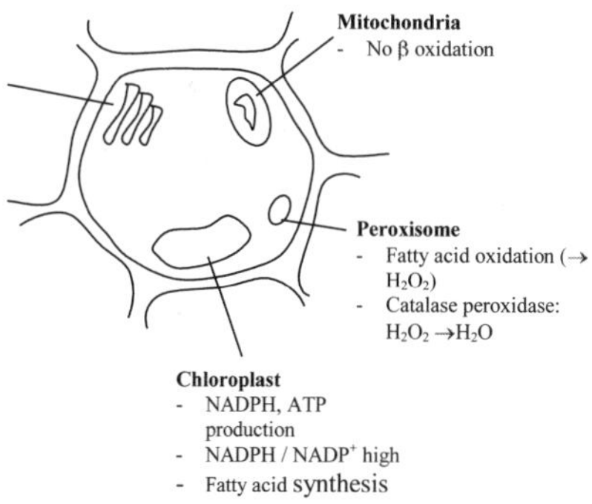


## Triacyl Glycerol and Phosphoglycerol Synthesis

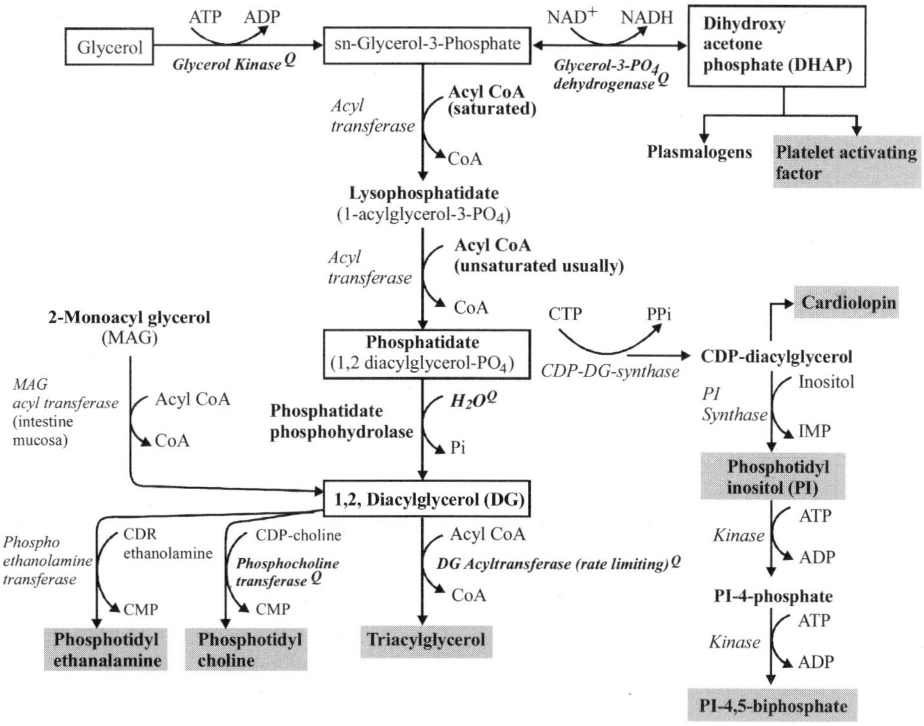

- So **2 molcules of acyl CoA**, combines with **glycerol 3 $PO_4$** to form phosphatidate in two steps catalyzed by glycerol 3 $PO_4$ acyltransferase and 1 acylglycerol-3-$PO_4$ acyl transferase. ***Phosphatidate is hydrolyzed by phosphorylase into 1, 2 diacyl glycerol***[Q]. **Diacyl glycerol acyl transferase,** ***rate limiting enzyme,*** **catalyzes the** ***only step specific for triacyl glycerol synthesis.***
- Choline & ethanolamine are first activated by *ATP phosphorylation followed by CTP linkage* to form CDP – choline or CDP – ethanolamine which reacts with 1, 2 – diacylglycerol to form either phosphotidyl choline or phosphotidylethanol-amine. Phosphotidyl serine is formed from phosphotidyl ethanolamine by reaction with serine, and decarboxylation reverses the reaction. In liver phosphotidyl ethanolamine gives rise to phosphotidyl choline by methylation.
- These are formed by acylation of triose phosphates; and **phosphatidate** is the common precursor of triacylglycerols, many phosphor-glycerols and cardiolipin. The biosynthesis is regulated by the availability of free fatty acids. Those that escape oxidation are preferentially converted to phospholipids, and when this requirement is satisfied they are used for triacylglycerol synthesis. Glycerol 3 $PO_4$ & DHAP are intermediates in glycolysis making connection between carbohydrate & lipid metabolism.

## Carnitine

### Chemistry & Synthesis

- Carnitine is β- OH Y Trimethy ammonium butyrate *[β- OHGTB]*
- It is found in meat diet or is endogenously synthesized from ***lysine***[Q] and *methionine* in liver (mainly) and kidney but not in skeletal or heat muscles.
- Skeletal muscle contains about *97% of all carnitine* in body.

### Functions

Carnitine is a carrier molecule. It facilitates transpost

**In mitochondria**
Transport long chain acyl – CoA in mitochondria for β-oxidation

**From mitochondria**
Transport acetyl CoA & acetoacetyl Co from mitochondria to cytosol

***Fatty acids must be first activated before they can be oxidized***[Q]. 'Active' FA (acyl – CoA) are formed in cytosol and for β- oxidation to occur it has to be transferred to mitochondrial matrix. Acyl CoA needs a transport system as it is impermeable to inner mitochondrial membrane.

| FA activation | FA transport across mitochondria |
|---|---|
| - Fatty acid is converted to an *'active fatty acid' or acyl CoA* in presence of ATP and co enzyme A by the enzyme acyl - CoA *synthetase (thiokinase).*<br>- Acy- CoA synthetase is present in endoplasmic reticulum, peroxisomes & mitochondria (inside & on outer membrane)<br>- This is the ***only step in FA degradation where ATP is used & form AMP***[Q]. | - Long chain acyl CoA is impermeable to inner mitochondrial membrane but bcome permeable by converting into 'acyl-carnitine' by the enzyme *carnitine palmitoyl transferase* 1 (CPMT1) which is present in the *outer mtochondrial membrane.*<br>- Now Acyl carnitine is transported inside the mitochondria by the enzyme *carnitine – acylcarnitine translocase* which also export one molecule of carnitine out.<br>- Acyl – carnitine is converted to acyl CoA in mitochondrial matrix by *Carnitine palmtoyl transfase II* (CPMT-2) located on the *inner membrane* |

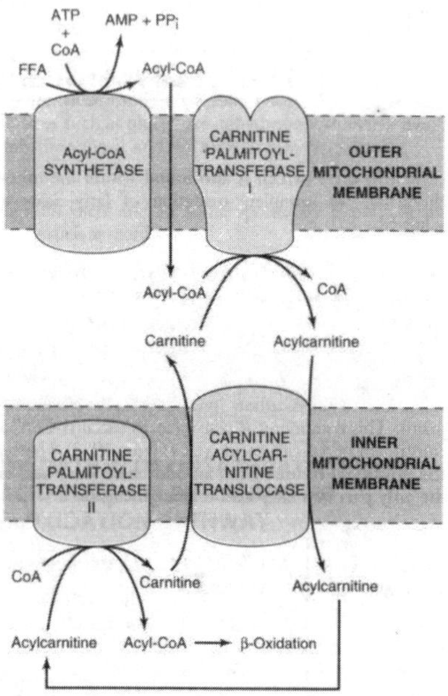


Role of carnitine in thetransport of long-chain faty acids through the inner mitochondrial membrane. Long-chain acyl-CoA cannot pass through the inner mitochondrial membrane, but its metabolic product, acylcarnitine, can.

# β - Oxidation of Fatty Acid

It involves successive cleavage of FA chain *between the α (2) and β (3) – carbon atom* (hence the name β- oxidation) with release of Acetyl CoA.

Oxidation of acyl CoA to acetyl CoA is catalyzed by *'Fatty acid oxidase complex'* in mitochondrial matrix

The successive steps are:
Dehydrogenation → Hydration → Dehydrogenation. In 1st Dehydrogenation reaction, 2H atoms are removed with the formation of *$FADH_2$ (2ATP)* in presence of acyl –COA dehydrogenase, and *Enoyl CoA* ($\Delta^2$ trans enoyl) is formed.

The hydration (addition of $2H_2O$) occurs in presence of enoyl CoA hydratase with the formation of *3-OH (hydro) acyl CoA*

↓

Further dehydrogenation (removal of $H_2$) catalyzed by 3 -OH- acyl CoA dehydrogenase to form ***keto acyl CoA & NADH (3ATP)***Q.

↓

Dehydrogenation f/b Hydration f/b Dehydrogenation = **Reactions**

Enoyl CoA f/b Hydroacyl CoA f/b ketoacyl CoA = **Products**

↓

Finally 3 – keto acyl CoA is split by *thiolase* and result in formation of:

| | |
|---|---|
| *One Acetyl CoA which enters* TCA cycle to form $H_2O$ & $CO_2$ | One Aceyl CoA containing 2 carbon less than original molecules & enters for reoxidation by acyl dehydrogenase. |

In this way a long chain fatty acid is degraded completely to acetyl CoA (C-2unit). Thus *palmitoyl – CoA ($C_{16}$) form 8 acetyl CoA from 7 cycles.*

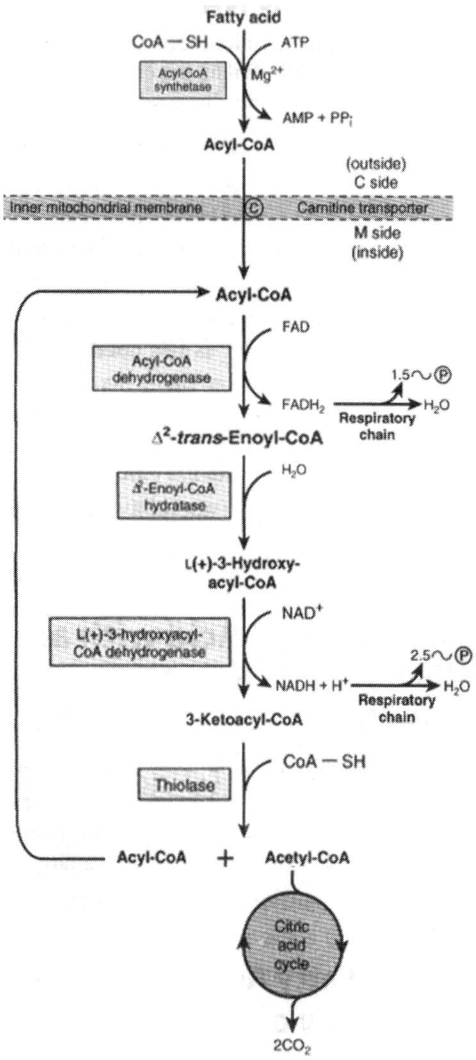


**Comparison of long chain, even numbered, saturated FA synthesis & B oxidation (degradation)**

| Feature | FA synthesis | Degradation |
|---|---|---|
| Occurs in | **Fed state** (after carbohydrate rich meal) | **Fasting & starvation** |
| Favouring hormone | **High insulin/** glucagon ratio | **Low insulin / glucagon ratio** |
| Primary site<br>Cellular site | **Liver**<br>**Cytosol** | **Muscle, liver**<br>**Mitochondria** |
| Acyl (acetyl) group carrier | **Citrate**<br>From mitochondria to cytosol | **Carnitine**<br>From cytosol to mitochondria |
| Phosphopant-etheine containing active carriers | Acyl carrier protein, coenzyme A | Coenzyme A |
| Coenzymers | **NADPH** (reduction) | **NAD+, FAD** (oxidation) |
| 2 Carbon donor / product | **Malonyl CoA** (donor of 1 acetyl group) | **Acetyl CoA** (product of beta oxidation) |
| Activator | Citrate | |
| Inhibitor | **Long chain fatty acyl CoA** (inhibits acetyl CoA carboxylase) | ***Malonyl CoA (inhibits CPTI)***Q |
| Product of pathways | Palmitate | Acetyl CoA |
| Repetitive 4 steps | **Condensation, reduction , dehydration, reduction (CRDR)** | **Dehydro-genation, hydration, dehydroge-nation, thiolysis (DHDT)** |

**β - Oxidation of fatty acid**

| Even Chain FA | Odd Chain FA |
|---|---|
| *2 carbons at a time* are cleaved from acyl – CoA in every cycle to form ***Acetyl – CoA (2carbon unit substance)***Q | With odd chain FA, β- oxidation produces *acetyl CoA*, until a ***three-carbon (propionyl –CoA) residue remains***Q.<br>**Propionyl CoA** is the ***only part of fatty acid that is glucogenic***Q [as it is converted to succinyl CoA, a consituent of TCA cycle] |

| Fatty Acid | Number of C atoms |
|---|---|
| *Acetic* | 2 |
| *Propionic* | 3 |
| *Butyric* | 4 |
| Valeric | 5 |
| Caproic | 6 |
| Lauric | 12 |
| Myristic | 14 |
| ***Palmitic***[Q] | **16** |
| ***Stearic***[Q] | **18** |

★ In any even numbered FA, the no, of β oxidation cycles would be $\frac{n}{2}-1$, and no. of TCA cycles would be n/2

★ So ATP produced by palmitic (no- 16) acid is

$$-\frac{16}{2}-1=7\times4=28 \text{ ATP}$$

$$-\frac{16}{2}=8\times10=80 \text{ ATP i.e. } 108 \text{ ATP} - 2 \text{ATP} = 106 \textit{ ATP}$$

**ATP Production in β-oxidation of Fatty Acids**

| Steps | Product | ATP formed Old concept | New concept |
|---|---|---|---|
| • **Each β oxidation cycle** | | | |
| - Acyl CoA dehydrogenase | **1 $FADH_2$** | 2 | 1.5 |
| - β-Hydroxyacyl-CoA dehydrogenase | **1 NADH** | 3 | 2.5 |
| • Total ATP produced | | **5** | **4** |
| • Each **acetyl CoA**, on **oxidation in TCA (citric acid cycle)** | | | |
| - Malate / Isocitrate/ Alpha (α) ketoglutarate dehydrogenase | **3 NADH** | 9 | 7.5 |
| - Succinate dehydrogenase | | | |
| - Succinyl CoA synthetase | | | |
| • Total ATP produced | **1 $FADH_2$** | 2 | 1.5 |
| | 1 GTP | 1 | 1 |
| | | **12** | **10** |
| • **Energy utilized in activation of FA** | **-2 ATP** | In all cycles | |

- Acording to **older concept 1NADH (Mitochondrial)** yields **3 ATP,** **1 NADH (cytosolic)** yields **3 or 2 ATP** depending upon shuttle system, and **1 $FADH_2$** yields **2 ATP**. So net gain of ATPs in **palmitic acid** (16 carbon) used to be **129 ATP** and in **stearic acid** (18C) **146 ATP**.

  For calculating this a formula derived by my friend is

  $$\text{Net ATP gain} = \frac{17\times \textit{no of carbon atoms}}{2}-7=\frac{7n}{2}-7$$

  (in even number fatty acid)

- But according to **new concept 1 NADH (mitochondrial)** yields **2.5 ATP, 1 NADH (cytosolic) yields 1.5 or 2.5 ATP depending** on the shuttle syste and **1 $FADH_2$** yields **1.5 ATP**. Therefore, net gain in **palmitic acid** would be ***106 ATP***[Q] and in ***stearic acid 120 ATP***[Q]. So now suggested formula is

  **Net ATP gain**
  (in even number fatty acid) = 7n- 6

  ★ The formulas are also valid for even numbered unsaturated fatty acids.

- 1 mol. Of palmitate involves net production of **106 mol of ATP** via β oxidation, whereas only **26 mol of ATP** are produced when acetoacetate is the end product and only **21 mol of ATP** when 3 hydroxybutyrate is the end product.

**ATP Production (old)**

| Stearic Acid | |
|---|---|
| **Stearic acid ($C_{18}$) is $C_{17}H_{31}COOH$**. In β- oxidation it will undergo *8 cycle* [2-C removed in each cycle +2 (C2) units remaining in last cycle], producing *9 acetyl CoA* | |
| - Each cycle produces | = 5 ATP. |
| ∴ 8 cycle produces | = 8x 5 = 40 ATP |
| - Each acetyl CoA produces | = 12 ATP |
| ∴ 9 acetyl CoA produces | = 12x 9 = 108 ATP |
| - Total ATP produced | = 148 ATP - 2 ATP |
| **Net gain** | **= 146 ATP** |

| Palmitic Acid |
|---|
| **Palmitic acid** is ***16 carbon compounds***[Q] and it will undergo ***7 cycles & produce 8 acetyl CoA***[Q] (for **citric acid cycle**) i.e. |
| - ATP from NADH & FADH2 in cycle = 7 x 5 = ***35 ATP***[Q] |
| - ATP from acetyl CoA in Citric acid cycle = 12 x 8 = ***96 ATP***[Q] |
| - ATP spend in activation = -2ATP |
| Net gain = ***129 ATP***[Q] |

## β- Oxidation

| In peroxisomes | In Mitochondria |
|---|---|
| • Facilitates oxidation of *very long chain FA* ($C_{20}$, $C_{22}$), do not attack shorter chain FA. | • Oxidation of *both long & short* chain FA. |
| • β - oxidation sequence *ends at octanoyl – CoA* & *acetyl CoA*. Both further oxidized in mitochondria. | • End product is acetyl CoA. |
| • **In 1st oxidation step**: (i.e. Ist dehydrogenation step; FAD linked) Flavoprotein dehydrogenase passes electrons to ***$O_2$ producing $H_2O_2$***[Q], which is broken down by catalase into $H_2O$ & $O_2$. *Energy released dissipates as heat* | • **In 1st oxidation step:** Electron removed from flavoprotein dehydrogenase passes through *respiratory chain to O2 to produce H2O* & this process is accompanied by *ATP synthesis*. |
| • This system is *not linked directly* to phosphorylation & ATP generation | • This system is directly linked to ATP generation. |
| • **Other functions:**<br>- *To shorten side chain of cholesterol* in bile acid formation.<br>- Synthesis of ether glycerolipids, cholesterol and dolichol. | |

## Impaired oxidation of Fatty Acids: l/t disease often associated with hypoglycemia

### Carnitine deficiencies

- Secondary deficiency occurs in
  - Decreased synthesis of carnitine in patients of *liver disease, malnutrition* or those on *strictly vegetarian* diets
  - Increased requirements as result of *pregnancy, trauma, severe burn, infection*
  - Increased losses d/t hemodialysis or renal leakage (eg in preterm infants).
- Genetic deficiency may be of 2 types
  - **CPT-1 deficiency *affects only liver***[Q], where an inability to use long chain fatty acid for fuel greatly impairs the tissues ability to synthesize glucose during a fast, resulting in reduced fatty acid oxidation and ketogenesis with hypoglycemia, coma and death.
  - **CPT II deficiency** affects ***primarily skeletal and cardiac muscles***[Q] and, when severe, the liver resulting in *cardiomyopathy, muscle weakness with myoglobinemia* following prolonged exercise
- *Sulfonylurea drugs (glyburide / glybenclamide, and tolbutamide*) used in tt of type 2 diabetes reduce fatty acid oxidation & therefore hyper glycemia by *inhibiting CPT-1*
- ***Malonyl CoA inhibits CPT-1 thus preventing long chain acyl group entery into mitochondrial matrix. The phosphorylation & inhibition of acetyl CoA carboxylase decrease malonyl CoA production, removing the break on fatty acid oxidation***[Q].

★ *Presence of methyl group on β-carbon* (eg in branched chain phytanic acid) *makes β oxidation impossible* and these fatty acids are catabolize in **peroxisomes by α oxidation**.

★ **ω oxidation** ( of ω cabon i.e. most distant from carboxyl group) occurs in **endoplasmic reticulum** of liver & kidney, and preffered substrates are fatty acids of 10-12 carbon atoms.

### Medium Chain fatty Acyl CoA Dehydrogenase (MCAD) deficiency

- *Autosomal recessive, most common* inborn error of fatty acid oxidation
- *Infants* are particularly affected because they rely on milk (which contains primarily medium chain FA) for their nourishment
- **Dicarboxylic auduria** is characterized by *excretion of C6 – C10 ω-dicarboxylic acids* & by non ketotic hypoglycemia, caused by MCAD deficiency.

### Jamaican Vomiting Sickness

- Eating of *unripe fruit of akee tree, containing hypoglycin toxin* causes JVS
- Toxin inactivates *medium & short chain acyl CoA dehydrogenase,* inhibiting β- oxidation and causing *hypoglycemia.*

### Zellweger's (Cerebrohepatorenal) syndrome

- Very long chain fatty acids (VLCFA) i.e. >20 carbons, undergo a preliminary β oxidation in peroxidomes. The shortend FA is then transferred to mitochondria for further oxidation
- So **absence of peroxisomes in all tissues (i.e. Zellweger syndrome)** or the inability to transport VLCFA across peroxisomal membrane (i.e. **X- linked adrenoleukodystrophy)** l/t accumulation of *VLCFA ($C_{26}$-$C_{38}$)*
- In ZS, accumulation of polyenoic acids in brain causes severe neurological symptoms & death in 1st year of life

### Refsum's Disease

- AR disorder caused by ***deficiency of phytanic -α oxidase / α hydroxylase / phytanoyl CoA hydroxylase***[Q] resulting in accumulation of phytanic acid d/t its decreased *α oxidation in peroxisome.*
- Phytanic acid impairs membrane function, protein prenylation and gene expression causing primarily neurological symptoms.
- Phytanic acid is found in *dairy products, & ruminant fat & meat.* It involves dietary restrictions.

## Ketogenesis: Synthesis of Ketone Bodies in Liver

- *Acetoacyetyl CoA* is the *starting material & this* can arise in two ways:
  - directly from terminal 4- carbon of fatty acid during β- oxidation
  - as a result of **condensation of two acetyl CoA molecule** (i.e. 2 C units) formed in β oxidation by ***reversal of thiolase reaction***.
- *Acetoacetate is the Ist ketone body to be formed.* It can be formed from Acetoacyetal in two steps:
  - Initially condensation of Acetoacyetyl with another acetyl CoA to form β -OH - β- methyl glutaryl CoA *(HMG CoA)* by enzyme HMG CoA synthesis.
  - Then HMG CoA is split into Acetoacetate and Acetyl CoA by the enzyme HMG CoA lyase. This is a commited step.
- Both **enzymes (HMG Co synthase & lyase) of ketogenesis** must be present in **mitochondria** for ketogenesis to take place. This occurs only in **liver** and **rumen epithelium. D(-) - 3 - Hydroxybutyrate** is quantitatively the predominant ketone body *present in blood stream* (ketonemia or hyper ketonemia) and urine (**ketonuria**) in ketosis.

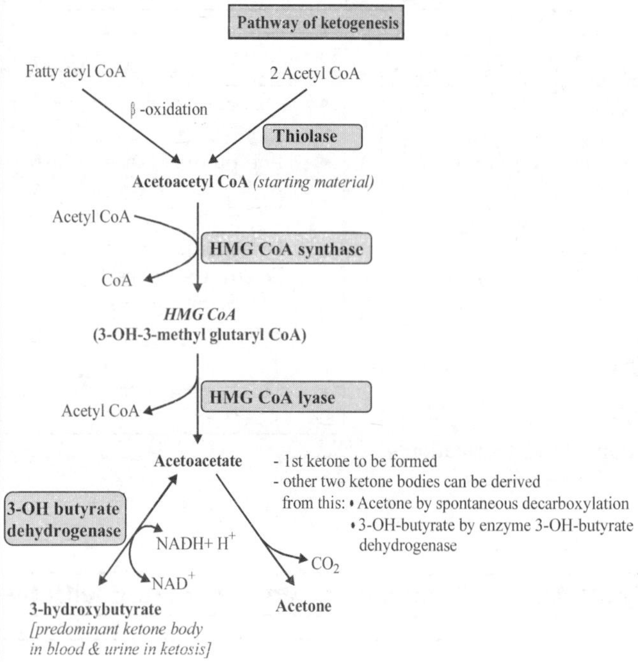


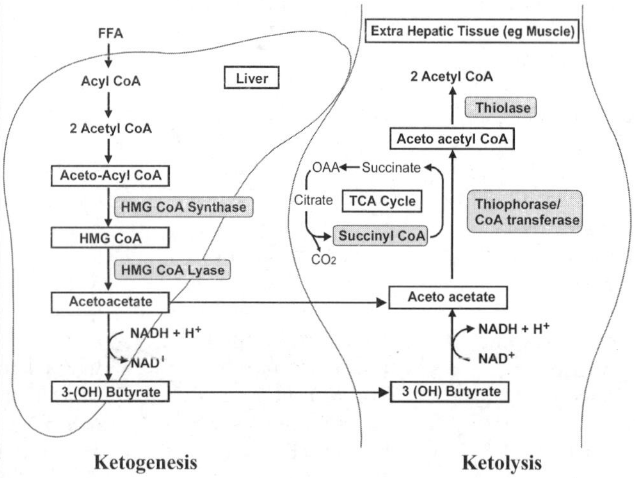


## Ketolysis: Use of ketone Bodies in Periphral Tissues as Fuel

- Although *liver constantly produces low levels of ketone bodies*, their production becomes much more significant during **fasting, starvation, type II diabetes mellitus**, twin lamb disease & in lactating cattle. Non pathological form of ketosis occurs under conditions of **high fat feeding & after severe exercise** in post absorptive state.
- Under certain metabolic conditions (depletion of available carbohydrate coupled with increased mobilization/lipolysis of FFF) associated with high rate of fatty acid oxidation, liver produces ketone bodies, which is used as respiratory substrate (fuel) by extrahepatic tissue. ***Ketone bodies is collective name given to 3 compounds***[Q]**: 1. Acetone 2. Acetoacetate 3. Beta hydroxybutyrate. In a well fed state, concentraton of ketone bodies in blood does not exceed** ***1mg/100ml***[Q].
- Extrahepatic tissues including brain but **excluding cells lacking mitochondria (RBC)** efficiently oxidize acetoacetate & 3(OH) butyrate. In contrast, ***liver actively produces ketone bodies but lacks thiophorase (Succinyl CoA : acetoacetate CoA transferase) and so is unable to use ketone bodies as fuel***[Q].
- Substrate utilized for energy production

| Organ | Fed | Fasting | Starvation |
|---|---|---|---|
| Brain | Glucose | Glucose | ***Ketone bodies***[Q] |
| Heart | ***Fatty acid***[Q] | Fatty acid | Ketone bodies |
| Liver | Glucose | Fatty acid | Amino acid |
| Muscles | Glucose | Fatty acid | Fatty acid |

*Heart utilizes F.A even in fed state. Resting muscles use FFA as fuel source while exercising muscle initially use glycogen reserve (glucose) and then FFF.*

- While **acetoacetate & 3(OH) butyrate** are oxidized by **extrahepatic tissue as fuel, acetone** is difficult to oxidize (in vivo) and is mainly **volatilized in lungs.** Both acetoaectate & 3(OH) butyrate are ***moderately strong acids*** and are buffered depleting alkaline reserve, thus causing **fatal ketoacidosis** (in very severe cases).

## Regulation of Ketogenesis

Ketogenesis is regulated at 3 crucial steps

1. During **mobilization of FFA (free fatty acids) from adipose tissue (lipolysis):** Liver extracts ~ 30% of FFA passing through it both in fed & fasting condition. **FFA are the precursors of ketone bodies in liver**. Therefore factors increasing /decreasing FFA mobilization from adipose tissue increase / decrease ketogenesis. So factors affecting **adipose tissue lipolysis, FFA release and ketogenesis** include

| Decreasing Factors | Increasing Factors |
|---|---|
| - **Insulin, Nicotinic acid, Prostaglandin $E_1$, Adenosine** & high concentration of **FFA** inhibit lipolysis *by inhibiting synthesis of c-AMP at adenylyl cyclase* site acting through Gi protein.<br>- *Lipolysis is more sensitive to changes in concentration of insulin than are glucose utilization & esterification*. Insulin also stimulates **phosphodiesterase** (removing c-AMP) and **lipase phosphatase** that inactivates hormone sensitive lipase (HSL). FFAs also inhibit HSL.<br>- **Perilipin** protein is involved in formation of lipid droplets in adipocytes and *inhibit lipolysis in basal condition* by preventing access of lipase enzyme to stored triacyl glycerol. | - **Epinephrine, norepinephrine, glucagon, ACTH,** alpha and beta **MSH (melanocyte stimulating hormone), TSH, GH and Vasopressin** increase lipolysis of triacyl glycerol by activating **hormone sensitive lipase** (through adenyl cyclase)<br>- For optimal effect most of these require **glucocorticoids and thyroid hormones as facilitatory or permissive lipolytic endocrinal factors.**<br>- On stimulation with lipolytic hormones, **perilipin** promote TAG degradation; thus regulating balance between TAG storage & lipolysis in adipocytes |

2. **During entery of FFAs for B oxidation pathway by CPTI (into mitochondria):** After uptake by liver, FFAs are either **beta-oxidized** (in fasting/ starving) **or esterified** to TAG & phospholipid (in fed state). The ***entery of FFAs into Beta oxidation pathway is regulated by CPTI (carnitine palmitoyl transferase I)***Q and the remainder of FA taken up by liver is esterified.

| In Fed State | In Fasting / Starvation |
|---|---|
| ↓ | ↓ |
| FFA enters liver in low concentration | Due to lipolysis FFAs entere liver in high concentration |
| ↓ | ↓ |
| **CPT I activity is low** as it is potently inhibited by **malonyl CoA** (the initial intermediate formed by *acetyl CoA carboxylase in fatty acid synthesis*) | *Acetyl CoA carboxylase enzyme in FA synthesis is directly inhibited* by acyl CoA (FFA) **decreasing malonyl CoA levels**; thereby **releasing the inhibition of CPT I** |
| ↓ | ↓ |
| Because of low CPT I activity, **fatty acid beta oxidation is depressed** and **nearly all FFA** entering liver is esterified to acyl glycerol and is transported out in **VLDL** | **More acyl CoA (FFA) enter beta oxidation by CPTI gateway into mitochondria** and balance of FFA uptake not oxidized is esterified |

3. **Acetyl CoA formed in beta oxidation is oxidized in citric acid cycle or it enters the pathway of ketogensis.**
   - Liver is unique as it synthesize ketone bodies, **primarily 3- hydroxybutyrate (beta-hydroxybutyrate)** *for use as fuel by peripheral tissues, but not by liver itself.* Ketogenesis is favoured when concentration of acetyl CoA produced from beta- oxidation, exeeds the oxidative capacity of TCA. So as the level of serum FFA is raised, proportionately more FFA is converted to ketone bodies & less is oxidized in TCA to $CO_2$. The fate of acetyl CoA between ketogenesis & TCA is regulated *so that the total ATP produced from the oxidation of FFA remains constant* as concentration of FFA in serum changes.
   - 1 mol of **palmitate** produces **106** mol of ATP via beta oxidation & $CO_2$ production in TCA, whereas only **26 ATP** are produced when **acetoacetate** is end product and only **21 ATP** when **3 hydroxybutyrate** is end product. **So ketogenesis allows liver to oxidize increasing quantities of FAs.** At the same time, ketogenesis releases CoA, ensuring its availability for continued fatty acid oxidation.

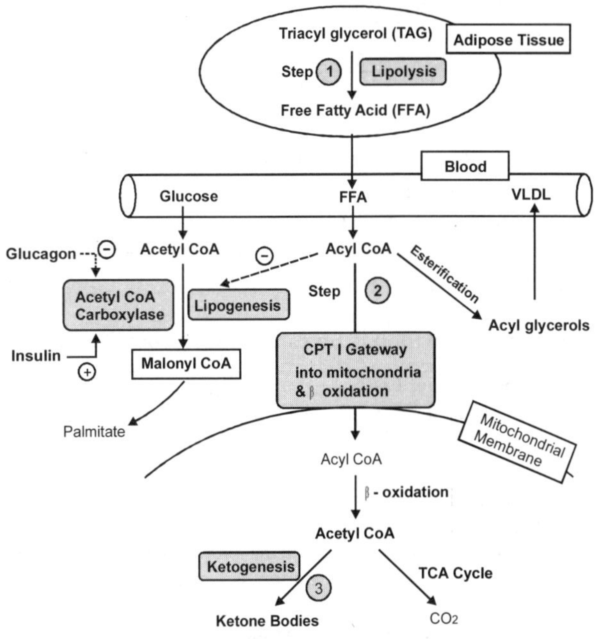

Regulation of Ketogenesis

## Metabolism In Fed & Fasting

**Brain Metabolism**

- **Brain tissue** uses ***glucose as an exclusive fuel*, *both during the fed state as well as in fasting state***[Q], except *during starvation* when it can adapt to ***use ketonebodies as an energy source***[Q].
- Brian does ***not utilize fatty acids as a fuel***[Q]. And brain contains ***no fuel reserves***[Q] and so must be continuously supplied with fuel from the blood. ***In brain 60% of total energy is utilized during the resting stage***[Q]

**Other Organs**

- ***Liver is the only source of ketone body production, but it does not utilize ketone bodies***[Q]
- **Liver** utilize *glucose in fed, fatty acid in fasting*, and *aminoacid in starvation*
- **Heart** utilize *fatty acid* as main substrate *in fed & fasting state;* and *ketone bodies* in *starvation.*
- ***Muscles do not utilize ketone bodies***[Q]. They utilize glucose in fed state and fatty acid in fasting and starvation.

## Effects of Starvation On Metabolism

**I[st] Stage**
(first **2 to 3 days** i.e. **48-72 hour**)

- **Glycogenolysis**: *liver glycogen* is first metabolized but d/t its limited storage it cannot last long
- **Gluconeogenesis**: initially from glucogenic amino acids ***(alanine glutamate***[Q]***)*** and then by glycerol & lactate

**Glucagon secretion** increases during starvation. It reaches a ***peak on 3[rd] day of fast at the time of maximal gluconeogenesis***[Q]. There after glucagons level declines as the ketones & fatty acids become the major source of energy. Ganong- 350

**II[nd] Stage** (last for *longest* period, usually *over 2 weaks*)

- 90% of energy requirement will be derived from fat & remainder 10% from protein
- Since the adipose tissue represents largest amount of stored fat 2[nd] stage will last for longest period
- Adipose tissue is broken into FFA which is oxidized for energy production and used for ketone body formation.
- The burning of fat is reflected by a lower RQ (~ 0.73) ↓

**IIIrd – Stage**

- When the fat stores are almost exhausted energy is derived from *breakdown of tissue protein*
- Digestive enzymes. Followed by muscle protein are first to be utilized, as these are least required
- This stage last for *less than one* week & leads to death.

## Metabolic Alterations During Fasting / Starvation

**Absorptive (fed) state** is **2-4 hours period** after ingestion of a normal meal. During this period, *transient increase in plasma glucose, amino acids and triacyl glycerol* (TAG; d/t increased chylomicron synthesis in intestinal mucosa) occur. The elevated insulin to glucagon ratio (in response to increased glucose) make it **anabolic phase** characterized by **increased synthesis of TAG, and glycogen to replenish fuel stores and enhanced synthesis of protein**. During absorptive phase, virtually all tissues use glucose as fuel.

**Fasting begins if no food is ingested after absorptive phase.** Metabolic changes include

| Features | During Brief Fasting | During Prolonged Fasting |
|---|---|---|
| Liver | - **Glycogenolysis (glycogen degradation)** maintains blood glucose level initially (a **transient early response**)<br>- **Gluconeogenesis** begins 4-6 hours after last meal and becomes fully active after depletion of liver glycogen stores. *Glucogenic amino acids & lactate from muscles and glycerol from adipose tissue* is utilized.<br>- **Beta-oxidation of fatty acids is increased** for energy production and **ketone body formation.** FAs obtained from adipose tissue lipolysis becomes the main fuel. However **RBC and brain continue to use glucose mainly**. Blood levels of ketone bodies (esp 3-hydroxy butyrate) increase gradually. | - Liver glycogen is nearly **exhausted after 10-18 hours of fasting**, therefore glycogenolysis can no longer maintain glucose level.<br>- **Rate of gluconeogenesis is decreased in prolonged fasting** to spare functional proteins and therefore less protein is degraded to provide glucogenic aminoacids<br>- **Beta oxidation of FA and production of ketone bodies** continue to be increased. **Ketone bodies** can **be used for fuel by most tissues (except liver) including brain**, once their level in blood is sufficiently high. |
| Adipose Tissue | - **Decreased FA & TAG synthesis** d/t decreased glucose transport by insulin sensitive GLUT-4 into adipocytes<br>- **Increased degradation of TAG** (by hormone sensitive lipase) resulting in **increased release of FFAs and glycerol**.<br>- **Decreased uptake of FA** (in adipocytes from circulating TAG of lipoproteins) d/t low lipoprotein lipase activity. | |

| | | |
|---|---|---|
| **Skeletal Muscle** | - **Rapid breakdown of muscle** protein providing aminoacids for gluconeogenesis<br>- Resting muscle use FFA and ketone bodies for fuel | - Rate of ***muscle proteolysis decreases paralleling a decline in the need for glucose as a fuel for brain which has begun using ketone bodies as a source of energy***[Q].<br>- FA is mainly used as source of fuel. ***The increased use of ketone bodies by the brain as a result of their increased concentration in blood is correlated with decreased use of ketone bodies by muscle***[Q]. |
| **Brain, RBCs** | - **Urea production d/t proteolysis increases**<br>- **Brain and RBC use glucose as fuel** | - **Urea production by liver decreases**<br>- Brain use of glucose decrease but **RBCs still need glucose as fuel** |

## Biochemical Tests for Detection of

### Ketone Bodies

- Ketone bodies (such as **acetone, acetoacetic acid/ diacetic acid,** and **betahydroxy butyric acid**) are produced ***exclusively in liver***[Q] as ***products of fat catabolism***[Q] usually in **diabetes mellitus** (ketoacidosis) & **starvation**.
- Ketone bodies serve as an *alternate source of energy especially in brain* (& other parts of CNS) providing **50-70% of brain energy needs** during starvation. This is an adaptation for survival during starvation.
- Ketone bodies in urine are detected by **Rothera's and Gerhardt's test**.

| Rothera's test | Gerhardt's test |
|---|---|
| Also called **Nitro prusside test** | Also called **ferric chloride test** |
| Detects **acetone** & **acetoacetic acid** | Detects **acetoacetic acid** |
| Urine (5ml) is saturated with *solid ammonium sulphate.* Adding few drops of *sodium nitroprusside f/b liquor ammonia* l/t appearance of **purple/pink permanganate ring** | $FeCl_3$ is added drop by drop to 3ml urine. And appearance of **red wine** color indicates presence of ketone bodies |

### Reducing Sugars

- **Benedict's test** and **Fehling's test** are used to detect reucing sugars like glucose in urine.
- So the patient with **diabetic ketoacidosis** will give ***positive Benedict's test and Rothera's test both***[Q], whereas urine of patient with **starvation** will give a ***negative Benedict's test but a positive Rothera's test***[Q].
- Benedict's reagent contain *copper sulphate, sodium carbonate & sodium citrate.*

**Reducing sugar** → Enediol ⤫ $Cu^{++}$ ← $CuSO_4$

Oxidized ⤫ **Reduced**

Sugar acid   $Cu^{++}$→$CuOH$→$Cu_2O$

Yellow   Red

- Benedict's is a semiquantitative test i.e. color roughly indicating concentration of sugar
  - blue (absence), green (0.5%), yellow (1%), orange (1.5%), and red (≥ 2% i.e. ≥ 2 gm/100ml reducing sugar)
- Any reducing sugar (like *glucose, fructose, lactose, galactose and pentose/xylulose*) will give positive Benedict's test. So Benedict's test is positive in
  - **Glucosuria** (diabetes mellitus)
  - **Fructosuria** (fructose intolerance/aldolase B deficiency, fructokinase deficiency)
  - **Lactosuria**
  - **Galactosuria** (galactose – 1-$PO_4$- uridyl transferase deficiency)
  - **Pentosuria (xylulosuria)**
  - Presence of non carbohydrate reducing substance in urine like *ascorbic acid (vitamin C), homogentisic acid, glucuronides and salicylate.*

★ Presence of **proteins** is detected by ***heat coagulation test, acetic acid test and Haller's nitric acid test***[Q]. Whereas **benzidine test** detects ***presence of blood (hemoglobin > myoglobin)***[Q].

### Bile salts

**Hay's test** detect bile salts *(sodium salts of taurocholic acid & glycocholic acid) in urine.* Positive test indicates obstruction in biliary passage.

### Bilirubin

- **Fouchet's** (barium sulphate) test, **Gmelin's** (nitric acid) test and **Vanden Bergh** (diazo/diazotized sulphanilic acid reagent) **tests** detect bilirubin.
- **Conjugated bilirubin** being water soluble gives **direct** Vanden Bergh test (immediate color); whereas **free bilirubin**, being water insoluble give **indirect** reaction (i.e. color after extraction with alcohol)

### Bile pigments

- **Uro & steco-bilinogens (UBG & SBG)** give positive **Ehrlich's** (para-amino benzaldehyde reagent) test to form red color.
- **Schlesinger's test** is positive for **Uro & Sterco-bilins** (UB & SB) to give brilliant green fluorescence with zinc ions.
- **Rosenbach's test**

| Bile pigments | Detection - Tests | | |
|---|---|---|---|
| | **Fouchet's; Gmelin; Vanden Bergh** | **Ehrlich's** | **Schlesingers** |
| **Bilirubin** | + | - | - |
| **Bilinogens (UBG, SBG)** | - | + | - |
| **Bilins (UB + SB)** | - | - | + |

# Chapter -3 STRUCTURE, FUNCTION AND REPLICATION OF INFORMATIONAL MACROMOLECULES

## QUESTIONS

### Purines and Pyrimidines

1. **Pyrimidine metabolism features a/e**
   A. Require CAD polypeptide chain ☐
   B. 6-azauridine l/t oritidinuria ☐
   C. DHOA-dehydrogenase is mitochondrial ☐
   D. Reye syndrome decrease cytosolic carbamoyl phosphate ☐
   E. Urea cycle is linked ☐
2. **What is involved in formation of d-TMP from d-UMP?**
   A. N5, N10-methylene tetra hydrofolate ☐
   B. Form imino folate ☐
   C. N5 formyl folate ☐
   D. Dihydro folate ☐
3. **End product of purine metabolism in non-primate mammals is:**
   A. Uric acid ☐
   B. Ammonia ☐
   C. Urea ☐
   D. Allantoin ☐
4. **Inositic acid is biological precursor of -**
   A. Uracil and thymine ☐
   B. Purines and thymine ☐
   C. Adenylic acid and guanylic acid ☐
   D. Orotic acid and uridylic acid ☐
5. **False regarding gout is** :
   A. Due to increased metabolism of pyrimidines ☐
   B. Due to increased metabolism of purines ☐
   C. Uric acid levels may not be elevated ☐
   D. Has a predilection for the great toe ☐
6. **Gout is a disorder of** :
   A. Purine metabolism ☐
   B. Pyrimidine metabolism ☐
   C. Oxalate metabolism ☐
   D. Protein metabolism ☐
7. **What is not true about gout**:
   A. Abrupt increase in serum urate levels is more common a cause for acute gout than an abrupt fall in urate levels. ☐
   B. Patient may be asymptomatic with high serum uric acid for years ☐
   C. Development of arthritis correlates with level of serum uric acid ☐
   D. Uric acid crystals are best seen by polarising light microscope ☐
8. **Specific test for gout is**:
   A. Raised serum uric acid level ☐
   B. Raised uric acid in synovial fluid of joint ☐
   C. Raised urea level ☐
   D. Raised urease enzyme level ☐
9. **A ten year old child with aggressive behavior and poor concentration is brought with presenting complaints of joint pain and reduced urinary output. Mother gives history of self mutilitative behavior stating that he tends to mutilate his fingers. Which of the following enzymes is likely to be deficient in this child**
   A. HGPRTase ☐
   B. Adenosine Deaminase ☐
   C. APRTase ☐
   D. Acid Maltase ☐
10. **The enzyme deficient is Lesch-Nyhan syndrome is**:
    A. GTRT ☐
    B. Glutaminase ☐
    C. Transcarboxylase ☐
    D. HGPRT ☐
11. **Lesch Nyhan syndrome is due to deficiency of**:
    A. Hypoxanthine phosphoribosyl transferase ☐
    B. Xanthine oxidase ☐
    C. Purine phosphorylase ☐
    D. Adenosine deaminase ☐
12. **A 12 year old child presents with mental retardation and history of self mutilation. Which of the following tests will help in determining the diagnosis**
    A. Serum Lead Levels ☐
    B. Serum Alkaline Phosphatase Levels ☐
    C. Serum Lactate Dehydrogenase Levels ☐
    D. Serum Uric Acid Levels ☐
13. **Which is common metabolic process in human as well as bacteria**:
    A. Purine synthesis ☐
    B. Nitrogen fixation ☐
    C. Mucolipid formation ☐
    D. Nonoxidative photophosphorylation ☐
14. **Apart from occurring in nucleic acids, pyrimidines are also found in**:
    A. Theophylline ☐
    B. Theobromine ☐
    C. Flavin mononucleotide ☐
    D. Thiamine ☐

### DNA Structure

15. **True statements about DNA structure:**
    A. All nucleotides are involved in linkage ☐
    B. Antiparallel ☐
    C. Parallel ☐
    D. Bases are perpendicular to DNA ☐
    E. Attached by hydroxy bond. ☐
16. **mRNA is a complimentary copy of -**
    A. TRNA ☐
    B. RRNA ☐
    C. Ribosomal DNA ☐
    D. Both strands of DNA ☐
    E. A single strand of DNA ☐
17. **Which is not found in DNA**:
    A. Adenine ☐
    B. Thymine ☐
    C. Guanine ☐
    D. Uracil ☐
18. **The two strands of DNA are held together by**:
    A. Van-der -Waal bond ☐
    B. Hydrogen bond ☐
    C. Covalent bond ☐
    D. Ionic interaction ☐

**19. True about DNA structure:**
- A. Purines are adenne and guanine & pyrimidines are uracil and cytosine ☐
- B. Watson and Crick discovered structure in 1973 ☐
- C. Deoxyribose-phosphate backbone with bases stacked inside ☐
- D. Mainly consists of left handed helix ☐
- E. 5′-3′ phosodiester bonding is present ☐

**20. Which form of DNA is predominantly seen:**
- A. A ☐
- B. C ☐
- C. B ☐
- D. Z ☐

**21. Triplex DNA is due to**
- A. Hoogsteen pairing ☐
- B. Palindromic sequences ☐
- C. Large no. of guanosine repeats ☐
- D. Polypyramidine tracts ☐

**22. Chargaff rule state that -**
- A. A+G = T+C ☐
- B. A/T = G/C ☐
- C. A = U= T= G= C ☐
- D. A + T = G + C ☐

**23. A nucleic acid was analyzed and found to contain 32% adenine, 18% guanine, 17% cytosine and 33% thymine. The nucleic acid must be:**
- A. Single-stranded RNA ☐
- B. Single-stranded DNA ☐
- C. Double-stranded RNA ☐
- D. Double stranded DNA ☐

**24. In a sample of DNA, if adenine is 23% what will be the amount of guanine present:**
- A. 23% ☐
- B. 25% ☐
- C. 46% ☐
- D. 27% ☐
- E. 54% ☐

**25. Triple bonds are found between which base pairs:**
- A. A-T ☐
- B. C-G ☐
- C. A-G ☐
- D. C-T ☐

**26. Thermo-stability in DNA is contributed mostly by:**
- A. A=T ☐
- B. G≡C ☐
- C. Molecular base ☐
- D. Parallel arrangement ☐

**27. In Hybrid RNA-DNA, DNA is 5CTTAAG3. The sequence of RNA will be:**
- A. 5CTTAAG3 ☐
- B. 5CUUAAG3 ☐
- C. 5GAATTC3 ☐
- D. 5GAAUUC3 ☐
- E. 5CTTUUG3 ☐

**28. Which one of the following is the complementary sequence of 5′ TTAAGCTAC 3′?**
- A. 5′ GTACGCTTAA 3′ ☐
- B. 5′ AATTCGCATG 3′ ☐
- C. 5′ CATGCGAATT 3′ ☐
- D. 5′ TTAAGCGTAC 3′ ☐

**29. True about coding strand of DNA:**
- A. Template strand ☐
- B. Minus strand ☐
- C. Runs at 5- - 3' direction ☐
- D. Runs at 3' – 5' direction ☐
- E. Plus strand ☐

**30. True a bout coding strand of DNA:**
- A. DNA acts as template for mRNA ☐
- B. Minus strand ☐
- C. Plus strand ☐
- D. Matches with RNA transcript hat encodes protein ☐

**31. 5′ TTACGTAC-3′ after transcription what will be the RNA:** *(PGI June 08)*
- A. 5-TTACGTAC-3′ ☐
- B. 3′- TTACGTAC-5′ ☐
- C. 5′ CATGCATT-3 ☐
- D. 3′- CATGCATT-5 ☐
- E. 5′- GUACGUAA-3′ ☐

**32. Bromodeoxyuridine is related to DNA in:**
- A. Uracil ☐
- B. Adenosine ☐
- C. Cytosine ☐
- D. Thymidine ☐

**33. At the physiological pH the DNA molecules are :**
- A. Positively charged. ☐
- B. Negatively charged. ☐
- C. Neutral. ☐
- D. Amphipathic ☐

**34. True about mitochondrial DNA:**
- A. Maternal inheritance ☐
- B. Same evolutionary origin ☐
- C. Not highly conserved & has high mutation rate ☐
- D. Mitochondrial disease is associated mostly with Mutation & some have deletion ☐
- E. Mostly encodes membrane protein ☐

**35. True about mitochondrial DNA**
- A. UGA codes for tryptophan ☐
- B. Codes for 13 protein ☐
- C. High content of untranslated sequences ☐
- D. Circular double stranded DNA ☐
- E. Mitrochondrial disease occur due to Point Mutations and Large-Scale Rearrangements ☐

**36. Intron is not found in which DNA?**
- A. Nuclear DNA ☐
- B. Mitochondrial DNA ☐
- C. B DNA ☐
- D. ZDNA ☐

**37. NARP syndrome is seen in**
- A. Lysosomal disorder ☐
- B. Glycogen storage disease ☐
- C. Mitochondrial disease ☐
- D. Lipid storage disease ☐

**38. Mitochondrial DNA is:**
- A. Paternally inherited ☐
- B. Maternally inherited ☐
- C. Horizontal inheritance ☐
- D. Vertical inheritance ☐

**39. Mitochondria gene (True statement):**
- A. Paternal transmission ☐
- B. Maternal transmission ☐
- C. Mendelian inheritance ☐
- D. Mitochondrial myopathy ☐

**40. Mitochondrial DNA is:**
- A. Closed circular ☐
- B. Nicked circular ☐
- C. Linear ☐
- D. Open circular ☐

**41. Circular DNA is found in:**
A. Virus ☐
B. Chloroplast ☐
C. Bacteria ☐
D. Mitochondria ☐
E. Fungus ☐

**42. Total number of genes in a human being is-**
A. 800,000 ☐
B. 50,000 ☐
C. 100,000 ☐
D. 30,000 ☐

**43. Cellular bearings of herediatary disease seen in:**
A. DNA ☐
B. Ribosome ☐
C. RNA ☐
D. Membrane ☐
E. Proteins ☐

**44. Highly repetitive DNA is seen in:**
A. Cloning of DNA ☐
B. Microsatelite DNA ☐
C. Telomere ☐
D. Centromere ☐

**45. True about telomerase or telomere is/are:**
A. They are present at the ends of eukaryotic chromosome ☐
B. Increased telomerase activity favours cancer cells ☐
C. DNA dependent RNA polymerase ☐
D. DNA polymerase ☐

**46. Action of 'Telomerase' is**
A. DNA repair ☐
B. Longetivity of cell – Ageing ☐
C. Breakdown of telomer ☐
D. None ☐

**47. Ends of chromosomes replicated by:**
A. Telomerase ☐
B. Centromere ☐
C. Restriction endonuclease ☐
D. Exonuclease ☐

**48. Which enzymatic mutation is responsible for immortality of cancer cells :**
A. DNA reverse transciptase ☐
B. RNA polymerase ☐
C. Telomerase ☐
D. DNA polymerase ☐

**49. All of the following cell types contain the enzyme telemerase which protects the length of telomeres at the end of chromosomes, *except*:**
A. Germinal ☐
B. Somatic ☐
C. Hemopoietic ☐
D. Tumor ☐
A.

**50. True about Histone protein:**
A. Ribonucleoprotein ☐
B. Present inside the nucleus ☐
C. Acidic ☐
D. Basic ☐
E. Glycoprotein ☐

**51. Histone acetylation causes?**
A. Increased Heterochromatin formation ☐
B. Increased Euchromatin formation ☐
C. Methylation of cystine ☐
D. DNA replication ☐

**52. Components of chromosome are:**
A. DNA ☐
B. tRNA ☐
C. m RNA ☐
D. r RNA ☐
E. Histones ☐

**53. The protein rich in basic amino acids, which functions in the packaging of DNA in chromosomes, is:**
A. Histone ☐
B. Collagen ☐
C. Hyaluronic acid binding protein ☐
D. Fibrinogen ☐

**54. Histone has post - translational modification by all/except.**
A. Acylation ☐
B. Methylation ☐
C. Phosphorylation ☐
D. Glycosylation ☐

**55. Euchromatin is the region of DNA that is relatively:**
A. Uncondensed ☐
B. Condensed ☐
C. Overcondensed ☐
D. Partially condensed ☐

**56. Nucleosome consists of:**
A. Histone ☐
B. DNA ☐
C. RNA ☐
D. DNA & RNA both ☐
E. Carbohydrate ☐

**57. True about nucleosome:**
A. Use only one type of histone protein ☐
B. Each complex is separated from each other by non histone proteins ☐
C. Regular repeating structure of DNA & histone proteins ☐
D. Reflect small nucleus ☐
E. Core of DNA with protein wrapped ☐

## DNA synthesis and replication

**58. True about prokaryotic DNA replication:**
B. Conservative ☐
C. Semi conservative ☐
D. Unidirectional ☐
E. Bidirectional ☐
F. Semi discontinuous ☐

**59. True about DNA supercoiling is all except**
A. Underwinding results in negative superhelical density & supercoiling ☐
B. Superhelical density depends on length of DNA ☐
C. Underwinding strain is normally accommodated by strand separation ☐
D. Topoisomerase II change linking number in increments of 2 ☐
E. Most cellular DNA is underwound ☐

**60. Okazaki segments are required for :**
A. DNA synthesis ☐
B. RNA synthesis ☐
C. Protein synthesis ☐
D. None of the above ☐

**61. Okazaki fragment helps in:**
A. DNA replication ☐
B. Translation ☐
C. Protein synthesis ☐
D. Transcription ☐

**62. Okazaki fragments are formed during the synthesis of**
A. ds DNA ☐
B. ss DNA ☐
C. m RNA ☐
D. t RNA ☐

**63. During replication of DNA, which one of the following enzymes polymerizes the Okazaki fragments?**
A. DNA Polymerase I ☐
B. DNA Polymerase II ☐
C. DNA Polymerase III ☐
D. RNA Polymerase I ☐

**64. True-regarding DNA-replication:**
A. Occurs in the M-phase of the cell cycle. ☐
B. Sister Chromatids are formed. ☐
C. Follow base pair rule. ☐
D. Semi conservative. ☐
E. Single strand breaknd. ☐

**65. Correct sequence of enzymes required for DNA formation is:**
A. DNA polymerase → Protein unwinding enzyme → DNA ligase → DNA Isomerase → Polymerase -1 ☐
B. Protein unwinding enzyme → Polymerase 1 → DNA ligase→ DNA Isomerase→ DNA polymerase ☐
C. RNA polymerase → DNA polymerase III → DNA polymerase I → DNA ligase ☐
D. RNA polymerase → DNA polymerase III → dNA ligase → Exonuclease → DNA polymerase I ☐

**66. False statements are:**
A. In leading strands DNA is synthesized continuously ☐
B. Multiple origins of replication are possible for bacteria ☐
C. DNA replication proceeds in one direction ☐
D. Lagging strand stick by RNA primase ☐
E. DNA polymerase III- processive leading strand synthesis ☐

**67. The gaps between segments of DNA on the lagging strand produced by restriction enzymes are rejoined sealed by:**
A. DNA Ligases ☐
B. DNA Helicase ☐
C. DNA topoisomerase ☐
D. DNA phosphorylase ☐

**68. DNA synthesis requires:**
A. DNA polymerase ☐
B. DNA ligase ☐
C. DNA topoisomerase ☐
D. Primase ☐
E. RNA polymerase ☐

**69. DNA supercoiling is done by:**
A. DNA polymerase I ☐
B. DNA polymerase II ☐
C. DNA topoisomerase ☐
D. DNA gyrase. ☐

**70. Which statements are true about E. coli chromosomal DNA in relation with eukaryotic chromosomal DNA:**
A. Circular ☐
B. Packed into nucleolus ☐
C. Positively Supercoiled ☐
D. Negatively sepercoiled ☐
E. Nucleoid present ☐

**71. Which DNA polymerase is/are involved in repair of mammalian DNA:**
A. α ☐
B. β ☐
C. γ ☐
D. ε ☐
E. δ

**72. True about DNA polymerase in eukaryotes:**
A. Components are α, β, γ, Δ, ε ☐
B. β associated with repair ☐
C. γ associated with repair ☐
D. Δ associated with synthesis of mitochondria DNA ☐
E. Alpha is abundant amount ☐

**73. DNA polymerase have:**
A. 3' → 5' polymerase activity ☐
B. 5' → 3' polymerase activity ☐
C. 3' → 5' exonuclease activity ☐
D. 5' → 3' exonuclease activity ☐

## DNA Damage, Repair and Protooncogene

**74. Nucleoside is made up of:**
A. Pyrimidine ☐
B. Histone ☐
C. Sugar ☐
D. Purine ☐
E. Phosphate ☐

**75. All of the following abbreviations are true except:**
A. AMP-Adenosine monophosphate ☐
B. CMP - Cytidine monophosphate ☐
C. GMP - Guanosine monophosphate ☐
D. TMP - Thymine monophosphate ☐
E. UMP - Uracil monophosphate ☐

**76. On complete hydrolysis of DNA, we will get all of the following except:**
A. Adenosine ☐
B. Purine base ☐
C. Phosphoric acid ☐
D. Dexose pentose sugar ☐

**77. What will happen to DNA if salt is added to it:**
A. Increase Melting point (Tm) ☐
B. Decrease Tm ☐
C. Not affect Tm ☐
D. Melting lead to denaturation of DNA ☐
E. Both increase & decrease in Tm depending on concentration of salt ☐

**78. What is meant by melting of double stranded DNA:**
A. Splitting of double strands into single strand. ☐
B. Splitting of DNA into fragments. ☐
C. Formation of triple helix ☐
D. Separation of bases. ☐

**79. Concentration of DNA is measured by:**
A. Absorption at 260 nm ☐
B. D-oxyribose estimation ☐
C. Infrared examination ☐
D. Ultrasound examination ☐

**80. Incorrect statement are:**
A. T4 DNA polymerase has 3'>5' exonuclese activity ☐
B. Klenow fragment of DNA polymerase I function is almost similar to T4 DNA polymerase ☐
C. Restriction endonuclease cut DNA chains at specific location ☐
D. Endonuclease cut DNA at 5' terminus ☐
E. Right handed helix of DNA is more common ☐

**81. Photolyase helps in -**
A. DNA repair ☐
B. DNA replication ☐
C. Protein synthesis ☐
D. None ☐

**82. Excessive ultraviolet (uv) radiation is harmful to life. The damage caused to the biological systems by ultraviolet radiation is by:**
A. Inhibition of DNA synthesis ☐
B. Formation of thymidine dimmers ☐
C. Ionization ☐
D. DNA fragmentation ☐

**83. The primary defect in Xeroderma pigmentosa is :**
A. Formation of thymidine dimmers ☐
B. Poly ADP ribose polymerase is defective ☐
C. Exonuclease is defective ☐
D. Formation of adenine dimers ☐

**84. Xeroderma pigmentation is caused due to a group of closely related abnormalities in:**
A. Mismatch repair ☐
B. Base excision repair ☐
C. Nucleotide excision repair ☐
D. SOS repair ☐

**85. Xeroderma pigmentosum is produced as a result of a defect in:**
A. DNA polymerase III ☐
B. DNA polymerase I ☐
C. DNA exonuclease ☐
D. DNA ligase ☐

**86. A child develops blisters on exposure to sunlight. Irregular dark spots on the skin are also found. He is very likely to have a defect in which of the following mechanisms?**
A. Nucleotide excision repair ☐
B. Mismatch repair ☐
C. Recombination repair ☐
D. Thymine dimmers ☐

**87. 5-methyl cytosine mutation of DNA (DNA methylation) leads to:**
A. Deamination to uracil ☐
B. Deamination to thymine ☐
C. Mispair with adenine ☐
D. DNA repair ☐
E. Methylation protects the host DNA from cleavage by its own restriction enzyme ☐

**88. DNA repair defect is seen in:**
A. Xeroderma pigmentatosa ☐
B. Bloom's syndrome ☐
C. Ataxia telangiectasia ☐
D. Li-Fraumani syndrome ☐
E. Retinoblastoma ☐

**89. The normal cellular counterparts of oncogenes are important for the following functions, *except*:**
A. Promotion of cell cycle progression ☐
B. Inhibition of apoptosis ☐
C. Promotion of DNA repair ☐
D. Promotion of nuclear transcription ☐

**90. True about Proto-oncogenes are:**
A. Normally involved in cell cycle proliferation ☐
B. Produces tumor ☐
C. Normally involved in suppression of tumour production ☐
D. Proto- oncogens on mutation causes cancer. ☐

**91. Anti –carcinogens are:**
A. Carotenoids ☐
B. Flavenoids ☐
C. Curcumoids ☐
D. Benzene ☐
E. Lignase ☐

**92. Following required for Normal growth:**
A. Protooncogenes ☐
B. Tumour suppressor genes ☐
C. Oncogenes ☐
D. DNA repair genes ☐

**93. Which is not a tumor suppressor gene?**
A. WT-1 ☐
B. Rb ☐
C. p53 ☐
D. RAS ☐

**94. Maximum damage to DNA is caused by:**
A. $\alpha$-rays ☐
B. $\beta$-rays ☐
C. $\gamma$-rays ☐
D. $\delta$-rays and UV rays ☐

## Genetic Code

**95. Amino acids not coded by triplet codon:**
A. Lysine ☐
B. Hydroxyproline ☐
C. Selenocysteine ☐
D. Pyrrolysine ☐
E. Ornithine ☐

**96. True about genetic code except:**
A. Degenerate ☐
B. Overlapping ☐
C. Ambigous ☐
D. Universal ☐
E. Commaless ☐

**97. Stop codons are:**
A. UAA ☐
B. UAG ☐
C. UGA ☐
D. UAC ☐
E. UCA ☐

**98. True about genetic code:**
A. AUA codes for methionine in mitochondria ☐
B. UGA codes for selenocysteine ☐
C. AUG codes for initiator codon in mammalian cell ☐
D. AGA & AGG act as chain terminator in mammalian mitochondria ☐
E. UAA, UAG & UGA are stop codon ☐

**99. If there are 4 nucleotides instead of 3 in codon, how many amino acids may be formed?**
A. 16 ☐
B. 21 ☐
C. 256 ☐
D. 64 ☐
E. 265 ☐

**100.Stop codon:**
A. UAG ☐
B. UCA ☐
C. UAC ☐
D. AUG ☐

**101.A codon consists of -**
A. One molecule of amono acyl-t RNA ☐
B. Two complementary base pairs ☐
C. 3 consecutive nucleotide units ☐
D. 4 individual nucleotides ☐

**102.All are true of the genetic code except -**
A. Degenerate ☐
B. Universal ☐
C. Punctuation ☐
D. Non overlapping ☐

**103.Chain initiation in protein synthesis is by-**
A. AUG ☐
B. GLA ☐
C. UGA ☐
D. UAG ☐

**104.Nonsense codons bring about-**
A. Elongation of polypeptide chain ☐
B. Pre-translational modificastion of protein ☐
C. Initiation of protein synthesis ☐
D. Termination of protein synthesis ☐

**105. A codon consists of -**
A. 2 complementary base pairs ☐
B. 3 complementary base pairs ☐
C. 4 complementary base pairs on RNA ☐
D. 4 individual nucleotides ☐

**106. A condon consists of -**
A. Two complementary base pairs ☐
B. Three consecutive nucleotide units ☐
C. An individual ribosome ☐
D. Four individual nucleotides ☐

**107. Which one is nonsense codon -**
A. UUA ☐
B. UAG ☐
C. UGA ☐
D. UAU ☐

**108. Same aminoacid is coded by multiple codons d/t following :**
A. Degeneracy ☐
B. Frame-shift mutation ☐
C. Transcription ☐
D. Mutation ☐

**109. Wobble hypothesis –regarding the variation true is:**
A. 3 - end of anticodon ☐
B. 5 – end of anticodon ☐
C. m-RNA ☐
D. t-RNA ☐

## Regulation of Gene Expression

**110. Steroids act via nuclear receptors which interact with DNA through**
A. Helix turn helix ☐
B. Zinc finger motif ☐
C. Histidine ☐
D. Leucine zipper ☐

**111. Zinc finger is :**
A. Nuclear receptor ☐
B. Membrane receptor ☐
C. Receptor associated kinase ☐

**112. Steroid receptor regulatory protein:**
A. Zinc finger ☐
B. Heliz-turn –helix ☐
C. Leucine zippor ☐
D. RNA ☐

**113. Proteins which is having DNA binding domain in its structure:**
A. Zinc finger ☐
B. β- sheet ☐
C. β-band ☐
D. helix-turn helix ☐
E. leucine zipper ☐

**114. In leucine zipper model, Leucine residue seen after every**
A. 3 amino acids ☐
B. 6 amino acids ☐
C. 9 amno acids ☐
D. 12 amino acids ☐
E. 7 amino acid ☐

**115. Binding of proteins to DNA is regulated by:**
A. Copper ☐
B. Zinc ☐
C. Selenium ☐
D. Nickle ☐

**116. Leucine-Zipper complex is**
A. DNA binding protein ☐
B. Membrane attack complex ☐
C. B cell epitomes ☐
D. Receptor ligand protein ☐

**117. Which is the smallest fundamental unit coding for DNA synthesis:**
A. Cistron ☐
B. Operon ☐
C. Replican ☐
D. Anticodon ☐

**118. True about genes**
A. Smallest functional unit of genome ☐
B. Not capable of independent expression ☐
C. Promoter & enhancer geens are typical example ☐
D. Cistron is single functional unit ☐

**119. CAP in Lac operon is an example of:**
A. Positive regulator ☐
B. Negative regulator ☐
C. Constitutive expression ☐
D. Attenuation ☐

**120. Which of the following are situated away from the coding region:**
A. Promoter ☐
B. Enhancer ☐
C. Operator ☐
D. Structural gene ☐

**121. House keeping genes are**
A. Inducible ☐
B. Required only when inducer is present ☐
C. Mutant ☐
D. Not regulated ☐

**122. True among all is**
A. Repressor is dimer and a positive regulator ☐
B. CRP is gratuitous inducer ☐
C. Lactose is positive regulator ☐
D. De-repression is d/t presence of glucose ☐
E. Catabolite repression is mediated by CRP ☐

**123. False statement is**
A. Repressor binds operator gene ☐
B. Regulator genes produce repressor subunits ☐
C. IP TG is inducer but not substrate ☐
D. Regulator gene is inducible ☐

**124. Lac operon transcription is induced by**
A. Glucose ☐
B. Glucose with inducer ☐
C. Inducer without glucose ☐
D. All ☐

**125. All of the following statements about Lambda phage are true, Except:**
A. In Lysogenic phase it fuses with host chromosome and remains dormant ☐
B. In Lytic phase it fuses with host chromosome and replicates ☐
C. Both Lytic and lysogenic phases occur together ☐
D. In Lytic phase it causes cell lysis and releases virus particles ☐

**126. In conversion of DNA to RNA, enzyme required:**
A. DNA- Polymerase I ☐
B. DNA Ligase ☐
C. DNA-Polymerase III ☐
D. RNA polymerase ☐
E. Primase ☐

## Transcription

**127. The sigma (σ) subunit of prokaryotic RNA polymerase:**
- A. Binds the antibiotic rifampicin
- B. Is inhibited by α-amanitin
- C. Specifically recognizes the promoter site
- D. Is part of the core enzyme

**128. The atachment site of DNA dependent RNA polymerase to a gene is the -**
- A. Operator
- B. Promoter
- C. Structural gene
- D. Regulatory gene
- E. Repressor

**129. RNA polymerase does not require :**
- A. Template (ds DNA)
- B. Activated precursors (ATP, GTP, UTP, CTP)
- C. Divalent metal ions (Mn2+, Mg2+)
- D. Primer

**130. R-RNA is mainly produced in -**
- A. Nucleus
- B. Nucleolus
- C. Ribosome
- D. Endoplasmic reticulum

**131. Part of eukaryotic DNA contributing to polypetide synthesis:**
- A. Exon
- B. Enhancer
- C. Leader sequence
- D. tRNA
- E. ncRNA

**132. Not true about eukaryotic gene:**
- A. Polycistronic mRNA
- B. Noncoding intron
- C. Contain nuclear gene & pseudogene
- D. Modification of mRNA before transportation from nucleus
- E. Noncoding exons

**133. The following is a generalized diagram of a typical eukaryotic gene:**

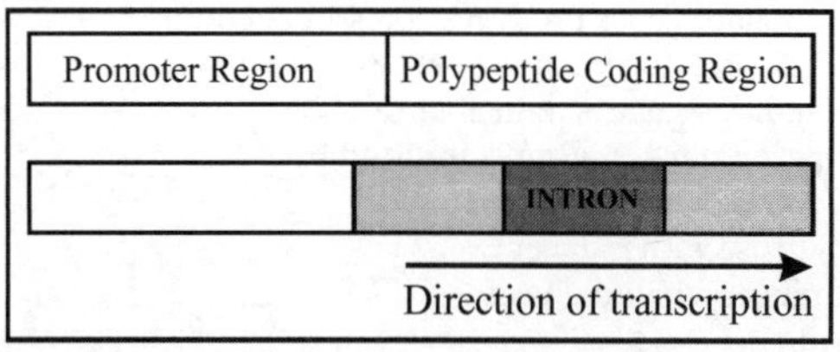


What is the most likely effect of a 2bp insertion in the middle of the intron?
- A. Normal transcription, altered translation
- B. Defective termination of transcription, normal translation
- C. Normal transcription, defective mRNA splicing
- D. Normal transcription, normal translation.

**134. Part of M-RNA removed during protein synthesis -**
- A. Interon
- B. Codon
- C. Exon
- D. Suistron

**135. Function of endonucleases -**
- A. Cut DNA at specific DNA sequences
- B. To point out the coding regions
- C. Enhancers
- D. To find out antibiotic resistance

**136. Replication and transcription are similar processes in mechanistic terms because both :**
- A. Use RNA primers for initiation.
- B. Use deoxyribonucleotides as precursors.
- C. Are semi conserved events
- D. Involve phosphodiester bond formation with elongation occurring in the 5' - 3' direction.

**137. In a DNA the coding region reads 5'-CGT-3'. This would code in the RNA as:**
- A. 5'-CGU-3'
- B. 5'GCA-3'
- C. 5'-ACG-3'
- D. 5'-UGC-3'

**138. True about eukaryotic initiation is a/e**
- A. Initiator sequence spans TSS (+1)
- B. Distal regulatory element (DRE) is exclusively found in eukaryotes
- C. Different σ subunits are responsible for recognition specificity
- D. Trans acting factors bind to CAAT/GC box – promoter proximal element.

**139. A young boy who has difficulty in getting up from sitting position was diagnosed to have Duchene's muscular dystrophy. Which one is true regarding the mutation in the dystrophin gene in promoter region:**
- A. Initiation of transcription of the dystrophin gene would be affected
- B. Capping of mRNA of dystrophin gene would be affected
- C. Tailing of mRNA of dystrophin gene would be affected
- D. Premature termination

**140. Non coding RNAs are:**
- A. siRNA
- B. miRNA
- C. tRNA
- D. mRNA
- E. rRNA

**141. Not product of transcription:**
- A. tRNA
- B. mRNA
- C. rRNA
- D. cDNA
- E. New strand of DNA

**142. Gene transmitted but not translated:**
- A. Glycosyl transferase
- B. t-RNA
- C. Keratin
- D. Histone

**143. Which of the following statements regarding mature cytoplsmic messenger RNA is true**
- A. Transcribed from Nuclear DNA
- B. Has Thiamine in place of Uracil
- C. Sugar is DeoxyRibose
- D. Its molecular weight is more than hn-RNA

**144. Nobel prize in 2006 (recently) was given for the discovery of**
- A. Lipoxins
- B. RNAI
- C. mt DNA
- D. β-transcription factor

**145. Micro RNA transcribed by:**
- A. RNA polymerase I
- B. RNA polymerase II
- C. RNA polymerase III
- D. DNA polymerase
- E. Drosha

**146. Normal role of Micro RNA is:**
A. Gene Regulation ☐
B. RNA splicing ☐
C. Initiation of Translation ☐
D. DNA conformational change ☐

**147. Poly(A) tail translates into (i.e. on translation give rise to):**
A. Polyproline ☐
B. Polylysine ☐
C. Polyalanine ☐
D. Polyglycine ☐

**148. Some mRNA has self splicing activity. The removal of introns is/are done by:**
A. Occur in intron that form Ribozyme ☐
B. Spliceosome ☐
C. Self-splicing introns ☐
D. sn RNA ☐
E. Lariats intermediates are formed

**149. Introns are exised by**
A. RNA splicing ☐
B. RNA editing ☐
C. Restriction endonuclease ☐
D. DNAase ☐
E. Helicase ☐

**150. A segment of a eukaryotic gene that is not represented in the mature messenger RNA is known as:**
A. Intron ☐
B. Exon ☐
C. Plasmid ☐
D. TATA box ☐

**151. Splicing Activity is a function of:**
A. mRNA ☐
B. sn RNA ☐
C. r RNA ☐
D. t RNA ☐

**152. Which is involve in processing of post-transcriptional modification of mRNA:**
A. Lariats formation ☐
B. Splicing ☐
C. Capping at 3′ end ☐
D. Poly tail(A) formation at 5′ end ☐
E. Methylation ☐

**153. Some mRNA has self splicing activity. The removal of introns is/are done by:**
A. Occur in intron that form Ribozyme ☐
B. Spliceosome ☐
C. Self-splicing introns ☐
D. sn RNA ☐
E. Lariats intermediates are formed ☐

**154. Cytoplasmic process during processing is**
A. 5′ capping ☐
B. Poly (A) tailing ☐
C. Methylation of tRNA ☐
D. Attachment of CCA in tRNA. ☐

**155. All are processing reactions in t-RNA except**
A. CCA tailing ☐
B. Methylation of bases ☐
C. Poly (A) tailing ☐
D. Trimming of 5′ end ☐

**156. Least post translational modification occurs in**
A. t-RNA ☐
B. Prokaryotic r- RNA ☐
C. Eukaryotic r – RNA ☐
D. Prokaryotic mRNA ☐

**157. Which of the following is not a post transcriptional modification of RNA?**
A. Splicing ☐
B. 5′capping ☐
C. 3′ polyadenylation ☐
D. Glycosylation ☐

**158. In RNA, gene during processing undergoes all, except**
A. Chemical hydrolysis ☐
B. Terminal addition ☐
C. Nucleoside *modification* ☐
D. Nucleoside cleavage ☐

**159. APO B48 & APO B100 is synthesized from the same mRNA; the difference between them is due to:**
A. RNA splicing ☐
B. Allelic exclusion ☐
C. Deamination of cytidine to uridine ☐
D. Upstream repression ☐

**160. Post transcriptional modification includes:**
A. All RNA undergo post transcriptional modification ☐
B. Capping of the pre-m RNA Involves the addition of 7-methylguanosine to the 5′end ☐
C. Poly A tailing occur at 3′end ☐
D. Intron excision by spliceosome ☐
E. Primarily occur in cytoplasm ☐

**161. True about ribozymes is:**
A. Cut DNA at specific site ☐
B. GTPase activity ☐
C. Peptidyl transferase activity ☐
D. Participate in DNA synthesis ☐

**162. True about ribozymes are A/E**
A. Catalytic activity ☐
B. Involved in transesterification ☐
C. Hammerhead metallo enzyme ☐
D. Peptidyl transferase ☐
E. Deamination ☐

**163. Acitomycin D interferes with enzyme induction by combining with -**
A. TRNA ☐
B. DNA ☐
C. R-RNA ☐
D. Repressor protein ☐
E. Negative feedback inhibition system ☐

**164. Which of the following blocks DNA replication with getting incorporated in DNA strand:**
A. Cytarabine ☐
B. Nalidixic acid ☐
C. Ciprofloxacin ☐
D. Paclitaxel ☐

**165. Transcripton is inhibited by:**
A. Actinomycin D ☐
B. Amanitin ☐
C. Chloramphenicol ☐
D. Streptomycin ☐
E. Puromycin ☐

**166. Inhibitors of DNA synthesis -**
A. Penicillin ☐
B. Polymyxin ☐
C. Chloramphenicol ☐
D. Actinomycin ☐

**167. hn RNA seen in :**
A. Spinal muscular dystrophy ☐
B. Sickle cell disease ☐
C. Hutchinson chorea ☐
D. αThallasemia ☐

**168. An enzyme that makes a double stranded DNA copy from a single stranded RNA template molecule is known as:**
A. DNA polymerase ☐

B. RNA polymerase ☐
C. Reverse transcriptase ☐
D. Phosphokinase ☐

**169. True about reverse transcriptase:**
A. Forms DNA from RNA ☐
B. Forms RNA from DNA ☐
C. Important for replication of HIV ☐
D. Amplification of DNA ☐
E. DNA dependent RNA polymerase ☐

**170. Which of the following require template for it's formation:**
A. Carbohydrate ☐
B. Protein ☐
C. Lipid ☐
D. Nucleic acid ☐
E. Phospholipid ☐

**171. The anticodon region is an *important* part of the**
A. r-RNA ☐
B. m-RNa ☐
C. t-RNa ☐
D. hn-RNa ☐

**172. In transcription anticodon is seen in -**
A. t-RNA ☐
B. m-RNA ☐
C. r-RNA ☐
D. DNA ☐

**173. Which of the following RNA has abnormal purine bases:**
A. t-RNA ☐
B. m-RNA ☐
C. r-RNA ☐
D. 16S RNA ☐

**174. About t-RNA, TRUE is:**
A. No intrabasal pairing ☐
B. Clover leaf pattern ☐
C. Inverted T appearance ☐
D. Each specific for one m-RNA ☐

**175. Which type of RNA has the highest percentage of modified base?**
A. mRNA ☐
B. tRNA ☐
C. rRNA ☐
D. snRNA ☐

**176. Thymidylated RNA present in:**
A. mRNA ☐
B. rRNA ☐
C. tRNA ☐
D. 16-s-RNA ☐

## Translation (Protein Synthesis)

**177. The cellular component for protein synthesis is :**
A. Smooth endoplasmic reticulum ☐
B. Rough endoplasmic reticulum ☐
C. Ribosomes ☐
D. Mitochondria ☐

**178. Translation occurs in :**
A. Ribosomes ☐
B. Mitochondria ☐
C. Nucleus ☐
D. Cytoplasm ☐

**179. True regarding aminoacyl t-RNA synthetase is A/E**
A. Isoaccepting t RNA ☐
B. Implement genetic code ☐
C. Attachment of amino group to 5′ end ☐
D. Editing function ☐

**180. Fidelity of protein translation depends on:**
A. RNA polymerase ☐
B. DNA polymerase ☐
C. MRNA polymerase ☐
D. Amino acyl t-RNA synthetase ☐

**181. In translation process, proof reading of tRNA is done by:**
A. RNA polymerase ☐
B. Amino - acyl-t - RNA synthetase ☐
C. Leucine zipper ☐
D. DNA ☐

**182. Which enzyme involved in translation is often referred to as 'Fidelity enzyme' :**
A. DNA polymerase ☐
B. RNA polymerase ☐
C. Amino acyl-t RNA synthetase ☐
D. Amino acyl-reductase ☐

**183. Polypetide chain termination is enhanced by:**
A. Stop codon ☐
B. Promoter ☐
C. Ribosomal unit ☐
D. Pepitdyl transferase ☐
E. UAA ☐

**184. The hydrolytic step leading to release of polypeptide chain from ribosomes in catalysed by:**
A. Stop codons ☐
B. Pepitidyl transferase ☐
C. Release factors ☐
D. AUG codon ☐
E. Dissociation of ribosomes ☐

**185. About peptidyl transferase true is**
A. Used in elongation & cause attachment of peptide chain to A-site of t RNA ☐
B. Used in elongation & cause attachment of peptide chain to P site ☐
C. Used in initiation and cause 43S complex formation ☐
D. Used in initiation & cause 48S complex formation ☐

**186. Termination is caused by all except**
A. RF-1 ☐
B. UAA ☐
C. Peptidyl transferase ☐
D. 48 S complex ☐

**187. Ribosome has following enzymatic activity?**
A. Peptidyl transferase ☐
B. Peptidase ☐
C. Aminoacyl tRNA synthetase ☐
D. GTPase ☐

**188. For 1 peptide bond formation how many high energy phosphate bonds are required:**
A. 0 ☐
B. 1 ☐
C. 2 ☐
D. 3 ☐
E. 4 ☐

**189. Which group of amino acid is responsible for peptide bond:**
A. Amino group ☐
B. Carboxyl group ☐
C. Side chain ☐
D. Aldehyde group ☐
E. Amide group ☐

**190. Termination process of protein synthesis is performed by:**
A. Releasing factor ☐
B. Stop codon ☐
C. Peptidyl transferase ☐

D. UAA codon ☐
E. AUG codon ☐

**191. Which of the following is not required for protein synthesis (in translation) of eukaryotes:**
A. RNA polymerase ☐
B. Ribosomes ☐
C. Peptidyl transferase ☐
D. Amino acyl tRNA synthetase ☐

**192. Amber codon refers to**
A. Mutant codon ☐
B. Stop codon ☐
C. Initiating codon ☐
D. Codon for more than one amino acids ☐

**193. Shine-Dalgarno sequence in bacterial mRNA is near:**
A. AUG codon ☐
B. UAA codon ☐
C. UAG codon ☐
D. UGA codon ☐

**194. tRNA$_f$ met would recognize:**
A. AUG ☐
B. UGC ☐
C. GUG ☐
D. GCU ☐
E. UUG ☐

**195. False about eukaryotic protein synthesis is:**
A. N formyl Met is the first–RNA to come into action ☐
B. mRNA read from 5′ to 3′ ☐
C. Ef2 shift between GDP to GTP ☐
D. Capping helps in attachment of mRNA to 40 S ribosome ☐

**196. Ragarding Cytosolic Eukaryotic gene expression false is :**
A. Capping helps in attachment of mRNA to 40 S Ribosome ☐
B. N formyl methionine tRNA will be the first t – RNA to come into action ☐
C. EF2 shifts between GDP & GTP ☐
D. Releasing factor releases the polypeptide chain from the P site. ☐

**197. True about translation of protein is**
A. It has 3 steps initiation, elongation & termination ☐
B. IF-2 prevent reassociation of ribosomal subunit ☐
C. IF-3 and 1A cause binding of initiating codon ☐
D. IF 2 has α and β units ☐

**198. 43S preinitiation complex include all except:**
A. IF3 ☐
B. IF1A ☐
C. IF2β ☐
D. IF-4F ☐

**199. IF4F include all except**
A. 4A ☐
B. 4G ☐
C. 4E ☐
D. 4S ☐

**200. Which of the following does not undergo phosphorylation by protein kinases in Eukaryotes:**
A. Threonine ☐
B. Tyrosine ☐
C. Serine ☐
D. Asparagine ☐

**201. Component of 50s subunit is/are:**
A. 23s ☐
B. 28s ☐
C. 5s ☐
D. 5.8s ☐
E. 16s ☐

**202. Components of 60 S subunit of ribosome are:**
A. 5.8 S ☐
B. 23 S ☐
C. 16 S ☐
D. 18 S ☐
E. 28 S ☐

**203. True about ribosomes:**
A. Conserved in nature ☐
B. Role is to bring t-RNA and m-RNA together ☐
C. DNA forms RNA and rotein are formed from RNA ☐
D. They are always free ☐
E. Have two subunits ☐

**204. Regarding ribosome all is true except**
A. 16 S ribosome identifies shine- dalgarno sequence ☐
B. Cytosolic ribosomes synthesize proteins of peroxisome ☐
C. Large subunit catalyzes peptide bond formation ☐
D. Binding of aminoacyl tRNA uses 2ATP ☐

**205. Vitamin required for post translational modification of coagulants is :**
A. Vitamin A ☐
B. Vitamin C ☐
C. Vitamin B6 ☐
D. Vitamin K ☐

## Immunoglobin

**206. Correct pair of Ig subclass with their heavy chain:**
A. IgM - α (alpha) ☐
B. IgG -γ (gamma) ☐
C. IgM - δ (delta) ☐
D. IgE- γ- (gamma) ☐
E. IgA -γ (gamma) ☐

**207. Correct order of switching of Ig:**
A. IgM to IgG ☐
B. IgA to IgG ☐
C. IgM to IgA ☐
D. IgM to IgD ☐
E. IgE to IgG ☐

**208. True about IgM**
A. Fix complement ☐
B. Increased in primary response ☐
C. Fab region is composed of variable region ☐
D. Fc is antibody –binding portion ☐

**209. True about Ig gene rearrangement & Ig diversity:**
A. Somatic mutations theory ☐
B. One loop and two loop joining theory ☐
C. DNA rearrangement ☐
D. Appropriate class switching ☐

**210. True about location of Ig chromosome:**
A. κ- 2 ☐
B. κ - 6 ☐
C. κ - 14 ☐
D. λ – 22 ☐
E. λ- 10 ☐

**211. What factor is responsible for deciding whether an antibody will remain membrane bound or get secreted?**
A. RNA splicing ☐
B. Class switching ☐
C. Differential RNA regulation ☐
D. Allelic exclusion ☐

**212. Synthesis of an immunoglobulin in membrane bound or secretory form is determined by:**
A. One turn to two turn joining rule ☐
B. Class switching ☐
C. Differential RNA processing ☐
D. Allelic exclusion ☐

## Intracellular traffic & Sorting

**213. Secretory proteins are synthesized in:**
- A. Cytoplasm ☐
- B. Endoplasmic reticulum ☐
- C. First in cytoplasm and then in Endoplasmic Reticulum ☐
- D. First in Endoplasmic Reticulum and then in cytoplasm ☐

**214. Signal peptides are synthesized in**
- A. ER ☐
- B. Free ribosomes ☐
- C. Membrane bound ribosomes ☐
- D. Golgi body ☐

**215. Elongation arrest occurs due to**
- A. SRP- R ☐
- B. SRP ☐
- C. Signal peptide ☐
- D. Docking protein ☐

**216. Sequence which is responsible for retaining proteins in membrane**
- A. Translocon ☐
- B. Sec 61 complex ☐
- C. Docking protein ☐
- D. Halt signal ☐

**217. Not true among the following is**
- A. Sec 61 translocon complex form passage way ☐
- B. SRP-R is docking protein ☐
- C. SRP blocks elongation ☐
- D. SRP-R releases elongation block ☐
- E. SRP-R is ATP bound ☐

**218. Which of the following groups of proteins assist in the folding of other proteins?**
- A. Proteases ☐
- B. Proteosomes ☐
- C. Templates ☐
- D. Chaperones ☐

**219. The primary role of chaperones is to help in:**
- A. Protein synthesis ☐
- B. Protein degradation ☐
- C. Protein denaturation ☐
- D. Protein folding ☐

**220. Folding protein are:**
- A. GLUT-1 ☐
- B. Calnexin ☐
- C. Cytochrome 450 ☐
- D. Insulin receptor ☐
- E. Protein disulfide isomerase ☐

**221. True statement about chaperones:**
- A. Belong to heat shock proteins ☐
- B. Wide range of expression ☐
- C. Present from bacteria to human ☐
- D. Ubiquitin is the most important chaperones ☐
- E. Also k/a stress proteins ☐

**222. Proteins targeted for destruction in eukaryotes are covalently linked to:**
- A. Clathrin ☐
- B. Pepsin ☐
- C. Laminin ☐
- D. Ubiquitin ☐

**223. Proteins are sorted by :**
- A. Golgi Bodies ☐
- B. Mitochondria ☐
- C. Ribosomes ☐
- D. Nuclear Membrane ☐

**224. Not a disorder of protein misfoldig?**
- A. Alzheimer's disease ☐
- B. Tuberculosis ☐
- C. Cystic fibrosis ☐
- D. CJD (Creutzfeld-Jakob disease) ☐

**225. The secondary structure of prion particles is:**
- A. Alfa helix ☐
- B. Beta bends ☐
- C. Beta sheets ☐
- D. Beta turns ☐

**226. Defect in folding of the protein result in which of the following clinical disease:**
- A. Kuru ☐
- B. Migraine ☐
- C. Hypothyroidism ☐
- D. Myopia ☐

**227. If cellular proteins do not fold into a specific conformation, their function are affected. Certain disorders arise, if specific proteins are misfolded. Which of the following disorders arises due to conformational isomerization:**
- A. Familial fatal insomnia ☐
- B. Hepatitis delta ☐
- C. Pernicious anemia ☐
- D. Lesch-Nyhan syndrome ☐

## Gene Duplication

**228. Gene duplication plays an important role in the evolution of**
- A. mRna ☐
- B. rRna ☐
- C. tRna ☐
- D. hn Rna ☐

## Mutation

**229. Small scale mutations include all except:**
- A. Substitution ☐
- B. Deletion ☐
- C. Paracentric inversion ☐
- D. Insertion ☐

**230. Base substitution of GAC (Asp) to GAG (Glu) is an example of:**
- A. Point mutation ☐
- B. Silent mutation ☐
- C. Non-sense mutation ☐
- D. Conserved mutation ☐
- E. Non-conserved mutation ☐

**231. Which of these is a conservative mutator:**
- A. Glutamic acid- glutamine ☐
- B. Histidine-glycine ☐
- C. Alanine- leucine ☐
- D. Arginine-aspartic acid ☐

**232. In sickle cell anaemia, the defect can be explained as having arisen from -**
- A. A base insertion in DNA ☐
- B. A base deletion in DNA ☐
- C. A base substitution in DNA ☐
- D. None of the above ☐

**233. Hbs has defect in aminoacid position -**
- A. 4 ☐
- B. 6 ☐
- C. 11 ☐
- D. 12 ☐

**234. One of the following mutation is potentially lethal -** a)
- A. Substitution of adenine for cytosine ☐
- B. Substitution of methylcytosine for cytosine ☐

C. Substitution of guanine for cytocine ☐
D. Insertion of one base ☐

**235.Sickle cell ancmia is the clinical manifestation of homozygous genes for an abnormal haemoglobin molecule. The event responsible for the mutation in the B chain is -**
A. Insertion ☐
B. Deletion ☐
C. Nondisjunction ☐
D. Point mutation ☐

**236.Null mutation is** :
A. Mutation occuring in Non Coding region. ☐
B. Mutation that does not change the amino acid or end product ☐
C. Mutation that codes for a change in progeny without any chromosomal change ☐
D. Mutation that leads to no functional gene product ☐

**237.A mutation in the codon which causes a change in the coded amino acid, is known as**:
A. Mitogenesis ☐
B. Somatic mutation ☐
C. Missense mutation ☐
D. Recombination ☐

**238.Somatic mutations involve**:
A. Deletion ☐
B. Plasmid mediated ☐
C. Frame-shift alteration in coding nucleotides ☐
D. Trinucleotide repeat mutations ☐
E. Non-sense alteration of DNA ☐

**239.Base substitution mutations can have be following molecular consequence except**:
A. Changes one codon for an amino acid into another codon for that same amino acid ☐
B. Codon for one amino acid is changed into a codon of another amino acid ☐
C. Reading frame changes downstream to the mutant site ☐
D. Codon for one amino acid is changed into a translation termination codon ☐

**240.Transition mutation of GATCCT is:**
A. GGTCCT ☐
B. GTTCCT ☐
C. GABCCT ☐
D. GrUGGT ☐
E. GTTUCT ☐

**241.Trinucleotie repeats are found in:**
A. Huntington's disease ☐
B. Spinocerebellar ataxia ☐
C. Amyotropic latera sclerosis ☐

**242.In a mutation if valine is replaced by which of the following would not result in any change in the function of protein**:
A. Proline ☐
B. Leucine ☐
C. Glycine ☐
D. Aspartic acid ☐

**243.Which of the following can be a homologous substitution for valine in hemoglobin?**
A. Isoleucine ☐
B. Glutamic acid ☐
C. Phenylalanine ☐
D. Lysine ☐

**244.True about silent mutation in gene:**
A. No change in mRNA ☐
B. No change in Amino acid sequence in protein ☐
C. No expression of protein ☐
D. No change in expression of protein ☐
E. Termination of protein synthesis ☐

**245.True about Sickle cell disease are all, Except:**
A. Single nucleotide change results in change of Glutamine to Valine ☐
B. Deoxygenated Hb l/t exposure of sticky end d/t replacement of nonpolar residue by polar residue ☐
C. HbS confers resistance against malaria in heterozygotes ☐
D. RFLP results from a single base change ☐

**246.In sickle cell anemia replacement is**:
A. Valbglu in b6 ☐
B. Glu by val in b6 ☐
C. Hist val b8 ☐
D. 6A ☐

**247.Sickling in 'HbS' disease is primarily caused by**
A. Decreased Solubility ☐
B. Decreased Stability ☐
C. Altered function ☐
D. Altered $O_2$ binding capacity ☐

**248.All of the following are true about Sickle cell disease, Except**
A. Single nucleotide change results in change of Glutamine to Valine ☐
B. RFLP results from a single base change ☐
C. 'Sticky patch' is generated as a result of replacement of a non polar residue with a polar residue ☐
D. HbS confers resistance against malaria in heterozygotes ☐

**249.Technique (s) used to detect Gene Mutation is/are**
A. RT-PCR ☐
B. Denaturing gradient gel electrophoresis ☐
C. DNA sequencing ☐
D. Restriction fragment polymorphism (RFLP) ☐
E. Single-strand conformational polymorphism ☐

**250.All the following can be used to detect mutation, except**:
A. Single strand conformational polymorphism ☐
B. Ligase chain reaction ☐
C. Polymerase chain reaction ☐
D. DNA Sequencing ☐

## Answers:

### Purines and Pyrimidines

1. **D i.e. Reye syndrome decrease cytosolic carbamoyl phosphate**
2. **A i.e. N5 – N10 methylene tetrahydrofolate**
   *[Ref: Harper's 28/e P- 298; Chattergea 7/e p. 214-17; Lippincott 5/e p. 302-5; Lehninger 5/e p. 892-94]*
3. **D i.e. Allantoin**
4. **C i.e., Adenylic & guanylic acid** 5. **A i.e. Due to increased metabolism of pyrimidines** 6. **A i.e. Purine metabolism**
7. **A i.e. Abrupt increase in serum urate levels is more common a cause for acute gout than an abrupt fall in urate levels**
8. **B i.e. Raised uric acid in synovial fluid of joint** *[Ref: Harper's 28/e p.292-99; Lippincott's 5/e P-294-302; Harrison 16/e P 2046]*
9. **A i.e. HGPRTase** *[Ref: Lehninger 5/e p. 893, 882; Lippincott 4th/e p 296-97; Harrison 17/ 2447-48; Nelson 18/e p-629-30; Harper 28th/ed pg- 298-99]*
10. **D i.e. HGPRT** 11. **A i.e. Hypoxanthine phosphoribosyl transferase**
12. **D i.e. Serum Uric Acid Levels**
13. **A i.e.Purine synthesis** *[Ref: Harper's 27/e P-301]*
14. **D i.e. Thiamine** *[Ref: Chatterjea 6/e P-159; Harper's 27/e P-496-97]*

### DNA Structure

15. **A i.e. All nucleotides are involved in linkage; B i.e. Antiparallel; D i.e. Bases perpendicular to DNA**
16. **E i.e. A single strand of DNA** 17. **D i.e. Uracil** 18. **B i.e. Hydrogen bond**
19. **C i.e. Deoxyribose-phosphate backbone with bases stacked inside**
20. **C i.e. B** *[Ref: Harper 28/ed 289-90, 302-304; Chattarjae 7/e 225-27; Lippincott 5/e 396-98; Lehninger 5/e 277-82]*
21. **A i.e. Hoogsteen pairing** *[Ref: Harrison 17th /1764; Harrison's 18th/2312]*
22. **A i.e. A+G = T+C** 23. **D i.e. Double stranded DNA**
24. **D i.e. 27%** *[Ref: Lehninger 5/e p. 278; Lippincott 6/e p. 291, 397; Satyanarayan 3/ e p. 73]*
25. **B i.e. C- G** 26. **B i.e. G ≡ C** *[Ref: Harper's 27/e P-311]*
27. **B i.e. 5CUUAAG3** 28. **A i.e. 5′GTACG CTTAA′** *[Ref: Harper 29/e p-343-46; Lippincott 5/e p 396-98]*
29. **C i.e. Runs at 5′- 3′ direction** *[Ref: Harper's 27/e P-348-350]*
30. **D i.e. Matches with RNA transcript that encodes protein.**
31. **E i.e. 5′- GUACGUAA-3′** *[Ref: Lippincott 4th/ed p. 419, 430]*
32. **D i.e. Thymidine** *[Ref: NMS 3/e P-222; Harper's 27/e P-298-99]*
33. **B i.e. Negatively Charged** *[Ref: Ronald Hofman hematology 2/e P-2202]*
34. **A i.e. Maternal inheritance; C i.e. Not highly conserved & has high mutation rate; D i.e. Mitochondrial disease is associated mostly with Mutation & some have deletion**
35. **A, B, D, E i.e. UGA codes for tryptophan, Codes for 13 protein, Circular double stranded DNA, Mitrochondrial disease occur due to Point Mutations and Large-Scale Rearrangements**
36. **B i.e. DNA** 37. **C i.e. Mitochondrial disease**
38. **B i.e. Maternally inherited** 39. **B i.e. Maternal tranmission, D i.e. Mitochondrial myopathy**
40. **A i.e. Closed Circular** *[Ref: Lehninger 5th/ed pg-738-42; Harper 28th/ed pg-319-20; Robbin's 7/e p. 185; Teitz 6th/ed pg-269; Eberhard: Colour atlas of genetics 3/ed pg-134; Acta Neuropathol (2006) 111: pg-610-16]*
41. **A i.e. Virus; B i.e. Chloroplast; C i.e. Bacteria; D i.e. Mitochondria** *[Ref: Greewood 16/e p 10-11; Ananthanarayana 8/e p 10-13; Jawetz 25/e p 2-4- 97- 100]*
42. **D i.e. 30,000** 43. **A i.e. DNA** *[Ref: Harper's 28/e P-316-18; Lehninger 5/e p. 950]*
44. **C i.e. Telomere; D i.e. Centromere; B ie. Microsatelite DNA** *[Ref: Harper 28/e 315-19; Lipincott 5/e 475; Lehninger 952-53]*
45. **A i.e. They are present at the ends of eukaryotic chromosome; B i.e. Increased telomerase activity favours cancer cells.**
46. **B i.e. Longetivity of cell- aging**
47. **A i.e. Telomerase** 48. **C i.e. Telomerase** 49. **B i.e. Somatic**
   *[Ref: Lehninger 5/e 1053-55, 953; Harper 28/e 315-19; Robbins 7/e p 308-9; Lippincott 5/e 408-7; Ganong 22/e p 20]*
50. **B i.e. Present inside the nucleus; D i.e. Basic** 51. **B i.e. Increased Euchromatin formation**
52. **A i.e. DNA; E i.e. Histones** 53. **A i.e. Histone** 54. **D i.e. Glycosylation**
55. **A i.e. Uncondensed** 56. **A, B i.e. Histone, DNA** 57. **C i.e. Regular repeating structure of DNA & histone proteins**
   *[Ref: Chatterjea 8/ p 83, 240; Harper 28/ed 312-13; Lehninger 5/e 963-66; Lippincott 5/e 409-11, 422; Satyanarayan 3/e p 79; Vasudevan 6/e 471-72]*

## DNA Synthesis and Replication

58. **B i.e. Semi conservative; D i.e. Bidirectional; E i.e. Semi discontinuous**
59. **B, C i.e. Superhelical density depends on length of DNA, Underwinding strain is normally accommodated by strand separation**
60. **A i.e. DNA synthesis**
61. **A i.e. DNA replication**
62. **A i.e. ds DNA**
63. **C i.e. DNA Polymerase III**
64. **B i.e. Sister chromatids are formed C i.e. Follows base pair rule D i.e. Semi conservative E i.e. Single strand breakend.**
65. **C i.e. RNA polymerase → DNA polymerase III → DNA Polymerase I → DNA ligase.**
66. **B i.e. Multiple origins of replication are possible for bacteria; D i.e. Lagging strand stick by RNA primase; C i.e. DNA replication proceeds in one direction**
67. **A i.e. DNA Ligases**
68. **A i.e. DNA polymerase, B i.e.DNA ligase, C i.e. DNA topoisomerase, D i.e. primase, E i.e. RNA polymerase**
69. **D i.e. DNA gyrase** *[Ref: Lippincott 5/e p 399-405; Lehninger 5/e p 954-58, 977-92; Harper 29/e p 365-72; John Baynes 3/e p 418]*
70. **A, D, & E i.e. Circular, Negatively sepercoiled & Nucleoid present** *Ref: Lehninger 5th/ed pg- 949-50; Greenwood 16/ed pg- 10-12*
71. **B, D i.e. β; ε** *[Ref: Lippincott 4th/ed pg- 407; Harper 29/367; Lehninger 5th/ed pg. 989]*
72. **A, B, & C i.e. Components are α, β, γ, Δ, ε, β associated with repair, & γ associated with repair**
73. **B i.e. 5′→ 3′ Polymerase activity; C i.e. 3′→ 5′ exonuclease activity; D i.e. 5′→ 3′ exonuclease activity**

## DNA Damage, Repair and Protooncogene

74. **A, C, D i.e. Pyrimidine, Sugar, Purine** *[Ref: Lehninger 5/e 271-75; Chatterjae 7/e 206-8; Vasudevan 6/e 457-59-296;*
75. **D, E i.e. TMP – Thymine monophosphate, UMP – Uracil monophosphate** *Lippincott 5/e 291-93; Harper 28/e 285-87]*
76. **A i.e. Adenosine**
77. **A & D i.e. Decrease Tm & Melting lead to denaturation of DNA**
78. **A i.e. Splitting of double strands into single strand.** *[Ref: Lippincott's 4/ 397-98, Harper's 28/ 303-4; Chatterjea 7/ 228-229; Lodish 6/e p. 117]*
79. **A i.e. Absorption at 260 nm** *[Ref: Harper 28/e 288; Lehninger 5/e 276]*
80. **D i.e. Endonuclease cut DNA at 5′ terminus** *[Ref: Lehninger 5/e 979-82; Harper 28/e 311-404; Vasudevan 6/e 475]*
81. **A i.e. DNA repair** *[Ref: Chattergea 7/e p. 239-40]*
82. **B i.e. Formation of thymidine dimmers**
83. **A i.e. Formation of thymidine dimmers**
84. **C i.e. Nucleotide excision repair**
85. **B i.e. DNA Polymerase I > D i.e. DNA ligase**
86. **A i.e. Nucleotide excision repair** *[Ref: Harper's 27/e P-345-46,343; Lehninger 5/e p. 1003]*
87. **B i.e. Deamination to thiamine; D i.e. DNA repair > E i.e. Methylation protects the host DNA from cleavage by its own restriction enzyme** *[Ref: Vasudeven 6/e p 477; Harper 29/e p 370-74; Lippincot 5/e p 398, 460-62, 422; Lehninger 5/e p 289-92, 302, 993-95]*
88. **A, B & C i.e. Xeroderma pigmentatosa, Bloom's syndrome & Ataxia telangiectasia**
*[Ref: Harper-28th/ed pg- 330-33; Chatterjea 7th/ed pg-239-41; Lehninger 5th/ed pg- 1003-992; Harrison 17/ed pg-396]*
89. **B i.e. Inhibition of apoptosis** *[Ref: Robbins 7th/293,295; ww.lungcancerbooksandnewsletter.com/what_is_cancer.htm]*
90. **A i.e. Normally involved in cell cycle proliferation; D i.e. Proto- onchogenes on mutation cause cancer**
91. **A i.e. Carotenoids** *[Ref: Casciato: Onchology 5/e p-22, 25; Harrison 16/e p- 1072, Robbins 7/e p. 100, 288, 292- 95]*
92. **A i.e. Proto-oncogenes; B i.e. Tumor suppressorgene; D i.e. DNA repair genes**
93. **D i.e. RAS** *[Ref: Robbins 7/e p. 289- 309]*
94. **A i.e. α-rays** *[Ref: Radiology; Grainger & Allison's diagnostic Radiology 4/e P-139; Park 17/e P-521; K.N. Sharma Chemistry]*

## Genetic Code

95. **B i.e. Hydroxyproline; E i.e. Ornithine**
96. **B, C i.e. Overlapping, Ambigous**
97. **A, B, C i.e. UAA, UAG, UGA**
98. **A, C, D, E i.e. AUA codes for methionine in mitochondria, AUG codes for initiator codon in mammalian cell, AGA & AGG act as chain terminator in mammalian mitochondria, UAA, UAG & UGA are stop codon**
99. **C i.e. 256**
100. **A i.e. UAG**
101. **C i.e. 3 consecutive nucleotide units**
102. **C i.e. Punctuation**
103. **A i.e. AUG**
104. **D i.e. Termination of protein synthesis**
105. **B i.e. 3 complementary base pairs**
106. **B i.e. 3 consecutive nucleotide unit**
107. **B i.e. UAG C i.e. UGA**
108. **A i.e. Degeneracy**
109. **B i.e., 5-end** *of* **anticodon** *[Ref: Lippincott 5/e p 432; Harper's 29/e P- 270; Lehninger 5/e p 1085*

## Regulation of Gene Expression

110. **B i.e. Zinc finger motif** 111. **A i.e. Nuclear receptor** 112. **A i.e. Zinc finger**
113. **A i.e., Zinc finger D i.e., Helix turn helix E i.e., Leucine zipper** *[Ref: Harper's 28/e p. 381-84; Lippincott's 5/e p. 423, 450, 18]*
114. **E i.e. 7 Amino acid** 115. **B i.e. Zinc** 116. **A i.e. DNA binding protein**
117. **A i.e. Cistron** *[Ref: Chatterjae 7/e 253; Vasudevan 6/e 473-561-60; Harrison 17/e p-385; Harper 28/e 370-71; Lehninger 271-477-948]*
118. **A, C, D i.e. Smallest functional unit of genome, Promoter & enhancer geens are typical example, Cistron is single functional unit**
119. **A i.e. Positive regulator**
120. **A i.e. Promoter; B i.e. Enhancer; C i.e. Operator** *[Ref: Harper's 28/e p. 370-373; Lippincott's 5/e p. 449-53; Chattergea 7/e p. 253-58]*
121. **D i.e., Not regulated** 122. **E i.e., Catabolite repression is mediated by CRP**
123. **D i.e., Regulator gene is inducible** 124. **C i.e. Inducer without glucose**
125. **C i.e. Both Lytic and lysogenic phases occur together** *[Ref: Harper 28th/ed pg- 373-76]*
126. **D i.e. RNA polymerase**

## Transcription

127. **C i.e. Specifically recognizes the promoter site** 128. **B i.e. Promoter**
129. **D i.e. Primer** 130. **B i.e., Nucleolus**
*[Ref: Lippincott's 5/e p. 419, 422, 424; Harper's 28/e p. 337, 345; Lehninger 5/e p. 1024-32; Chatterjea 7/e p. 242-43]*
131. **A i.e. Exon > B i.e. Enhancer** 132. **A i.e. Polycistronic mRNA; E i.e. Non coding exon**
133. **D i.e. Normal transcription, normal translation** 134. **A i.e. Interon** 135. **A i.e. Cut DNA at specific DNA sequence**
*[Ref: Harper 29/e p 360-64]*
136. **D i.e. Involve phosphodiester bond formation with elongation occurring in the 5′- 3′ direction.**
*[Ref: Harper's 27/e P-348; Chatterjea 6/e P-232]*
137. **A i.e. 5′ - CGU - 3′** *[Ref: Harper's 28/e p. 336-46; Lippincott 5/e p. 418-22]*
138. **C i.e. Different σ subunits are responsible for recognition specificity**
139. **A i.e. Initiation of transcription of the dystrophin gene would be affected**
*[Ref: Lippincott 5/e 430-423; Harper 28/e 553-54; Harrison 17/e 2682-83; Chattarjae 7/e 243; Robbins 7/e p-1337]*
140. **A, B, C, E i.e. siRNA, miRNA, tRNA, rRNA** *[Ref: Harper 28/e 307-10; Lehninger 5/e 1146-1060-33-1076]*
141. **D i.e. C-DNA; E i.e. New strand of DNA** 142. **B i.e. t RNA**
143. **A i.e. Transcribed from Nuclear DNA**
144. **B i.e. RNAI** 145. **B & E i.e. RNA polymerase II & Drosha** 146. **A i.e. Gene Regulation**
*Ref: Harper 28th/e p. 348-50, 306-10,366; Lehninger 5th/ed pg- 1030-33, 1145, 1045-46,1146; Lippincott 4th/ed pg- 422-24; Lodish-Molecular Biology 6/ed pg-348*
147. **B i.e. Polylysine** *[Ref: Harper's 27/e p. 366; Lippincott's 4/e p. 432, 424-27 ; Genes & development 21 : 519- 524, 2007]*
148. **A i.e. Occur in intron that form Ribozyme; C i.e. Self-splicing introns; E i.e. Lariats intermediates are formed**
149. **A i.e. RNA splicing** 150. **A i.e. Intron**
151. **B i.e. snRNA** *[Ref: Harper 28th/ed pg- 307, 346-48; Lippincott 5th/ed pg- 426-27; Lehninger 5th/ed pg- 1146, 1043-44]*
152. **A i.e. Lariats formation; B i.e. Splicing; E i.e. Methylation**
153. **A i.e. Occurs in introns that form ribozyme; C i.e. Self splicing introns; E i.e. Lariat intermediates are formed**
154. **D i.e. Attachment of CCA in tRNA.** 155. **C i.e. Poly (A) tailing** 156. **D i.e. Prokaryotic mRNA**
157. **D i.e. Glycosylation** 158. **A i.e. Chemical hydrolysis**
159. **C i.e. Deamination of cytidine to uridine** *[Ref: Vasudevan 6/e p 485-86; Harper 29/e p 389-94; Lippincott 5/e p 427, 457-58; Lehninger 5/e p 1036-49]*
160. **A i.e. All RNA undergo post transcriptional modification; B i.e. Capping of the pre-m RNA Involves the addition of 7-methylguanosine to the 5′end; C i.e. Poly A tailing occur at 3′end; D i.e. Intron excision by spliceosome**
161. **C i.e. Peptidyl transferase activity**
162. **E i.e. Deamination** *[Ref: Harper 29/e p. 68, 348]*
163. **B i.e. DNA** 164. **A i.e. Cytarabine** 165. **A i.e. Actinomycin D - B i.e. Amanitin** 166. **D i.e. Actinomycin**
*[Ref: Chatterjea 7/e p. 245, 252; Lippincott's 4/e p. 424, 397; Harrison 16/e p. 479, 794, 635, Harper 27/e p. 351, 378]*

167. **A i.e.Spinal muscular dystrophy** *[Ref: Lippincott 5/e 425-26; Harper 28/e 317-348-49-308; Lehninger 5/e 1035-40; Vasudevan 6/e p. 484-85]*
168. **C i.e. Reverse transcriptase** *[Ref: Harper's 27/e P-316, 410; Lippincott's 3/e P- 405]*
169. **A i.e. Forms DNA from RNA; C i.e. Important for replication of HIV**
170. **B i.e. Protein; D i.e. Nucleic acid** *[Ref: Harper's 27/e P-314, 316]*
171. **C i.e. t - RNA** 172. **A i.e. t - RNA** 173. **A i.e. tRNA** 174. **B i.e. Clover leaf pattern**
175. **B i.e. t-RNA**
176. **C i.e. t RNA**

## Translation (Protein Synthesis)

177. **C i.e. Ribosomes** 178. **A i.e. Ribosome** 179. **C i.e. Attachment of amino group to 5′ end**
180. **D i.e. Amino acyl t-RNA synthetase** 181. **B i.e. Amino acyl t-RNA synthetase**
182. **C i.e. Amino acyl t- RNA synthetase**
183. **A i.e. Stop Codon; E i.e. UAA; D i.e. Peptidyl** 184. **B i.e. Peptidyl transferase; C i.e. Release factors**
185. **A i.e. Used in elongation & cause attachment of peptide chain to A-site of t RNA**
186. **D i.e. 48 S complex** 187. **A i.e. Peptidyl transferase** 188. **E i.e. 4**
189. **A i.e. Amino group; B i.e. Carboxyl group**
190. **A, B, D i.e. Releasing factor, Stop codon, UAA codon**
191. **D i.e. Amino acyl tRNA synthetase** *[Ref: Harper 29/e p 400-408; Lippincott 5/e p 438-45; Lehninger 5/e p 1075-95]*
192. **B i.e Stop Codon** 193. **A i.e. AUG Codon** 194. **A i.e. AUG**
195. **A i.e. N formyl Met is the first - RNA to come into action**
196. **B i.e. N formyl methionine t RNA will be first t RNA to come into action.**
197. **A i.e. It has 3 steps initiation, elongation & termination; D i.e. IF-2 has α and β units**
198. **D i.e. IF-4F** 199. **D i.e. 4S**
200. **D i.e. Asparagine:** *[Ref: Lehininger 5/e p 1096-97, 224-26; Smith 8/e p 96-221]*
201. **A i.e. 23s; C i.e. 5s** 202. **A, E i.e. 5.8 S, 28 S**
203. **A, B, C, E i.e. Conserved in nature, Role is to bring t-RNA and m-RNA together, DNA forms RNA and rotein are formed from RNA, Have two subunits** *[Ref: Lehninger 5/e 3, 1076-79; Harper 28/e 308-10; Lippincott 5/e 436; Vasudeven 6/e 493-487]*
204. **D i.e. Binding of aminoacyl tRNA uses 2ATP**
205. **D i.e. Vitamin K**

## Immunoglobin

206. **A i.e. IgG -γ (gamma)** 207. **A, C i.e. IgM to IgG, IgM to IgA**
208. **A, B, C i.e. Fix complement, Increased in primary response, Fab region is composed of variable region**
209. **A, C, D i.e. Somatic mutations theory, DNA rearrangement, Appropriate class switching**
210. **A, D i.e. κ- 2, λ - 22** *[Ref: Lehninger 5/e 1014-16, 1040-41, 170-73; Harper 28/e 349, 361, 322, 576-80; Lippincott 5/e 461-62-426; Vasudevan 6/e 561-62, 554-58; Anantnarayan 7/e p 96; Harrison 17/e p 2036; Chattarjae 7/e 256]*
211. **C i.e. Differential RNA regulation**
212. **C i.e. Differential RNA processing** *Ref: Lehninger 5th/ed pg- 1014-16; Tasuku: Immunoglobulin genes 2/e pg-237*

## Intracellular traffic, sorting and folding

213. **B i.e. Endoplasmic reticulum** *[Ref: Vasudevan 6/e p. 493; Harper 28/e p. 487-91]*
214. **C i.e. Membrane bound ribosomes** 215. **B i.e. SRP** 216. **D i.e. Halt signal**
217. **E i.e. SRP-R is ATP bound** 218. **D i.e. Chaperones**
219. **D i.e Protein folding** 220. **B, E i.e. Calnexin, Protein disulfide isomerase**
221. **A, B, C, E i.e. Belong to heat shock proteins; Wide range of expression; Present from bacteria to human; Also k/a stress proteins** *[Ref: Harper 28/e p- 39, 496-97; Devlin Biochemistry 5/e p- 255; Ganong 22/e p.25, 297-96, Chatterjea 8/e p 269-270]*

222. **D i.e. Ubiquitin** *[Ref: Lippincott's 3/e P-244; NMS 4/e P-375; Harper 28/e p. 497-987; Ganong 22/e p. 296-98, 25]*
223. **A i.e. Golgi bodies**
224. **B i.e. Tuberculosis** *[Ref: Harper 28/e p 497-98, 493; Vassudevan 6/e 590, 495]*
225. **C i.e. Betasheets** *[Ref: Harper's 28/e p. 39; Lippincott's 4/e p. 22; Harrison 17/e p. 2646]*
226. **A i.e. Kuru** *[Ref: Harper's 28/e P-39, 496-97; Lippincott's 3/e P- 21- 22]*
227. **A i.e Familial fatal insomnia**

## Gene Duplication

228. **A i.e. mRna** *[Ref: Lehninger 5/e p. 1060-61, 325, 34, 30]*

## Mutation

229. **C i.e. Paracentric inversion**
230. **A i.e. Point mutation; D i.e. Conserved mutation** 231. **C i.e. Alanine - leucine**
232. **C i.e. A base substitution in DNA** 233. **B i.e. 6** 234. **D i.e. Insertion of one base**
235. **D i.e. point mutation** 236. **D i.e. Mutation that leads to no functional gene product** 237. **C i.e. Missense mutation**
238. **C i.e. Frame shift alteration in coding nucleotide; D i.e. Trinucleotide repeat mutation; E i.e. Nonsense alteration of DNA**
239. **C i.e. Reading frame changes down stream to the mutant site**
240. **A i.e. G G T C C T** 241. **A i.e. Hutingtoris disease B i.e. Spinocerebellar ataxia**
242. **D i.e. Aspartic acid** 243. **B i.e. Glutamic acid**
244. **B, D i.e. No change in amino acid sequence, No change in expression of protein** *[Ref: Harper 28/e 355-58; Lippincott 5/e 433-34, 460, 427; Chattarjae 7/e 258-60; Lehninger 5/e 29-289,947,993; Vasudevan 6/e 501-503-262; Harrison 16/e p 370]*
245. **B i.e. Deoxygenated Hb l/t exposure of sticky end d/t replacement of nonpolar residue by polar residue**
246. **B i.e. Glu by val in b6** 247. **A i.e. Decreased Solubility**
248. **C i.e. 'Sticky patch' is generated as a result of replacement of a non polar residue with a polar residue**
*[Ref: Harper 28th/ed pg-49, 357, 397-98; Lippincott 5/e p. 475-77; Robbins 7th/ed pg- 402, 628; Eichler medical Biochemistry (2006) p-44; Gribben-Molecular hematology (2009) pg-9; John Baynes & Marek Dominiczak medical Biochemistry 3/rd pg-53-55,438,475; Lehninger 5th/ed pg 168-69]*
249. **ALL i.e. (RT-PCR, Denaturing gradient gel electrophoresis, DNA sequencing, Restriction fragment polymorphism (RFLP), Single-strand conformational polymorphism**
250. **B i.e. Ligase chain reaction**
*[Ref: Harrison's 18th/508-7; Harrison 17th/e/d p406; Eming's Elemens of Medical Genetics by Muller & Young P-63].*

# STRUCTURE, FUNCTION AND REPLICATION OF INFORMATIONAL MACROMOLECULES: REVIEW NOTES

## Pyrimidine Synthesis & Catabolism

- Unlike purine ring, which is constructed on a preexisting ribosome 5 $PO_4$, (derived from PRPP) the pyrimidine ring is synthesized from **aspartic acid** (contributing $N_1$, $C_4$, $C_5$, & $C_6$ atoms), **amine $N_2$ of glutamine** (source of $N_3$) and **$CO_2$** (source of $C_2$ atom of ring). Although both purine & pyrimidine synthesis require glutamine, aspartic acid & PRPP as essential precursors.

  The steps are Mn- **"GAS CAP AA CAA DHOA OA OMP UMP UDP"** see the rhythm AA, OA, MP, DP

- It uses 2 *multifunctional-multicatalytic polypeptides*, which ensures efficient channeling of carbamoyl phosphate to pyrimidine synthesis.
- First 3 enzymes (i.e. CPS II, Aspartate trans carbamoylase and Dihydroorotase) are **three different catalytic domain of single CAD polypeptide chain** (name derived from 1st letter of each domain).
- Next (4th) non multifunctional enzyme **DHOA dehydrogenase** is the ***only mitochondrial enzyme***[Q]
- ***Orotate phosphoribosyl transferase and Orotidylate (OMP) decarboxylase***[Q] are also catalytic domains of a single polypeptide chain of bifunctional enzyme **UMP synthase. Orotic aciduria** is caused by defect of single (type II) or both (type I) domains and result in poor growth, megaloblastic anemia & excretion of large amounts of orotate in urine. *Uridine administration* improves condition.
- **Allopurinol & 6-azauridine** drugs may precipitate oritic aciduria & oritidinuria by ***inhibiting OMP decarboxylase (i.e type II orotic aciduria)***[Q]. This enzyme is actually blocked by product of allopurinol & enzyme OPRT and 6-azauridylate.
- Orotic aciduria occurs in **deficiency of liver mitochondrial ornithine transcarbamoylase enzyme of urea cycle** and **Reye syndrome** (in which severly damaged mitochondria is unable to utitize carbamoyl phosphate). ***Excess carbamoyl phosphate exits to cytosol***[Q] and becomes available for cytosolic over production of orotic acid (by stimulating pyrimidine biosynthesis).

| | Carbamoyl Phosphate Synthetase | |
|---|---|---|
| | I | II |
| Occur in | Mitochondria | Cytosol |
| Used in | Urea cycle | Pyrimidine synthesis |
| Activator | N-acetyl glutamate | PRPP |
| Nitrogen source | Ammonia | γ-amide group of glutamine |

- Unlike purine ring, which is not cleaved in human cells, the pyrimidine ring is opened & degraded by **dihydropyrimidine dehydrogenase** (DHPD) & Beta-ureidopropionase to highly water soluble products *Beta-alanine (from uracil) and Beta-aminoisobutyrate (from thymine)*, with production of $NH_3$ & $CO_2$. DHPD deficiency results in *Beta-hydroxybutyric aciduria; a disorder of pyrimidine catabolism (and also of Beta amino acid metabolism* since formation of Beta-alanine & Beta-amine iso butyrate is also impaired) is also k/a **combined uraciluria-thyminuria**. High water solubility of end products results in few clinical features.

- d-UMP (deoxy-uridine monophosphate) is converted to d-TMP (deoxy-thymidine monophosphate) ***which uses N5, N10 – methylene tetra hydrofolate as a source of methyl group (1 carbon & 2 hydrogen)***[Q].). This is an unusual reaction in that THF (tetrahydrofolate) contributes not only 1 carbon unit but also 2 hydrogen atoms from pteridine ring , which causes oxidation of THF to DHF. Disorders of **folate & vitamin $B_{12}$** metabolism cause deficiency of TMP.
- Thymine analog, antitumor drug **5-flurouracil** (**5Fu**) is converted to *5-F dUMP*, which becomes ***permanently bound to the inactive thymidylate synthase***[Q]. So 5FU is a **suicide inhibitor.** ***Methotrexate (Mtx) and antibacterial trimethoprim inhibits dihydrofolate reductase, an enzyme which reduces DHF to THF***[Q].

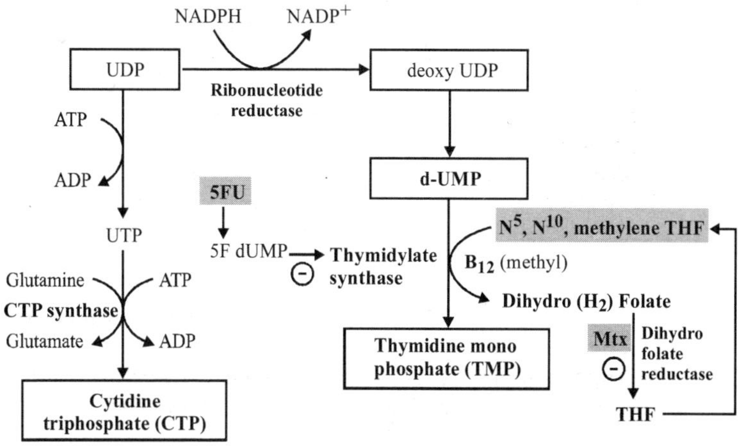

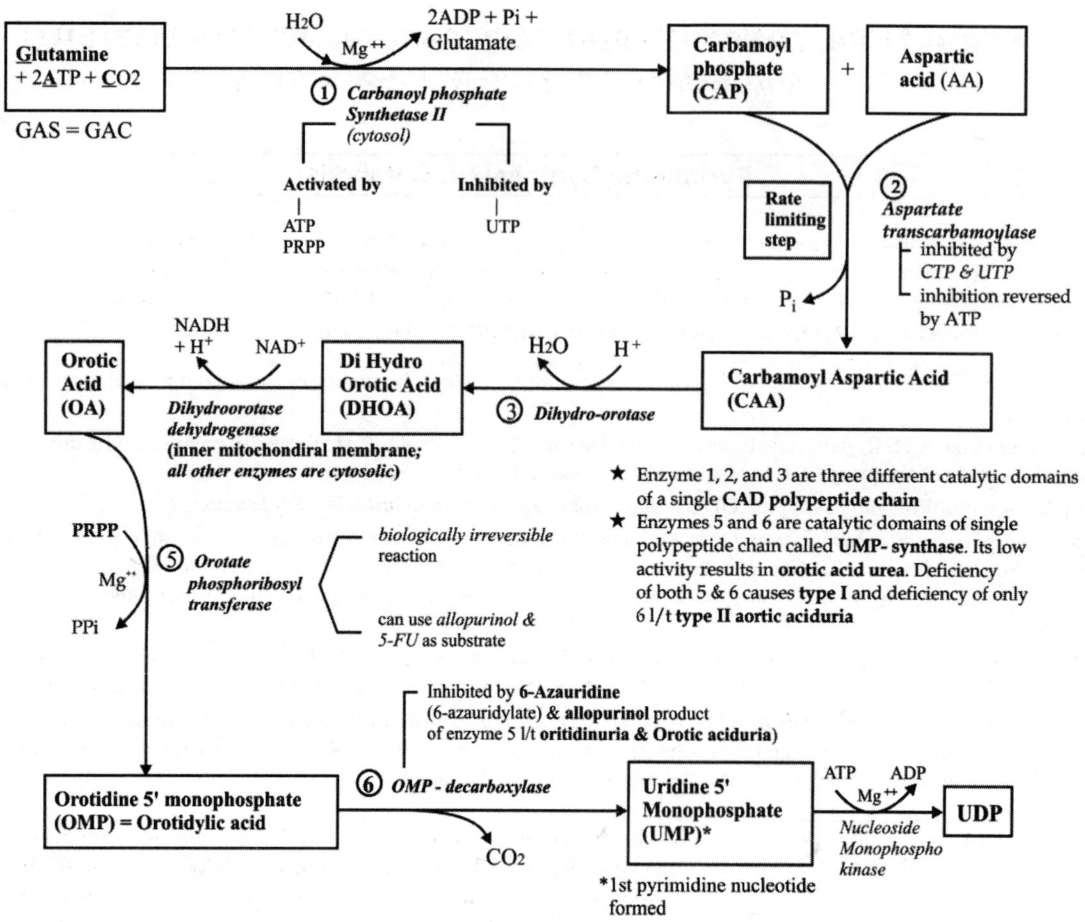


## Purine Synthesis

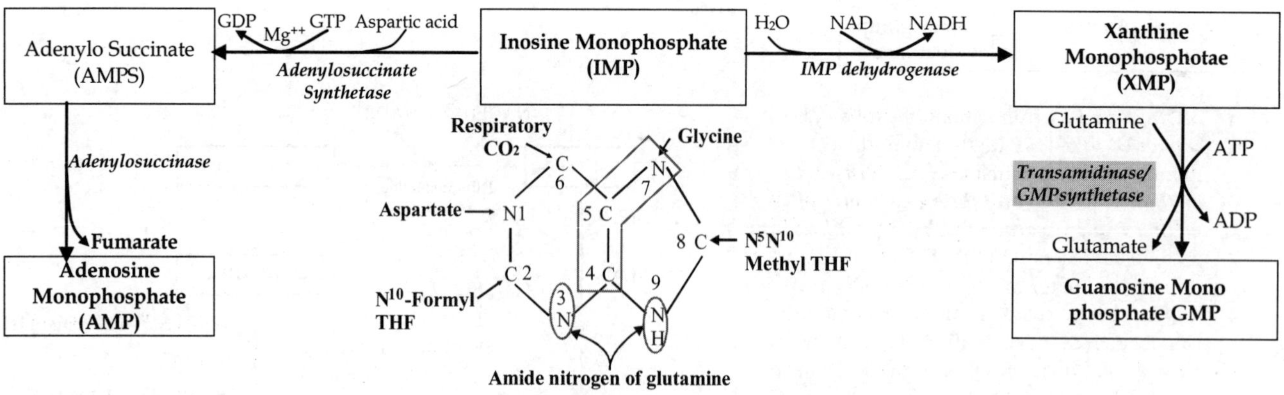


Sources of atoms in purine ring

★ **Mycophenolic acid** is reversible, uncompetitive *inhibitor of IMP dehydrogenase.* It deprives rapidly proliferating T & B cells of nucleic acids and used to prevent *graft rejection.*

## Uric Acid Synthesis (Purine Catabolism)

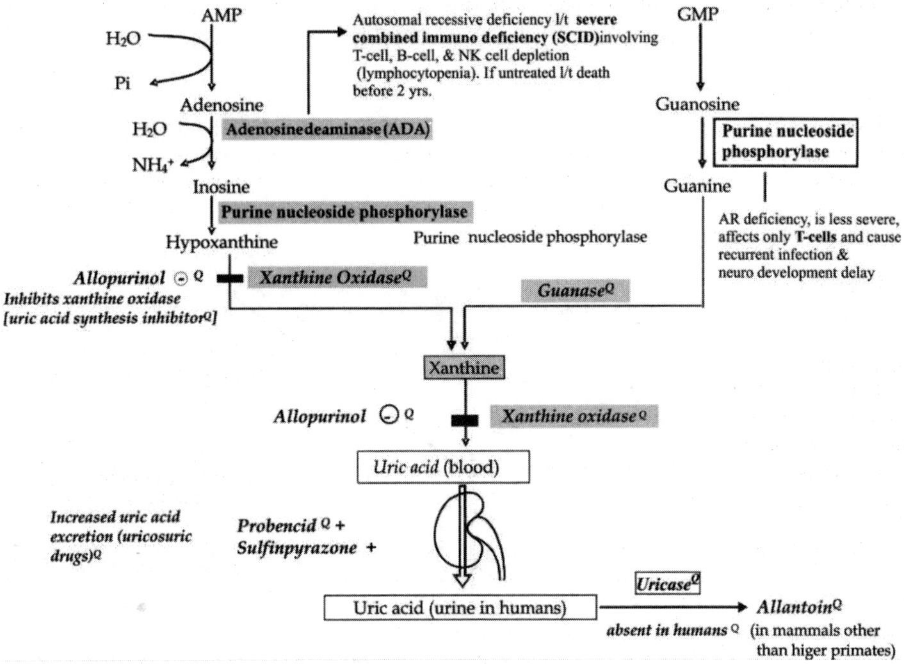


★ Hyperuricemia result in deposition of sodium urate crystals in kidney and joints

★ *Hyperuricemia does not always lead to gout,* but *gout is usually preceded by hyperuricemia.*

## Gout

This is characterized by *hyperuricemia* with *recurrent attack of acute arthritic joint inflammation*, caused by *deposition of uric acid crystal.*

### Types

- **Primary gout (hypeuricemia):** Due to inborn error of metabolism and is caused by
  - most often d/t urate crystal
  - less often d/t ↑ urate synthesis
- **Secondary hypeuricemia:** Caused by other disease eg:
  - Cancer
  - Chronic renal insufficiency
  - Myeloprofiferative disorder
  - Drugs

### Clinical Features

- The vast *majority of hyperuricemic patient are asymptomatic.* Any factor that cause ***either an abrupt increase or decrease in the serum urate levels may provoke an acute attack, the best correlations being factors that cause an abrupt fall***Q.
- Mostly affecting *middle- aged to elderly men* and *postmenopausal women.*
- Usually only one joint is affected, ***1st metatarsophalangeal joint is M.C involved***Q
- *Polyarticular acute gout* is seen in – male hypertensive patient with ethanol abuse & postmeno pausal women
- The Ist episode *frequently begins at night with dramatic joint pain and swelling*
- Joint becomes warm, red & tender
- ***Tophi***Q: aggregate of monosodium urate monohydrate (MSU) crystals form in extraarticular & articular structures, cause deformity and destruction of hard and soft tissue.

### Lab Diagnosis

- *Serum uric acid* level can be ***normal or low at the time of acute attack***Q.
- Serum uric acid is ***almost always elevated at some time***Q & can be used to follow cource of hypouricemic therapy.
- Radiologically:
  - ***Tophi***Q: eccentric soft tissue selling which may calcify
- **Definitive diagnosis**
  - **Aspiration of synovial fluid of affected joint**
  - **Aspiration of Tophaceous deposits in tissue**

***Strongly birefringent needle shaped MSU crystals with negative elongation under polarized light***Q.

### Treatment

**In Acute Gout**

- **NSAIDS** : eg. ***Indomethacin***Q , Naproxen , Piroxicam
  - strong anti inflammatory action
  - ***effective in terminating the attack***Q
- **Colchicine**
  - It has ***no effect on blood uric acid level***Q
  - It does not inhibit the synthesis or promote the excretion of uric acid.
  - It ***inhibits release of glycoprotein***Q which aggravates inflammation by increasing lactic acid production [Lactic acid → ↓ pH → urate crystals precipitated]
- **Corticosteroids:**
  - In refractory cases &
  - Those not tolerating NSAIDs / Colchicine

**In Chronic Gout**

- **Uricosuric drugs** : *Probencid*Q and ***sulfinpyrazone***Q promotes uric acid excretion & reduce blood level.
- ***Allopurinol***Q inhibits uric acid synthesis by ***inhibiting xamthine oxidase***Q. [an enzyme responsible for uric acid synthesis]

# Purine Nucleotide Biosynthesis

**The total- body urate level** is the net result between urate production and excretion. Urate production influenced by, dietary intake of purine, pyrimidine, de novo synthesis of purine, nucleic acid turnover and salvage by phosphoribosyl transferase activity.

## De novo biosynthesis

- It begins with their metabolic precursors amino acids, ribose 5 phosphate, $CO_2$ & $NH_3$.
- Purine ring is contributed by number of compounds
  - A.A [Glycine, Aspartic acid, glutamine]
  - $CO_2$
  - $N^{10}$ – Formyltatrahydrofolate
  - Ribose -5 $PO_4$ [Product of HMP shunt]
- Ribose -5- $PO_4$ is activated by ATP to form phosphoribosyl pyrophosphate (PRPP) by PRPP synthetase.
  - *PRPP concentration is major determinant of purine synthesis*
  - PRPP acts as a substrate in salvage pathway
  - *PRPP synthetase is inhibited by AMP. & GMP* (end product inhibition)

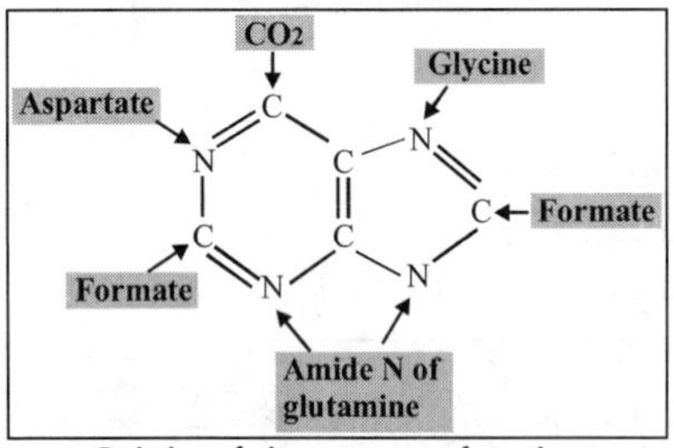


**Origin of ring atoms of purine**

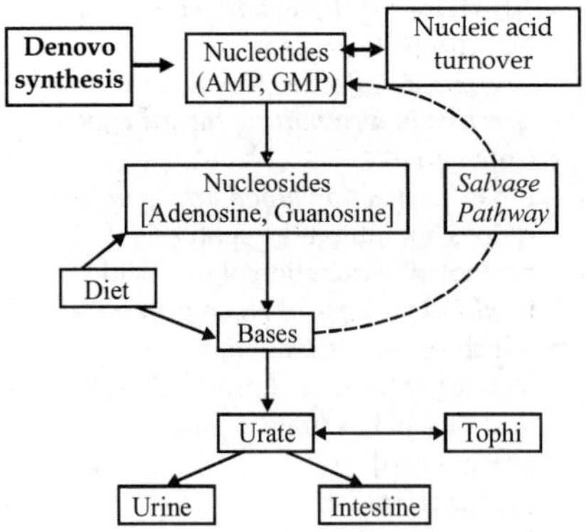


★ **Adenosine deaminase deficiency** l/t immunodeficiency d/t dysfunctional T cells and B cells causing fatal infectios in infants **Purine nucleoside phosphorylase deficiency** is a/w severe deficiency of T cells but apparently normal B cell function.

## Salvage Pathway

- It recycles the free bases & nucleotides released from nucleic acid breakdown.
- Purines that result from normal turnover of cellular nucleic acids or obtained from diet and not degraded, can be reconverted into nucleoside triphosphates and used by the body.

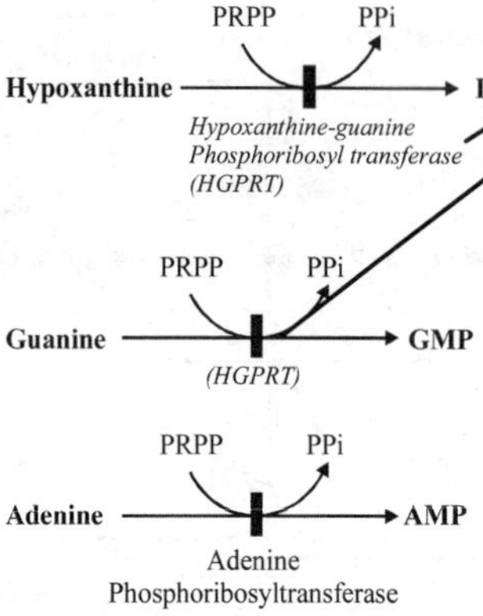


Inherited deficiency of HGPRT

Result in increased level of PRPP and ↓ed level of IMP and GMP causing↑ed de novo purine synthesis

| Complete deficiency of HGPRT | Partial deficiency of HGPRT |
|---|---|
| *Lesch- Nyhan syndrome*[Q] | *Kelley-Seegmiller syndrome*[Q] |

**Lesch-Nyhan syndrome**

- *X linked recessive disorder* of purine metabolism which becomes manifest by the **age of 2 years** and seen almost exclusively in **male children**.
- Homozygous males are affected & carrier females are asymptomatic
- It demonstrates the importance of salvage pathways. Hypoxanthine & guanine arise constantly d/t breakdown of nucleic acids. In absence of HGPRT-ase, PRPP level rises & purines are produced by denovopathway resulting in high levels of uric acid production and gout like damage to tissue.
- The brain is especially dependent on salvage pathway and this is the reason for central nervous system damage in Lesch-Nyhan syndrome

**Kelley-Seegmiller syndrome**

- Hyperuricemia
- Gout
- No CNS manifestation

| Hyper Uricemic Symptoms | Neurological (CNS) Symptoms |
|---|---|
| - ***Hyperuricemia, Hyperuricosuria***<br>- ***Gouty arthritis l/t joint pain***[Q]<br>- Uric acid crystaluria<br>- Nephrolithiasis (urate nephropathy, urinary tract stones)<br>- ***Obstructive uropathy (l/t reduced urinary out put)***[Q] | - ***Mental retardation***[Q] (intellectual disability)<br>- **Poor coordination** (spasticity, choreoathetosis & dystonia)<br>- ***Compulsive aggressiveness (extremely hostile)***[Q]<br>- Show **compulsive self-destructive tendencies** & ***self mutilating behaviour is characteristic feature***[Q] and occurs despite intact sensory (including pain) modalities. Mostly *fingers, mouth & oral mucosa are mutilated*. They mutilate themselves by biting off their fingers, toes and lips. |

**T/t**

Early diagnosis + Allopurinol

- Prevent or eliminate all the problem d/t hyperuricemia
- No effect on neurological abnormalities

## Structure of DNA

- **Erwin-Chargaff** in late *1940s* postulated **Charagaff rules** that in a DNA, - Number of adenosine (A) residues is equal to number of thymidine (T) residues **(A=T)** and number of cytidine (C) residues is equal to number of guanosine (G) residues (**C=G**)
- Hence sum of **purine residues (A + G)** = Sum of **pyrimidines residue (T + C)**
- **Rosalind Franklin & Maurice Wilkins** analyzed DNA by **X-ray diffraction** and deduced that DNA molecules are *helical*, with *2 periodicities* along their long axis, a primary one of *3.4A°* and a secondary one of *34A°*.
- **James Watson & Francis Crick in 1953 postulated 3 dimensional model of DNA** with following features
- 2 **helical** , **antiparallel** and **complementary** DNA chains *wound around the same axis* to form a *right handed double helix*.
- **Hydrophillic backbone** formed of alternating **deoxy ribose sugar and phosphate groups** (linked by **3′-5′ phosphodiester bond**) lie on the outside of double helix facing, the surrounding water. Whereas the ***purine & pyrimidine bases of both strands are stacked inside***[Q] the double helix, with their hydrophobic & nearly planar ring structures lying very close together & *perpendicular to long axis*.
- Each nucleotide base of one strand is paired with the base of other strand in **same plane**. The *offset pairing* of 2 stands l/t formation of major & minor grooves. Original model had **10 base pairs or 34A° (3.4 nm) per turn of helix** but subsequent measurements revealed **10.5 base pairs or 36 A° (3.6 nm) per turn.**
- **3 hydrogen bonds link C and G (C≡G) and 2 link A and T**. So separation of strands is difficult in DNAs with higher C≡G concentration.)

### Primary structure

- Each DNA is a polymer of about $10^{10}$ *deoxyribo nucleotide* monomers. These deoxynucleotides are of 4 types – deoxy **adenylate** (containing **adenine**), deoxy **guanylate** (containing **guanine**), deoxy **cytidylate** (containing **cytosine**) and deoxy **thymidylate** (containing **thiymine**).
- These monomeric nucleotides are held in polymeric form in each strand by covalent ***3′, 5′ – phosphodiester linkage***[Q].
- Phosphodiester bond joins 3′- hydroxyl group (OH) of deoxypentose (2′- deoxy D- ribose) sugar of one nucleotide to the 5′- hydroxyl group of deoxy pentose sugar of an adjacent nucleotide through a phosphate group.
- The end of strand which bears 5- hydroxyl or phosphate terminal is called **5 end**. And the opposite end with free 3′ OH or 3′ phosphate group is k/a **3′ end**. ***So the polymer show polarity***[Q]. ***The nucleotides are always written and read in 5′ → 3′ direction***[Q].
- So the primary structure consists of *linear back bone of deoxyribose sugar and phosphate*. While the ***purine or pyrimidine bases project laterally from the backbone at 90° (perpendicular***[Q]***).***

**Bases** (Adenine, thymine, cytosine & guanine) | **Deoxyribose sugar** | **Phosphate in diester linkage**

**Bases** + **Deoxyribose sugar** → **Deoxyribonucleoside**

**Deoxyribonucleoside** + **Phosphate in diester linkage** → **Deoxyribonucleoside**

### Secondary structure

- It consists of **2 helical, antiparallel** and **complementary** chains that wound around the same axis to form a double helix. Anti parallel orientation means that the 3′→5′ phosphodiester bonds of both chains run in opposite direction.
- The chains are paired in **antiparallel manner** i.e. 5′ end of one strand pairs with 3′ end of other strand and thus the phosphodiester bonds in two interwoven strands run in opposite direction. In other word one strand run in 5′ ti 3′ 'direction and other in 3′ to 5′ direction. (analogous to a highway carrying traffic in opposite directions).
- 2 Antiparallel chains are not identical in either base sequence or composition. Instead they are complementary i.e. ***Adenine (A) is always paired with thymine (T) by 2 hydrogen bonds and cytosine (C) is always paired with guanine (G) by 3 hydrogen bonds***[Q]***. The base pairs are perpendicular to the axis of helix***[Q]. A = T; C ≡ G
- This specific base pairing l/t **Chargaff's rule** i.e. in any sample of ds DNA (double stranded DNA) the amount of **adenine equals** the amount of **thymine** and the amount of **cytosine equals** the amount of **guanine**. So the ***total amount of purine equals the total amount of pyrimidine***[Q]
  $(A+G/T+C \approx 1)$
- Each of the two chains (strands) of double helix are coiled around a common central axis called the **axis of symmetry.**
- *Hydrophillic deoxyribose- phosphate* backbone of each strand is on the *outside* whereas *hydrophobic bases* are stacked inside. The structure resembles twisted ladder.
- **Two strands are held together** by both
  1. ***Hydrogen bonds between purine & pyrimidine bases***[Q]
  2. Vander walls and hydrophobic interaction between stacked adjacent base pairs.
- In ds DNA, **genetic** information resides in the sequence of nucleotides on **3′ → 5′ strand, the template strand** which is copied during m-RNA synthesis. It is also k/a **non coding strand**. The opposite strand with *5′ to 3′ polarity* is considered ***coding strand, because it matches the sequence of RNA transcript (but containing uracil in place of thymine)***[Q]***.***
- One polypeptide strand of ds DNA is ***always complementary***[Q] of the other. So the **m-RNA transcript** with a 5′ to 3′ polarity is ***complementary to the template strand with its 3′ to 5′ polarity, and matches the coding strand***[Q]. (Harper)
- The glycosidic bonds b/w sugar & bases are not directly opposite each other and two grooves of unequal width are formed. The edge of helix that measures >180° from glycoside bond to glycoside bond is called **major groove**, and if **< 180°**, it is called **minor groove**.
- The hydrogen atoms (proton) in the bases can shift from one ring nitrogen or oxygen atom to another k/a **tautomerisation** – thus interconverting the position that can severe as hydrogen bond donor & acceptor

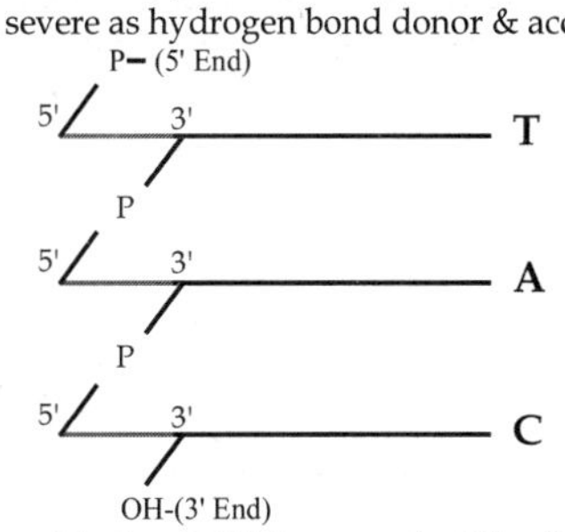


★ RNA is far less stable than DNA because the **2[1]-hydroxyl group** of RNA (absent from DNA) functions as *nucleophile* during hydrolysis of 3′→5′ phosphodiester bonds. However in absence of phosphodiestreases, hydrolysis of phosphodiester bonds of DNA occur only over long periods of time, despite an extremely favourable ΔG. and so DNA even persists in fossils.

**DNA Strands**

Coding -5′ – TGGAATTGTGAGCGGATAACAATTTCACACAGGAAACAGCTATGACCATG - 3′
Template- 3′- ACCTTAACACTCGCCTATTGTTAAAGTGTGTCCTTTGTCGATACTGGTAC - 5′
RNA transcript 5′- p AUUGUGAGCGGAUAACAAUUUCACACAGGAAACAGCUAUGACCAUG - 3′

## Unusual Structures Variations In DNA (Chromosome)

### Bending of DNA Helix

**DNA helix bends** whenever **≥4 adenosine (A) residues** appear sequentially in row in one strand (6 A produce 18° bend).

### Triplex DNA & Hoogsteen Pairing

- Nucleotides participating in Watson-Crick base pairing can form additional hydrogen bonds, particularly with functional groups arrayed in the **major groove**. For example protonated cytidine residue ($C^+$) can pair with guanosine residue of a G ≡ C nucleotide pair; and a thymidine (T) can pair with adenosine of A = T pair.

C ≡ G • $C^+$ T = A • T

- **Hoogsteen (non Watson-Crick) pairing** at $N^7$, $N^6$ and $O^6$ positions of purines (**Hoogsteen positions**) allow the **formation of triplex DNAs**. The triplexes are formed **most easily within long sequences containing only pyrimidines or only purines in a given strand**; or in **DNAs containing 2 pyrimidine & 1 purine or 2 purine & 1 pyrimidine strands**. The triplexes are most stable at **low pH** because the C ≡ G • C+ triplet requires **protonated cytosine residue** (≡ is WC hydrogen bond & • is Hoogsten hydrogen bond). Normally **pKa** of cytosine is 4.2, which is altered to **> 7.5** in triplex. It is important to understand that Hoogsteen pairing is essential for triplex DNA formation, whereas other factors like long polypyramidine / polypurine only sequences in a strand, 2 + 1 purine / pyramidine strands, **low pH, increased pKa & protonated cytosine** are facilitatory.

### Tetraplex / Quadruplex - DNA & G/Guanosine Tetraplex

- **Four stranded DNA (tetraplex or quadruplex)** occurs only for DNA sequences with **very high proportion of guanosine residue** (or very stable **guanosine /G tetraplex**).
- Guanosine (G) tetraplex is very stable over wide range of conditions

### Palindromes & Hairpin or Cruciform (Cross shaped) Structures

- Palindrome word / phrase / sentence /sequence is identically read either forward or backward; such as ROTATOR and NURSES RUN.
- Palindromic sequences of DNA have **twofold symmetry over two strands of DNA** and in order to superimpose one repeat on the other, it must be rotated 180° about the horizontal axis then 180° about the vertical axis.

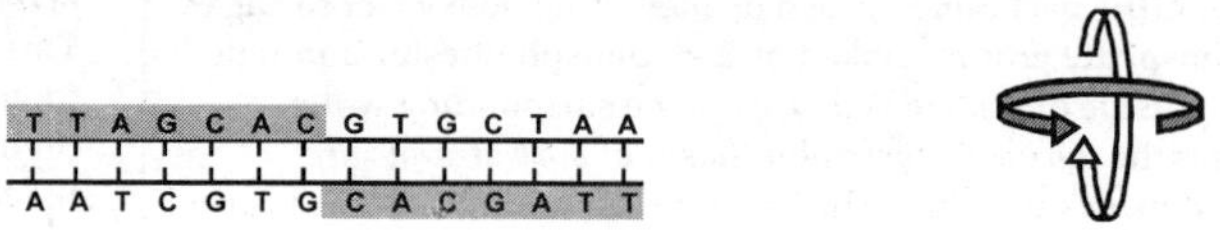


- Palindromic sequences are **self complementary within each strand** and therefor can form **hairpin or cruciform (cross shaped) structures** with **intrastrand** base pairing. When only **one strand** of DNA (or RNA) is involved the structure is called hairpin and when **both strands** of a duplex DNA are involved it is called cruciform.

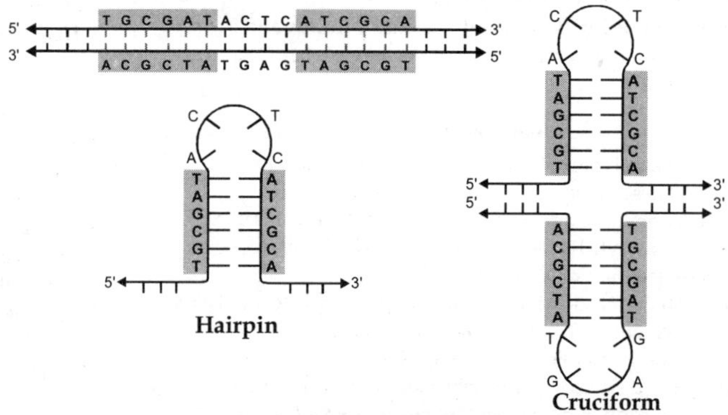


Hairpin

Cruciform

### Mirror Repeats

- Mirror repeat has **symmetrical inverted repeat sequence within each strand**. So super imposing one repeat on the other requires only a single 180° rotation about the vertical axis.

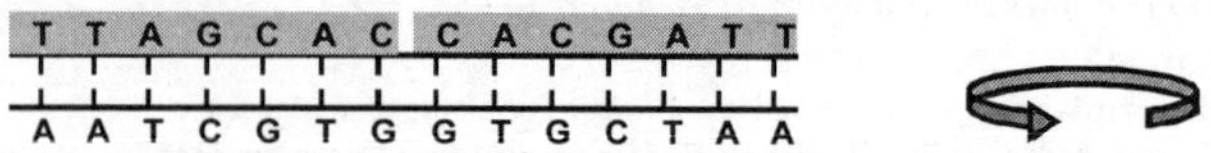


- Mirror repeats **donot have complementary sequences with in the same strand and so cannot form hairpin or cruciform structures.**

## Human Mitochondrial DNA (mt DNA)

- Mitochondria contain their own genome which is *a closed circular piece of double stranded DNA*Q that is composed of heavy (H) and light (L) strands or chains.
- Mt DNA is double stranded for most of its length *except at the replication and transcription control region (the D-loop)*, It is *not packaged in nucleosomes*
- **Genetic code of mt DNA differs slightly** from standard code: mt RNA reads 4 codons differently

| Codon | Normal | Mt DNA |
|---|---|---|
| AGA | Arginine | Terminator or stop codon |
| AGG | Arginine | Terminator or stop codon |
| **UGA** | Terminator | **Trypthophan** |
| AUA | Isoleucine | Methionine |

- Human mt DNA contains *16,569 base pairs (16.599 kb) in length and 37 genes* that encode ***13 protein complexes of respiratory chain, 2r RNAs and all 22 mt tRNAs* required for mitochondrial protein synthesis**[Q]
- However the great majority of mitochondrial proteins – about 900 different types (of which about 54 out of 67/ 66 but of 79 proteins of respiratory chain)- are encoded by nuclear genes, synthesized on cytoplasmic ribosomes, then imported into & assembled in the mitochondria.
- 1% of cellular DNA is in mitochondria as each mitochondria contains 2-10 copies of mt DNA. Each human cell contains variable number of mitochondria depending on the energy requirement of a particular cell. So each cell has large number of mt DNA owing to the fact that mt DNA replication is not limited to one per cell cycle as it is in nuclear genome. This greater abundance, compared with that of nuclear DNA, makes mt DNA attractive for testing applications in which sample DNA is limited (eg crime scene investigation, pathogen detection, & paleontology)
- Mt DNA is transmitted between generations by **non mandalian maternal inheritance**, with the mitochondria coming from oocytes and not (usually) from sperm
- Mitochondrial and nuclear DNA are located in different places in the cell. During fertilization, the sperm and egg cell nuclei fuse to form an embryo. The egg cell is very large compared to the sperm, so although the cells' nuclei fuse, the rest of the cell mass in the embryo comes from the egg only. *Nuclear DNA is therefore co-inherited but the mitochondrial DNA, which is located outside of the nucleus, is always maternally inherited because all mitochondria in a foetus and later adult are derived from the mitochondria in the mother's egg. All children from affected mother will inherit the disease but it will not be transmitted from an affected father to his children.*
- Mt DNA is ***not highly conserved & has high mutation rate*** *(5-10 times that of nuclear DNA) which accumulate through out the life* of organism. It is because
  - Mt DNA suffers *greatest exposure to reactive oxygen species* produced in respiratory chain
  - It has less effective proof reading system at correcting mistakes made during replication and at repairing DNA damage
  - ***It contains no (or very few) introns (or untranslated sequences)***[Q]
- Rapid accumulation of mutation provides sufficient data, to allow the comparison of closely relatede species or population with in the same species providing **evidence about evolutionary origins** of primates & other species.
- It can be used to study **evolutionary relationship (phylogeny) of organisms** & build evolutionary tree as well as for **genealogical research into person's maternal line** (eg prince Williams has Indian origin maternal line).

- **Proteins & structures encoded by mt DNA**
  - Encodes 2 *mitochondrial ribosomal RNAs large (16s) and small (12S) units*
  - Encodes all *22 mt tRNA molecules*
  - Encodes **13 protein** subunits of respiratory chain (of a total of about 67-Harper/ 79- Lehninger)

| Respiratory chain protein complex | Total no. of subunits | No. of sub units encoded by mt DNA |
|---|---|---|
| I NADH dehydrogenase | 43 | 7 |
| II Succinate dehydrogenase | 4 | 0 |
| III Ubiquinone: cytochrome C oxidoreductase (cytochrome b) | 11 | 1 |
| IV Cytochrome oxidase | 13 | 3 |
| V ATP synthase | 8 | 2 |
| Total | 79 | 13 |

- Disorders due to (*point mutation, large scale rearrangements & some deletions*) defect in mt DNA: (Mn- **"Pearson No Progressive Leigh Deaf Labour Kissed Me Adequtely"**)

| **Disease & Phenotype** | **Mt DNA Mutation & Inheritance (mostly)** |
|---|---|
| **Pearson (PEAR) syndrome** i.e. pancreatic & bone marrow failure | Large deletion , Heteroplasmic, Sporadic somatic mutations |
| **NARP syndrome** i.e. neurogenic muscle weakess (with sensory or sensory motor neuropathy), ataxia, retinitis pigmentosa due to mutation in MT-ATP 6 gene.<br>**Leigh syndrome** i.e. progressive neurological disease with motor & intellectual developmental delay, signs & symptoms of basal ganglia / or brain stem disease and raised lactate concentration in blood and CSF. | Point mutation in **ATPase subunit 6 gene**, Heteroplasmic; Maternal |
| **Progressive** external opthalmoplegia (CEOP) | **Single deletion / duplication**; Heteroplasmic; Sporadic somatic mutations |
| **Deafness:** Progressive sensorineural deafness induced by amino glycoside antibiotics. | A 1555 G mutation in **12 s RNA; Homoplasmic**; Maternal |
| **LHON syndrome** i.e. **Leber's** hereditary optic neuropathy (atrophy) | G17778 A, G 3460A, T 14484 C; **Homoplasmic** (±); Maternal |
| **Kearns- Sayre Syndrome (KSS)** i.e. opthalmoplegia, pigment degeneration of retina and cardiomyopathy | 5Kb **common deletion**; Heteroplasmic; sporadic somatic mutation |
| **MELAS syndrome** i.e. mitochondrial myopathy with encephalopathy, lactic acidosis and stroke | Point mutation in **tRNA leu**; Heteroplasmic; Maternal |
| **MERRF syndrome** i.e. myoclonic epilepsy and ragged red fibres disease d/t mutation in mitochondrial gene that encodes t RNA specific for lysine (t RNA Lys) | Point mutation in **t RNA lys**; Heteroplasmic; Maternal |
| **MMC syndrome** i.e. **M**aternally inherited **m**yopathy and **c**ardiomyopathy | |
| **ADMIMY syndrome** i.e. **a**utosomal **d**ominant **m**itochondrial **i**nherited **my**opathy with mitochondrial deletion. | |
| Somatic mutations in cytochrome complex III deficiency, muscle pain, ragged red fibers | |

★ *Deafness & LHON are homoplasmic* and others are heteroplasmic usually. All have *maternal inheritance* except Pearson syndrome, KKS and chronic progressive external opthalmoplegia (CPEO) which are sporadic somtic mutations mostly.

## Types of DNA

| Feature | A- DNA | B- DNA | Z- DNA |
|---|---|---|---|
| Prevalence | Not found under physiological conditions. When B DNA crystals are dried, the long thin B-DNA becomes short stubby A- DNA | ***Most common***[Q] | Occurs *in region* that have a sequence of alternating purines & pyrimidines eg poly GC *rich in guanine & cytosine base pairs.* |
| Helix handedness | Right | *Right*[Q] | *Left*[Q] |
| **Sugar pucker** conformation | C-3' endo | C-2' endo | **C-2' endo for pyrimidines** and **C-3' endo for purines** |
| **Glycosyl bond** confirmation | Anti | Anti | Anti for pyrimidines; Syn for purines |
| Deoxyribose – phosphate backbone | Linear | Linear | ***Zigzag***[Q] |
| Major groove | Present | Present | Non existing or convex |
| Minor groove | Present | Present | Deep cleft |
| Repeating unit base pairs<br>**Base pairs /turn** | 1<br>11 | 1<br>10.5 | 2<br>12 |
| Inclination of base pair to axis of helix | ~ 20° (19°) | ~1° (1.2°) | ~ 10° (9°) |
| **Base tilt** normal to helical axis | 20° | 6° | 7° |
| Rotation / base pair | ~ 33° | ~ 35° | 30° |
| Pitch (nm)<br>Diameter (nm) | 2.46<br>2.55 | 3.40<br>2.37 | 4.56<br>1.84 |
| **Helical Rise** / base pair along helix axis (nm) | 0.26 | 0.34 | 0.37 |

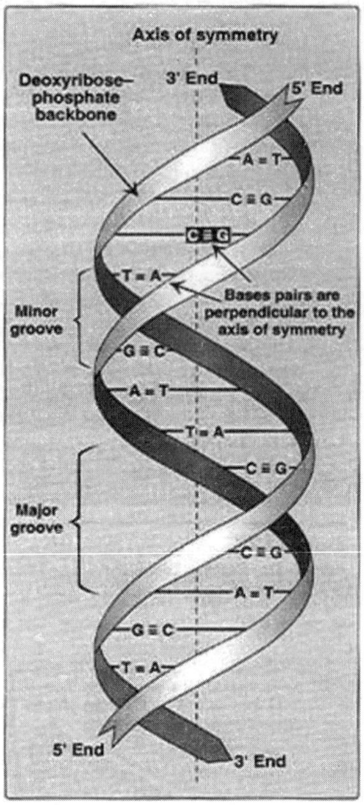


## In Human genome

- Haploid genome of each human cell consists of **$3 \times 10^9$ base pairs (3000 mega bases)** of DNA and about **$1.7 \times 10^7$ nucleosomes** subdivided into 23 chromosomes (chromatids). Each of these 23 chromatids would contain on the average **$1.3 \times 10^8$ nucleotides** in one ds DNA molecule.
- Entire haploid genome contains sufficient DNA to have nearly 1.5 million average sized genes but studies suggest that humans have < 1 lakh proteins encoded by ~1% of human genome composed of exonic DNA containing ≤ 25,000 protein coding genes (previously 30-35 thousand). This means most of the DNA is non-protein coding i.e. its information is never translated into an aminoacid sequence of a protein molecule.
- Pathologic effects of genetic diseases are expressed at levels:
  i) DNA ii) RNA iii) Protein iv) Cell & organ consequences.

## Eukaryotic DNA: Human Genome

- > 50% of eukaryotic DNA is **unique** or **non repetitive** and at least (i.e. >) 30% consists of **repetitive** sequences, About 30% of genome is genes (for protein) but only 1.5% is **coding sequences (or exons)** carrying information for RNA or protein products.
- **Non coding (non-translated) DNA** segments in genes are called **intervening sequences** or **introns** (28.5%), and the coding segments are called exons. Genes for histones have no introns and genes for muscle protein titin have 178 introns.
- 1% of cellular DNA is in mitochondria. **Repetitive sequence DNA** can be classified as

### Highly Repetitive Sequence (HRS)

- Also called **simple sequence DNA** or **simple sequence repeats (SSR)** and constitute 3% of human genome
- SSR is also called **satellite DNA** because its unsual base composition often causes it to migrate as *satellite bands (separated from the rest of DNA)* when fragmented cellular DNA samples are centrifuged (in cesium chloride density gradient).
- Are usually **<10 basepair long** and sometimes repeated millions of times per cell. But may be 5-500 bp long, repeated many times in tandem
- **VNTR (variable number of tandem repeats)** are short sequences of DNA at scattered locations in genome, repeated in tandem (i.e. one after another). The number of these repeat units varies from person to person, but is unique for any given individual and, therefore, **serves as a molecular finger print**. Microsatellites are a type of VNTR.
- **Microsatellite repeat sequences (MiRS)** consist of 2-6 bp repeated upto 50 times as both dispersed and grouped tandem arrays. It most commonly is found as dinucleotide repeats of AC on ones strand and TG on opposite strands-occuring upto 1 lack times in genome. Several other repeats may be CG, CA and AT. It produces **polymorphism** (i.e. *clinically harmless DNA variation that does not affect phenotype*) & is a *heritable trait*. Because of their unique number (for an indvidual), usual association with most genes and ease of detecting them using PCR, MiRS are useful in constructing genetic linkage map.
- **Microsatellite instability** (i.e. *increased tri nucleotide repeats*) can lead to diseases like *fragile X syndrome* d/t unstable p(CGG)n, **myotonic dystrophy (CTG)** and Hutington's chorea, spinobulbar muscular atrophy and Kennedy disease (all d/t unstable CAG).
- HRS-DNA is *transcriptionally inactive (i.e. does not encode proteins or RNA)* but (unlike transposons) have an *identifiable functional importance in cellular metabolism*, because much of it is associated with – **centromeres & telomeres**. It may play a *structural role* also.

#### Centromere

- It is **adenine- thymine-(A-T) rich** region containing repeated DNA sequences from $10^2$ – $10^6$ bp size (i.e. thousands of tandem copies of short segments in same orientation) which *connects sister chromatids*.
- Metazoan centromere is bound by nucleosome containing CEN P-A (a H3 histone variant protein & other centromere binding proteins, forming **Kinetochore** which *provides the attachment for mitotic spindle*.
- This anchoring is essential for equal & orderly chromosomal segregation (distribution) during mitosis.

#### Telomere

- Telomeres are **short T-G rich repeats** at the ends of eukaryotic chromosomes that *help stabilize the chromosome*.
- Human telomeres have variable number of **'5' - TTA GGG-3"** repeats which may extend upto several Kb.

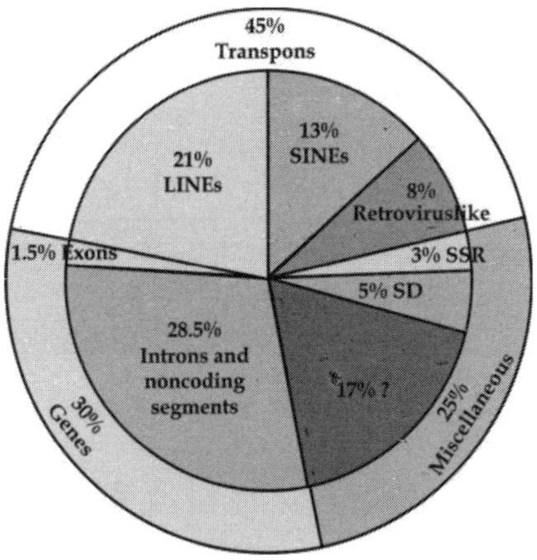


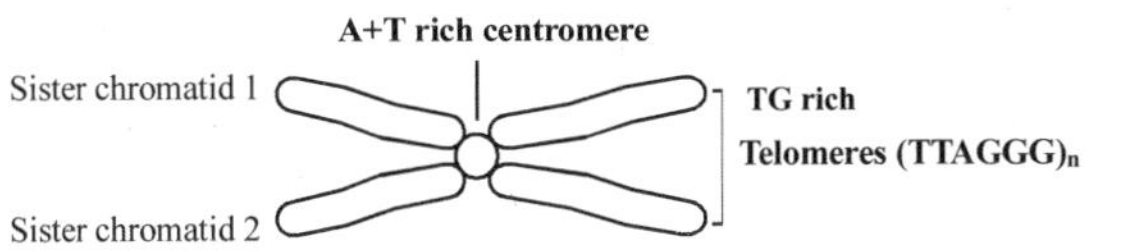


### Moderately Repititive Sequences

- Defined as being present in numbers of <$10^6$ *copies per haploid genome, are not clustered but are interspersed* with unique sequences.
- About half (45%) of human genome is made up of MRS which is derived from **transposable elements (transposons) – a kind of molecular parasite,** efficiently *making a home (or trapped) with in the host genome* during evolution.
- These DNA segments range from few *hundred to several thousand bp* long, that can *move from one location to another* in the genome (**transposition**) through an RNA intermediate by action of reverse transcriptase (i.e. **retroposons**).
- Many transposons have genes transcribed by RNA polymerase II encoding m-RNA (containing indistinguishable caps) and proteins that catalyze transposition process.
- Although these do not encode RNA or proteins used in human cells, they have played a major role in human evolution –as movement of transposons can l/t redistribution of other genomic sequences.
- Most transposons are **inactive**, evolutionarily altered by mutations, however, some may be active moving (transcribing) at a low frequency.
- Depending on their length MRS can be

**1. Long interspersed repeat sequences (LINEs):**

- **6 – 8 Kbp** (1 kbp = 1000bp) long and have 20-50 thousand copies (Harper)/8.5 lack LINEs (Lehninger) in human genome.
- It is species specific families of repeat element.

**2. Short interspersed repeat sequences (SINEs)**

- Are shorter (70-300 bp long) and have >1 lack copies per genome (Harper)
- Of 1.5 million in human genome >1 million are **Alu family**, so called because they generally have one copy of recognition sequence for AluI, restriction endonuclease (Lehninger).
- Alu elements (family) a/f 5-6% human genome (i.e. 5 lack copies per haploid genome). Harper it is **highly conserved** *within as well as between mammalian species.*
- SINEs are **mobile elements**, capable of jumping from one region to another region of genome and can l/t disastrous events as insertion of Alu sequences may cause *neurofibromatosis*.

**3. Retrovirus like transposons**

- 1.5 – 11 kbp long, 4.5 lack copies of these are present in human genome.
- Although evolutionarily related to retrovirus they are trapped & cannot move from one cell to another.

**4. Transposon remnants** that differ greatly in length

## Telomeres

- Telomeres are complexes of **non-coding DNA & protein** located at the ends of **linear eukaryotic chromosome**. (Greek telos = end).
- It consist of **many tandem** (one after another) **repeats** (> 20 to > 1500) **of short DNA sequence /oligo nucleotide** (dimeric to octameric). Telomere usually has **TG rich** *longer strand* and **AC rich** *shorter complementary strand*. The general formula is

| | |
|---|---|
| 5′- ($T_x$ $G_y$)n<br>3′ – ($A_x$ $C_y$)n | where x & y = Between 1 & 4 and number of telomere repeat **n** range from 20 -100 in single cell eukaryotes to >1500 in mammals |

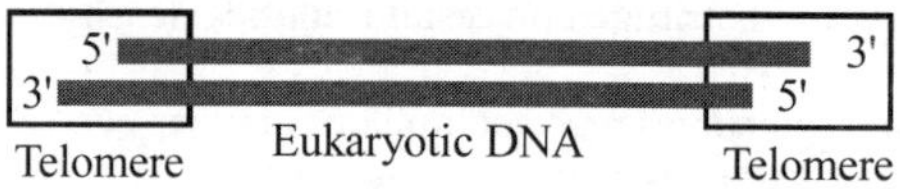


- Telomeres very in length from few dozen bp in protozoa to several thousands bp in mammals (humans). In humans, **non coding hexameric sequence $AG_3T_2$** base paired to complementary CA sequence forms telomere.

| Species | Telomere Repeat Sequence |
|---|---|
| **Human** | **(TTAGGG)n** |
| Thermophilic ciliated protozoa | **(TTGGGG)n** |
| Yeast | [$(TG)_{1-3}$ $(TG)_{2-3}$]n |
| Plant | (TTTAGGG)n |

- The **TG strand is longer** than its AC complement, leving a region of single stranded *(ss) DNA of few hundred nucleotides in length at the 3′ end.*
  Single stranded region (end) is folded back on itself, and paired with its complement in ds portion of telomere, forming a **T-loop structure**. The looped DNA is bound (stabilized) by several **telomere binding proteins**, including **TRF-1 & TRF-2 (telomere repeat binding factor)** with the latter protein involved in formation of T loop. It maintains the **structural integrity** and **confer stability** to chromosomal ends. T-loops *protect 3′ end*, making them *inaccessible to nucleases and enzymes* that repair double strand breaks, and allow repair system to *distinguish a true end from a break in ds DNA*. So telomeres *protect* chromosomal termini *from fusion & degradation.*

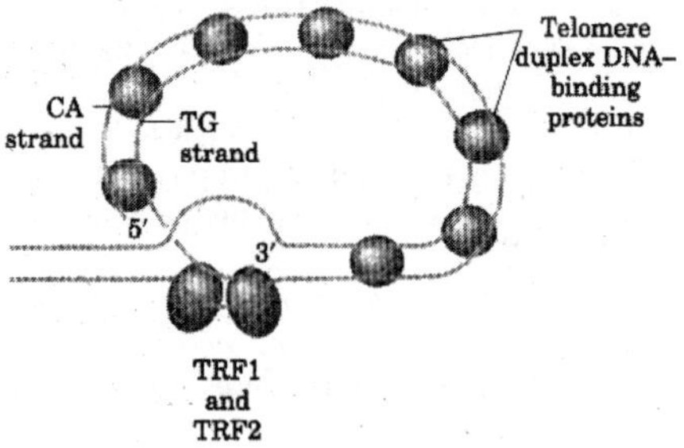


- Because DNA replication (by DNA polymerase) requires a template & primer, and beyond the end (extreme 5′ end) of lagging strand there is *no DNA template available for pairing of an RNA primer*. So **telomeres are not readily replicated by DNA polymerase** and consequently telomeres **shorten with each cell division** in most normal **somatic** human **cells.**
- There is a linear, inverse relationship between telomere length and cell senescence (cessation of cell division) or age. So telomerase is a **mitotic clock** in that their length in most cells is inversely related to the number of times cells have divided.
- Once the telomeres are shortened beyond a certain point, the loss of telomere function leads to activation of p53 dependent cell cycle check points, causing proliferation arrest & apoptosis. Thus *telomere shortening functions as a clock that counts cell divisions.* In germ cells, telomere shortening is prevented by the sustained function of enzyme telomerase, which maintains their ability to self replicate extensively. *Cancer cells show reactivation of telomerase activity* and maintenance of telomere length.

### Telomeres Repeats

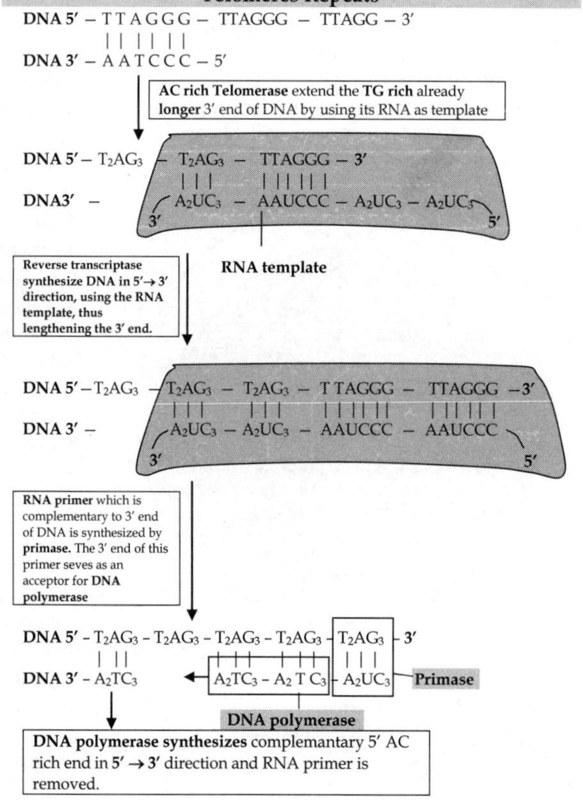


## Telomerase Enzyme

- It is a *multisubunit RNA containing-protein complex* with a **RNA dependent DNA polymerase** (i.e. **reverse transcriptase)** activity.
- It is responsible for **telomere synthesis and maintenance of telomere length.**
- Prevention of telomere shortening with every cell division, d/t activity of telomerase enzyme is the cause of **cellular immortality in cancer cells, germline cells and stem cells** as it protects from cellular aging & apoptosis.
- **Somatic cells lack telomerase** and *undergo cellular aging, senescence* ***(i.e. no longer able to divide) and death (apoptosis)***[Q] after 40-60 replications when telomeres become critically short or gone. So cells.

| With telomerase activity | Without telomerase activity |
|---|---|
| - *Germinal (Germline) cells*[Q]<br>- *Cancer (tumor)/ neoplastic cells*[Q]<br>- *Stem cells like hemopoetic cells*[Q] | *Somatic cells*[Q] |

- Telomerase contains a **protein** that acts as **reverse transcriptase and a short piece of (~150 nucleotide long) AC rich RNA** that acts as a **template** for synthesis of already longer TG (3′) strand.
- **CA-rich RNA template** (containing ~ 1.5 copies of Cy Ax telomere repeat) base pairs with *GT rich single stranded 3′ end of telomeric DNA*. The extra overhanging length of this RNA acts as a template for synthesis (lengthening) of already longer Tx Gy strand of telomere. **Reverse transcriptase** uses this RNA template to synthesize DNA in **5′→ 3′ direction**, extending the already longer 3′ (TG) end. However, unlike retroviral reverse transcriptase, telomerase copies only a small segment of RNA that it carries with itself.
- Having synthesized one copy of the repeat, the *telomerase repositions (translocates) to the newly synthesized end and the process is repeated* further lengthening already longer 3′ end (rich in TG).
- Once the GT rich 3′ end (strand) is appropriately lengthened, **primase** can use it as a template to synthesize a complementary **RNA fragment (primer)** opposite to TG strand. The RNA primer is extended by **DNA polymerase** & primer is removed.
- **This means 3′ TG rich end is synthesized by telomerase and complementary 5′ AC rich end is synthesized by DNA polymerase.**

## Structure of Chromosome & Chromatin

- Chromatin is the *chromosomal material in the nucleus* of eukaryotic cells. It is of 2 types – euchromatin & heterochromatin.

> - ***Less condensed (more open) & weakly staining, transcriptionally active***[Q] regions of chromatin are called **euchromatin**. So the euchromatin is the **dispersed (uncondensed)** portion of chromatin that is *transcriptionally active during interphase* (when RNA transcription occurs). In other words, *euchromatin contains genes capable of transcribing genetic information into proteins* that are necessary for young cells maturation, metabolic function or DNA repair.
> - Wheres, **highly condensed** & **strongly staining heterochromatin** is defined as a (chromotin) structure that does not alter inits condensation throughout the cell cycle (in contrast to euchromatin that decondense during interphase)

- Chromatin consists of *fibers containing (histone) protein and DNA in nearly equal proportions (by mass)*. Chromatin contains

> - Double stranded (ds) DNA ⎤ - Form **nucleosomes**
> - Small **basic proteins** k/a **histones** ⎦
> - Mostly acidic and larger (than histones) **non histone proteins**, that include enzymes involved in DNA replication & repair, and proteins involved in RNA synthesis, processing and transport to cytoplasm in smaller amounts
> - **RNA** (small quantity)

- DNA (in transcriptionally or potentially transcriptionally) active chromatin has larger regions (~ 1 lack bases long) that are relatively *more sensitive to digestion by nuclease* (like **DN ase I**, a *low sequence specific nuclease* that makes *single strand cuts* in nearly any segment of DNA that is not protected , or bound by protein into its component deoxynucleotides). The **sensitivity to DNase I** digestion reflects *only a potential for transcription rather than transcription* itself and can be associated with a relative **lack of 5-methyl deoxycytidine (meC)** in DNA and particular *(phosphorylation, acetylation etc) covalent modification of histones.*
- Shorter (100-300 nucleotides long), **Hypersensitive (10 times more sensitive)** sites to DN ase I exist in larger active chromatin. It is formedby *binding of non-histone regulatory transcriptional factor proteins* and proteins involved in maintaining access to template strand and result in structural conformation that favours access of nuclease to DNA. Hypersensitive regions are often **located immediately upstream from the active gene** that is capable of being transcribed.
- **Inactive chromatin** is *high in meC content in DNA and lower in covalent modifications of histones*. It can be of 2 types
  - **Constitutive hetero chromatin**, found in *centromere and telomeres* (i.e. chromosomal ends), is *always condensed* and thus *essentially inactive*.
  - **Facultative heterochromatin**, is at times condensed but at other times is uncondensed (appears as euchromatin) and is actively transcribed. Like *X chromosome* of females that is active only during gametogenesis.
- Approximately 1 m long DNA of 46 chromosomes is packed in small nucleus of each cell. This becomes possible only b/o multi levels of DNA compaction, condensing it to > 10000 ($10^4$) folds.

| **Chromatin form** | **Packing (Condensation) Ratio** | **Dia-meter** | **Features** |
|---|---|---|---|
| Nacked double helical DNA | 1 | 2 nm | |
| **10 nm chromatin fibrils** of **nucleosomes** | 7-10 | 10 nm | **Beads on string** form of chromatin |
| **30 nm chromatin fiber** of superhelical nucleosomes | 40-60 (Harper) /100 (Lehninger) | 30 nm | 10 nm fibril is further supercoiled with *6-7 nucleosomes per turn* to form 30 nm chromatin fiber: $H_1$ histones stabilize it and faces of nucleosome of successive turns would be nearly parallel to each other. |

## Nucleosomes

- Nucleosomes are *functional or originational units of chromatin* and appear as a **"beads on a string"** arrangement on electron microscopy.
- Flat protein cylinder consisting of **histone octamer** containing **2 molecules each of H3, H4, H2A & H2B** form tine **structural core of** individual **nucleosome beads**
- **(H3-H4)2 tetramer** itself can confer nuclesome like properties on DNA and so has a central role in nucleosome formation. Addition of **2 (H2A-H2B) dimmers** stabilize the primary particle & firmly binds two additional half turns of DNA previously bound only loosely to $(H_3\text{-}H_4)_2$.
- **Around the surface of disc shaped histone octamer (i.e. nucleosome protein core), the 1.75 superhelical turns** of DNA are wrapped (wound), forming **left handed solenoidal supercoil** (or **underwound** or **negatively supertwisted helix**), protecting 146 bp of DNA from digestion by a nuclease and forming the **nucleosome core particle.**
- Neighboring nucleosome core particles (beads) are linked by approximately 30 bp (Harper)/50 bp (Lippincot)/**54 bp** (Lehninger) long DNA segment termed as **linker. Histone H1** binds to the linker DNA. The bead plus the connecting DNA that leads to the next bead form the **nucleosome**. So nucleosomes are ***repeating units containing histones & 200 bp DNA (146 bp bound to core & 54 bp linker)***[Q].
- Tight wrapping of DNA around histone core *requires removal of 1 helical turn* in DNA, but because this process does not break the DNA (or change the linking number), the formation of a negative solenoidal supercoil must be accompanied by a compensatory positive super coil in unbound region of DNA. ***Eukaryotic topoisomerase*** *relax the unbound positive supercoil* (leaves the negative supercoil fixed to histone core) and results in an overall decrease in linking number. This is how eukaryotic DNA is underwound even through eukaryotic cells lack enzymes that underwind DNA.
- Majority of *core histone proteins interact with the DNA* on the inside of supercoil without protruding *except their amino terminal tails* which extend outside and are available for covalent modification.
- Nucleosome (histone) core exhibit **non random preferential binding (phasing)** to specific DNA sequence that has a local abundance of **A=T base pairs** in DNA where it is in contact with histones facilitating the compression of minor grooves that is needed for tight wrapping. Nucleosomes bind well to sequences where **AA** or **AT** or **TT** dinucleotides are staggered at 10 bp intervals. Phasing is d/t physical flexibility of certain sequences that are able to accommodate the regions of kinking within the supercoil.

| Loops (Domains) | 8000 | 300 nm | - 20-100 kbp (X 1000 bp) anchored in a **scaffolding (supporting) matrix** with in the nucleus (i.e. **nuclear matrix**) *containing $H_1$ histone and topoisomerase II, organize to form loops.*<br>- Looped domains contain a set of related genes corresponding to one or more separate genetic functions, containing both coding & non coding regions of cognate gene or genes. |
|---|---|---|---|
| **Rosette** | 6 loops | condense to form 1 rosette | |
| **Coil** | 30 rosettes | condense to form 1 coil | |
| **Chromatids** | 10 coils | condense to form each chromatid (of 1400 nm diameter) | |

## Chromatin Proteins

**1. Histone proteins**

- Histones are **small, basic proteins**Q, which package the DNA into structural units called **nucleosomes.**
- Carboxy terminal (2/3) of histone molecules are hydrophobic, while amino terminal (1/3) is rich in basic' amino acids.
- Histone proteins are *most abundant chromatin protein*. These are **positively charged** at physiological pH because of their **high content of basic amino acids arginine and lysine** and hence form **ionic bonds** with negatively charge DNA. Histones, along with positively charged ions like $Mg^{++}$ neutralize the negatively charged DNA phosphates.
- There are five classes of histones: *H1, H2A, H2B, H3, H4.* H1 histones are least tightly bound to chromatin and are, therefore, easily removed with salt solution, after which chromatin becomes soluble. The organizational unit of this soluble chromatin is the nucleosome. ***Nucleosome*** contains four type of histones- *H2A, H2B, H3, H4*; collectively called ***core histones.***
- The **histones interact** with each other in a very specific ways. H3 and H4 form a tetramer containing two molecules of each **(H3-H4)$_2$**, while **H2A and H2B form dimmers (H2A-H2B).** Under physiological conditions, these histone oligomers associate to form the **histone octamer (H3-H4)2 - (H2A-H2B)2.**
- **H3** and **H4 histones** are most conserved among eukaryotes f/b other core histones (H2A, H2B). This indicates that function of histones is identical in all eukaryotes and that the entire molecule is involved in carrying out this function.
- H1 histone is most tissue specific & species specific of histones. It facilitates the packing of nucleosoe into more compact structure.
- The four core histones are subjected to at least *six types* of covalent modification. Mn: **"RUPAM"** i.e. **R**ibosylation, **U**biquitin binding, **P**hosphorylation, **A**cetylation, **M**ethylation.

| Covalent Modification | DNA Repair |
|---|---|
| **ADP-Ribosylation** | - DNA repair |
| **Covalent linkage to Ubiquitin** | |
| - **Monoubiquitylation** | - Gene activation, repression, and heterochromatic gene silencing |
| - **Sumoylation** (SUMO; small ubiquitin – related modifier) | - Transcription repression |
| - Phosphorylation of $H_1$ | - Condensation of chromosomes during replication cycle |
| Acetylation | |
| - of core histones | - Chromosomal assembly during DNA-replication |
| - of H3 & H4 histones | - Activation & inactivation of gene transcription |
| Methylation | - Activation & repression of gene transcription |

- **Histone acetylation (by histone acetyl transferase = HAT)** causes ***increased (trancriptionally active) relatively uncondensed euchromatin formation***Q. Acetylation or phosphorylation of lysine residue at aminoterminal **decreases positive (+) charge of basic histone protein**, there by decreasing their association with negatively (-) charged DNA, thus releasing nucleosomes and allowing access to DNA. **Histone deacetylation (by histone deacetylase = HDAC)** removes acetyl group, restores positive charge and causes **increased formation of transcriptionally inactive hetero chromatin (relatively condensed).**

- Nucleosomes are deposited on DNA in a stepwise manner (during replication or other process that require a transient displacement) mediated by **RCAF** *(replication coupling assembly factor)* which includes acetylated H3 & H4, chromatin assembly factor-1 / **CAF1** and anti silencing factor / **ASF-1**). $(H_3\text{-}H_4)_2$ tetramer binds first f/b (H2A – H2B) dimmer.

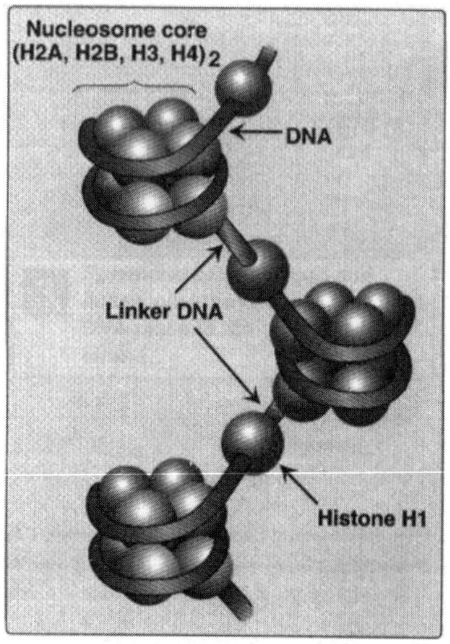


Organization of human DNA illustrating the sequence of nucleosomes

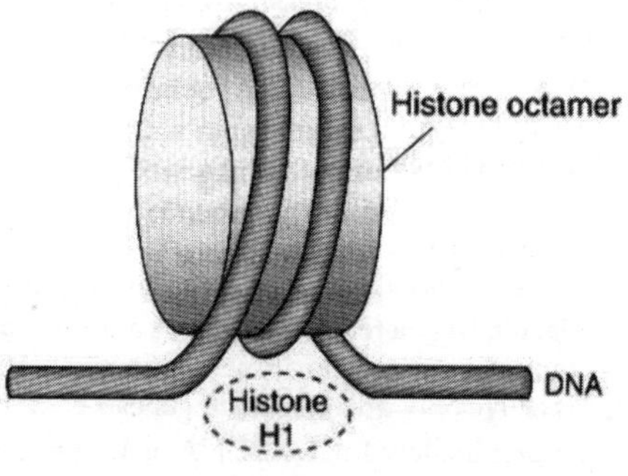


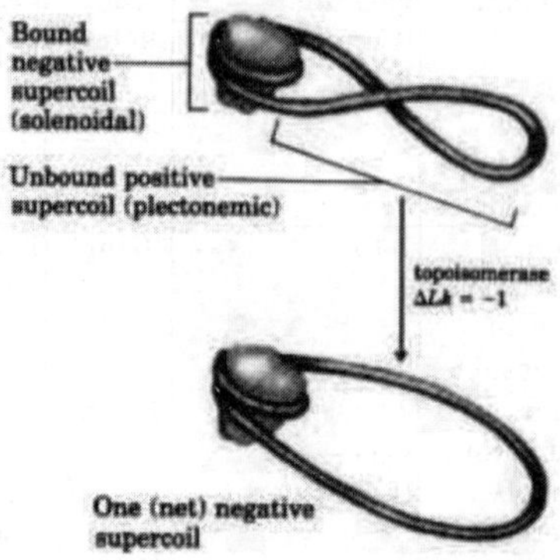

**2. Topoisomerase**

It relax *the compensatory positive plectonemic supercoil* in unbound region of DNA produced d/t negative solenoidal supercoiling of DNA around histone core.

**3. SMC (Structural maintenance of chromosomes) proteins**

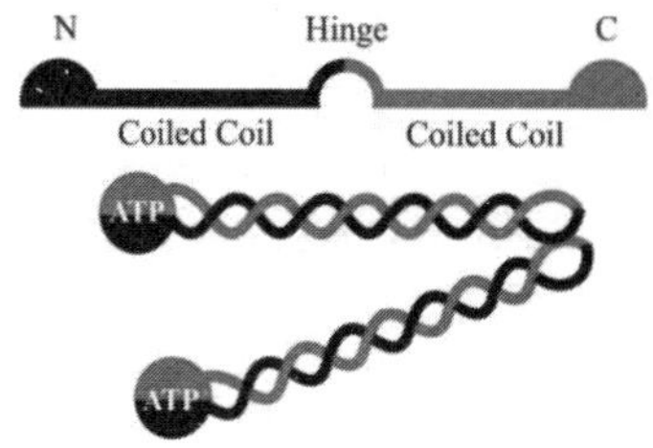


- SMC proteins *maintain structures of condensed chromosomes* and consist of 5 domains globular amino (N) & carboxy (C) terminals *with partial ATP hydrolytic site (on each* and becomes complete on joining). These 2 N & C terminals are joined by *2α-helical coiled coil motifs* joined by a hinge domain.
- **Cohesins** & **Condensins** are 2 SMC proteins. Condensins bind to DNA and *creates positive super coils* (i.e. DNA becomes **over wound** in contrast to underwinding introduced by binding of nucleosomes). So condensins are essential to chromosomal condensation as cell enters mitosis.
- **Cohesins** link sister chromatids together immediately after replication & keep them together as chromosomes condense to metaphase – a process essential for proper segregation of chromosomes at cell division. **Cohesin & Kleisin** form a ring around replicated chromosomes that tie them together (expand & contract in response to ATP hydrolysis) until separation is required at cell division.

## Supercoiling & Linking Number

- **Supercoiling** means the coiling of a coil. DNA is coiled in form of a double helix, with both strands of DNA coiling around an axis. The further coiling of that axis upon itself produce DNA super coiling, which is a *manifestation of structural strain*. When there is no net bending of DNA axis upon itself, the DNA is said to be in relaxed state.
- Supercoiling is an *intrinsic property* of DNA *tertiary structure* which is requied for DNA compaction. Replication & transcription of DNA also affect & are affected by supercoiling. It is studied in topology, a branch of mathemetics.

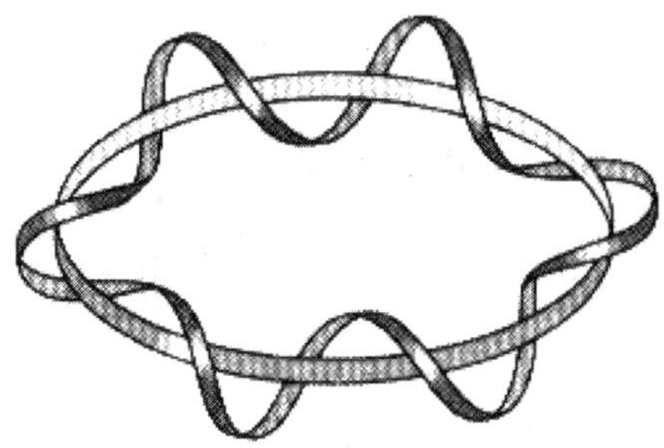

$Lk = 6$

- Closed circular (B form) DNA with **one turn of double helix per 10.5 base pair** is relaxed. Supercoiling is a manifestation of structural strain. And in almost every instance, the strain is a result of **underwinding** of DNA double helix in the closed circle. In other words, *DNA has fewer helical turns than would be expected for the B form* structure. An 84 bp segment of a circular DNA in relaxed state would contain 8 double helical turns, or 1 of every 10.5bp. If one of these turns were removed, there would be (84 bp) / 7= 12 bp / turn rather than 10.5 bp/ turn in B- DNA. This deviation from most stable form would result in a thermodynamically strained DNA
- In principle, the strain could also be accommodated by separating the two DNA strand over a distance of about 10 bp. But in isolated circular DNA the strain introduced by ***under winding is generally accommodated by supercoiling rather than strand seperation***[Q], because coiling the axis of DNA usually requires less energy than breaking the hydrogen bonds that stabilize paired bases. However underwinding represents a *form of stored energy and makes separation of DNA strands easier*
- ***Most cells maintain DNA in under wound state to facilitate its compaction by coiling***[Q].
- **Linking number**, is a topological property of ds DNA, because it does not vary when DNA is bent or deformed, as long as both strands remain intact. Linking number can be defined as the number of times the 2nd strand pierces the surface of 1st strand which is visualized as circle. It is defined **as positive (+ve)** if strands are interwound in *right handed helix and* ***negative (-ve)*** *in left handed helix* (not encountered).

$$\text{Linking number} = \frac{\text{Number of base pairs}}{\text{Number of base pairs per turn (which is 10.5 in relaxed form)}}$$

So linking number is number of turns.

- **Superhelical density** or **specific linking difference (σ)** is a measure of number of turns removed relative to the number present in relaxed DNA. It is ***independent of the length of DNA molecule***[Q]. The **negative** sign indicates that the change in linking number is d/t ***underwinding of DNA***[Q]. So the supercoiling induced by underwinding is called **negative supercoiling**. Over wound results in positive superwinding (which is a mirror image of negative supercoiling).

$$\sigma = \frac{\Delta Lk\,(\text{number of turns removed})}{Lko\,(\text{number of turns present in relaxed DNA})}$$

σ = - 0.01 means that 1% of helical turns present in B form of DNA has been removed. The degree of underwnding in cellular DNAs generally falls in range of 5-7%, that is σ = - 0.05 to - 0.07.

- Linking number (Lk) can be changed by $\pm 1$ by breaking one DNA strand, rotating one of the ends 360° about the unbroken strand, & rejoining the broken ends. This change has no effect on no. of base pairs. Lk can be broken down to **twist (Tw)** and **writhe (Wr)**, which are geometric rather than topological properties, because they may be changed by deformation.

$$Lk = Tw + Wr$$

- Writhe is a measure of coiling of helix axis and twist (Tw) determines the local twisting or spatial relationship of neighbouring base pairs.
- **Topoisomerase** *enzymes increase or decrease the extent of DNA underwinding* and so the linking number
  - **Topoisomerase type I**, act by transiently breaking one of the two strands, passing the unbroken strand through the break & rejoining the broken end; they ***change Lk in increments of 1***[Q].
  - **Topoisomerase type II** ***break both DNA strands & change linking number in increments of*** 2[Q].

## DNA Replication (Initiation, Synthesis, Elongation and Termination)

### Initiation of DNA Synthesis

- It ***follows base pair rule and is semiconservative***[Q] because, although the parental double strands are separated into two halves & therefore is not conserved as entily, each of the individual parental strands remains intact in one of the two daughter chromatids. Each strand of double helix (strand) serves as template for constructing a complementry daughter strand (**semiconservative strand**).
- The site at which the DNA replication is initiated is termed the **origin of replication (Ori)**. In prokaryotes, **Dna A** (a DNA binding protein) binds to **repeated nucleotide consensus (highly conserved) sequences** located within the origin. Binding of 20-30 Dna A molecules to ori induces unwinding, which separates strands in AT rich region adjacent to Dna A- binding sites, that is easy to unwind and is called **DNA unwinding element (DUE)**. The E coli replication origin is called **ori C**. Functionally similar **autonomously replicating sequences (ARS) or replicators** occur in **yeast cells**. The ARS contains degenerate 11 bp sequence, **origin replication element (ORE)** that binds to set of protein analogous to dna A of E.coli and form **origin recognition complex (ORC)**.
- Now the **hexameric protein Dna B** – binds to separated DNA strands. **Dna B has helicase activity** that catelyzes ATP mediated unwinding of DNA helix. DNA gyrase also participates in separation of strands. As this complex continues unwinding DNA strands in both direction from Ori, **SSBP (single stranded DNA- binding protein)** coat the separated strands to ***inhibit their reassociation (i.e. prevent premature reanneiling)***[Q]. DNA replication ***begins at origin of replication (ori) in S phase. The strands are seperated locally forming 2 replication forks***[Q]. Double stranded DNA's replication is **bidirectional. Helicase** *unwinds, seperates the double helix,* which produces *positive supercoil in the region of DNA ahead of replication fork.* **DNA topoisomerase I & II** remove suprecoils.

### Elongation Phase of Replication (Chain Elongation)

- Two strands of double stranded DNA molecules are **antiparallel**. The **DNA replication** in eukaryotes & prokaryotes ***occur on both strands simultaneously by a single asymmetric DNA polymerase III dimer***[Q]. Because , an enzyme capable of polymerizing DNA in 3′ to 5′ direction does not occur in nature, *so both of newly replicated DNA strands cannot grow in the same direction simultaneously.*
- **Replication exhibits polarity** because DNA polymerases responsible for copying the DNA templates are only able to **read** parental nucleotide sequences **in 3′ → 5′ direction and** they **synthesize** the new DNA strands **only in 5′ → 3′ (antiparallel) direction**
- Because of **unidirectional (5′ → 3′) synthetic activity** of polymerase and the antiparallel nature of two strands, the synthesis of DNA along the two strands is different and in **opposite direction**. **DNA polymerase** synthesize new DNA strand only in **5′ → 3′**direction, which is *towards (in the direction of advancing) replication fork* in **leading** strand and *away from replication fork* in **lagging** strand. DNA polymerase require **primer** (a short stretch of RNA), synthesized by **DNA primase**. The leading strand only needs one, whereas lagging strand needs *many primers*. The **leading strand** is ***replicated in a continuous fashion***[Q]. However, for the **lagging strand**, ***RNA primers are periodically added by DNA primase***[Q] along the strand. DNA polymerase III elongates these RNA primers to form Okazaki fragments.
- So the **leading strand** is produced as a **single, long continuous strand** (in 5′→ 3′ direction) **from a single primer** with the same overall forward direction. But the **lagging strand** is synthesized in **small fragments** (1000-5000 bp length) termed **Okazaki fragments** in a **discontinuous manner**, in 5′→ 3′ direction, but at the same time it faces towards the back end of the preceding RNA primer rather than toward the unreplicated portion. So overall DNA synthesis is **semi discontinuous (continuous in leading & discontinuous in lagging strand**).
- Replication proceeds from **single origin (ori) in prokaryotic** bacterial chromosome. In eukaryotic metazoan (mammals etc), the replication is **bidirectional (ie occurs in both directions)** and replication **proceeds from multiple origins** in each chromosome (~ 100 in humans). Thus replication **occurs in both directions and both strands are replicated simultaneously** generating **replication bubbles**.

**Proteins Required to Initiate Replication**

| Protein | No of sub units | Function |
|---|---|---|
| Dna A protein | 1 | - **Recognizes replication origin (ori) sequence** and opens duplex at specific sites in origin.<br>- This member of **AAA + AT pase protein** family has ATP bound active & ADP bound inactive forms. It has higher affinity for **R sites** (5 repeat of 9 base pair consensus sequence = TT (A/T) TNCACC) than I sites in ori. R-sites can bind to both active & inactive Dna A protein whereas, *I sites bind only the active ATP bound Dna A allowing* discrimination.<br>- **8 molecules of ATP bound (active) Dna A proteins form a helical complex and bind at R and I sites in origin (ori)** Tight right handed helical wrapping of DNA around this complex produces **a positive supercoil**. The resultant strain in near by DNA l/t **denaturation in A=T rich DUE (DNA unwinding element) region of ori** (ie tandem array of three 13 bp consensus sequence GATCTNTTNTTTT). |
| **HU, FIS*, IHF**<br><br>* = Identical sub units | 2 | - **Histone like bacterial protein (HU) or factor U, factor for inversion stimulation (FIS) and Integration host factor (IHF) are DNA binding proteins** which stimulate initiation by *facilitating formation of helical Dna A complex.*<br>- FIS & IHF have specific binding site in ori whereas HUS does not have a specific site. 2 subunits of FIS are identical (not of IHF and HU) |
| **Dna C protein** | 6* | - An AAA – ATPase protein **required for Dna B (helicase) binding or londing onto separated DNA strands** in the denatured region at origin. (**keystep** in initiation)<br>- Hexamer of Dna C (with ATP bound to each subunit) forms tight complex with hexameric, ring shaped Dna B helicase. This interaction **opens the ring of Dna B and results in loading of 2 ring shaped Dna B hexamers in DUE, one onto each strand**. The ATP bound to Dna C is hydrolyzed, releasing the Dna C and leaving Dna B (helicase) bound to DNA. |

- Entire protein complex at replication fork k/a **DNA replicase system or replisome** come into action. **Parental DNA is unwound by DNA B helicase** and **resulting topological stress is relieved by topoisomerases (I, II, gyrase).** Each **separated strand is stabilized by SSB (or RPA)** protein. Dna B helicase and Dna G primase form functional unit within replication complex k/a **primosome. Dna B helicase** bound in front, unwinds the DNA at replication fork as it moves **along the lagging strand template in 5′ → 3′ direction** and the primer is synthesized by **Dna G primese in 5′ → 3′ direction** but the direction **opposite to that in which Dna B helicase is moving**. However the first primer laid down serves to prime leading strand DNA synthesis in opposite direction.
- Once the strands are sufficiently unwound (seperated) by helicase, the DnaG primase (of primosome) synthesize RNA oligo nucleotides complementary to each parental DNA strand which serves as primer for DNA synthesis. Once each RNA primer has been laid down, two DNA polymerase III **core subunit** complexes are assembled, one at each of the primed site.
- **Both leading and lagging strands are produced by a single asymmetric DNA polymerase III dimer** tethered to the lagging strand. This is accomplished by **using one set of core subunits (core polymerase)** to synthesize the leading strand, while the other set of core subunits cycles from one Okazaki fragment to the next on the looped lagging strand (ie core subunits are attached to both strands). **Looping of lagging strand** brings together the two points of polymerization.
- Prokaryotic DNA chain elongation is catabolized by **DNA polymerase III** using *5′ deoxyribonucleoside triphosphate as substrate.* It ***proof reads & has 3′→ 5′exonuclease activity. RNA primers are removed by DNA polymerase I using its 5′→3′ exonuclease activity***[Q]. *It fills the gap with DNA and proof reads* (during synthesis). So **DNA polymerase I** ***removes the RNA primer, replaces it with DNA and eventually join Okazaki fragments***[Q]. Finally, ***DNA ligase seals nick and join the lagging strand DNA fragments to form a continuous strand***[Q] by catalyzing *final phosphodiester linkage.*
- Eukaryotic DNA has 5 types. **Pol $\alpha$** is a multisubunit enzyme with **primase & 5′ → 3′polymerase activity**. It adds a short piece of DNA to RNA, primer. **Pol $\delta$** completes DNA synthesis on leading strand and elongates each lagging strand fragment using 3′ → 5′exonuclease activity to *proof read.* **Pol β & pol ε** are involved with *DNA repair.* **Pol** *$\gamma$ replicates mitochondrial DNA.* Eukaryotes have many more ori and contain a **licencing factor** to insure that excess amount of unfinished replicating DNA do not accumulate.
- When the 3′ end of elongating Okazaki fragment, reaches the 5′ end of previously synthesized, DNA polymerase III release the template & find another primer further back along lagging strand synthesizing another okazaki fragment.
- Proteins of replisome include **Dna B helicase, DnaG primase, DNA gyrase (topoisomerase II), SSB, DNA polymerase III & I and DNA ligase.**

| | |
|---|---|
| **DNA Polymerase** | - Polymerize deoxyribonucleotide (DNA) and share 3 comon properties<br>1. **Chain elongation**: It is d/t **5′ -3′ polymerase activity** accounting for the rate (in nucleotides per second = ntd/s) at which polymerization occurs<br>2. **Processivity** : It is an expression of number of nucleotides added to nascent (new) chain before the polymerase disengages from the templet.<br>3. **Proof reading:** It is d/t **3′ – 5′ exonuclease** activity that identifies copying errors & corrects them. |
| **DNA polymerase I** | - Gap filling in lagging strand, proof reading & repair<br>- Mostly involved in *host clean up functions* during replication, recombination & repair (d/t 5′ → 3′ exonuclease activity)<br>- It *locates space (nick) between 3′ end of DNA newly synthesized (by polymerase III) & 5′ end of adjacent RNA primer.* |

| | | |
|---|---|---|
| **DnaB protein (Helicase) & MCM helicase** | 6* | - Helicase (Dna B) binds to single strand DNA near replication fork (V) and then **move along the SS DNA (that becomes lagging strand) in 5′ → 3′** direction into the neighboring double stranded region, forcing them apart –in effect **processive unwinding the ds DNA** to provide ss DNA as it travels. It requires energy provided by ATP. Dna B is principal helicase of E.coli.<br>- Thus **both Dna B halicases** loaded on to the two strands of DNA **travel in opposite directions, creating 2 replication V or Y forks.**<br>- All other proteins at replication fork are linked directly or indirectly to Dna B. pol III holoenzyme is linked through τ subunit.<br>- In eukaryotes, a heterohexameric, ring shaped complex of **minichromosome maintenance (MCM) helicase** (MCM 2 to MCM 7) functions like prokaryotic Dna B helicase. MCM is loaded on to DNA by a hexameric protein complex **ORC (origin recognition complex)** = Key step |
| **Stabilizing proteins: Single stranded DNA Binding protein (SSB) & Replication Protein A (RPA)** | 4* | - Seperation of DNA double helix is promoted by **single stranded DNA binding protein** (SSB) in prokaryotes and **replication protein A (RP-A)** in eukaryotes.<br>- These bind co-operatively & stoichiometrically to SS DNA with out interfering with the abilities of neucleotides to serve as template. So these **stabilizes the single stranded structure as replication fork progresses.**<br>- These proteins (not enzymes) ***keep the two strands of DNA separated by preventing premature reanneiling of ds DNA***[Q].<br>- *Protect DNA from nuclease that cleaves ss DNA*<br>- Bind to ss DNA created by helicase **cooperatively** – i.e., the binding of one molecule of SSB protein makes it easier for additional molecules of SSB protein to bind tightly. |
| **DNA Grayse** | 4 | - A **DNA topopscmerase II relieves torsional strain / topological stress (positive super coil or suprtwist)** induced ahead of replication fork by the helicase induced unwinding process. |

| | |
|---|---|
| | - Next, it removes RNA nucleotides (primer) ahead of itself moving in 5′→ 3′ direction (by its **(5′ → 3′ exonuclease activity)** and synthesizes DNA/chain elongation (by its **5′ → 3′ polymerase activity)**. During synthesis it also *proofreads* the new chain using **3′ → 5′ exonuclese activity**.<br>- This **removal – synthesis – proofreading** continues one nucleotide at a time, until the RNA is totally degraded & replaced with DNA<br>- The *5′ → 3′* ***exonuclease activity is specific to DNA polymerase I and is responsible for Nick translation***[Q]<br>- 5′→ 3′ exonuclease can remove *1 or upto 10, properly base paired or altered,* nucleotides (either ribonucleotides or deoxyribonucleotides) of RNA or DNA at a time. This ability is important in repair of damaged DNA.<br>When 5′ →3′ exouclease domain is removed the remaining large fragment is k/a **Klenow fragment** |
| **DNA polymerase II** | - DNA proof reading & repair |
| **DNA polymerse III** | - ***Processive leading strand and okazaki fragment synthesis***[Q].<br>It is a *assembly of 13 protein subunits (of a different types)* |

| | Subunit | No. per holo-enzyme | Gene | Function | |
|---|---|---|---|---|---|
| **Core polymerase** | α | 2 | pol **C** (dna **E**) | **Polymerization activity** | |
| | ε | 2 | mut **D** (dna **Q**) | **3′ → 5′ Proof reading exonuclease** | |
| | θ | 2 | hol **E** | Stabilization of ε subunit | |
| **Clamps** | β | 4 | dna **N** | DNA **donut shaped sliding clamps** required for optimal processivity (one dimer clamp per core subassembly). | |
| **Clamp loading (γ) complex** | τ | 2 | dna **X** | Stable template binding; core enzyme dimerization | |
| | γ | 1 | dna **X*** | Clamp loader | *Clamp loading (γ) complex loads β subunits on lagging strand at each okazaki fragment. It has 5 subunits cf 4 different types $\tau^2\ \gamma\ \delta^1\delta$ |
| | $\delta^1$ | 1 | hol **B** | Clamp loader | |
| | δ | 1 | hol **A** | Clamp opener | |
| | χ **(Chi)** | 1 | hol **C** | Interacts with SSB | |
| | ψ **(Psi)** | 1 | hol **D** | Interacts with γ and χ | |

| | |
|---|---|
| **DNA ligase** | - **Nick sealing enzymes** that **seals (ligates) nick created by removal of DNA polymerase I in lagging strand** (backbone of DNA in form of broken phosphodiester bond) by **using ATP**<br>- Forms final phosphodiester linkage b/w 5′ PO4 group on nascent DNA chain synthesized by DNA polymerase III & 3′ OH group on chain mede by DNA polymerase I |

★ ψ subunit is generated by translational frame shifting (of portion of gene for τ subunit) that l/t premature translational termination

### Termination of DNA Synthesis

- 2 replication forks of circular prokaryotic DNA meet at **terminus region containing multiple copies of 20 bp sequences called Ter**. Ter sequences function as **binding sites for protein terminal utilization substance (Tus) and create a trap that a replication fork can enter but cannot leave**.
- Tus – Ter complex can arrest a replication fork **from only one direction**. Only one Tus-Ter complex functions per replication cycle – the complex **first encountered by either** replication fork.
- Because opposing replication forks usually halt when they collide, Ter sequences would not seem essential, but they may **prevent over replication by**

| | | |
|---|---|---|
| | | - A *type II topoisomerase* that has unusual property of being able to ***introduce negative supercoils into relaxed circular DNA by using energy (ATP)***[Q]. This *facilitates the future replication of DNA* because negative supercoiling neutralize positive supercoils introduced during opening of ds DNA. Also aids *transient strand separation.* |
| **DnaG (Primase)** | 1 | - DNA primase is a specific **RNA polymerase** that **synthesize** short (~ 10 nucleotide long) stretches of RNA that are complementary and antiparallel to DNA template and are k/e **RNA primer**<br>- As with DNA synthesis the direction of primer synthesis is **5′ → 3′. One primer (& primase) is required for leading strand and many for lagging strand**.<br>- Helicase associates with primase to provide it proper access to the template. This mobile complex of helicase & primase is called **primosome**.<br>- Primer synthesis is important since, DNA polymerase cannot initiate DNA synthesis denovo (without primer). |
| **Hda** | - | - **Homologous to Dna A** (or **Hda**) is a AAA + ATPase that *binds to beta subunit of DNA polymerase III* and interacts with Dna A to stimulate hydrolysis of its bound ATP. This ATP hydrolysis **disassembles the Dna A complex at origin**. That is why, *loading of DNA pol III beta subunits on to the DNA signals completion of initiation* phase |
| **Dam Methylase** | 1 | - Methylates N 6 position of adenine within the palindromic sequence (5′) G ATC at origin (in Ecoli). **Dam stands for DNA adenine methylation** and **it affects timing of replication initiation**.<br>- Immediately after replication, DNA is hemimethylated at ori ie parent strands methylated but newly synthesized strand do not. The DNA **must be fully methylated before** it again binds Dna A and initiates new replication eg cycle. |

**one fork in the event** that the other is delayed or hated by an encounter with DNA damage or other problem. So, ***when either replication fork first encounters a Tus-Ter complex, it halts; the other replication fork halts when it meets the first arrested fork.***

- Final few hundred bps are replicated by unknown mechanism completing two **topologically interlinked (catenated)** circular chromosomes (k/a **catenanes**). The circles are not covalently linked, but because they are inter wound and each is covalently closed, they cannot be separated. Separation of catenanes requires **topoisomerase IV (a type II topoisomerase)** which transiently breaks both DNA strands of one chromosome and allowing the other chromosome to pass through the break.
- In eukaryotes, telomeres are synthesized.

| | |
|---|---|
| **Topoisomerase** | - ***Relieves torsion strain (supercoiling or supertwisting) that result from helicase induced unwinding***[Q] in the region of DNA ahead of replication fork. The swivel function is provided by introducing nicks in strand, thereby allowing unwinding & then resealing the nicks. These are of 2 types |
| **Type I topoisomerase** | - Have both **nuclease (strand cutting)** and **ligase (strand/nick sealing)** activity. They *do not require ATP*, but rather appear to *store the energy* for phosphodiester bond they cleave, reusing the energy to reseal the strand.<br>- It *reversibly creates a transient nick (cut) in one strand* of ds DNA. The intact DNA strand is passed through the break before it is resealed, thus relieving (relaxing) accumulated supercoils.<br>- Type I topoisomerase *relax negative supercoils in E. coli, and both negative & positive supercoils in eukaryotes*. (**Positive supercoil** is produced by twisting *in the direction of tightening* of strands so the DNA would contain more turns of helix than relaxed DNA. Whereas, the **negative supercoil** is produced by twisting *in the direction of loosening* the strands; so the negatively super twisted DNA would contain fewer turns of helix than relaxed DNA). |
| **Type II topoisomerase** | - Make *transient break in both strands* and *relieve both positive & negative supercoils* by utilizing *ATP*<br>- Required in both prokaryotes & eukaryotes for separation of interlocked molecules of DNA following chromosomal replication. |

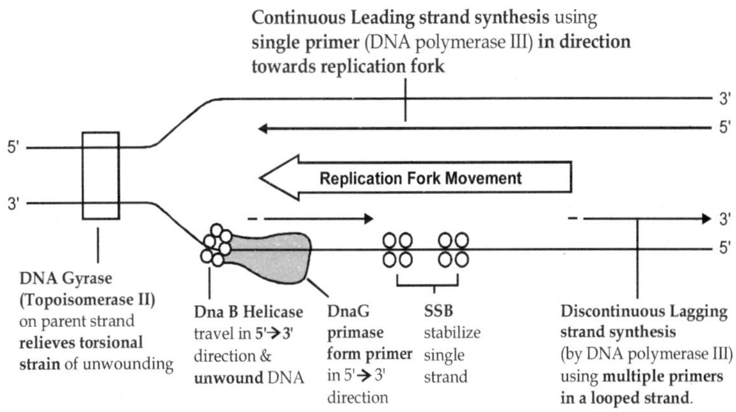

## Steps in DNA Replication

**Identify origin of replication** (ori)

- Specific site where replication start.
- *A + T rich region* adjacent to 'ori'

**Formation of Replication fork**
**By locals seperation of strands**

Leads to

**Positive supercoils** in the region of DNA ahead of replication fork which is removed by

***DNA topoisomerase I & II*[Q]**

- They have both *nuclease* (strand cutting) & ligase activity.
- First a transient nick is created in one strand, which relieves super coils, then it is resealed.

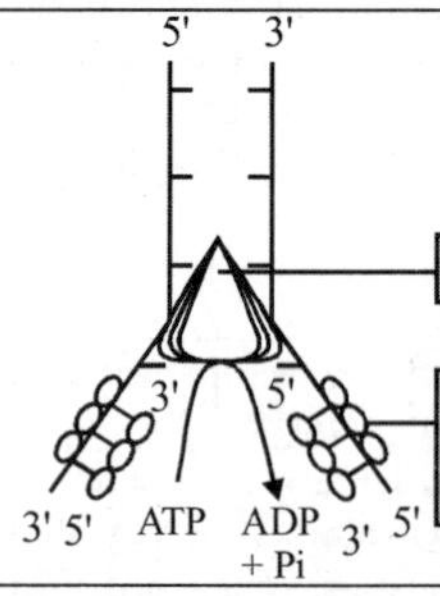


Helicase
- ***Unwinds the double helix*[Q]**
- Requires energy by ATP.

Single strand DNA binding Protein
- ***Keep the two strands of DNA separate*[Q].**

**RNA Primer**
- Required for initiation of DNA synthesis by DNA polymerase
- It is short strech of RNA that are complementary & antiparallel to DNA template
- Synthesized by ***Primase a specific RNA polymerase*[Q]**

**Replication fork**

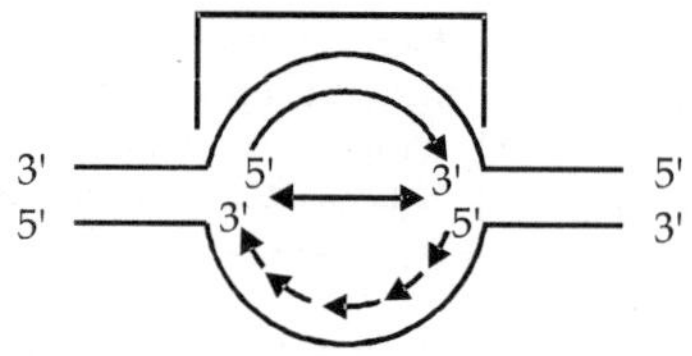


**Bidirectional - Replication Bubble**

**Initation of DNA synthesis and elongation** by

**DNA polymerase III**

- Recognizes primer & ***synthesizes DNA in 5'→3' direction*[Q]** (read template in 3' →5' direction) by 5'→3' polymerase activity
- *Proof reading* of newly synthesized DNA by its ***3→ 5' exonuclease activity*[Q]**.

Both strand of double helix serve as template for constructing tow complementary strands

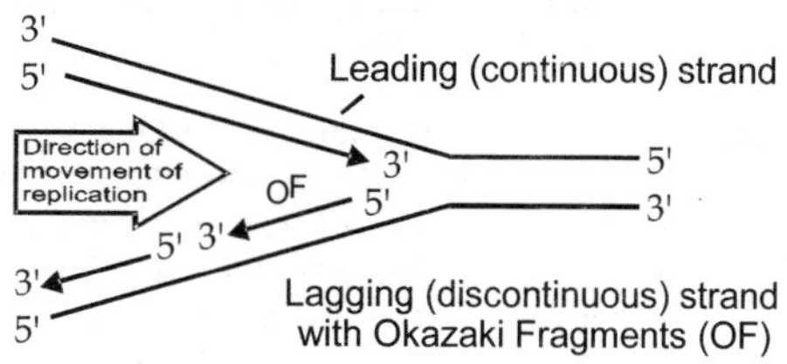


New **DNA strands** consisting of

**One leading strand**
- Synthesized in 5'→3' direction *towards the replication fork.*
- Requires *only one RNA primer*

**One lagging strand**
- Synthesized in 5'→3' direction *away from the replication fork in discontinuous manner.*
- Short stretches of discontinuous DNA called ***okazaki fragments.***
- Requires many RNA primer

***DNA polymerase I*[Q]**
- **5'→3' exonuclease activity** (degrade/excise primer)
- 5'→3' polymerase activity fill the gap produced by primer excision
- 3'→5' exonuclease activity is for proof reading.

**Excision of RNA primer and their replacement by DNA (Nick translation )**

***DNA ligase*[Q]**

**Joining of two stretches of DNA** & fill the gap produced by removal of DNA polymerase I. So it seals the nick on lagging strand **(Nick sealing)**

## DNA Polymerase Complex

### Prokaryotic DNA Polymerase

- **DNA polymerases III (pol III) catalyzes the highest rate of chain elongation (polymeriztion)** and is the **most processive** (polymerizing 0.5 Mb DNA in one cycle on leading strand).
- Pol III is > 1MDa (large), multi (13) subunit protein complex. Its association with 2 identical **beta subunits of DNA sliding clamp** markedly increases the **stability, rate of chain elongation** (20-50 nt/s) **and processivity** (100 to > 50 thousand nucleotides) of DNA polymerase III enzyme.
- **DNA polymerase I & II (pol I & II)** are mostly involved in **proof reading and DNA repair**.

| Feature | DNA Polymerase | | |
|---|---|---|---|
| | I | II | III |
| ***5′→3′ Polymerase activity***[Q] | + | + | + |
| ***3′→5′ Exonuclease activity (Proof reading)***[Q] | + | + | + |
| ***5′→3′ Exonuclease activity***[Q] **(Excision – repair/nick translation)** | +[Q] | - | - |
| Repair | + | + | - |
| **Polymerization rate** (nucleotide/s) | 16-20 | 40 | 250-1000 |
| **Processivity** (nucleotides added before polymerase dissociates) | 3-200 | 1500 | ≥5 lacs |
| Subunits | 1 | 7 | ≥10 |
| Structural genes | pol A | pol B | **pol C (dnaE)** |

**Endonucleases** are enzymes that ***cleaves internal bonds in DNA & RNA***[Q].

### Eukaryotic DNA Polymerase (Lippincott)

- At least of 5 type & are designated by Greek letter rather than roman numbers (i.e. α, β, γ, δ, ε)
- **α is a multi subunit enzyme.**
  - One subunit has **primase activity**, which initiates strand synthesis on leading strand & at beginning of each Okazaki fragment on lagging strand.
  - Primase subunit synthesizes a short RNA primer that is extended by **α5′ → 3′ polymerase** activity, which adds a short piece of DNA
  - **Pol δ** is then recruited to complete DNA synthesis of leading strand & elongate each Okazaki fragment, using 3′→5′ exonuclease activity to proofread the newly synthesized DNA
  - DNA polymerase δ associates with proliferating cell nuclear antigen protein, which serves as a **sliding DNA clamp** (similar to β subunit of DNA polymerase III ensuring high processivity).

| DNA polymerase | Function | Proof Reading |
|---|---|---|
| **Pol α** | Contains **primase Initiates DNA synthesis** | - |
| **Pol β** | **Repair** | - |
| **Pol ε** | **Repair** | + |
| **Pol γ** | **Replicates** mitochondrial DNA | + |
| **Pol δ** | **Elongates** leading strands & okazaki fragment | + |

### Comparison (Harper)

All DNAP complex share 3 features

1. **Chain Elongation**: accounts for nucleotide per second rate (nt/s) at which **polymerization** occurs
2. **Processivity**: is number of nucleotides added to nascent chain before the DNA polymerase disengages from the template.
3. **Proof reading**: is *identification of copying errors and correcting them.*

| E.coli | Eukaryotic | Function |
|---|---|---|
| I | | **Gap filling (synthesis) of lagging strand** following DNA replication, repair & recombination |
| II | | DNA proof reading & repair |
| | β | ***DNA repair***[Q] |
| | γ | ***Mitochondrial DNA synthesis***[Q] |
| III | ε | Procssive, leading strand synthesis |
| DNA G | α | Primase |
| | δ | Processive, lagging strand synthesis. |

## Components of Nucleic Acid

### Nitrogen -Bases

- Purines & pyrimidines are *nitrogen & carbon containing heterocyclic aromatic compounds with a planar character* (i.e. two or more bases are positioned with the planes of their rings parallel like a stack of coins)- a feature that facilitates their close association or stalking that stabilizes double stranded DNA.
- Larger purine molecules and smaller pyrimidine molecules are numbered in opposite direction for their 6 atom main ring i.e. *clockwise for pyrimidine & anteclockwise for purine.*
- Free purines and pyrimidines with – $NH_2$ group are **weak bases**. Physiological pH strongly favour **oxo and amino groups** of purine and pyrimidine exhibiting *Keto-enol and amine- imine tautomerism.*

### Pentose Sugar : Nucleoside

- Addition of pentose sugar to nitrogenous base produces a **nucleoside**
- Sugar is **D-ribose** in ribonucleoside (of RNA) and **2-deoxy-D-riobse** in deoxy ribionucleotide (of DNA).
- Carbons of pentose sugars are prime numbered $1^1$ to 5′ distinguishing them from those of heterocycles. Hence, 5′ carbon of nucleoside (or nucleotide) means a carbon atom in pentose ring rather than atom in base.
- All bases are attached to pentose sugar by a **β-N- glycosidic bond** between $1^{st}$ carbon of pentose sugar and almost always to the **N-1 of pyrimidine or N-9 of purine**.
- **Nucleosides** are *N-glycosides* formed by addition of **pentose sugar (D-ribose or 2 deoxy D-ribose)** to a **purine (adenine, guanine) or pyrimidine (cytosine, thymine & uracil) bases**. Nucleosides with purine bases (A, G) have – **'sine'** suffix viz – ***adenosine, guanosine***[Q], whereas pyrimidine nucleosides have '**dine**' suppix viz – ***cytidine, thymidine and uridine***[Q].

| Purine Bases | Pyrmidine Bases | Present in |
|---|---|---|
| **Adenine = A**<br>**Guanine = G** | **Cytosine = C** | Both DNA & RNA |
| | **Thymine = T** | **DNA** |
| | **Uracil = U** | **RNA** |
| **Hypoxanthine** (6 oxopurine)<br>**Xanthine** (2, 6-dioxopurine)<br>**Uric acid** (2, 6, 8-trioxopurine) | - | **Minor bases** formed in catabolism of purines |
| N6, N6 dimethyl adenine | N4 acetyl cytosine<br>Dihydro uracil | **Unusual Bases** |

★ Methylation acetylation, glycosylation or reduction in some viral DNA & tRNA bases forms unusual buses which may aid in its recognition by specific enzymes or protect it from being degraded by nucleases.

★ T and U differ in that only T has a methyl group.

**Phosphate / Phosphoric Acid: Nucleotide**

- Nucleotides are **phosphorylated (i.e. phosphate esters of) nucleosides.**

**Nuceotide = Nucleoside + Phosphate or Phosphoric acid = Purine / Pyrimidine Base + Pentose (D-ribose / 2 deoxy D-ribose) sugar + Phosphate / Phosphoric acid**

- Nucleotides may contain 1, 2 or 3 phosphate groups and are called mono, di or tri phosphate nucleotides (i.e. MP, DP, or TP)
- 1st phosphate (phosphoryl) group is attached (esterified) to hydroxyl (OH) group of pentose sugar by ester linkage on 5' (mostly) or 3' (rarely) position. Since most are 5'-nucleotides or nucleoside 5′ phoshate (i.e. have phosphate at 5' position) the prefix "5'" is usually omitted when naming them.
- Suffix "**- sine/- nylate/- nylic acid**" for purine nucleotides & "**-dine/- dylate/-dylic acid**" for pyrimidine nucleotides are used.

| Pentose Sugar | Nitrogenous Base | Nucleoside | Nucleotide (Mono /Di /Tri- phosphate), Mono phosphate (MP) | NDP | NTP |
|---|---|---|---|---|---|
| **D-ribose** sugar forming simple nucleosides & nucleotides in RNA and **2-deoxy ribose** sugar forming **deoxy (or d-) nucleosides & nucleotides** in DNA. | **Adenine (A)** | Adenosine | **Adenosine /Adenylate /Adenylic acid**-mono phosphate (**AMP**) | ADP | ATP |
| | **Guanine (G)** | Guanosine | **Guanosine /Guanylate /Guanylic acid** - monophosphate (GMP) | GDP | GTP |
| | **Cytosine (C)** | Cytidine | **Cytidine /Cytidylate /Cytidylic acid** mono phosphate (CMP) | CDP | CTP |
| | **Thymine (T)** | Thymidine | Thymidine / Thymidylate / Thymidylic acid mono phosphate (TMP) | TDP | TTP |
| | **Uracil (U)** | Uridine | **Uridine /Uridylate /Uridylic acid** mono phosphate (UMP) | UDP | UTP |

★ Xanthine base form **Xanthosine** nucleoside and hypoxanthine base forms **inosine** nucleoside of RNA.

## Denaturation / Melting of DNA and $T_m$

- The ds-DNA can be separated into two strands (melted) in solution by *increasing the temperature or decreasing the salt concentration.* Denaturation is also called **a helix to coil transition.**
- Not only do the two stacks of bases pull apart but the bases themselves unstack while still connected in the polymer by the phosphodiester backbone.
- **Concomitant with the denaturation of DNA molecule** is *an increase in the optical absorbance of purines & pyrimidine bases* – a phenomenon referred to as ***hyperchromocity*** of denaturation. DNA loses its viscosity on denaturation .
- The denaturation (melting) is used to analyze the structure of DNA. Denaturation & renaturation of DNA are basis of **nucleic acid hybridization.**
- Separate strands of DNA will renature or reassociate when appropriate physiological temperature & salt conditions are achieved; this **reannealing** process is often referred to as **hybridization.** If melted sample of DNA is slowly cooled the absorbance of solution decreases, which is an indication of complementary strands being pulled again. Annealing can occur at a temperature below Tm of DNA (i.e. 70°c). It is fastest at 20°c below Tm (i.e. 50°c)
- Hybridization when combined with **gel electrophoresis (that separate nucleic acids by size)** & radioactive or fluorescent labeling resulting analytic technique is called **southern (DNA-DNA) & Northern (RNA - DNA) blotting.**

**Tm & Factors affecting Tm**

- It is the *temperature at which DNA is half denatured.* In other words, the strand of a given DNA molecule separate over a temperature range. The midpoint is called the **melting temperature** or **Tm**. It is calculated by nearest neighbour method.
- At Tm, the absorbance of DNA at **260 nm** is increased by **18.5%** i.e. half of **37%** increased in absorbane when DNA is completely denatured. It is called **hyperchromicity phenomenon or hyperchromic effect**.
- It is in influenced by
  - Both *length of DNA molecule & specific nucleotide sequence.* DNA rich in C ≡ G base pairs with 3 H bonds melts at higher temperature than that rich in **A = T base pairs with 2 hydrogen bonds.**
  - **Salt concentration of solution** influence the Tm because negatively charged PO4 in two strands are *shielded by positively charged ion (cation).* Decreased ionic concentration decrease the shielding effect, thus increase the repulsive forces b/w strands and reducing Tm.
  - So ***a ten fold increase in movalent cation concentration increase the Tm by 16.6°C*** Q
  - ***Formamide***, which is commonly used in recombinant DNA experiments and **urea** both of them destabilizes hydrogen bonding between bases, thereby lowering Tm. This allows the strands of DNA or DNA hybrids to be separated at much lower temperatures and minimizes the phosphodiester bond breakage that can occur at higher temperatures.

**Applications of Tm**

- Estimate amount of G & C content
- In PCR
- To detect sequence differences b/w strands & different DNAs
- As a proxy for equalizing the hybridization strength of molecule eg oligonucleotide probe of DNA microarray.

## Ultraviolet Spectrophotometry of Nucleic Acids

- *Electron delocalization* among atoms in aromatic rings of purine & pyrimidine bases give most of the bonds *partial double bond character*. **All nucleotide bases** (d/t conjugated double bond of purine / pyrimidine) ***absorb ultraviolet light***[Q] and nucleic acids (DNA /RNA) are characterized by a strong absorption at near **260 nm** wavelengths.
- *Mutagenic effect* of UV light is d/t its absorption by nucleotides in DNA l/t chemical modification.
- Although spectra is *pH dependent*, all nucleotides of DNA /RNA absorb light at wave length close to 260 nm, at pH 7. So **concentration of nucleotides & nucleic acids** are often expressed in terms of "**absorbance at 260 nm**".
- **DNA purity (quality) measurement** is based on the fact that the *clean/pure DNA has twice (1.8 -2 times more) optical density (OD) at 260 nm then at 280nm.* So if OD-260/OD-280 is lesser, it indicates *contamination*, which decreases OD ratio. Hence purify the DNA again.

### Gene Expression in eukaryotes can be regulated / influenced through modifications to DNA in form of

1. **Availability** or **access of transcriptional apparatus to DNA**. Transcriptionally active, relatively relaxed & decondensed euchromatin differs from inactive, highly condensed hetero chromatin in 2 main ways.
   a. Euchromatin contains histone proteins covalently modified by **acetylation** or **phosphorylation of lysine residue at amino terminal**. This modification **decreases positive charge** of basic histone protein , thus decreasing their strength of association with negatively charged DNA; thus relaxing nucleosomes and allowing access to DNA. **Histone acetyl transferases (HAT)** mediates acetylation (removal of positive charge) and **histone deacetylase (HDACs)** removes acetyl group (restoring positive charge). This chromatin inter conversion from eu to hetero-chromatic is called **chromatin remodeling.**
   b. **Transcriptionally active genes are hypomethylated (less methylated) at cytosine base in CG rich region (CpG island) in promoter region** of gene than their inactive counter parts. This suggests **DNA hypermethylation silences gene expression.**
   c. **DNA methylation at C5 of cytosine** by DNA **methyl transferase (MTase) use S-adenosyl-methionine (SAM) as methyl donor** and is associated with **gene silencing** contributing to **X-chromosome inactivation, genomic imprinting** (selective silencing of paternal or materanal alleles) and transcriptional regulation of tissue specific genes during cellular differentiation. Degree of methylation differs in normal & cancer cells - *ROS (reactive oxygen species or free radicles) cause hypermethylation.* Aberrant methylation is observed in cellular senescence & age related diseases like Type 2 DM. So the **DNA maintains the same sequence**, when cytosine is methylated **but the expression of methylated gene is altered (Epigenetics)**. This epigenetic information which modifies genetic information is called **writings with nature's pencil** that can be erased & rewritten.
2. **Amount of DNA** (eg **gene amplification** of di hydrofolate reductase = DHFR enzyme required for thymidine triphosphate = TTP synthesis in pyrimidine biosynthesis pathway result in

### Resultant DNA Damages

**I. Single base alteration**
- **Depurination** (rarely depyrimidination)
- **Deamination of cytosine (C) to uracil (U)** and adenine (A) to hypoxanthine
- **Alkylation** of base
- Base-analog incorporation
- Insertion or deletion of nucleotide

**II. 2 - Base alteration**
- UV induced **thymine- thymine (pyrimidine)** dimer
- Bifunctional **alkylating cross linkage**

III. **Chain breaks** d/t ionizing radiation, oxidative free radicle formation or radioactive disintegration of backbone element

IV. **Cross linkage** between
- Bases in same & opposite strands
- DNA & protein molecules eg histone

### DNA Repair Mechanism

| DNA Damaging Agents | DNA lesion produced | DNA Repair Pathway | Fidelity of Repair | Procedure |
|---|---|---|---|---|
| **Replication (copying) errors** | **Base** (single or 2-5 base unpaired loops) **mismatch**; Insertions; Deletions | **Mismatch Repair (MMR)** | +++ | Corrects a single mismatch base pair (eg C to A rather than T to A) or short region of unpaired DNA. The **defective region in newly synthesized unmethylated strand is recognized by (mut H) endo nuclease** that makes a single strand cut at an adjacent **methylated GATC palindrome sequence** (present in opposite orientation on two strands) . The defective DNA strand is removed through mutation (by **exonuclease**), replicated or replaced (by **DNA helicase II, SSB, DNA polymerase III**) and relegated (by **DNA ligase**). Dam methylase methylates $N^6$ adenines within ($5^1$) GATC sequence of parent (template) strand. Replication mismatches in vicinity of hemimethylated GATC sequence are then repaired according to information in methylated template strand. **If both strands are methylated** (in vitro) at GATC, **few mismatches are repaired and if neither strand is methylated repair occurs but does not favor either strand.** |
| Oxygen radicles ; Hydrolysis; Alkylating agents | Abnormal bases like uracil, hypoxanthine, xanthine, alkylated bases, small pyrimidine dimmers, Abasic sites; | **Base Excision Repair (BER)** | + + + | Base removal by N-glycosylase, a basic sugar removal, replacement |

methotrexate drug resistance, which an inhibitor of DHFR).

3. **Arrangement / Rearrangements (recombination) of DNA** such as seen *in formation of unique variable region of immunoglobulins (antibodies) by B-lymphocytes*. This allows generation of $10^9$-$10^{11}$ different immunoglobulins from a single gene, providing the diversity needed for recognizing enormous numbers of antigens.
4. **Transposons (Tn) or mobile DNA elements** that move in random manner from one site to another on same or different chromosome. This molecular parasitic movement is mediated by **transposase** enzyme encoded by Tn itself. Movement can be
   a. **Direct** in which transposase cuts out and then inserts Tn at new site. or
   b. **Replicative** in which the Tn (also called **retrotransposon**) is copied involving RNA intermediate and the copy inserted elsewhere while the original remains in place.

Transposition expands genome, may alter gene expression and cause human diseases like *hemophilia A, Duchenne muscular dystrophy and antibiotic resistance* in bacteria.

## Nonenzymatic Transformations of Nucleatides & Nucleic Acids

Purines and pyrimidines, along with the nucleotides of which they are a part, under go spontaneous alterations in their covalent structure at very slow rate. But these mutations are physiologically significant because of the cells very low tolerance for alteration in its genetic information. Examples include.

1. **Spontaneous loss of exocyclic amino group (De amination):** converts ***cytosine to uracil; 5 methyl cytosine to thymine***Q; adenine to hypoxanthine; and guanine to xanthine. Although slow, the cytosine deamination rate is maximum (1 in every $10^7$ C residue = 100 events per day) and is the **reason why DNA contains thymine rather than uracil**. The product of cytosine deamination (uracil) is easily recognized by DNA repair system as foreign in DNA and removed. If DNA normally contained Uracils, recognition of uracils resulting-from cytosine deamination would be more difficult and unrepaired uracils would lead to permanent sequence changes as they were paired with adenine during replication – thus gradually *causing decrease in G = C base pairs* (almost eliminating in millinia) and **increasing A = U base pairs**. Therefore establishing thymine as one of 4 bases in DNA may well have been a *crucial turning point in evolution that prevented elimination of G = C base pairs and genetic code depending on them ; thereby making long term storage of genetic information possible*.
2. **Depurination / Depyrimidination**: in which a purine / pyrimidine is lost by hydrolysis of *N-beta – glycosyl bond* between the base and pentose. This creates a DNA lesion in which the deoxyribose is present but the base is not is called an **abasic site or AP site (apurinic / apyrimidinic site)**. *Depurination occurs at higher rate* (1 in $10^5$ purine = 10000 per mammalian cell in 24 hrs) than depyrimidination. Depurination can be accelerated by dilute acid; pH 3

| | single strand breaks; 8 oxoguanine lesions | | | |
|---|---|---|---|---|
| UV light, chemicals | Large structural DNA lesions like **pyrimidine dimmers**, Bulky adducts | **Nucleotide Excision Repair (N E R)** | +++ | Removal of an approximately 30-nucleotide oligomer and replacement |
| Ionizing radiation, X-rays, Antitumor drugs | Double / Single strand breaks; intra / inter strand cross links | **Double strand break repair.**<br>- **Homologous recombination (HR)**<br>- **Non Homologous End Joining (NHEJ)** | <br>++<br>+ | Synapsis, unwinding, alignment, ligation |
| Any | | **Direct Repair** | | |
| | **Pyrimidine dimmers** | **DNA photolyases** | | |
| | $O^6$ methyl guanine | $O^6$ methyl-guanine – DNA methyl transferase | | |
| | **Alk B protein** | 1 methyl guanine 3 methyl cytosine | | |

### Mismatch Repair (MMR)

- **Mut L protein** forms complex with **Mut S protein** and the complex binds to all mismatched bases (except C-C). **Mut H** binds to Mut L and unmethylated GATC (encountered by Mut L- Mut S complex).
- *DNA on both sides of mismatch is threaded (looped) through Mut L- Mut S complex* and both legs of loop move through complex simultaneously (equivalent to complex moving in both directions along DNA). Mut H attached to complex has site specific **endonuclease activity** which is activated on encountering hemimethylated GATC sequence and cleaves unmethylated strand on 5′ side of G in GATC.
- When mismatch is on **5′ side (right)** of cleavage site the unmethylated strand is unwound (by helicase II) and cleaved in 3′ → 5′ direction from cleavage site by **exonuclease I** or **exonuclease X** (both of which degrade DNA strand in 3′ → 5′ direction).

### Base Excision Repair (BER)

- **DNA glycosylases** remove purine / pyrimidine created by spontaneous deamination and create **AP (abasic or apurinic) site**. eg uracil DNA glycosylase removes the uracil created by spontaneous deamination of cytosine in DNA (it does not remove T from DNA or U from RNA).
- Humans have **4 types of DNA uracil glycosylase**: most abundant **UNG** is a/w replisome & *removes occasional U* inserted in place of T during replication; **h SMUG1** removes any U residues that occur in ss DNA during replication or transcription; **TDG & MBD 4** ***remove either U or T residues paired with G, generated by deamination of cytosine or 5 methyl cytosine respectively***Q.
- **AP endonuclease** cut DNA strand containing the AP site and a segment of DNA containing AP site is removed.
- **Repair polymerase (DNA polymerase I)** replaces DNA and fills the defect and **DNA ligase** seals the remaining nick (ligates the space created by DNA polymerase I removal )

causing selective removal of purine bases resulting in derivative called **apurinic acid.** *Depurination in ribonucleotide & RNA is slower & physiologically insignificant.*

3. UV or near UV light (200-400nm) induced formation of **pyrimidine dimmers (PD) which introduces a bend or kink into DNA. PD** may be of 2 types

a. **Cyclobutane pyrimidine dimer:** UV light induced condensation of 2 ethylene groups between adjacent pyrimidine bases in nucleic acids form cyclobutyl ring involving C5 & C6 of adjacent pyrimidine residues
b. **6-4 photoproduct**: a pyrimidine dimer with a linkage between C6 of one and C4 of its neighbor pyrimidine.

4. **Ionizing radiation** (cosmic rays, radiation emitted from radioactive elements, X-rays & gama rays) induced ring opening, fragmentation of bases and breaks in covalent backbone of nucleic acid.
5. **Deaminating agents nitrous acid ($HNO_2$) and bisulfite** used as preservatives in processed foods to prevent growth of toxic bacteria. Nitrous acid precursors are nitrosumine, nitrate & nitrite salts.
6. **Alkylating agents** such as **S-adenosyl methionine,** nitrogen mustard, dimethylnitrosamine, dimethyl sulfate can alter DNA bases. For example dimethyl sulfate can methylate guanine to yield $O^6$ methyl guanine.
7. **Oxidative stress (free radicles)** is most important source of mutagenic alterations in DNA.

## Methylated DNA Bases

*Adenine & cytosine* are methylated more often than guanine & thymine. All known *DNA methylases (methyl transferases / MTase)* use *S-adenosylmethionine (S A M) or S adenosyl L methionine (Ado.Met)* as a methyl group donor. Functions of methylation (in Ecoli) are

1. In **host cell's DNA** the sequence that would be recognized by its own restriction endonuclease is **protected from cleavage/ digestion by methylation of DNA** catalyzed by DNA methylase. So methylation helps the cell to distinguish its DNA from foreign DNA by marking its own DNA with methyl group and **destroying foreign DNA** (*eg of infecting virus) with out methyl group* (K/a **restricted DNA**). The restriction endonuclease & corresponding methylase are referred to as **restriction-modification system**.
2. **Dam (DNA adenine methylation) methylase** methylates adenosine residues with in the sequence (5') GATC (3') to $N^6$ methyl adenosine. This **system repairs mismatched base pairs** formed occasionally during DNA replication.

In eukaryotes, 5% cytidine residues in DNA are methylated to 5' methyl cytidine most commonly at CpG sequence, producing methyl CpG symmetrically on both strands of DNA.

Whereas mismatch or **3' side (left) use** either **exonuclease VII** (which degrade ssDNA in 5' → 3' or 3'→ 5' direction) or **Rec J nuclease** (which degrade ss DNA in 5'→3' direction).

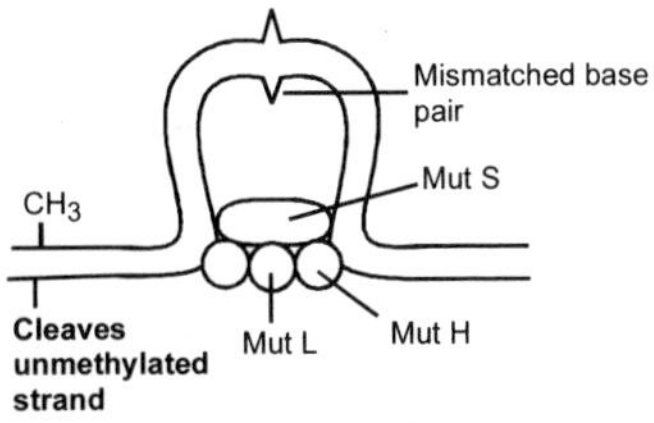


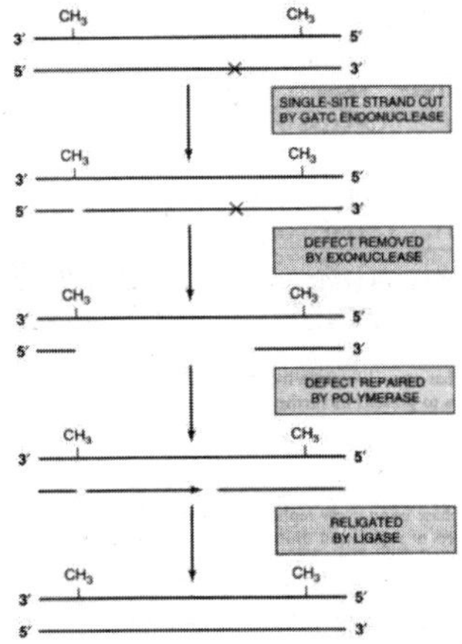


## Double Strand Break Repair

The protein Ku and DNA-dependent protein kinase combine to approximate the two strands and unwind them. The aligned fragments form base pairs; the extra ends are removed, probably by a DNA-PK-associated endo-or exonuclease, and the gaps are filled in; and continuity is restored by ligation.

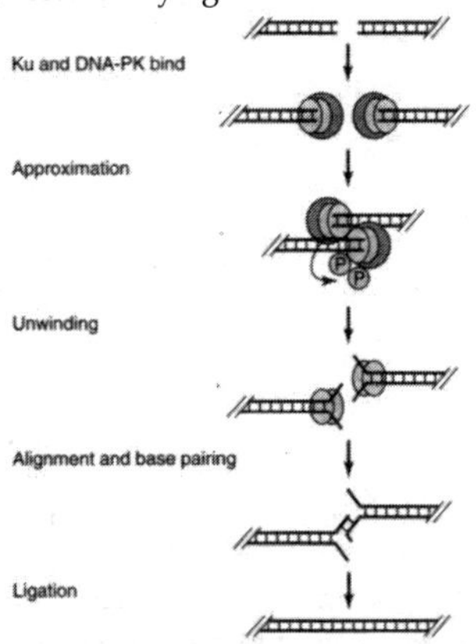


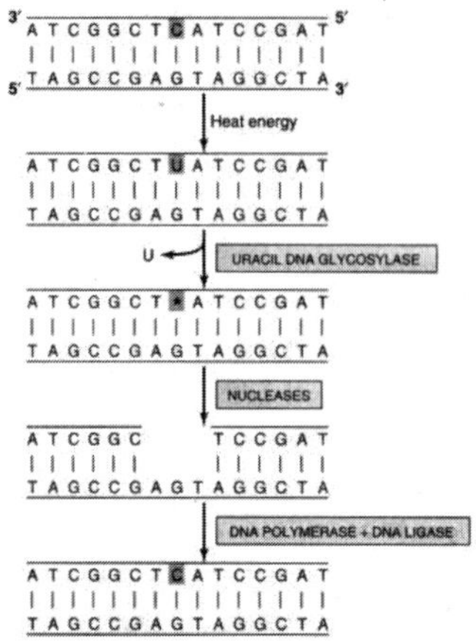


## Nucleotid Excision Repair (NER)

- Larger DNA defects that cause large distortion in DNA helix are repaired by NER.
- A multisubunit **excinuclease enzyme** hydrolyze 2 phosphodiester bonds one on either side of distortion. This corresponds in E.coli & bacteria to 5th phosphodiester bond (PDB) on 3' side & 8th PDB on 5' side creating 12 to 13 nucleotide fragment; and in humans to 6th PDB on 3' & 22nd on 5' side producing a fragment of 27-29 nucleotides.
- **Excinuclease** is a endonuclease with a unique capacity to catalyze 2 specific endonucleolytic cleavages. Following the **dual incision** the excised oligonucleotide are replaced from duplex and resulting gap is filled by **DNA- polymerase I** in E.coli and **DNA polymerase ε/δ** in humans. **DNA ligase** seals nick.
- In E.coli **ABC excinuclease** has 3 subunits **Uvr A, Uvr B** ($A_2B$ complex of both units scans DNA and binds to site of lesion; Uvr $A_2$ dimer then dissociates leaving a tight Uvr B- DNA complex) and **Uvr C** (binds to B subunit and Uvr B makes an incision at 5th PDB on 3' side whereas Uvr C makes an incision at 8th PDB on 5' side of lesion).

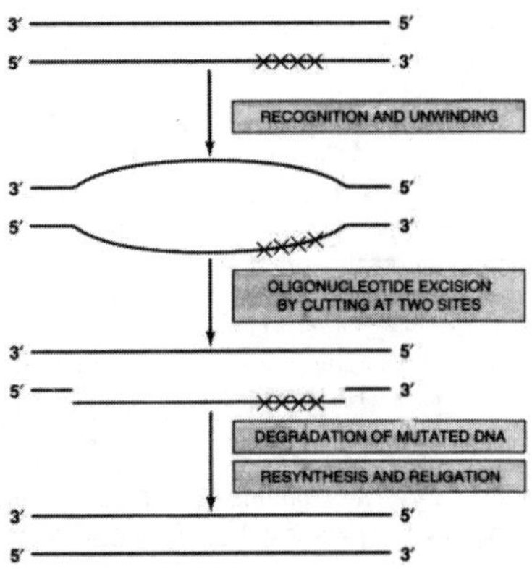

| Disease | Defect in DNA repair | Feature |
|---|---|---|
| **Xeroderma pigmentosa** | **Nucleotide excision repair** *pathway* specilly thymine dimmers cannot be incised d/t *deficiency of enzyme nicking endonuclease* (m.c), DNA polymerase I or DNA ligase, helicase (Subunits of transcription factor TFIIH) | - Autosomal recessive (AR)<br>- Marked sensitivity to sunlight (UV rays) l/t multiple skin cancers and premature death |
| **Ataxia telangiectasia** | | - Autosoml recessive (AR)Q<br>- Cerebellar ataxia, lymphoreticular neoplasms, increased sensitivity to damage by x-ray, oculo cutaneous telangiectasia & IgE deficiency. |
| **Fanconi's anemia** | Chromosomal instability & *defective repair of cross linking damage* | - Autosomal recessive (AR)<br>- Anemia & increased frequency of cancer<br>- Defective gene located on chromosome 20q & 9q |
| **Bloom's syndrome** | Chromosomal breaks & rearrangements are seen d/t *defective DNA ligase* | - Facial erythema, photosensitivity and telangiectasia |
| **Heridiatary non polyposis colon cancer (HNPCC)** | **Faulty mismatch repair** due mutation in **hMSH 2** gene (located inchromosome 2) that encodes human analog of E.coli ***Muts protein*** that is involved in mismatch repair. | - Most common inherited cancer<br>- Cells which harbour hMSH2 (50-60% cases) or hMSH-1 mismatch repair enzyme, are unable to remove small loops of unpaired DNA, & the *microsatellite* DNA thus *increase in size*. It affects either expression or function of a protein critical in surveillance of cell cycle in colon cells. |

## Normal Cell Cycle & Growth

**Protooncogene** | **Tumor suppressor genes** | **Genes regulating apoptosis** | **Genes involved in DNA repair**

### Protooncogene

- Are physiological regulators of cell proliferation & differentiation. On mutation protooncogene becomes oncogene, which is responsible for cancer (i.e., abnormal growth)
- **Cyclin D - CDK4 complex** phosphorylates *RB*, allowing the cell to progress through the *$G_1$ restriction point*. Further *progression through S phase and initiation of DNA replication* involve formation of active complex between **cyclin E & CDK2** in late $G_1$ stage. **CDK-2** forms complex with cyclin A, at the S phase that facilitates *$G_2M$ transition* and regulates events at *mitotic prophase*. **Cyclin B-CDK1** complex, activated by protein phosphatase (Cdc 25) propel the cell beyond prophase & initiate mitosis. Exit from mitosis requires inactivation of cyclin B- CDK1.

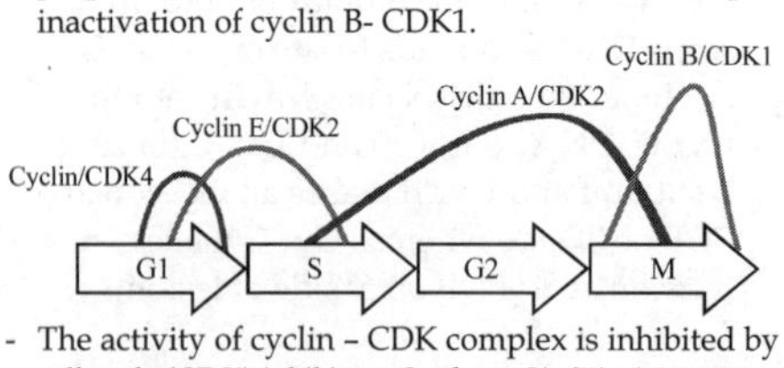


- The activity of cyclin - CDK complex is inhibited by *cell cycle (CDK) inhibitors*. Such as *Cip/Kip (p21, p27, and p57) and INK-4/ARF* (inhibitor of kinase 4/ alternative reading frame) families.
- The cell cycle has two check points - G1/S & $G_2$/M. The S phase is point of no return. The G1/S check point checks for DNA damage & prevents replication of cells that have defects in DNA. The $G_2$/M check point monitors the completion of DNA replication. The **sensor & transducers** of DNA damage are similar for both check points. The sensor are *proteins of RAD family & ataxia telangiectasis mutated (ATM)* and transducer is **CHK-kinase family**. The check point effector molecules differ - in **G1/S** checkpoint it is through *p53* (which induces cell cycle inhibitor p21) and in G2/M check point, arrest of cell cycle involves both p53 dependent & independent mechanism.

### Tumor suppressor genes

- These form proteins that *apply brakes to cell proliferation* & regulate cell growth. Eg. **RB gene, *p53, NF1/2, BRCA 1/2* & *WT-1*Q** etc.
- **P53** is located on *17 p13.1 chromosome* & acts as **molecular policeman** (or **guardian of genome**) by preventing the propogation of genetically damage cells in part by upregulating the synthesis of *CDK inhibitor p21*, GADD45 & BAX
- Main activities of p53 protein are *cell cycle arrest and initiation of apoptosis in response to DNA damage.* It upregulates transcription of

### Genes regulating apoptosis

- Normal cells require continuous survival signals (eg signaling through PI-3 kinase / AKT pathway) which prevents the activity of apoptotic machinery.
- MYC triggers proliferation & **BCL-2** *prevents cell death by a poptosis of tumor cells* (even if growth factors become limiting). On the otherhand cells in culture undergo *apoptosis if MYC activation occurs in absence of survival signals* (growth factors).
- P53, increases transcription of pro-apoptotic genes such as BAX

### Genes involved in DNA repair

**CDK inhibitor p-21** → G1 arreste

**GADD45** → DNA repair

CDK inhibitor p-21 / GADD45 → **Successful repair**

**BAX**: **Apoptosis** inducing gene which binds to & *antagonize apoptosis inhibiting protein BCL-2*

DNA repair **fails** → BAX → Promote cell death

- P53 has a short life (20 minutes) d/t ubiquitin- mediated proteolysis, hence in contrast to RB, it does not police the normal cell cycle. RB and p53' induced cell cycle arrest occurs in late $G_1$ phase.
- **Li - Fraumeni syndrome**, has one mutant p53 allele & are 25 times more prone to malignant tumors.

## Genetic Code and Codons

Genetic code is a dictionary that identifies a correspondence b/w a sequence of nucleotide bases and a sequence of amino acids. And **codon** is each individual *genetic word* of this dictionary that is ***composed of 3 nucleotide bases***Q.

- Condons are present in m- RNA in language of **A** (adenosine), **G** (guanine), **C** (cytsine), and **U** (uracil) nucleotides.
- There nucleotide sequences are always written *from 5′ to 3′* end. Each codon consist of a ***sequence of 3 nucleotides***Q i.e. it is a **triplet code**.
- Since there are only **4 different nucleotides** (A, G, U,C) in m- RNA and codon consists of sequence of 3 nucleotides; each codon must consist of >1 *purine or pyrimidine* nucleotide and there are **64 ($4^3$)** ***different combinations of codon***Q.
- 61 of 64 genetic codons code for 20 common amino acids – **phenylalanine (Phe), leucine (Leu), isoleucine (Ile), methionine (Met), Valine (Val), serine (Ser), proline (Pro), threonine (Thr), alanine (Ala), tyrosine (Tyr), histidine (His), glutamine (Gln), asparagine (Asn), lysine (Lys), aspartic acid (Asp), glutamic acid (Glu), Cysteine (Cys), tryptophan (Trp), arginine (Arg), and glycine (Gly).** ***AUG designating methionine is initiating codon***Q.
- 3 codones – **UAA, UAG, UGA** do not code for any amino acid and are known as **stop (termination or nonsence) codon**. When one of these appear in m-RNA sequence, it ***indicates that syntrhesis of protein coded by that mRNA is completed***Q.

| If codon consisted of | Number of codons |
|---|---|
| 2 nucleotide sequence eg. AU | $(4)^2$ = **16**Q |
| 3 nucleotide sequence eg AUG | $(4)^3$= **64**Q |
| 4 nucleotide sequence eg AUG | $(4)^4$= **256** Q |

| 5′ or First Base | Middle Bas U | C | A | G | 3′ or Third Base |
|---|---|---|---|---|---|
| U | Phe | Ser | Tyr | Cys | U |
| | Phe | Ser | Tyr | Cys | C |
| | Leu | Ser | Stop | Stop | A |
| | Leu | Ser | Stop | Trp | G |
| C | Leu | Pro | His | Arg | U |
| | Leu | Pro | His | Arg | C |
| | Leu | Pro | Gln | Arg | A |
| | Leu | Pro | Gln | Arg | G |
| A | Ile | Thr | Asn | Ser | U |
| | Ile | Thr | Asn | Ser | C |
| | Ile | Thr | Lys | Arg | A |
| | Met | Thr | Lys | Arg | G |
| G | Val | Ala | Asp | Gly | U |
| | Val | Ala | Asp | Gly | C |
| | Val | Ala | Glu | Gly | A |
| | Val | Ala | Glu | Gly | G |

### Natural Expansion (Evolution) of Genetic Code

- There are **actually 22 rather than 20 amino acids specified by known genetic code. The 21st amino acid selenocysteine** (Sec) **is coded by UGA and 22nd amino acid pyrrolysine (Pyl) is encoded by UAG.** So in effect, UGA and UAG doubles as a codon for both termination and (very occasionally) selenocysteine (in bacteria with *formate dehydrogenase* or in mammals with *glutathione peroxidase* protein) and **pyrrolysine (in methanogens** or methane producing anaerobic archaea).
- ***Unlike hydroxyl lysine or hydroxyproline, selenocysteine arises cotranslationally*** during its incorporation into peptides. Unlike selenocysteine -pyrrolysine was attached directly to a dedicated tRNA by a cognate *pyrrolysyl tRNA synthetase.*

### Characteristics of Genetic Code

- **Specificity (Unambiguous)**: which means *a particular codon always codes for the same amino acid.*
- **Universal**: which means the specificity of genetic code is conserved from very early stages of evolution to mammals (between species) and among different tissues in a species. The exceptions are
  - *Mitochondrial* translational machinery reads *four codons differently* from t-RNA molecules in cytoplasm of even same cell. So mitochondria requires only *22 t- RNA* molecules to read their genetic code, where as cytoplamic translation system has a full complement of *3′ tRNA.*

| Codon | Cytoplasm | Mitochondria |
|---|---|---|
| AUA | Ile | Met (**Methionine**) |
| UGA | Termination codon | Trp (**Tryptophan**) |
| **AGA** **AGG** | Arginine | **Stop** or **chain termination codon** |

- **Degeneracy (Redudancy):** which means ***some aminoacids are coded by multiple codons***Q. For example six diffrent codons specify serine as well as arginine
- **Non overlapping, non punctuated and commaless**: which means the code is read from a fixed starting point as a continuous sequence of bases taken 3 at a time *without any overlapping or comma (punctuation)* between the codons. For example ABCDEFGHI is ABC/DEF/GHI.

### Unnatural Expansion of Genetic Code

- **Codon UAG** is the best target (of scientific research) for encoding a new aminoacid as it is least used of the three termination codons and strains with tRNAs selected to recognize UAG do not exhibit growth defects.
- Over 30 unnatural aminoacids with a unique reactive chemical group like ketone, azide, photocrosslinker (a functional group designed to form a covalent bond with a nearby group when activated by light), a highly florescent amino acid, aminoacid with a heavy atom (Br) for use in crystallography and aminoacid with long chain cysteine analog that can form extended disulfide bonds have been added to genetic code.

### Induced Variation in Genetic Code: Nonsense Suppression

- **Nonsense mutation** produce a termination codon in interior of gene, prematurely halting translation, producing inactive incomplete polypeptide. The gene can be restored to normal function if a 2nd **restorative mutation (k/a nonsense suppressors)** either suppresses the effects of termination codon or converts the misplaced termination codon to a codon specifying an aminoacid.
- Mostly nonsense suppressors involve mutations in t-RNA genes to produce **altered (supprssor) t RNA** (mostly *with a single base substitution in their anti codon) that can recognize the termination codon and insert an aminoacid at that position.*
- A cell usually has several copies of each tRNA. Nonsense suppression does not completely disrupt normal information transfer in cell because these suppressor mutations usually involve minor (weakly expressed) t RNA, leaving the normal tRNA to read its codon normally. However nonsense suppression can produce enough full length active protein from a gene with nonsense mutation to allow the cell to survive.
- Nonsense suppression *does not always lead to abnormally long proteins or creation of suppression t-RNA with mutation in anticodon*. Eg suppression of UGA nonsense codon generally involves tRNA trp that normally recognize UGG and inserts Trp at that position. Alteration of G to A at 24 position in arm of tRNA allows it to read both UGA and UGG (& insert Trp).

## Wobble Hypothesis

- It *explains the degeneracy of genetic code*, a mechanism by which *t RNAs can recognize more than one codon* for a specific aminoacid, in which the **base at 5′ end of anticodon ( = 1st base of anticodon)** is not as spatially defined as the two other bases.
- Movement of this *1st base of anticodon (5′ end)* allows non traditional (i.e., not according to watson- Crick rule) base pairing with the *last base of codon (at 3′ end)*. This is called wobble and allows single t RNA to recognize more than one codon.
- So there need not be 61 tRNA types to read 61 codons. For example **two codons for arginine, AGA & AGG, bind to same anticodon** having uracil at 5′ end (UCU), or 3 codons for glycine - GGU, GGC, and GGA can bind to one anticodon CCI. (I = inosine nucleotide)

★ Codon of mRNA is recognized by anticodon of tRNA and it follows the rule of **complimentary & antiparallel binding**, i.e. the **mRNA codon is read 5′ →3′** by an **anticodon** pairing in the flipped **3′→5′ orientation.** When writing the sequences of both codons & anticodon, the nucleotide sequence must always be listed in the 5′→3′ order.

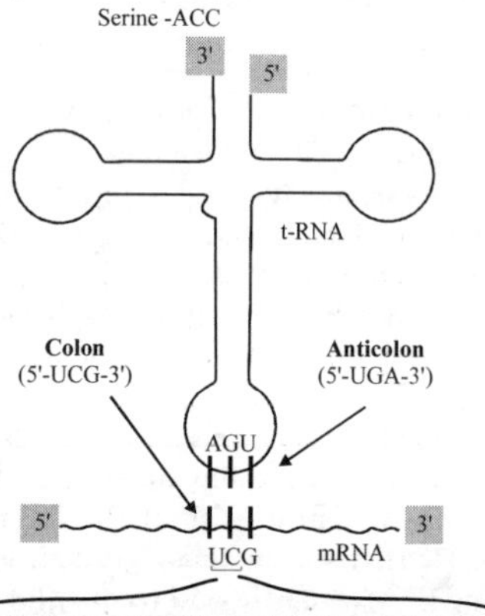


| **Traditional base pairing** observed in **1st & 2nd position of codon:** | |
|---|---|
| tRNA | m- RNA |
| A | U |
| G | C |
| U | A |
| C | G |

| Non traditional base pairing b/w **3rd (3′) position of codon and 1st (5′) positin of anticodon: Wobble** | |
|---|---|
| t- RNA | mRNA |
| A | U |
| G | C, U |
| H | C,U,A |
| U | A,G |

★ H = hypoxanthine (base of inosine)

## Characteristics of Motif Containing Proteins

- ***Control of transcription requires high affinity and specificity in binding of regulatory proteins to the correct region of DNA, which is provided by motifs***Q. Binding must be high affinity to specific sites and low affinity to others. Binding must be *high affinity to specific sites and low affinity to others*. The DNA – protein interactions are maintained by *hydrogen bonds & vander waals forces*. The presence of motifs in unknown protein *suggest that the protein may bind to DNA*.
- *Small regions of motif make direct contact with DNA*. The rest of protein may provide ligand binding sites, trans activation domains, or contact surface for formation of hetero dimers, & interaction with coactivatior or corepressor. It may be involved in dimerization of monomers of binding ***protein. Proteins with helix turn helix & leucine zipper motifs form symmetrical palidromes and their DNA binding sites are symmetrical palindromes***Q. Whereas, ***in proteins with zinc finger motif, the binding site is repeated 2- 9 times***Q.

### Helix turn helix motif

- Each monomer consist of *three antiparallel β- sheets & three α- helix.*
  - β3 sheets for dimmer.
  - α3 helices form DNA recognition surface.
- Examples of transcription regulatory proteins containing helix turn helix motif

| Regulatory protein | Organism |
|---|---|
| lac repressor, CAP | E. Coli |
| Cro, λ cl, tryptophan & 434 represor | Phage |
| Homeo box proteins, pit 1, Oct1, Oct2 | Mammals |

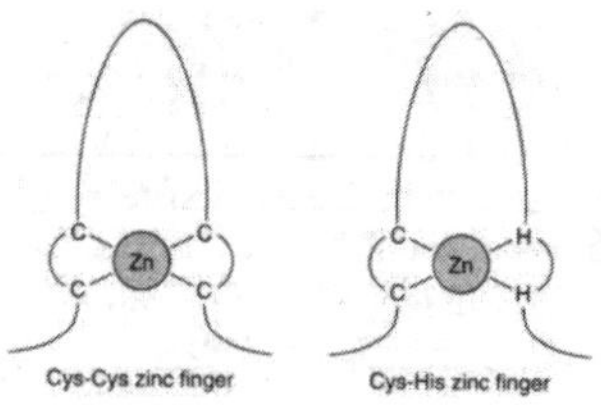


Zn finger motif

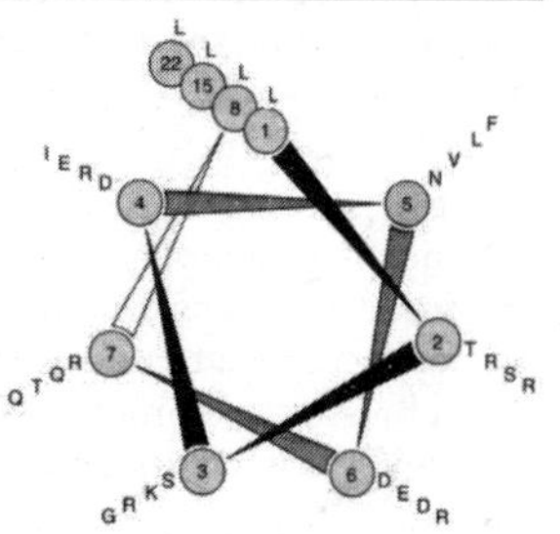

Leucine Zipper motif

### Zinc- finger motif

- They are series of *repeated domains (2-9)* in which each is centered on a tetrahedral coordination ***with Zn***Q.
- In TF III A (transcription regulatory protein) *9 zinc* ions present in repeating Co0 ordination complex formed by *pair of cystine (C) separated by 12-13 amino acid from a pair of histidine residue.*
- Transcription regulatory proteins containing Zn-finger motif

| Regulatory protien | Orgainsm |
|---|---|
| Gene 32 protein | E. coli |
| Gal 4 | Yeast |
| **Serendipity, Hunch back** | Drosophila |
| TF III A | Xenopus |
| ***Steroid receptor family***Q, Sp1 | Mammals |

### Leucine- zipper motif

- Carboxyl terminal of DNA binding protein C/EBP, forms an α- helix in which ***there is periodic repeat of leucine residue at every 7th position***Q.
- This structure allow two identical monomer or hetero dimer (eg, fos- Jun or Jun- Jun) to 'Zip together' in a coiled coil & form tight dimeric complex.
- This enhance association of separate DNA binding domain with their target
- Transcription regulatory containing leucine zipper motif

| Regulatory protein | Organism |
|---|---|
| GCN-4 | Yeast |
| C- myc, n- myc, l-myc<br>CRE binding protein<br>C/EBP<br>Fra 1, fos<br>Jun | Mammals |

★ Gene expression is controlled by **regulatory sequences of DNA** that lie in *non coding regions* of genome *flanking a coding gene*. These are **Cis - acting**, if they influence expression of gene only *on same chromosome* and **transacting** if influences the expression of gene on other chromosome (that is different from its site of origin).

### Gene

- A *segment of DNA* molecule that *contains the information* required for *synthesis* of a functional biological product, whether *protein or RNA,* is referred to as a *gene*
- Edward **Tatum** & George **Beadle** proposed molecular definition of gene in 1940 a/t which a gene is a *segment of genetic material that determines or codes for one enzyme" the* ***one gene-one enzyme*** **hypothesis**. Later this concept was broadened to **1 gene-1 polypeptide**, because many genes code for a protein that is not an enzyme or for one polypeptide of a multi subunit protein.
- A/t modern biochemical definition, a gene is *all the DNA that encodes the primary sequence of some final gene product*, which can either be polypeptide or an RNA with a structural or catalytic function.
- **Gene** is a **functional unit** that *encodes a RNA* product which is *mostly (but not always) translated into a protein*, which exerts activity within or outside the cell. (Harrison-385). Gene is regulated by transcription & corresponds to a *unit of inheritance*
- **Inducible genes**, with relatively *low basal rates of transcription* are upregulated (i.e. expression increased) in response to an **inducer** or **activator** (a **positive regulator**). By contrast repressible genes, with high basal rate of transcription are often down regulated by **repressor** (negative regulator).
- **Housekeeping genes** are **constitutively** expressed meaning that they are expressed at a reasonably constant rate & not known to be subject to regulation. A mutation resulting in constitutive expression of what was formerly a regulated gene is k/a **constitutive mutation.**
- **Care taker** (or **stability) genes** encodes proteins that function in *repair of major genetic defect* that result from aberrant DNA replication, environmental carcinogens or ionizing radiation. So mutation in these genes *l/t mutation* (unrepaired damage) in other genes including protoonchogenes & tumor suppressor genes and thus to cancer. Examples include ATM gene, XP gene (l/t Xeroderma pigmentosa), BRCA1 gene (l/t breast cancer), and p53 gene (l/t *Li Fraumeni cancer syndrome.*)

### Cistron

- As we know; some enzymes & proteins are composed of 2 or more *non identical subunits. Thus 1 gene- 1 enzyme concept is not always valid.*
- **Cistron** is the ***smallest unit of genetic expression***[Q]. It is the basic genetic unit ***coding for one polypeptide chain/ structure of subunit of a protein molecule***[Q].
- So one gene- one enzyme concept might more accurately be regarded as **one cistron-one subunit** concept.
- A single mRNA that encodes >.1 sepeatily translated proteins is referred to as **polycistronic m RNA**. Eg polycistronic lac operon m-RNA.
- But this concept is also changing as many cistrons could be spliced & rearranged. In other words, **many genes together can produce one peptide chain by** means of **transposition** of genes or **gene rearrangement** or **somatic recombination of DNA or gene shuffling** (described by Susumu Tonegawa for antibodies).

## Jacob & Monod's Operon Concept for Prokaryotic Gene

In prokaryotes, genes involved in a metabolic pathway are often present in a linear array called an **operon**. The **cistron** is the smallest unit of genetic expression coding for subunit of a protein molecule (One cistron - one subunit concept). **Polycistronic mRNA,** predominantly found in prokeryotes is a m-RNA that encodes more than one seperately translated proteins. Operon (transcription unit of prokaryotes) consists of

#### Structural (coding) genes

- Carries the codon that code for proteins involved in a particular metabolic pathway
- In lac operon of E coli (responsible for lactose metabolism), 3 structural genes **lac Z, lac Y,** & **lac A** code respectively for *β*-galactosidase, (hydrolyze lactose or *β- galactoside* to galactose & glucose), *permease* (responsible for permeation of galactose into cell), and *thiogalactoside transacetylase*.

| Inducible regulated genes | Constitutive (house keeping) genes |
|---|---|
| - Their expression *increases in response to an* **inducer** or **activator** (a positive regulatory signal)<br>- In general, inducible genes have relatively *low rates of transcription* | - They are expressed at ***a reasonably constant rate and are not subjected to regulation***[Q]<br>- The *product* of these genes are ***required all the time***[Q] in a cell.<br>- A mutation resulting in constitutive expression of what was formerly a regulated gene is called **constitutive mutation** |

#### Regulatory region consisting

##### Promoter (P) gene

- It is situated on the upstream (5′- side of transcription start site b/w operator & regulator gene.
- It is the site, where ***DNA dependent – RNA polymerase (RNP) binds to form preinitiation complex (PIC)***[Q], and commence transcription.
- **Catabolite gene activator protein (CAP)** in **conjunction with c-AMP** (als k/a c-AMP regulatory protein = **CRP**) is required for efficient formation of PIC. So it is a **positive regulator**. Adenylate cyclase which forms c-AMP from ATP, is activated by *absence of glucose*. So the lac operon ***transcription only occurs in absence of glucose***[Q] (**catabolite repression**). And presence of glucose prevents it by depleting c-AMP.

##### Operator (O) genes

- It is a segment of ds DNA (i.e., gene) that *regulates the activity of the structural genes.*
- In lac operon, it is 27 bp long segment situated *between promoter site* (at which RNAP binds) *and lac Z* (transcription initiation site) and show a **twofold rotational symmetry** and **an inverted palindrome** in 21 bp long region as shown below

```
5′ - AATTGT →        G ----------- 3′
3′ ------------ C ----- TGTTAA 5′ ←
```

When attached to operator (o) gene, the **repressor** (LacI) acts as a **negative regulator** and prevents transcription of operator and structural (lac /Y/A) genes.

##### Regulator (I) genes

- It is a *constitutive gene, that forms subunits* of lac repressor (MW 38,000), A lac repressor molecule (**Lac I repressor protein**) is formed by union of *4 subunits* and has ***high affinity for operator locus***[Q].
- At any time only *2 subunits* of repressor *binds to operator* , mostly in its *major groove without interrupting the base paired double helical nature of operator DNA.*
- Normally 20-40 repressor tetramers, occupy > 95% of lac operator, thus ensuring a low (but not zero) lac operon transcription in absence of inducer.
- **Presence of lactose or gratuitous inducer** (i.e., lactose analog which induces lac operon but is not a substrate) such as **isopropylthio galactoside (IPTG)** on bacteria growing on poorly utilized carbon source (eg succinate) results induction of lac operon enzymes by **de-repression.** This occurs because lactose /IPTG bind to free & attached repressor & decrease its affinity $10^3$ times for operator by inducing coformational change.

- ★ The first base at transcription start site (of DNA) is assigned a position of **+1**. There is **no** base designated "**O**". A base is assigned a **negative number**, if it occurs *upstream* ( i.e., *prior* to or on *left side* or towards the *5′end* of) the transcription start site. And in the same way **more positivity** indicates *more downstream* (i.e., *after to* or on the *right side* or *towards 3′-end*) distance from +1 position.
- ★ **Enhancer** and **repressor (silencer)**, can either increase or decrease the rate of transcription initiation of eukaryotic gene respectively. They ***can be located upstream or downstream of transcription start site (+1) and even within transcribed portion of some genes***[Q]. **In contrast to** proximal & upstream **promoters**, these *can exert their effect when located even hundreds or thousand bases away* from transcription unit on same chromosome and function in *orientation independent fashion*. Enhancers are promiscuous, they can stimulate any promoter (homologous or hetrologus). Enhancers work by binding one or more proteins and by facilitating binding of basal transcription complex to promoter.

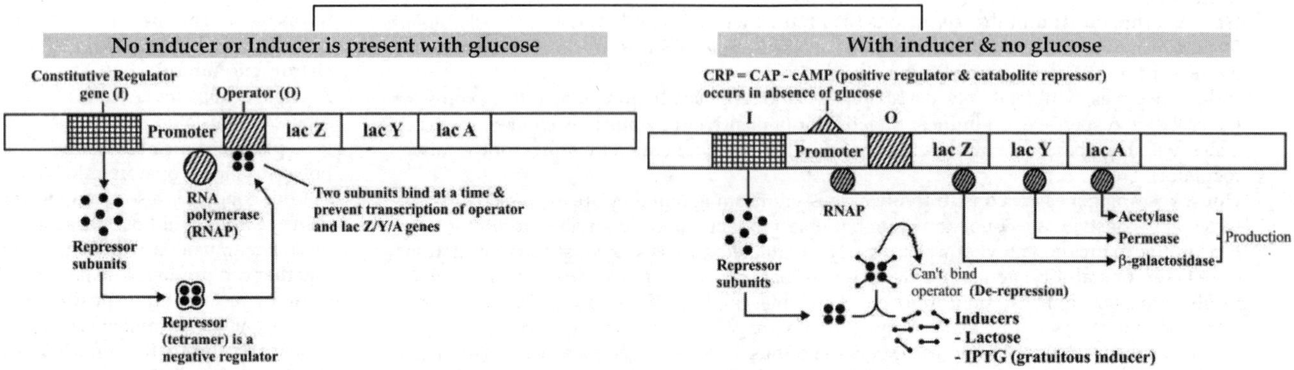


## Bacteriophage Lambda (λ) : Gentetic Switch & Lysogenic and Lytic Pathways

- Bacteriophage lambda (λ) is a temperate virus that infects E. coli bacteria and injects its 45, 000 -bp- ds linear - DNA genome into the cell.
- Depending upon the nutritional state of host , the (λ) virus will ***enter either lysogenic or lytic pathways***[Q] depending on which of 2 sets of viral genes is turned on

**Lysogenic Pathway**

- *Poor growth conditions* favor lysogeny
- In lysogenic pathway, the viral DNA becomes integrated into bacterial chromosome where it *replicates passively as the bacterial DNA and cell divides.*
- This **dormant genomically integrated** virus is called **prophage** and the cell that horbours it is called a **lysogen**.
- A prophage can be induced by DNA damaging agents such as ultraviolet rays to enter lytic phase by turning on different set of genes (genetic switch)

**Lytic Pathway**

- *Good growth conditions* promote lytic pathway
- In lytic pathway, *viral DNA replicates* itself and direct synthesis of viral proteins
- About 100 new complete protein packed viral particles are formed. And the proliferating viruses induce the lysis of cell

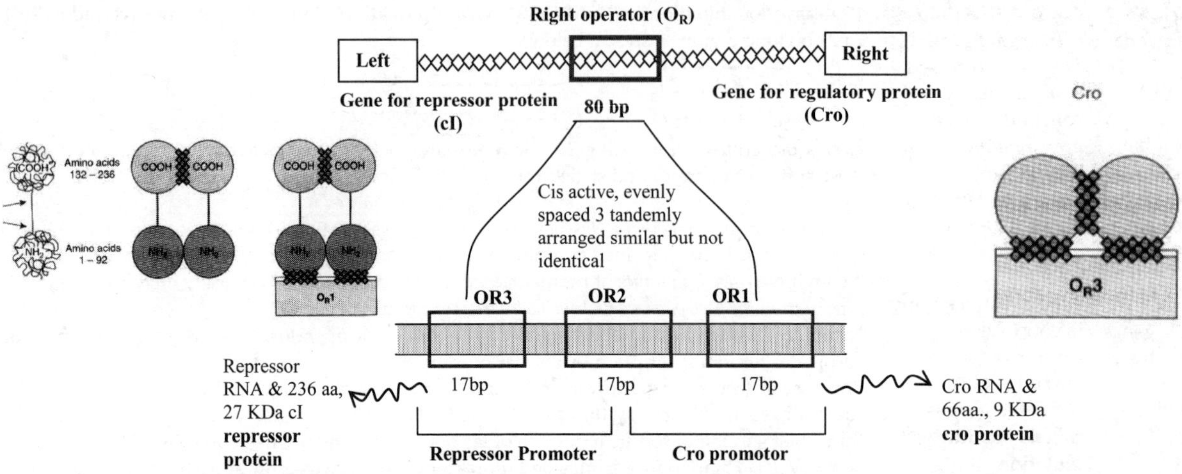

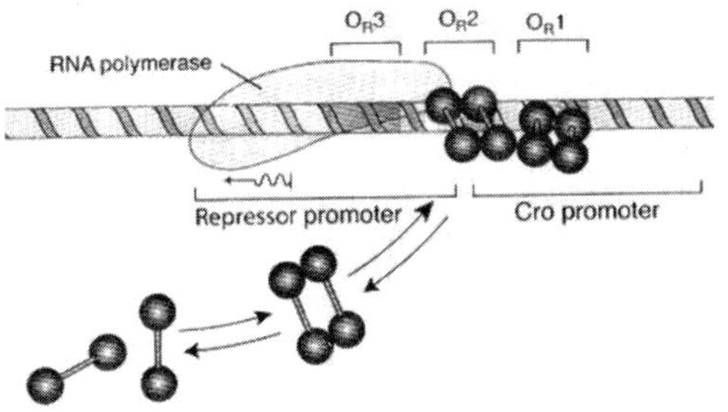


Prophage

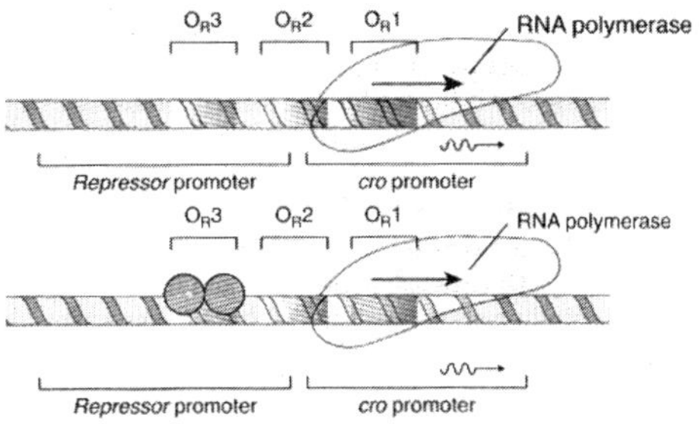


Early lytic phase

- The lytic – lysogenic genetic switching in (λ) is centered around 80 bp ds DNA **right operator ($O_R$) genome** which is flanked on its **left side** by **gene for repressor protein (cI)** and on its **right side** by genes encoding regulatory protein **cro** (Mn *"R is not on right side"*)
- $O_R$ can be subdivided into 3 discrete, evenly spaced, tandemly arranged, similar but not identical, 17 bp cis active DNA elements termed **operators $O_R1$, $O_R2$, $O_R3$**. These can be bound by either cI or cro proteins, however *by different binding affinities*, a feature that regulates molecular switch.
- DNA between cro & repressor genes also contain **2 promoter sequences** that over lap the recognition ($O_R$) sites and direct binding of RNA polymerase in either **right ward** direction (& so transcribing **cro protein**) or **leftward** direction (& so transcribing **cI protein**)
- **Repressor protein (cI)** is a 236 aminoacid, 27 kDa product of repressor gene. It exists as two domain molecule in which the amino terminal domain binds to operator DNA (preferably $O_R1$) and carboxy terminal domain promotes the association of one repressor protein with another to form a dimer. A dimer of repressor molecules binds to operator DNA much more tightly than does the monomeric form.
- **Cro protein** is a 66 aminoacids, 9 kDa product of cro gene. It has a single domain that operates both operator binding (preferably to $O_R3$) and dimerization. It also binds to operator DNA more tightly as dimer.
- When the (λ) is in its **lysogenic- prophage – dormant state**- the **cI repressor gene** is the only gene that is expressed. *When bacteriophage is in* ***lytic state*** *– cro gene is expressed. So when the repressor gene is on, cro gene is off,* and when the cro gene is on, the cI repressor gene is off – a paradigmatic example of a **molecular transcription switch.**

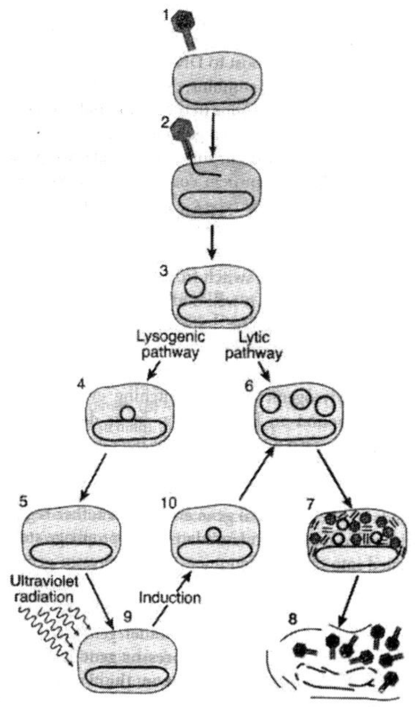


- In lysogenic (dormant- prophage) lambda, the **repressor (cI) dimer protein binds preferentially to $O_R1$** and and enhances binding (by a factor of 10) of another cI dimer to $O_R2$. The affinity of repressor for $O_R3$ is least
- $O_R1$ occupancy *blocks the binding of RNA polymerase to right ward promoter* & in that way prevent cro formation **(negative regulation).**
- Binding of repressor to $O_R2$ *enhances the binding of RNA polymerase to leftward promoter* that overlaps $O_R3$ and there by enhances transcription & expression of repressor (cI) gene **(positive regulator)**
- This dual regulation is responsible for stable state of dormant lambda bacteriophage. When intracellular cI protein concentration becomes very high, this *excessive repressor will bind to $O_R3$ and by doing so diminish transcription of repressor gene* from leftward promoter until the cI concentration drops & repressor dissociates itself from $O_R3$

When a DNA damaging signal (eg UV rays) strike lysogenic host bacteria, fragments of single stranded DNA are generated that activate a specific **coprotease rec- A** coded by bacterial gene

- Rec A protease hydrolyze portion of repressor protein that connects the amino terminal to carboxy terminal
- Such cleavage of repressor domains causes the repressor dimers to dissociate, which in turn cause dissociation of repressor (cI) from $O_R2$ & eventually from $O_R1$
- RNA polymerase immediately has acess to the rightward promoter & commences transcribing the cro gene
- Newly synthesized **cro protein** binds to operator region, but its order of preference is opposite to that of repressor i.e. **Cro binds most lightly to $O_R3$** but there is no co operative effect of Cro at $O_R3$ on binding of Cro to $O_R2$. At increasing concentrations of Cro, the protein will bind to $O_R2$ and eventually $O_R1$
- Occupancy of $O_R3$ by Cro immediately turns off transcription from the left ward cI promoter & so preventing any further expression of repressor gene. Molecular switch is thus completely thrown in lytic direction. The cro is expressed and repressor gene is fully turned off irreversibly
- In very high concentrations Cro occupy $O_R1$ and reduce expression of its own gene in the final stages of lytic cycle.

# DNA Dependent – RNA – Polymerase (RNAP)

It is the ***key enzyme in transcription***[Q]. In both, prokaryotes & eukaryotes, RNA polymerase ***does not require primer & has no proof reading activity***[Q].

## Prokaryotic RNA polymerase (Bacterial DNA dependent)

**RNAP lacks a separate proof reading 3′ → 5′ exonuclease active site** (as of DNA polymerase) & so **error rate for transcription is higher than that for DNA replication.** Because many copies of RNA are produced from single gene and eventually all are degraded, so a mistake in RNA is of less significance to cell as compared to DNA which is permanently stored.

### Structure & Function

- It *recognizes promoter nucleotide sequence*[Q] at the begining of length of DNA that is to be transcribed.
- It ***makes a complementary RNA copy of DNA templete (antisense) strand, which is identical to coding (sense) strand***[Q]; with U replacing the T. RNA is synthesized from its 5′ end to its 3′ end, antiparallel to its DNA template strand.
- And then it *recognizes the termination region* (i.e., the end of DNA sequence to be transcribed).
- It is a multisubunit- enzyme, with ~400 kDa **core complex** consisting of *two identical $\alpha$ subunits, similar but not identical $\beta$ and $\beta'$ subunits and a $\Omega/w$ subunit* **($\alpha\beta\beta'\omega$). β subunit binds $Mg^{++}$** and composes **catalytic** subunit.
- It is *multi subunit metalloenzyme* containing 2 *zinc molecules* and

### Requirements

RNA polymerase holoenzyme reuires:

1. *Template* of double stranded DNA (or occasionally single stranded DNA)
2. ***Four ribonucleotide triphosphates GTP, UTP, ATP, CTP***[Q].
3. *$Mg^{++}$* or *$Mn^{++}$*[Q]

### Type

Only one type of RNAP ***synthetizes all of RNAs (i.e. m-RNA, t-RNA, & r-RNA) except for the short RNA primers needed for DNA replication***[Q]. RNA primers are synthesized by **primase** enzyme.

### Core- complex (E)

It is ~ 400 kDa complex formed by 5units **($\alpha_2\beta\beta'\omega$)**

#### Coreenzyme

- Consists of two ***identical $\alpha$ subunits, similar but not identical $\beta$ and $\beta'$ subunits ($\alpha_2\beta\beta'$***[Q]***, and possess 5′→ 3′ polymerase activity***[Q]
- It *lacks specificity* and *cannot recognize promoter region*

#### ω/Ω subunit

Function of this 5th subunit is unclear

### Sigma ($\sigma$) subunit

- Sigma factor binds **transiently** to core & directs the enzyme to specific binding sites on DNA. ***It enables RNAP to recognize promoter regions on DNA***[Q] and to form the preinitiation complex (PIC).
- It *decreases RNAP's affinity for non promoter regions, while simultaneously increasing holoenzyme affinity for promoter* DNA (dual role)
- It is responsible for **promoter recognization specificity** of RNAP as bacteria has multiple σ factors recognizing different genes. **$\sigma^{70}$** is the most common type
- Sigma (σ) unit plus the core enzyme makes up the **holoenzyme ($\alpha_2\beta\beta'\omega$+σ)**.

★ Termination of transcription requires termination factors, such **ρ factor** of E. coli.

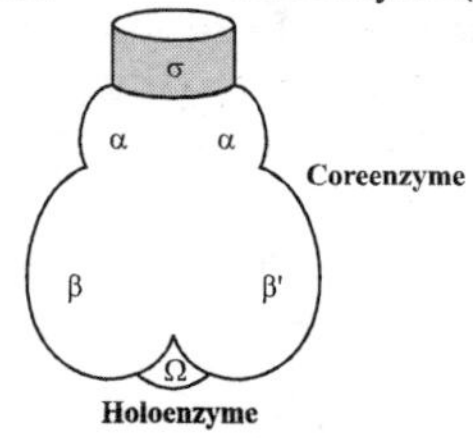


## Eukaryotic (Mammation) RNA Polymerase (Nuclear DNA dependent)

- Eukaryotes have **3 types** of RNA polymerases (RNAPs) with size ranging from 5 lack to 6 lack MW and all having **2 larger and multiple** (upto 14 in pol-III) **smaller** subunits. However, these subunits do **exhibit extensive amino acid (& 3 dimensional structure) homologies** with prokaryotic RNA polymerase.
- α- Amantin obtained from **Amanita phalloides (death cap)** is a specific **differential inhibitor** (i.e. differentiates different types) of eukaryotic RNAP. ***It blocks translocation of RNAP during phosphodiester bond formation***[Q]. Different forms/types of eukaryotic RNAPs are

| RNAP-type | α-Amantin sensitivity | Product | |
|---|---|---|---|
| | | Main | Detailed |
| I/ Pol I | Insensitive | r-RNA | Synthesize only one type of pre-r **RNA (pre ribosomal RNA)** in nucleolus which forms 28S, 18S and 5.8S rRNAs |
| II (Pol II) | High | m-RNA, mi-RNA, sn RNA | Synthesize **nuclear precursor of m-RNA** and certain small non coding (nc) RNAs such as **mi-RNA, sn RNA and sno RNA** |
| III (Pol III) | Intermediate | t-RNA, 5S r RNA | Forms small RNAs including **t-RNA, 5S rRNA** and some **sn RNA and sno RNA** |

- Pol II, responsible for transcription and eukaryotic gene expression consists of **12 subunits**. The two largest subunits **RBP1** (190 KDa) and **RBP 2** (150 kDa) are **structurally similar (homologous)** to prokaryotic **β′** and **β subunits** respectively. *RBP 3 and 11* are homologous to *prokaryotic α- subunits.*
- Largest subunit has characteristic **long carboxy tail** consisting of many **repeats of consensus 7 (hepted), aminoacid sequence – Y SPT SPS – (i.e. Tyro – Ser – Pro – Thr – Ser – Pro - Ser). This carboxy terminal repeat domain (CTD)** has 27 repeated units (18 exactly matching the consensus) in yeast and **52 (21 exact)** in mammalian (mouse & human) pol II. The CTD is separated from main enzyme by unstructured linker sequence.
- **Phosphorylation of Ser & Thr** aminoacids of CTD **activates** and **dephosphorylation** of these residues **deactivates** pol II (i.e. increasing & decreasing activity respectively). The phosphorylation & dephosphorylation is essential for *promoter clearance, elongation, termination and even appropriate RNA processing*. So cells with pol II lacking CTD tail are *incapable of activating transcription* and hence are *inviable.*
- CTD is both a *substrate for various kinases (including kinase of TF II H) and binding site for many RNA processing enymes* as well as nuclear transport proteins – thus serves to *couple transcription initiation with m-RNA splicing, 3′ end formation and transport to cytoplasm.*
- Pol II can a/w **Mediator** or **Med** proteins to form **pol II holoenzyme**. Meds are essential for *activating & repressing (i.e. regulating) transcription*. Since mediators (like **TF IID**) are required for actions of activators, they are also called **coactivators /co regulators**. Over 30 meds (Med 1- Med 31) are described in human cells.

★ **Mitochondrial RNA polymerase** more closely resembles bacterial (than eukaryotic) enzyme and is *single* (1 in number).

★ **RNA polymerase leaves its footprints on a promoter**. Foot printing analysis tells the precise location of protein, binding site (like that for RNAP) in a DNA by showing *missing bands (gaps i.e. foot prints)* corresponding to that location. In this 2 identical radioactively labeled DNA (one with and other without RNAP) are cut with DNase and separated by **polyacrylamide gel electrophoresis** (side by side) – the missing bands / gaps in DNA bound to RNA indicate the prescise location of protein binding site.

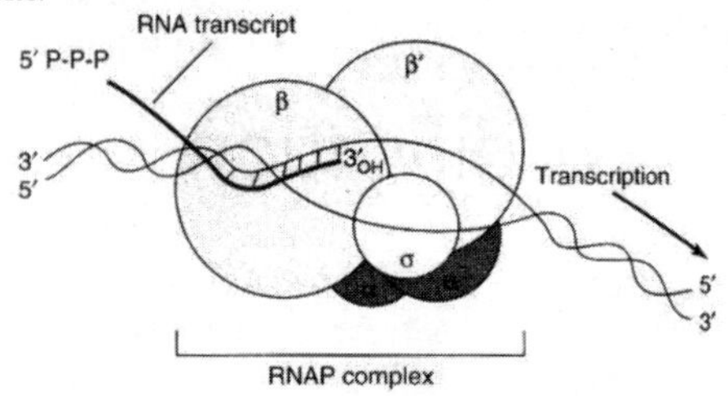


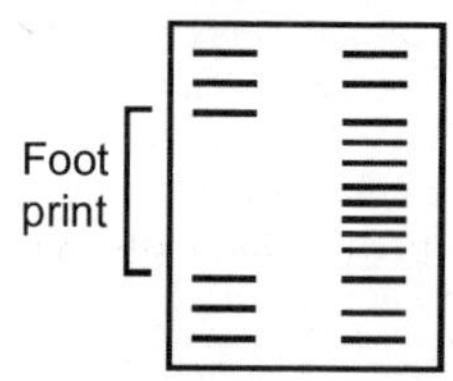

## Comparison Between DNA-Replication and Transcription

Similarities:
1) The general steps of initiation, elongation and termination occurs in *5′- 3′ direction*[Q]
2) Both involve large, multi component initiation complex.
3) Adherence to Watson – Crick base pairing rule (i.e. Hydrogen bonding between A= T & between C ≡ G)

| DNA Replication | Differences | Transcription |
|---|---|---|
| In this process *DNA molecule serves as a template for the formation of daughter DNA molecule* | Definition | In this process *mRNA is synthesized from a DNA template* |
| *Deoxyribonucleotides* are used in DNA synthesis | **Nucleotides** | *Ribonucleotides* are used in RNA synthesis |
| ---- | **Bases** | 'U' replaces 'T' as the complementary base pair for 'A' |
| *Entire genome* is copied. | **Copied Genome** | Only a *small portion of genome* is transcribed. |
| Proof reading occurs. | Proof Reading | No proof reading |
| *Present* in DNA polymerase | Endonuclease & Exonuclease activity | ***Absent***[Q] in RNA polymerase |
| Initiation of DNA synthesis ***requires Primer***[Q] [a short length of RNA, about 10-200 nucleotides] | *Primer*[Q] | ***Not needed***[Q] |

**Semiconservative Replication**: When the two strands of DNA double helix are separated, each can serve as template for replication of new complementary strand producing two daughter molecule. This process is called semiconservative replication because ***although the parental duplex is separated in two halves (& therefore not conserved as an entity), each of individual parental strands remains intact in one of the two new duplexes***[Q].

## Transcription

- DNA constitutes the genetic master plan of an organism, which is however, expressed through RNA – "the working copie of DNA" – This copying process (i.e. synthesis of mRNA from DNA) in which a DNA strand serves as a template is called **transcription**. The 2 complementary DNA strands (of ds DNA) have different roles.

**Template Strand**

- Template strand of DNA is **transcribed or copied** into an m-RNA molecule. In other words it **is used as a template to make the copy** of that part of DNA (i.e. gene).
- The ***information of template strand is readout in 3′ to 5′ direction***[Q].
- So **template strand is complemantary to mRNA transcript** in nucleotide / base sequence.

**Non-template or Coding Strand**

- The opposite DNA strand (which is complementary to template strand) is called **non template strand.**
- Non template DNA strand is also called **coding strand** because **with the exception of T for U changes**, it **corresponds exactly to the sequene of mRNA** primary transcript , which encodes the protein product of that gene.
- So **Coding (non-template) strand of DNA is identical to mRNA transcript (except T for U)**

- This means that the information for protein to be produced is encoded in (or is identical to) coding / non template strand of DNA (oriented 5′ to 3′). But the opposite DNA strand acts as template for transcription and is read in 3′ to 5′ direction.
- In ds DNA containing many genes the template strand for each gene will not necessarily be the same strand. So any strand can serve as a *template strand for some genes and coding strand for other genes*. So genes can be transcribed off both strands of DNA.

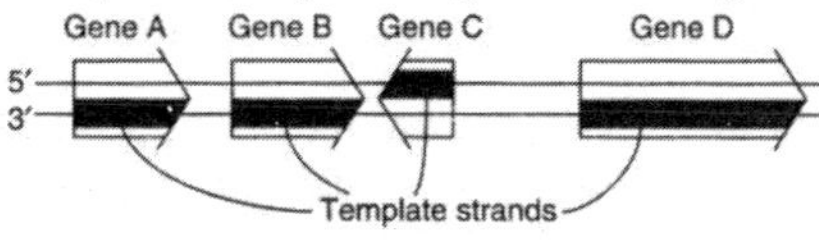


**Arrow indicates direction (polarity) of transcription**

| | |
|---|---|
| (5′) CGC **T**A**T**AGCG**TTT** (3′) | DNA **coding strand** |
| (3′) GCGA TAT CGCAAA (5′) | DNA **template strand** |
| (5′) CGC **U**A**U** AGCG **UUU** (3′) | **mRNA transcript** |

- **Regulatory sequences** that control transcription are designated by the sequences in the **coding strand**.

- **Transcription unit** (TU) is the region of DNA that includes signals for all 3 phases of transcription i.e. **initiation, elongation & termination**. TU extends *from promoter to termination region* and the initial RNA product of RNA polymerase (RNAP) which is synthesized in 5′ to 3′direction is called **primary transcript**.
- The **stranting point of transcription in DNA (usually) corresponds** to the 5′ nucleotide of m-RNA. The **base at the transcription start site** is assigned **+1 (first positive) position**. There is **no** base designated "**O**". By convention, DNA base pairs that corresponds to the beginning of an RNA molecule are given positive numbers & those preceding the RNA start site are given negative numbers. In other words, a base is assigned a **negative number** if it occurs **prior to (towards the 5′ end** or **upstream** of or to the **left** of) transcription start site (+1) and these bases are called **5′ flanking sequences.** Whereas the bases situated **after / down stream / towards 3′ end & right of TSS (+1)** are assigned **positive** numbers in increasing order (i.e. + 10 is more distal to +3). The sequenes down stream of transcription termination site are termed **3′-**

**Flanking sequences**. Although all regulatory sequences function only in ds DNA, by convention, these elements (eg TATA box etc) are **described in 5′ to 3′ direction as being on coding strand**.

### Initiation

- Transcription begins with the **assembly/binding of RNA polymerase (RNAP) holoenzyme** to (the template strand of) **promoter region** of DNA – forming a **pre-initiation complex (PIC)**. The RNAP can bind with low affinity to many regions of DNA, but instead it scans DNA at a rate of $10^3$ **bp/s** to find a specific DNA region to which it binds with **higher affinity**. These higher affinity binding, non-transcribing zones are termed **promoters** and it is the binding of RNAP with promoters that **ensures accurate initiation (fidelity)** of transcription.
- Promoter contains characteristic consensus sequences (i.e. ideal sequences in which the base shown at each position is the base most frequently but not necessarily always encountered at that position). Because these sequences are on the same molecule of DNA as the gene being transcribed, they are called **Cis-acting elements**. No one consensus sequence (CS) is found in all core promoters i.e. different bacteria /organism have slightly different CS, but all promoter have 2 common features.
  - These tend to be in the *same position relative to transcription start site (+1).*
  - *Sequences b/w 2 promoters have no similarity* but still provide **critical spacing functions** that facilitate recognition.
- Promoter regions *can be located upstream & downstream both.* (eg it extends b/w - 70 and +30 in E.coli). **Prokaryotic promoters (-35 sequene, -10/pribnow box)** are recognized by **σ (sigma) subunit** of RNAP holoenzyme. **Eukaryotic** promoters **(TATA box, Inr, DPE** etc) are recognized & assembled to RNAP by **general transcription factors (GTF) like transcription factor II** (i.e. TF required by RNAP II) A to H (except C & G) Because these TFs are encdoded by different genes, synthesized in cytosol, and must transit to their site of action – they are called **trans acting factors.**

### Elongation

- Beginning of elongation phase is defined when,
  - Primary transcript (characteristically starting with purine is **> 10 nucleotides** in length)
  - **Sigma (σ)** subunit is **released** and protein **NusA** binds to elongating RNAP competitively
  - **Core enzyme** forming elongation complex is able to leave /clear the promoter sequence and move along the template strand in a processive manner (i.e. **promoter clearance**)
- Prokaryotic RNAP has an intrinsic unwindase activity l/t formation of **transcription bubble** (DNA unwinding) of about **20 bp/ RNAP molecule** which remains constant through out transcription (i.e. initiation & elongation). Its size is **determined by RNAP** & is independent of **DNA sequene.**
- Elongation proceeds at a rate of **50-90 nucleotides per second.** Because DNA is a helix, movement of transcription bubble requires considerable strand rotations. So movement of RNAP along DNA tends to generate a **positive superoil (i.e overwound DNA) in front** of transcription bubble and **negative supercoil (underwound DNA) behind** it. This topological problem in cells is relieved by action of **topoisomerases** which rapidly eliminates positive supercoils & regulate the level of negative supercoiling.
- So **topoisomerases both preceeds & follows progressing RNAP** to prevent formation of superhelical tensions that would increase the energy demand to unwind the DNA in front of RNAP.
- RNAP requires, **DNA template**, all 4 nucleotide 5′ triphosphates **(ATP, GTP, CTP and UTP),** $Mg^{++}$ and $Zn^{++}$ for synthesis (elongation) of RNA strand – by adding ribonucleotide units to 3′ hydroxyl end, building RNA in **5′→3′ direction.**
- Just like DNA replication, transcription (RNA elongation) is in **5′ to 3′ direction antiparallel to its template strand** (which is read & copied in 3′ to 5′ direction). But unlike it , RNAP **does not require primer** for initiation & has **no proof reading** activity
- Bases are added a/t Watson-Crick base pairing rule and **pyrophosphate (PPi) is released** after each addition (except of 1st initiating purine base, which remains intact throughout transcription). PPi is rapidly degraded to 2 mol of inorganic phosphate (Pi) by ubiquitous pyrophosphatases, making over all reaction irreversible.
- Growing end of newly synthesized RNA strand base pairs temporarily with DNA template strand to form short **8 bp long RNA-DNA double helix** in the transcription bubble.
- RNA hybrid duplex peels off shortly after its formation & DNA duplex reforms.
- In **eukaryotes**, TF IIF remains associated with pol II throughout elongation. **Elongation factors** like Ell; pTEFb, SII (TF IIS) and elongin (S III)- greatly enhance the activity of pol II. pTEFb phosphorylates pol II within CTD and suppress pausing.

### Termination

- RNAP is **highly processive** (i.e. adds) great number of bases before dissociation)- necessarily so because if it gets detached prematurely, it would have to start from beginning again. So *elongation of SS-RNA continues until termination signal is reached.*
- 2 types of termination are

**1. Spontaneous / Intrinsic Rho (ρ) independent termination.**

- In mot **prokaryotic genes** a sequence in DNA template strand is spontaneously terminating which produces
  - Nascent (newly formed) RNA transcript with self complementary sequences, permitting the RNA to fold back on itself forming a **hair pin structure** centered **15 to 20 nucleotides before** the projected end of RNA strand. This hair pin has **GC rich stem** stabilized by hydrogen bonds and *loop of non complementary bases.*
  - Highy conserved string of 3′ 'A' in template DNA is transcribed into a **string of 'U's at the 3′ end just beyond hair pin.**
- RNAP pauses on reaching termination site with this structure. The bonding of string of Us to complementary As of DNA template is weak. Dissociation of RNA transcription from DNA template in this area is facilitated by formation of hair pin structure and zipping up of DNA double helix behind RNAP.

**2. Rho (ρ) dependent termination**

- Termination site (in template strand of DNA) **lacks repeated A string** but usually includes **CA-rich** sequence k/a **rut (rho utilization) element**
- This requies addition **ρ protein** that is a **hexameric ATPase** (adenosine triphosphatase ) **with helicase activity**.
- Rho binds to **C rich-ρ-recognition site** near the 3′ end of nascent RNA and migrates in **5′ → 3′ direction,** along RNA using its ATPase activity until it reaches the transcription complex (RNAP) that is paused at termination site.
- **ATP dependent RNA-DNA helicase** activity of ρ- protein separates the RNA-DNA hybrid helix-causing the release of RNA. (this enz also promotes translocation along RNA-Lehninger.)

- On completion of transcription NusA dissociates from RNAP, which itself dissociates from DNA. The σ- factor can now bind to RNAP to initiate new transcription – in a cycle called **sigma (σ) cycle.**

- Summary: Transcription initiates with **binding of RNAP to promoter region** of DNA (on **template strand**) to form **PIC** – a process which is guided by **σ- subunit** in prokaryotes & **TFs** in eukaryotes. This l/t formation of **closed (wound DNA) f/b open complex** (with unwound DNA) or **transcription bubble.** Nucleotides are added (i.e. RNA is synthesized) in **5'→ 3' direction antiparalled to temlate strand** a/t base pairing rule. In both prokaryotes & eukaryotes 1st nucleotide is usually purine and its 5′ triphosphate end is maintained (not degraded) in mRNA.

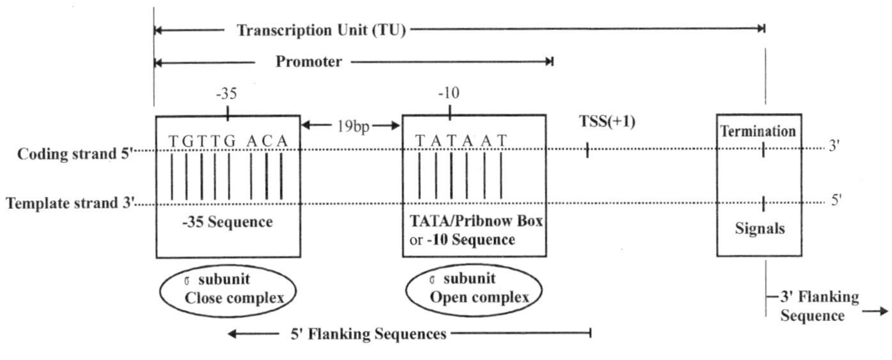


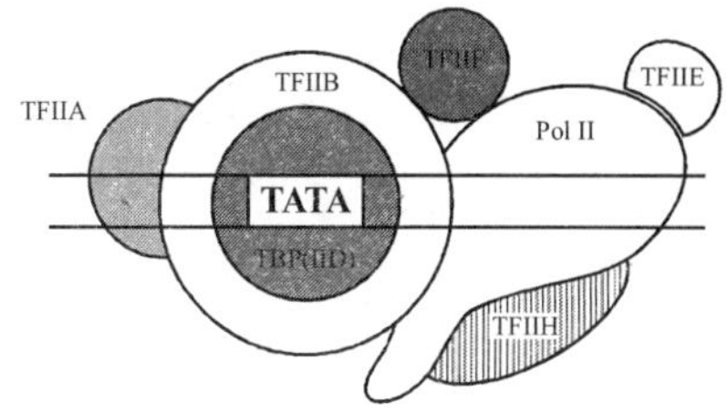


Prokaryotic TU

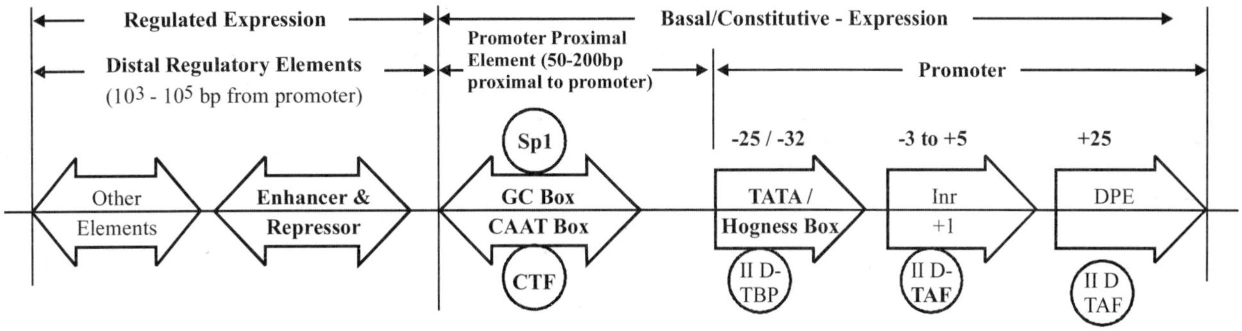


Eukaryotic TU

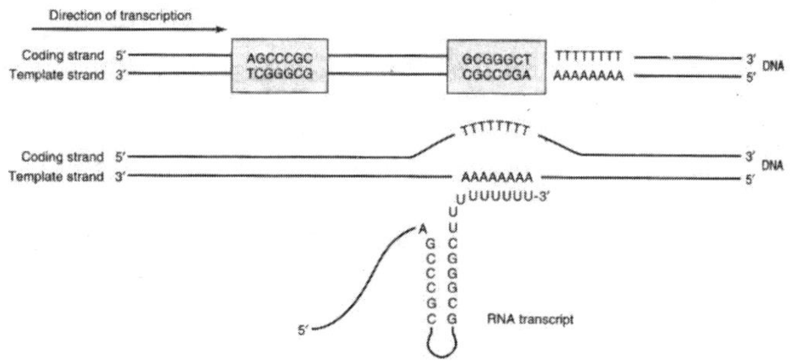


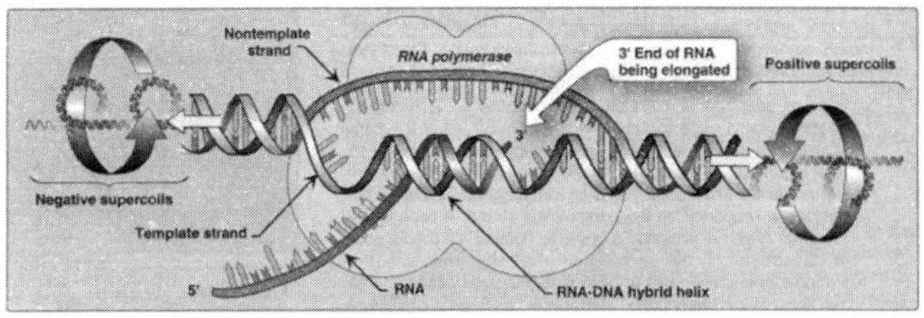


Local unwinding of DNA caused by RNA polymerase

| | Prokaryotes | Eukaryotes |
|---|---|---|
| **Promoters (Cis-acting element):** Named & positioned a/t location of **5′to3′** base sequence in **coding/non-template strand** | 1. **"-35 sequence"**: It is a consensus sequence of **8 nucleotie pairs** (5′-TGTTG-ACA-3′) centered approximately **35 bp upstream (left)** of transcription start site (+1). RNA binds & forms **closed complex**.<br>2. **"-10 sequence"** or **Pribnow/TATA-box**: It is a **6 nucleotide** pairs of A+T rich consensus sequence (5′-**TATA-AT-3′**) centered more proximally about **10 bp upstream (left)** to TSS (+1). Closed f/b **open complex** (k/a **transcription bubble**) is formed d/t melting /unwinding of short stretch (~14 bases) of DNA-as TATA box lack GC base pairs.<br>3. **UP (Upstream promoter):** It is AT rich recognition element occurring b/w **-40 & -60** in highly expressed genes. It is bound by **α-subunit** of RNAP. | 1. **Hogness/TATA-box (-25 or -32 sequence):** It is the major assembly point usually located 25 bp upstream from TSS (+1). This region has a sequence of TATAAAG and the consensus sequene is 5′ – **TATA-AA-3′**, which is recognized by **TATA- binding protein (TBP)** subunit of TF IID It is functionally similar to prokaryotic TATA box<br>**2. Initiator sequence (Inr): It spans the transcription start site (from-3 to +5)** and consist of **CS**<br>**"Y Y A N T Y Y"**, where N is any nucleotide and<br>**A** Y is pyrimmidine (Lehninger)<br>**T C A+1 G T T** , where A+1 is first transcribed<br>**T C** nucleotide. (Harper).<br>TSS is very near or usually within Inr hence forming open complex with unwound DNA. **TBP associated factor (TAFs) subunit of TFIID** recognize & help binding it to pol II.<br>3. **Downstream promoter element (DPE):** It is located **25 bp downstream (+25)** of TSS and has CS - (5'-A G A **CGTG** - 3') which is recognized by **TAF subunit of TF IID**<br>G T |

**Promoter proximal elements** (located b/w **50-200 bp** proximal to promoter)

- This **cis acting upstream element** located **proximal** to promoter is **not found in prokaryotes**
- It long with (a/w) promoters is required for **basal (Constitutive) expression** of gene.
- It **determines frequency** of even and **function in both direction**.
- PPEs bind to trans elements (proteins/activators) through **DNA binding domains (DBD)** and others (eg TF, pol II, coregulators) through activation domain (AD)

**1. CAAT box:**
It is located between 70 & 80 bp upstream (**-70 to -80**) of TSS (+1) and has CS (**CCAATC**) which is recognized & bound by **trans acting transcription factors** like **CTF** (als called **C/E PB, NF-1, NFY**)
2. **GC box** with CS (GGGCGG) recognized by Sp1

| Element | Consensus Sequence (CS) | Activator/Factor that bind to them |
|---|---|---|
| GC | $G_3CG_2$<br>CAACTGAC<br>TGGAN$_5$GCCAA<br>C C | **Sp1**<br>**MyoD**<br>**NF-1** |
| AP1 | T G A G T C A<br>C A | Jun, Fos, ATF |
| Ig Octamer | A T G C A A A T | Oct 1, 2, 4, 6 |
| Heat Shock | $(NGAAN)_3$ | HSF |
| Serum response | GATGCCCATA | SRF |

**Distal Regulatory Elements – Enhancer & Repressor (Silencer) Only found in eukaryotes**

- These are **cis acting** (i.e. located on same chromosome) DNA sequences that **regulate** (i.e. **increase or decrease**) the rate of initiation of transcription by Pot IIin eukaryotes. These are **not found** in these **prokaryotes.** These are usually located distally (i.e. **$10^3$ to $10^5$** from promoter site. However they can
1. be located **upstream** (to 5′ end) **or down stream** (to 3′ end) of transcription start site and even **within the transcribed protein coding portions.**
2. function in **orientation independent manner** (in both direction).
3. occur on **either strand** of DNA.
4. exert effects when *located close to or even tens of thousands of bp away* from promoter/TU.
5. be of 2 types – **enhancer (response elements)** and **repressor (silencer)** that bind TFs to increase & decrese transcription initiation respectively. So these are required for **regulated expression.**
- These enhancer / silencer – binding TFs can interact with other TFs bound to promoter with RNA pol II by **bending & looping the DNA.**

**Factors for promoter specific binding**

- **Sigma (σ) subunit** of prokaryotic RNAP is responsible for promoter **recognition specificity** of enzyme and its binding to promoter l/t formation of PIC
- Functions of different sigma subunits are

| | |
|---|---|
| **σ 70** | **House keeping** |
| σ54 | Modulations of cellular *nitrogen levels* |
| σ38 | Stationary phase gene |
| **σ32** | **Heat shock gene** |
| σ28 | Chemotaxis & flagella genes |
| σ24 | Extracytoplasmic functions like *heat shock functions* |
| σ18 | Extracytoplasmic functions like *ferric citrate transport* |

- Various **general transcription factors (GTFs)** like transcription factor for pol II i.e. **TF II from A to H (except C & G)** are required for PIC formation as RNAP II alone cannot discriminate b/w promoter & other regions of DNA. GTFs in order of binding assembly (i.e. basal components of transcription and their functions) are

| Components | Function |
|---|---|
| **TF II D** | - It consists of 1 **TATA binding protein (TBP)** & **14** TBP associated factors **(TAFs)**<br>- It is the only factor that is **independently capable of recognizing & specific, high affinity binding** to **(TATA box) promoter DNA** through its TBP subunit.<br>- TBP binds to TATA box **in minor groove** of DNA (whereas most TFs bind in **major groove**) causing around **100° kink/bend** in DNA helix, which facilitates the interaction of TAFs with other components of transcription initiation complex (TIC).<br>- Because of various TAFs, TF-II D is also an important *component of TIC of pol I and II, even if they do not contain TATA box.*<br>- All transcription factors (including **TBP** of **IID**) are **basal components** i.e. they *support basal transcription* but not augmented /enhanced transcription. However , **TAFs** (of **IID**) are essential for activator (like Sp 1 etc) **enhanced /augmented transcription** – and so are **coactivatior /coregulator**: (Coregulators are required for action of activators and examples include – *TAFs, Meds, chromatin modifiers and remodelers).* |
| **TFIIB** (subunits **1**) | **It binds to TBP** (of II D) and to **DNA** on either side of TBP (of II D) and recruits (+ binds) RNA **polymerase II** – TFIIF complex. |
| **TFIIA** (3 sub units) | - It **stabilizes** the **TF II and TBP (II D) on promoter** DNA, resulting in a ternary complex that is more tightly bound & more precisely located on TIC. This TBP- promoter IIA-IIB complex then attracts & tethers pol II- IIF complex.<br>- Its binding is *not always essential* but is very *important at non consensus promoters* where TBP binding is relatively weak. IIA binds prior to IIB |
| **TF II F (2** sub **units)** | **It binds tightly to pol II and targets/brings it to promoter** both by binding with **TF-IIB** and by *reducing the binding of polymerase II to non specific sites on DNA.* |
| **TF II E (2** sub **units)** | Recruits TF **II H** and has **ATPase & helicase** activities |
| **TF II H (12** subunits) | - After binding of IIH, **closed complex** of 60 bp (-30 to + 30) size is formed – as binding of each TF has increased the size.<br>- **Helicase activity** of II H **melts /unwinds DNA** (a process requiring ATP) near TSS there by creating an **open complex.**<br>- **Kinase activity** of II H **phosphorylates pol II** (within the CTD) allowing it to clear the promoter.<br>- It recuruits nucleotide excision repair protein. So the repair of damaged DNA is more efficient in template strand (than non template strand) of actively transcribing (than inactive genes.) |

| Promoter Acessibility | - Transcription machinery cannot access promoter of **eukaryotic genes** b/o their *wrapping up in nucleosomes*. Binding of TFs to enhancers causes recruitment of **chromatin remodeling & modifying coregulatory factors** (like Swi/Snf, SRC-1, p300 /CBP or P/CAF) – ultimately l/t **nucleosome eviction (removal)** and opening of promoter to become accessible.<br>- **Interconversion of hetero chromatin** (i.e. highly condensed, most inactive segments of DNA) and **euchromatin** (i.e. relatively relaved, highly transcribing genes) is k/a **chromatin remodeling. Acetylation**, mediated by **HATs (histone acetyl transferases)** *removes positive* charge on **lysine** residues at amino terminal of histone and thus decreases the interaction b/w histones and negatively charged DNA – ultimately converting hetero chromatin to euchromatin and removing nucleosomes. **HDACs (histone deacetylase)** *restores positive charge* building stronger interactions b/w histones & DNA thus forming nucleosomes.<br>- So this **epigenetic code of histone – protein modifications** can increase or decrease gene transcription. Mutations in **code writers** (proteins that catalyze) or **code readers** (proteins that differentially bind) modified histones l/t diseases. |
|---|---|

## Micro- RNA (mi-RNA), si RNAs, st RNAs, sRNAs & RNA interference

- Micro-RNAs are *non coding (nc RNA* i.e. they do not encode protein) *RNAs about 22 (21-25) nucleotide long*, found in *multicelluar eukaryotes* (eg worms, flies, plants & mammals).
- Upto *1% of human genome* may encode *mi RNAs & mi RNAs may target upto 1/3rd of human m-RNAs*
- mi – RNAs are synthesized from much larger precursors in several steps. The transcription units of pri-mi RNAs are located *either in introns (intronic DNA) of other genes* or (and coexpressed with) host genome. Therefore mi *RNA encoding genes must possess a distinct promotor , coding region, and polyadenylation / termination signals.*
- Most mi RNAs are transcribed by **RNA polymerase II** into **primary transcripts (pri-mi RNAs)** which is **5′ – capped & 3′ – polyadenylated**. pri-mi RNA is 500-1000 nucleotide long single stranded RNA with extensive intramolecular 2° (double stranded hair pin) structure, which is maintained following processing by **Drosha – DGCR8 nuclease.** A nuclear RN ase for double stranded (d/t 2° structure) RNA called **Drosha** acts with a nuclear double stranded RNA binding protein called **DGCR8** in humans (**Pasha** in drosophila) and cleaves the hair pin region out of long precursor RNA generating a 70-80 nucletide long **pre- mi RNA**
- pre – mi RNA is exported through nuclear pore by **exportin 5** into cytoplasm, where **dicer nuclease** (ds RNA specific RNA ase called Dicer act with cytoplasmic ds RNA binding protein called TRBP) in humans to form mi- RNA duplex. Ultimately one of the 2 strands (21-22 nucleotide long) is selected for loading into RISC or RNA induced silencing complex to form a mature functional mi RNA.
- mi RNA is *complementary in sequence* to particular regions of m RNA. So mi RNAs typically hybridize, via the formation of **imperfect RNA-RNA duplexes** within the 3′ untranslated regions (3′ UTRs) of specific target m-R NAs leading to either translational arrest (near perfect match) or mRNA degradation (partal match). In either case, the mRNA and thus the **gene** that produces it is **silenced.**
- Micro (mi) RNA are non coding regulatory RNAs that play ***important role in gene expression***Q. These **inhibit gene expression** by **RISC mediated gene silencing**. It is used as a mechanism to protect against invading RNA viruses (esp important in plants which lack an immune system) & to control the activity of transposons & developmental timing.
- Many mi RNAs are present only transiently during development , & are referred to as **small temporal RNAS (st RNAs)**.
- If an investigator introduces into an organism a duplex RNA molecule corresponding in sequence to virtually any mRNA,

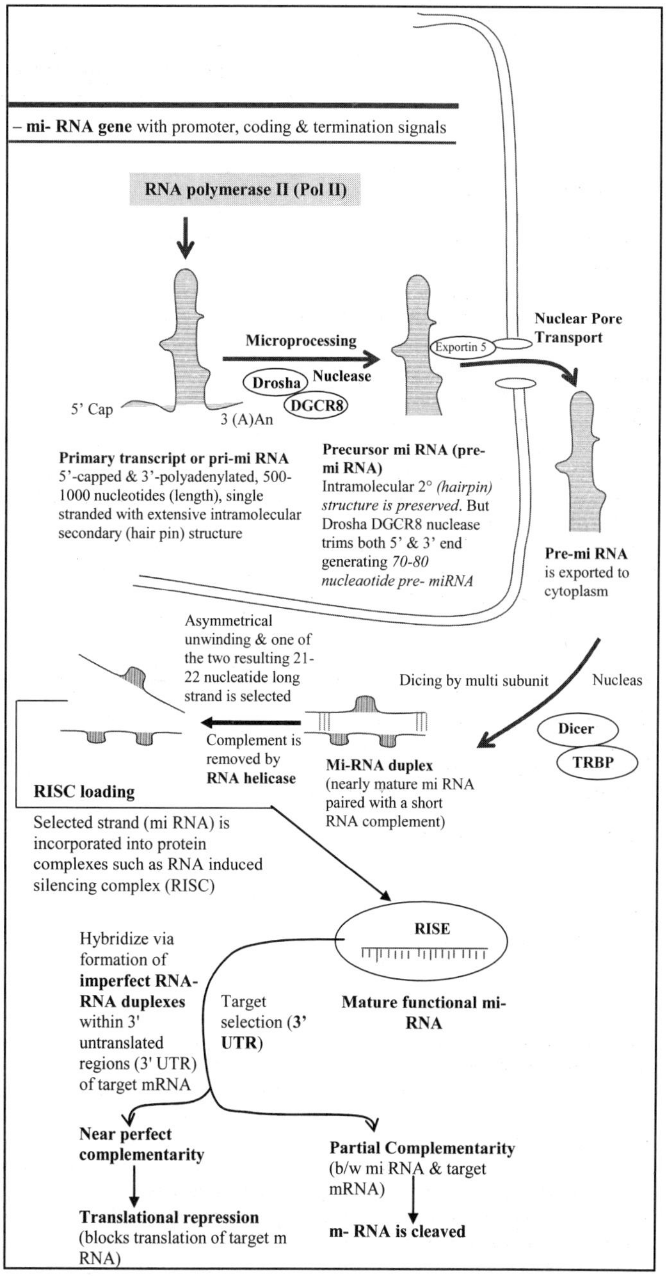

Dicer nuclease cleaves the duplex into short segments, called **small interfering RNAs (siRNAs).** These short (21-25 nucleotide long) si RNAs usually form **perfect RNA-RNA hybrid** with their targets potentially anywhere within the length of m RNA where the complementary sequence exists. Formation of such RNA-RNA duplexes between si RNAs and mRNA results in reduced specific protein production because the si **RNA – mRNA complexes are degraded**, mostly in specific cytoplasmic organelles termed **P- bodies**. The process is k/a **RNA interference RNAi** for which **Nobel prize** was given to Andrew Fire & Craig Mello in 2006.

- **RNAi** is activated when RNA molecule occurs in double stranded pairs in cell. Ds RNA activates biochemical machinery which degrades those mRNA that carry a genetic code identical to that of ds RNA. When such m RNA molecules disappear, the corresponding gene is silenced and no protein of encoded type is made.
- So **RNA i** is extremely useful research tool as it allows genetic researchers to **knock out specific genes**, observe the consequent disruptions, and so determine exactly what the gene does. It has already revealed genes responsible for diabetes and muscle problems. In lab it has been used to block HIV and polio virus infections.
- **Nearly all mi RNAs and si RNAs cause inhibition of gene expression**. Bacteria also contain small hetrogenous regulatory RNAs called sRNAs. Bacterial sRNAs range in size from 50-500 nucleotides, and like eukaryotic mi RNA / si RNA also control a large array of genes. Similary sRNAS often repress, but some times activate protein synthesis by binding to specific m RNA
- *Mi RNAs are considered to be endogenously expressed counterparts of Si RNAs*

## Mechanism &Types of Splicing

There are 4 classes of introns

### 1 & 2 Self Splicing Introns (SSI)

- It **function as ribozyme,** does *not require protin enzymes and high energy cofactors* (such as ATP) for splicing
- Splicing mechanism involves **two transesterification** reactions in which a new phosphodiester bond *(5' – 3' PDB in group I and 5'-2' PDB in group II) is formed at the expense of old bond* maintaining the balance of energy. These reactions are very similar to DNA breaking and rejoining reactions promoted by topoisomerase and site specific recombinases.
- Self splicing introns may be of 2 types

| Group I SSI | Group II SSI |
|---|---|
| Found in some nuclear, mitochondrial and chloroplast genes that code for r RNAs, mRNAs & t-RNAs; and some introns in bacteria | Found in primary transcript of mitochondrial or chloroplast m RNAs in fungi, algae & plants; and some introns in bacteria |
| - Nucleophile in first transesterification reaction is **3'-hydroxyl group of guanine nucleoside or nucleotide (guanosine, GMP, GDT, or GTP)**<br>- 3' → 5' phosphodiester bond is formed but **lariat (loop) like intermediate is not formed** | - **2' hydroxyl group of adenosine (A) residue** (known as **branch site**) in intron is nucleophile.<br>- **2'→ 5' phosphodiester bond and branched lariat (loop) like intermediate structure is formed.** The excised intron is released as a lariat, in which adenosine has 3 phosphodiester bonds. Lariat is degraded. |
| 2 Transeterifications reactions include<br>- **3' (OH) of G (guanosine, GMP, GDP, GTP cofactors)** is used for nucleophile attack (not energy). It **attacks the phosphate at 5' splice site (junction of 5' exon & intron = 5' end of intron = splice donor site) forming a normal 3'- 5' phosphodiester bond** with 5[1] end of intron.<br>- 3'(OH) of 5' exon that is displaced in this step then acts as nuceophile and triggers 2nd transesterification reaction by attacking **5' phosphate** at **splice acceptor site (3' end** of **intron** or **3' splice site**) forming 3'→5' phosphodiester bond. This results in precise excision of introns & ligation of exons. | 2 Transesterification reactions are<br>- **2' (OH) group of A (adenosine)** in the branch point sequence of intron act as nucleophile, attacking the phosphate at 5' splice site forming ***unusual 2' → 5' phosphodiester bond and creating a lariat (loop) like structure***[Q].<br>- Newly freed 3' (OH) of 5' exon attacks 5' phosphate at splice acceptor site (3' end of intron or 3' splice site) forming 3' → 5' phospodiester bond, resulting in excision of introns & ligation of exons. |

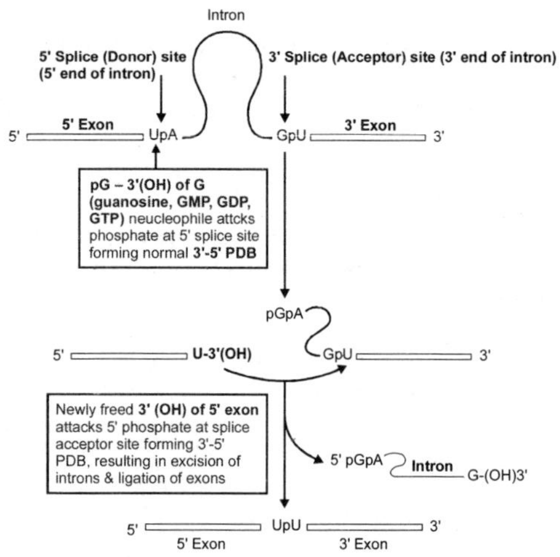


**Group I SSI**

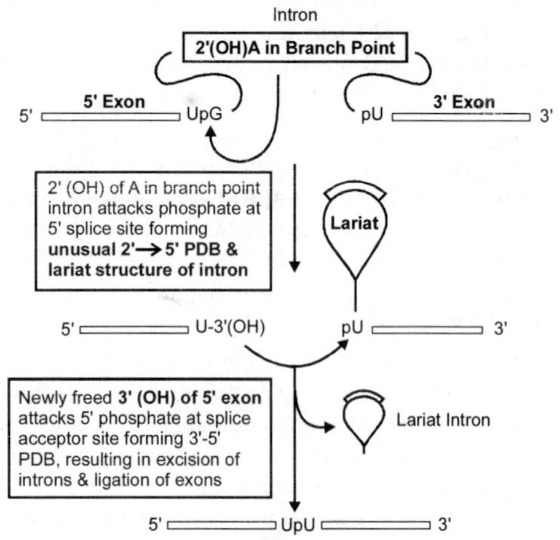


**Group II SSI**

### 3. Splicesomal Introns

- Most introns are not self **splicing**. This *largest class* of introns includes those *found in nuclear mRNA primary transcripts*
- These are called splicesomal introns, *because their removal occurs within and is catalyzed by large protein complex called* ***splicesome****. Within the splicesome,* the introns undergo splicing by same ***lariat (loop) forming mechanism as group II introns***[Q].
- Splicesomal introns have **dinucleotide sequence GU at 5' end and AG at 3'** end and these **mark the site where splicing occurs**. The GU and AG sequences at the beginning and end respectively, of introns are invariant.

- **U1 sn RNA** contains a sequence complementary to sequences near the **5′ splice site of nuclear mRNA introns**; and **U1** binds to this region of primary transcript. **U2** is paired *to intron at a position encompassing the A residue that become nucleophile.* This adenyl residue in branch point sequence is typically located 20-40 nucleotides upstream from 3′ end of intron being removed. *The branch site identifies the 3′ splice site.* Base pairing of U2 causes a bulge that displaces and activate **adenylate (of branch site in intron), whose 2′ (OH) will form the lariat structure through a 2′- 5′ phosphodiester bond**.
- After $U_1$ and $U_2$, the remaining sn RNPs ($U_4$ – $U_6$ complex and $U_5$) bind to form an inactive spliceosome. Internal rearrangements activate complex in which $U_1$ & $U_4$ have been expelled and U6 is paired with both U2 and 5′ splice site. This is followed by catalytic steps similar to and group II SSI. **ATP is required for the assembly of spliceosome, but not for RNA cleavage - ligation**
- Some less common spliceosomes contain **$U^{11}$ and $U_{12}$ snRNPs** in place of $U^1$ and $U^2$. Whereas **U1 and U2** containing spliceosome remove introns with **(5′) GU and AG (3′) terminal sequences**, the $U^{11}$ and $U^{12}$ containing spliceosome remove rare class of introns that have **(5′) AU and AC (3′) terminal sequence** to mark the intrionic splice site.
- Splicing apparatus is tethered to *CTD of RNA polymerase III* coordinating splicing & transcription and providing a mechanism for bringing 2 splice sites together. **After splicing introns (lariat) remains in nucleus and is degraded.**

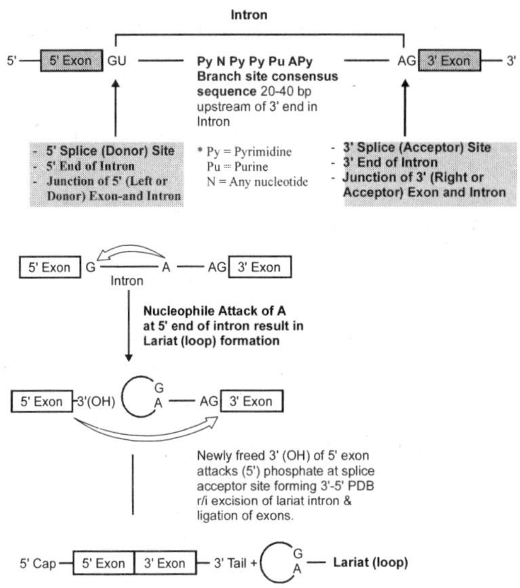


**4. Class 4 Introns are found in t RNAs**

- Distinguished from group I and group II introns in that the splicing reaction **requires ATP and endonuclease**
- **Splicing endonuclease (ribonuclease) cleaves the phosphodiester bond** at both ends of introns and two **exons are joined by** a mechanism similar to DNA **ligase** reaction.

## Splicing and sn RNAs

- Uracil rich Small nuclear RNAs (sn RNAs) are **non coding RNAs** that play pivotal ***role in RNA processing and splicing***[Q] by forming **small nuclear ribonucleo protein particles (SnRNPs or "snurps")**
- SnRNAs vary in size from *90-300 Nucleotides*. Some example include.

| Name | Length (nucleotides ) | Localization | Molecules per cell |
|---|---|---|---|
| U1 | 165 | Nucleoplasm | $1\times10^6$ |
| U2 | 188 | Nucleoplasm | $5\times10^5$ |
| **U3** | 216 | **Nucleolus** | $3\times10^5$ |
| U4 | 139 | Nucleoplasm | $1\times10^5$ |
| U5 | 118 | Nucleoplasm | $2\times10^5$ |
| **U6** | 106 | **Perichromatin granules** | $3\times10^5$ |
| 4.55 | 95 | Nucleus & cytoplasm | $3\times10^5$ |
| 7 SK | 280 | Nucleus & cytoplasm | $5\times10^5$ |

- Besides its role in splicing, the **sn RNA U1** directly binds to transcription factor TF II H and may regulate TF II H or affect the *coupling between transcription & splicing.*
- **$U_1$, $U_2$, $U_4$, $U_5$ & $U_6$** – SnRNAs are involved in intron removal and processing of mRNA precursors into mRNA. **$U_7$** - snRNA is involved in **production of correct 3′ ends of histone mRNA**, which lacks a poly (A) tail.
- A 331 nucleotide nc RNA called **7SK**, abundant in mammals, binds to *pol II transcription elongation factor P-TEFb* (that modulates mRNA gene transcription elongation by RNA polymerase II) and repress transcriptase elongation.
- In **SLE**, autoantibodies develop against their own nuclear proteins like SnRNPs.

## sno RNAs and r RNA modification

- Small nucleolar RNAs (sno RNAs) are nc RNAs that guide nucleoside modification and cleavage reactions in pre- rRNAs.
- In yeast about 70 and in humans > 200 sno RNAs are found
- sno RNAs are *60-300 nucleotides* long and many are encoded with in the *introns of other genes.*
- Each sno RNA includes a *10-21 nucleotide* sequence that is perfectly *complementary to some site in rRNA.* The conserved sequence elements in the remainder of sno RNA fold into structures that are bound by sno RNP proteins.
- The most common nucleoside modification in eukaryotic r RNAs are, again, conversion of uridine to pseudouridine and ado met dependent nucleoside methylation (often at 2′ –OH groups). These reactions rely on **sno-RNA protein complexes** or **sno RNPs**, each consisting of a sno RNA & 4-5 proteins
- There are 2 classes of sno RNPs, both defined by *Key conserved sequence elements referred* to as lettered boxes.

1. **Box C/D** sno RNPs function in *2′ – O – methylations*
2. **Box H/ACA** sno RNPs are involved in *pseudouridylylation*

## Splicing of Primary Transcript

- **Primary transcript** contains 2 types of sequences

| **Introns (Intervening) sequence** that do not code the genetic information | **Exon (Expressed) sequence** that contain genetic information & code for various amino acids |
|---|---|

- It undergoes extensive processing **(RNA splicing)** to convert into functional RNA which involves **cleaving out of introns** and **splicing together of exons,** facilitated by **Sn RNP or snurp of spliceosome.** This process occurs in nucleus and mature m RNA is then transported to cytoplasm where it is translated into protein.
- *The process of removing introns (RNA sequences which do not code for proteins) and joining exons (RNA sequences that code for proteins) is called 'Splicing'.*
- ***The process of splicing is mediated by Small nuclear ribonucleoprotein particles (sn RNP) or 'Snurps' which are formed from sn RNA***
- *The molecular machinery that accomplishes splicing is called a* **spliceosome** *which is formed when the primary transcript combines with the Sn RNP.* **Spliceosome** consists of *primary transcript,* ***five (Sn-RNA) small nuclear RNAs (U1, U2, U4, U5, U6)*** and > 60 proteins collectively these form a **small nuclear ribo**

### Splice Site Mutation & Alternative Splicing

- Splice site mutation can l/t improper splicing & production of aberrant proteins. 15% of all genetic disease are caused b/o **faculty splicing** and example includes beta thalassemia (with defective beta -globin protein)
- **Alterantive patterns of mRNA splicing** result from *tissue specific developmental & adaptive control mechanism (such as chromatin epigenetic markers). This produces diverse set of proteins from a limited set of genes and example includes multiple isoforms of* ***tropomyosin protein.***
- Tissue specific regulation of gene expression can be provided by alternative splicing by control elements in promoter or by use of alternative promoters. Example, **insulin & cAMP control glucokinase (GK) gene transcription in liver while glucose controls GK expression in pancreatic beta-cells.**

**nucleoprotein (Sn RNP) complex** or **snurp.**

- *The binding of sn RNP brings the sequences of neighboring exons into correct alignment for splicing.*

| | |
|---|---|
| $U_1$ | 1[st] binds to 5′ **exon-interon boundary** |
| $U_2$ | Binds to **branch site** and this **expose the nucleophilic A residue** |
| $U_5/U_4/U_6$ | Mediate an ATP dependent protein mediated **unwinding** that results in disruption of the base paired U4-U6 complex with the release of U4. U6 is then able to interact first with U2, then with U1. This approximate the 5′ splice end, the branch point with its reactive A, and 3′ splice site. This alignment is enhanced by U5. This process also results in formation of **loop or lariat** structure. |
| $U_2$-$U_6$ | **Two ends are cleaved**, by U2-U6 with in the SnRNP complex. |

*U6 is essential* since yeast deficient in this are not viable.

## Primary Transcript and Post Transcriptional Modification of hn-RNA

- The RNA formed and released from DNA template is known as **primary transcript**. The **primary transcript** of m-RNA is **hn-RNA** (and of mi-RNA is **pri-miRNA**).
- A **primary transcript** is a linear, RNA copy of a trancriptional unit – i.e., segment of DNA between initiation & termination sequence. The primary transcripts of both **prokaryotic & eukaryotic t-RNA and r-RNA** as well as **eukaryotic m-RNA**, 55 RNA, Sn RNAs, RNA processing mechinary are inactive and undergoes modifications for activation. In contrast, ***prokaryotic mRNA is generally identical to its primary transcript***[Q].
- ***Nearly all eukaryotic & prokaryotic RNA (except prokaryotic m-RNA) are extensively processed primariy with in the nucleus (for eukaryotes) before they become functional***[Q]. The processes of transcription, RNA processing & RNA transport from nucleus are highly co-ordinated by – **SAGA** (in yeast) & **P/CAF** (in humans) and **TREX** (transcription export). Transcriptional co-activator (SAGA or P/CAF) link *transcription activation to RNA processing* by recruiting TREX that links *transcription elongation complex, RNA splicing machinery and nuclear export.*

### Modification of Eukaryotic mRNA

- All primary transcript synthesized in nucleus by **RNA polymerase II** is k/a **heterogenous nuclear (hn)** RNA. This **pre-mRNA** (primary transcript) the immediate product of gene transcription, is very heterogenous and can be > *10-50 times longer* than mature m-RNA. This hn RNA is very unstable, exists as hn RNP (ribonucleoprotein) and must undego post transcriptional modification (processing) to appear in cytoplasm as m-RNA.
- Addition of **7-methylguanosine cap** at 5′ terminal, **poly (A) tail** at 3′ terminal; secondary **methylation** of **2′ hydroxy** and **$N^7$ adenyl** residues and **splicing** (introns removed & exons joined) converts hn-RNA to m-RNA.

- **Capping**

- It is the 1[st] *processing reaction* for hn-RNA occuring in the ***nucleus***[Q].
- ***Cap structure (7 methyl guanosine) is attached backwards to 5′ end of hn RNA***[Q] forming unusual *5′ → 5′ triphosphate* linkage.
- *Nuclear guanylyl transferease* enzyme is required for creation of GTP (guanosine triphosphate) part of cap.
- **Secondary methylation** of 2′ hydroxy (of 1[st] & 2[nd] nucleotide) & $N^7$ of adenylyl residues of terminal guanine occurs in ***cytosol***[Q], and is catalyzed by *guanine-7 methyl transferase.* S-adenosylmethionine is the source of methyl group.
- ***5′ capping is required for recognization of mRNA by translation machinery, efficient translation initiation and protection of 5′ end of m-RNA from attack by 5′ → 3′exonuclease***[Q]. Cap ***facilitates binding of m-RNA to 43 S initiation complex***[Q] (Harper) / ***40 S ribosome unit***[Q] (Lippincot).
- The **guanine** of cap is methylated at **$N^7$** position, and **Ist & 2[nd] nucleotides** adjacent to cap (of m RNA) are methylated at $2^1$ – OH position. So the 7-methyl guanosine triphosphate cap is linked to 5′ end (at 5′-hydroxyl position of 2′ – O – methyl ribonucleoside) through three phosphate *(i.e. triphosphate linkage).*

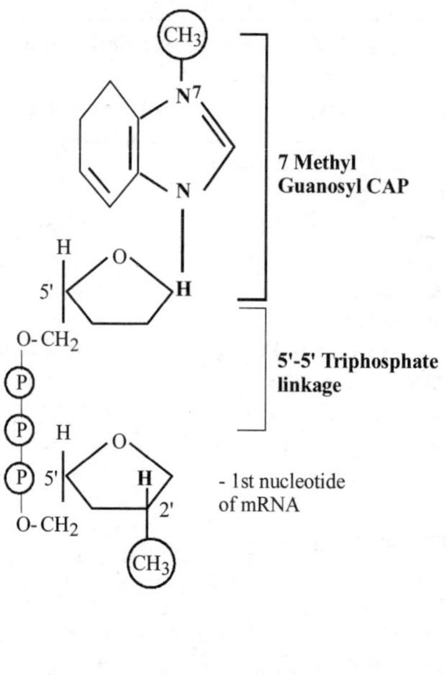


### Modification of Transfer (t) RNA

Both eukaryotic & prokaryotic t-RNA precursor molecules are modified by

- *Removal of introns from anticodon loop*
- **Trimming of sequences both at 5′ and 3′ end.** 16 nucleotide sequence at 5′ end is cleaved by RNase P (a ribozyme).
- ***Replacement of uracil residues at 3′ end by CCA sequence***[Q], catalyzed by *nucleotidyl transferase.* 3′ OH of A ribose is point of attachment
- Many bases are converted to modified unusual bases including ***Dihydrouracil (D), pseudo uracil (Ψ) and methylated bases (m)***[Q] by methylation, reduction, deamination, rearranging glycosidic bonds & nucleotide alkylation
- ***Methylation occurs in nucleus whereas cleavage & attachment*** **of CCA are cytoplasmic functions.**

- **Addition of poly (A) tail at 3′ end**

- The m-RNA is cleaved ***about 20 nucleotides down stream of a consensus recognition sequence, called the poly adenylation signal sequence (AAUAAA)***[Q] found near 3′ end.
- Poly (A) tail is added to new 3′ end by ***nuclear enzyme polyadenylate polymerase***[Q], using ATP as the substrate. This tail is not transcribed from DNA and contain *40-200 adenine nucleotide.*
- Tail helps stabilize the m-RNA, facilitate their exit from nucleus and protects 3′ end from attack of 3′ → 5′exonuclease[Q].
- The presence of poly (A) tail does not necessarily means that the precurssor mRNA will appear in cytoplasm, ***because all poly (A) taild hnRNA do not contribute to hn-RNA***[Q]. Similarly ***not all cyto plasmic m-RNA have poly A tails (although most have)***[Q]; m-RNA *coding for histones & some interferons* do not have poly (A) tails
- Poly (A) tail is gradually shortened as m-RNA enters cytoplasm.

- **Removal of introns & joining of exons (splicing)**

- Maturation of m-RNA involves ***removal of non- coding (introns or intervening sequences***[Q]) from primary transcript and ***joining of remaining coding sequenes (or exons)***[Q]
- The process of removing introns & joining exons is called **splicing** and the molecular machine accomplishing the task is k/a **spliceosome.** The splicing occurs in nucleus &serves to bring the actual aminoacid coding sequences (exons) together.
- Primary tanscript from histone genes contain no interons
- A hn RNA can be spliced in >2 ways to produce multiple variations of m-RNA & therefore proteins.

- **RNA Editing**

- It *changes the coding information at m-RNA level,* so that coding sequence of mRNA diffes from that of cognate DNA (exception to central dogma)
- **APo B gene** transcribes *100 kDa apo B-100 protein in liver and 48 kDa apo B-48 protein in intestine;* because **cytidine deaminase** converts a *CAA codon* in m-RNA *to UAA* at single specific site. So rather than coding *glutamine* this becomes *termination codon.*
- In **parasitic protozoa (trypanosomes)** large regions of m-RNA are synthesized without uridylate and U residues are inserted later by RNA editing.

**Modification of Ribosomal (r) RNA**

- Both prokaryotic (5S, 16S & 23S) & eukaryotic (5.8S, 18S, & 28S) rRNA are synthesized from long precursor molecule
- All ribosomal (r) RNA molecules except 5S r-RNA, are processed from a single **45 S precursor RNA** molecule in nucleolus
- ***Eukaryotic 5S rRNA is synthesized by RNA polymerase II & modified seperately***[Q].
- The ***r-RNA genes are located in nucleoli (in eukaryotes)***[Q]. Because of *lack of amplification,* large number of genes and high transcription rate is required to synthesize sufficient copies of rRNA to form the $10^7$ *ribosomes* required for each cell replication.
- The precursor (pre ribosome RNA) are cleaved in nucleolus by **ribonucleases** to yield intermediate size pieces of RNA, which are further trimmed to produce required rRNA

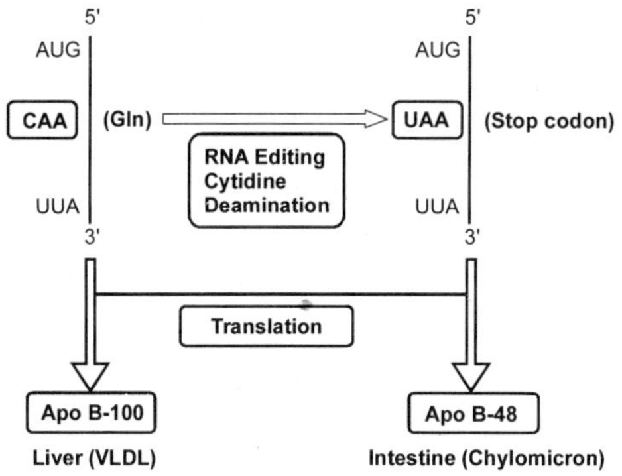


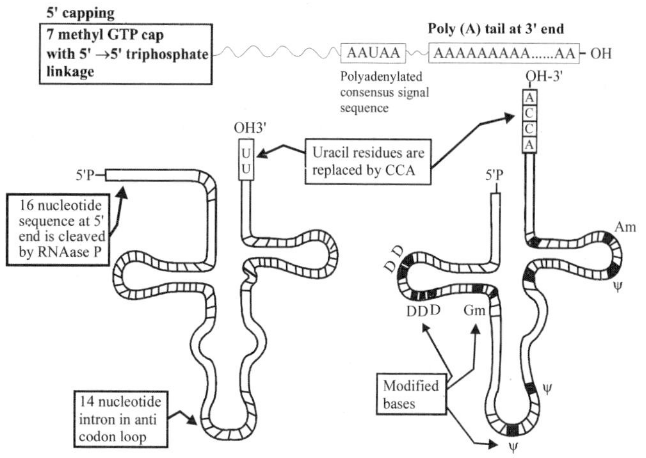


## Ribozymes

- Ribozymes are **RNA molecules with enzymatic /catalytic activity**. Examples include **peptidyl transferase**[Q], **self splicing group I introns, RN ase P,** and **hammerhead ribozyme**. Most of the activities of these ribozymes are based on 2 fundamental reactions: **transesterification** and **phosphodiester bond hydrolysis (cleavage)**. The substrate for ribozyme is often an RNA molecule and it may even be part of ribozyme itself; so most ribozyme are concerned with RNA metabolism (**splicing & endoribonuclease**). Recently a r-RNA component has been implicated in *hydrolyzing an aminoacylester &* ***plays a central role in peptide bond formation (peptidyl transferases)***[Q].
- Ribozymes vary greatly in size (40 nucleotide hammer head to 400 nucleotide SS group I intron). 3-dimensional structure is important for function. Ribozymes are inactivated by melting, or by addition of denaturing agents or complimentary oligonucleotides which disrupt normal base pairing patterns or by changing essential nucleotides.
- Certain virusoids (virus like elements) have small RNA genomes and usually require other virus to assist in their replication and /or packaging. **Hammer head ribozymes** are small segments of virusoidal RNAs, that *promote site specific RNA cleavage reactions associated with*

*replication*. Hammerhead ribozyme is a *metalloenzyme requiring Mg++ ions* for activity and their secondary structures is shaped like a head of hammer.

- **Sidney Altman & Thomas Czech** were awarded Nobel Prize (in 1989, Chemestry) for discovering catalytic property of RNAs. And this discovery changed the central dogma (DNA→RNA→protein) that RNAs are not just the transmitters of genetic information but can also act as enzyme.

## Inhibitors of

### Transcription

| | |
|---|---|
| **Refamycin, Streptovaricin** | Binds with β-*subunit of polymerase to block initiation of transcription* |
| **Actinomycin D** | Forms a *complex with double stranded DNA* & prevents movement of core enzyme & thus ***inhibiting process of chain elongation***[Q] |
| **Streptoglydigin** | Binds with β-subunit of prokaryotic polymerase & thus *inhibiting elongation* |
| **Heparin** | Binds to β-subunit & inhibits transcription in vitro |
| **α-Amanitin (Death cap, destroying angel)** | - ***Blocks m-RNA formation by inhibiting RNA polymerase II***[Q]<br>- Blocks translocation of RNA polymerase during transcription. |

### DNA replication

| | |
|---|---|
| **Cytarabine** (cytosine arabinoside) | - Cell cycle S phase specific antimetabolite that becomes phosphorylated intracellularly to an active triphosphate form which ***inhibits DNA polymerase and blocks DNA synthesis by incorporating into DNA***[Q]<br>- 1- $\beta$ - D-arabinofuranyl cytosine- triphosphate is active metabolite |
| **Anthracyclins** (eg daxaorubicin) | DNA inter calaters, *inhibiting topoisomerase II*, leading to DNA breaks |
| **Etopaside** | - Arrest cell growth in $G_2$ phase<br>- Causes DNA breaks by affecting *DNA topoisomerase II function* |
| **Nalidixic acid** | Inhibits *bacterial DNA gyrase* |
| **Ciprofloxacin** | Inhibits *bacterial DNA gyrase*, which nicks the double stranded DNA, induces negative supercoil and reseals the nicked ends |

### Translation (protein synthesis)

| | |
|---|---|
| **Streptomycin** (highly basic trisaccharide) | - Interferes with binding of f-met t RNA to ribosomes & thus inhibiting initiation process<br>- Leads to misreding of m- RNA |
| **Puromycin** | Release nascent polypeptide chains before their synthesis is complete. It binds to A site on ribosome and inhibits the entry of aminocyl t-RNA (both in bactarial & mammalian cells). |
| **Tetracycline** | Binds to 30 S subunit & inhibits binding of aminoacyl t-RNA & so inhibiting initiation process. |
| **Chloramphenicol** | Inhibits the peptidyl transferase activity of 50s subunit, thus inhibiting process of elongation. |
| **Cycloheximide** | - Inhibits peptidyl transferase activity of 60S ribosomal subunit in eukaryotes<br>- Also inhibits elongation. |
| **Erythromycin** | Binds to 50s subunit & inhibits translocation |
| **Diptheria toxin** | Binds EF-2 in eukaryates & blocks its capacity to carryout translocation |
| **Ricin & abrin** (lectins) | - Prevent aminoacyl t-RNA from binding to A site<br>- Inactivates eukaryotic 28 s ribosomal RNA |
| **Sparcomycin** | - Inhibits peptidyl transferase & release factor dependent termination |
| $\alpha$ - **Sarcin** (toxic RNA ase) | - Prevents aminoacyl t- RNA binding by cleaving a single phosphodiester bond in 28 S r- RNA |

★ **Paclitaxel** *enhances polymerization of tubulin*; a mechanism opposite to that of vinca alkaloids

★ **Actinomycin D (dactinomycin)** intercalates into the *narrow groove* of DNA double helix, thus ***interfering with DNA and RNA synthesis***[Q].

## RNA structure

consists of

- Ribose sugar
- Phosphate in diester linkage
- Bases → consisting of - Adenine - Guanine - Cytosine - Uracil

Producing ↓ Ribonucleotide ↓ Polymers of which form

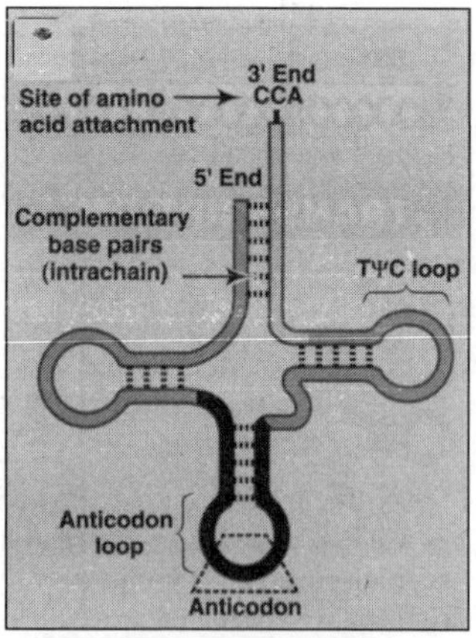


Characteristic tRNA structure

| rRNA | tRNA | mRNA |
|---|---|---|
| - ***80% of RNA in cell***[Q]<br>- Associates with protein<br>- Four size species in eukaryotes (28S, 18S, 5.8S and 5S)<br>- *Sructural component of ribosomes* | - *15%* of total RNA<br>- *Smallest* of the three species of RNA<br>- ***Contains unusual bases (pseudouridine, thymine)***[Q]<br>- ***Extensive intrachain base pairing***[Q] | - *5%* of total RNA<br>- *Most heterogenous* type<br>- *5' 'Cap'* of 7- methyl guanosine<br>- *3' Poly- A 'tail'* |

| | | |
|---|---|---|
| - Serve as site *for protein synthesis*[Q].<br>['S' - Svedberg unit, related to molecular wt & shape of compound] | - *Clover leaf pattern*[Q]<br>- At least *one specific type of molecule for each of 20 amino acids found in portein*[Q].<br>- Serve as adaptor molecule that carries a specific a.a. to ribosome / mRNA complex | - Used as *template for protein synthesis*[Q]. It carries genetic information from DNA to cytoplasm. |

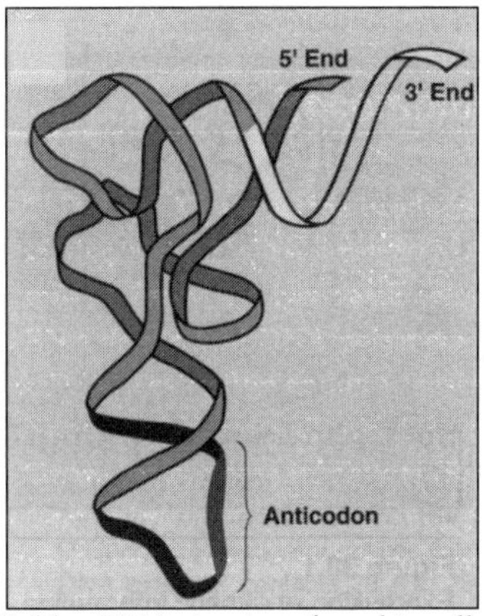


Folder tRNA structure found in cells

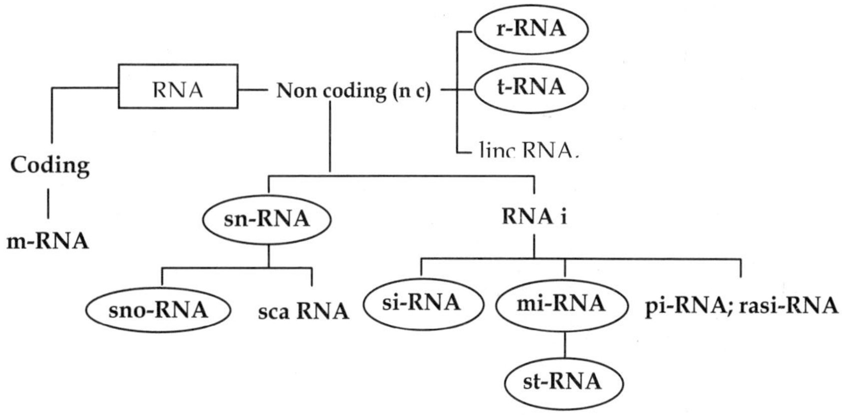


## Translation (Protein Synthesis)

***The translation of mRNA commences near its 5' terminal. The message is read from 5' to 3', concluding with the formation of carboxyl terminal of the protein***[Q]. Occurs in three phases: Initiation, Elongation & Termination

### Initiation Sequence

| Shine Dalgarno Sequence | Kozak Consensus Sequence |
|---|---|
| • Present in *prokaryotes.* **Shine Dalgarno sequence** is a ***sequence of nucleotide bases (5' - UAGGAGG-3') located 6-10 base upstream of AUG codon on mRNA molecule***[Q]. It helps ribosomes in recognizing the nucleotide sequence that is *essential for initiation of translation.*<br>• Sequence of nucleotide base (5'- UAGGAGG-3') located 6- 10bp upstream of AUG codon on mRNA at its 5' end.<br>• The 16 S ribosomal RNA component of 30 S ribosomal subunit has a nucleotide sequence at its 3' end, that is complementary to all or part of shine Dalgarno sequence<br>• Thus mRNA 5' end & 3' end, of 16 S rRNA can form complementary base pair & *facilitating binding of mRNA on 30 S ribosomal subunit.* | • Present in *eukaryotes*<br>• This sequence *surrounds AUG and determines the initiating codon of mRNA.*<br>• In this sequence *–3 and +4* positions relative to AUG are *occupied by purine* (A&G)<br><br>GCCA$^{-3}$ / GCC**AUGG**$^{+4}$ |

### Initiation Codon

- Although amino acid **methionine (Met)** has only one codon **AUG**, all organism have 2 types of t RNA for methionine tRNA $^{fMet}$ incorporating **N-formyl methionine (f-met)** in response to **initiation codon** AUG and **tRNA$^{Met}$** incorporating **methionine (Met)** in response to AUG codon in **internal position.**

Codon - **AUG**

**In prokaryotes**

| At-Initiation site | At Internal site |
|---|---|
| **N-formyl methionine** (f-Met) is incorporated by **t RNA$^{fMet}$** | **Methionine (Met)** is incorporated by **t-RNA $^{Met}$** |

**In Eukaryotes**

| Mitochondria & Chloroplast | Cytosolic Ribosomes |
|---|---|
| **N-formyl methionine** (f-Met) is incorporated by **t RNA$^{fMet}$** | Polypeptide synthesis begin with **Methionine (rather than f-Met)** but again cells use *specialized initiating t-RNA* that is distinct from tRNA$^{Met}$ used at AUG codons at interior positions of m-RNA. |

- Initiating amino acid **N-formyl - methionine (f-Met)** arrives with **tRNA $^{f-met}$** at ribosome as **N-formyl methionyl tRNA$^{f-Met}$ (f-Met - t RNA $^{fMet}$)**, which is formed in 2 steps.

- **Met -tRNA synthetase** aminoacylates (attaches) aminoacid methionine to tRNA $^{fMet}$ (and also tRNA $^{Met}$) with the help of ATP

**Methionine + t-RNA$^{fMet}$ +ATP** —**Met-tRNA Synthetase**→ **Met-tRNA$^{fMet}$ + AMP + PPi**

- More selective & specific (for only Met residue attached to tRNA$^{fMet}$) - **transformylase** transfer a formyl group from N$^{10}$-formyl tetrahydrofolate to amino group of met residue.

**Met-tRNA$^{fMet}$ + N$^{10}$ - f-THF** —**Transformylase**→ **fMet–t RNA$^{fmet}$ + THF**

- **Methionine** having anticodon **UAC** is the first amino acid required in binding to the initiation codon AUG on mRNA. In **bacteria (prokaryotes)** & **mitochondria** the ***initiator t-RNA carries an N - formylated methionine aminoacid***[Q], whereas in **eukaryotes**, the ***initiator tRNA carries a methionine that is not formylated***[Q].
- Formyl group is added to methionine by enzyme transformylase which uses N$^{10}$ formyl THF as carbon donor.
- The initiator t-RNA is the only t - RNA to be recognized by eIF2 (in eukaryotes) / IF2 (in prokaryotes) and the only t RNA to go directly to P site.

## I. Steps of Initiation of Protein Synthesis

It can be divided into 4 steps (for ease of writing eukaryotic initiation factor i.e. eIF is written as IF)

1. **Ribosomal dissociation into 40s & 60s subunits.** IF (i.e. e IF) 1A and 3 binds to 40 s subunit which delays its reassociation.
2. **Formation of 40s/43 S preinitiation complex by binding of ternary complex & 40s** subunit

- **GTP** binds to **IF2** to form binary complex & then to **met t RNAi** (a t RNA that binds initiation codon AUG & code methionine) to form **ternary complex**
- Ternary complex binds to 40 s subunit to for 43 s preinitiation complex, which is stabilized by IF 1A & 3
- IF (eIf)2 is one of the two **control points** for protein synthesis initiation in eukaryotes and ***consists of α, β & γ subunits***[Q]. **IF2α** is phosphorylated (on serine 51) by at least 4 different protein kinase (HCR, PKR, PERK & GCN2) that are activated when a cell is under stress and energy expenditure required for protein synthesis would be deleterious. Phosphorylated IF-2α binds tightly to and **inactivates the *GTP-GDP recycling protein e IF-2B***. Thus *preventing formation* of 43 s preinitiation complex & blocking protein synthesis.

3. **Formation of 43/48 S initiation complex** by binding of 40/43s preinitiation complex to mRNA.

- *MGTP (methyguanosyl triphosphate) cap at 5′ terminal of most eukaryotic m RNA facilitate its binding to 43S preinitiation complex*[Q].
- **Cap binding protein IF 4F** (which consist of 4A, 4G, 4E units) binds to the cap through 4E protein and to 40 S ribosome subunit through 4G component. IF (eIF)3 is a key protein because it binds to 4G component of 4F with high affinity and it links this complex to 40 S ribosomal subunit (in 43 S preinitiation complex)

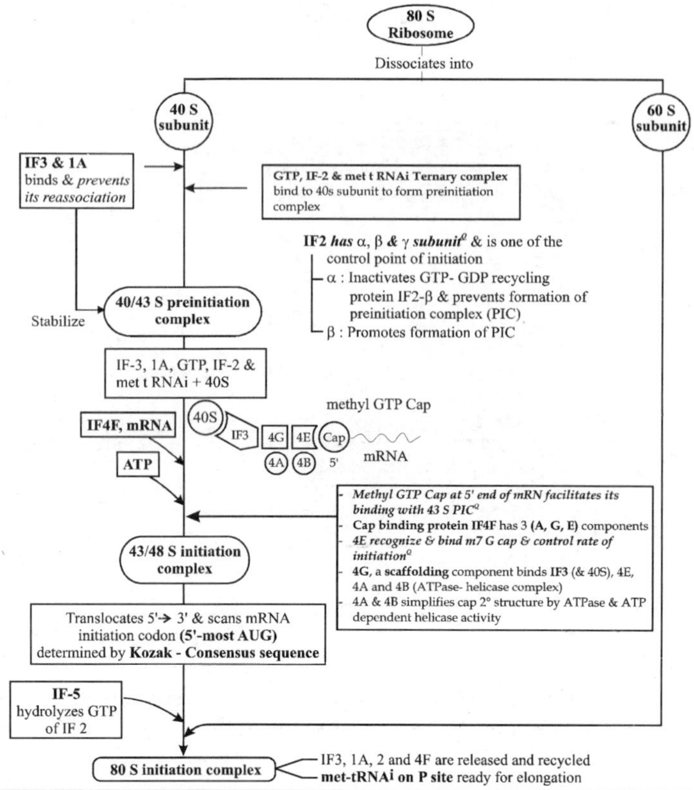


- **IF 4B (4B)** binds & reduces (melts) the complex 2° structure of 5′ end of mRNA through **ATPase & ATP dependent helicase activity**. Formation of 48 s initiation comlex require ATP hydrolysis
- **4E** is responsible for recognition & binding of m7 G cap structure at 5′ end of m RNA, ***a rate limiting step in translation. So 4E control rate of initiation***[Q]. **4G** is a *scaffoiding rotein*[Q] which binds to 4E, 4A and 4B (i.e. ATP ase- helicase complex that unwinds RNA) and to eIF3, which links the complex to 40 s ribosomal subunit.

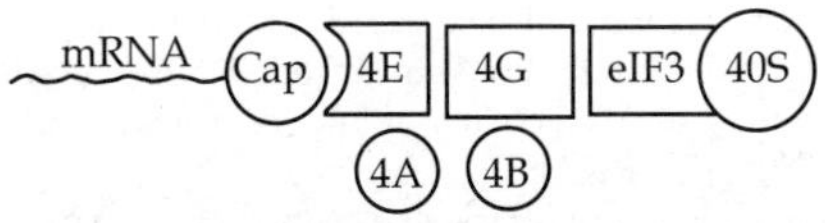


- After binding of 43 S preinitiation complex with m RNA cap, and melting of 2° structure near 5′ end of mRNA through the action of 4B helicase and ATP, the 43/48 S initiation complex translocates 5′ – 3′ & scans mRNA for suitable initiation codon. Generally this is 5′- most AUG, precisely determined by **Kozak- consensus sequence** that surround AUG (i.e. *purine at – 3 and + 4 positions relative to AUG*).

```
  -3     -1     +4
   |      |      |
GCCA / GCC AUG G
```

4. **Formation of 80 S initiation complex** by combination of 43 S initiation complex with 60 S ribosomal subunit

- Involves hydrolysis of GTP bound to IF2 by IF5, resulting in release and recycling of initiation factor bound to 48 s initiation complex and rapid association of 40S & 60S subunits to form 80 S ribosome.
- met – t RNAi is on P site ready for elongation.

| Difference | Prokaryotes | Eukaryotes |
|---|---|---|
| **m- RNA** | **Polycistronic** i.e. have several coding regions; each with its initiation & termination codon producing a seperate polypeptide | **Monocistronic** with one coding region |
| **Amino acid incorporation rate** | **18 aa/sec** | **6 aa/sec** |
| **Initial amino acid** | *Formylated methionine* (f-met) | *Methionine*[Q] (Met) |
| **Initial t-RNA** | **t-RNA $^{fMet}$** | **$tRNA^{Met}$** |
| **Transcription & translation** | Translation starts before transcription is ended (coupled) | Uncoupled |
| **Initiation factors (IF)** | 3 i.e. IF1, IF2, IF3 | >10 designated eIF |
| **Determination of initiating codon** | - *Shine Dalgarno sequence*[Q]<br>- Facilitated by IF-2 bound to GTP | *Kozak consensus sequence*[Q]<br>Facilitated by eIF-2 bound to GTP (plus additional eIF) |
| **Elongation: Delivery of aminoacyl t-RNA to A site** | - Facilitated by EF-Tu & EF- Ts | Facilitated by EF1 α and EF 1 βγ |
| **Nucleotide exchange factors** | - EF – Ts (as it exchanges its GTP for GDP on EFTu) | EF 1βγ (as it exchanges its GTP for GDP on EF 1α |
| **Peptidyl transferase activity catalyzing peptide bond formation** | *23 S rRNA of 50 S* ribosomal subunit (ribozyme) | *28 S rRNA of 60 S* ribosomal subunit (ribozyme) |
| **Translocation** | Requires EF-G & GTP | Requires EF-2 & GTP |
| **Termination** | - **Release factor (RF) 1** recognizes UAA & UAG, **RF2** recognizes UAA & UGA<br>- **RF-3** (bound to GTP) causes release of RF-1 or RF-2 as GTP is hydrolysed | - **eRF** recognizes all 3 UAA, UAG and UGA and release nascent polypeptide chain<br>- **eRF-3** (bound to GTP) function like prokaryotic RF-3 & release eRF |

## II. Elongation

It involves the addition of aminoacids to carboxy end of growing chain and movement of ribosome from 5′ end 3′ end of mRNA that is being translated (translocation)

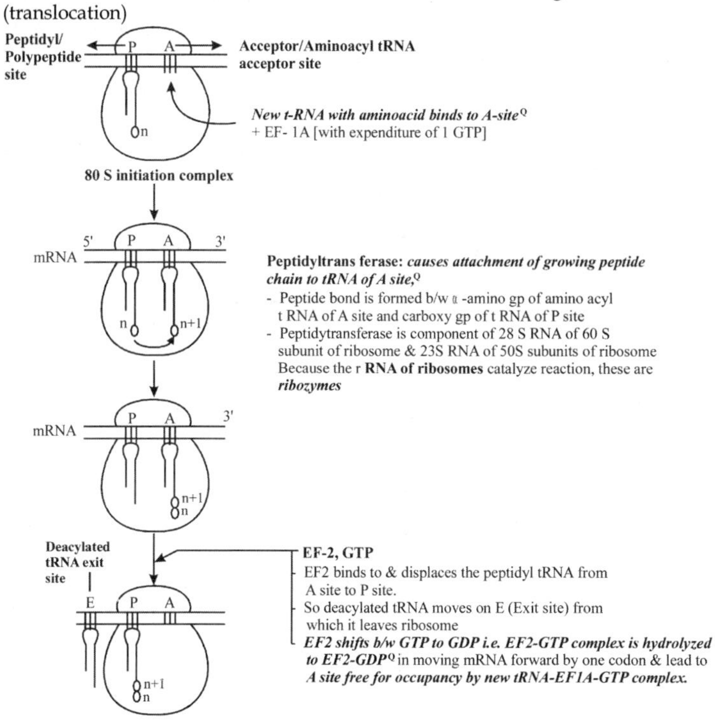


* **Total energy expenditure**: tRNA+A.A= 2ATP
- 2 GTP in elongation } 4ATP

## III. Termination

**Termination of protein synthesis** occurs when *a stop codon of m-RNA (UAA, UAG, UGA) appears in 'A' site.* These codons are recognized by release factors (RF-1, RF-3). ***RF with GTP & peptidyl transferase promotes hydrolysis of bond between the peptide & t RNA occupying the 'P' site***[Q].

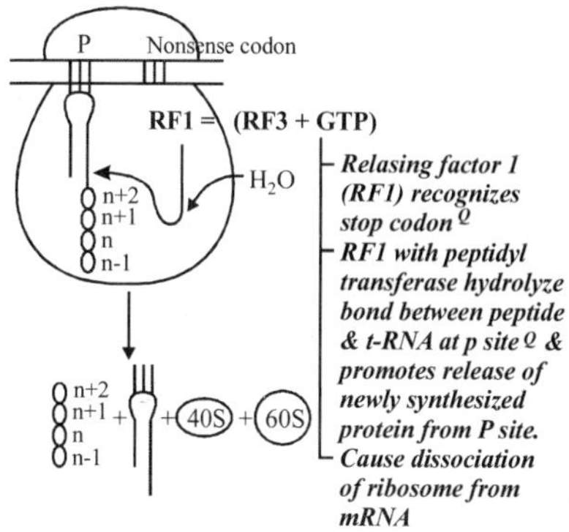


**Sites: Function**

| A site | P site | E site |
|---|---|---|
| Donor tRNA carrying appropriate amino acid on its acceptor stem, is positioned before that aa. is incorporated in protein. | Contains tRNA with growing peptide chain | Deacylated tRNA moves once the peptide bond is formed & it will soon be exiting the ribosome. |

## Peptide Bond Formation & Translocation

- **Peptidyl transferase** activity (of ***23S rRNA of 50 s or 28 S rRNA of 60 S ribosome)***[Q] is responsible for peptide bond formation.
- This **ribozyme** catalyzes the reaction between the amino group of aminoacyl t RNA at A site and carboxy carbon of peptidyl tRNA in the P site, forming a peptide bond from an ester bond.
- Because the amino acid on aminoacyl t RNA is already activated *no further energy is required for this reaction*
- The reaction *result in attachment of the growing peptide chain to the t RNA in the A site,* the which makes t RNA of P site to become deacylated.
- The **recently deacylated tRNA** is attached to P site by its anticodon and to an exit (E) site by the open CCA tail.
- **Elongation factor (EF)-2** binds and ***shifts between GTP to GDP (i.e. EF2 GTP is hydrolyzed to EF2 GDP)***[Q] to move the ribosome down one codon on m RNA, so that
  1. A site is vacant & ready to receive next charged t RNA
  2. P site contain peptidyl tRNA that has been translocated (displaced) from A site
  3. Deacylated t RNA is on E site, from which it leaves the ribosome.

## Evidence that rRNA is Peptidyl Transferase

- Ribosomes can *form peptide bonds even when proteins are removed* or inactivated
- *Few r RNA sequences are highly conserved* in all species
- These conserved regions are *on the surface of RNA molecule*
- RNA can be catalyst
- Mutations that result in antibiotic resistance at the level of protein synthesis are more often found in r RNA than in protein component of ribosome
- X-ray crystal structure of large subunit bound to tRNA suggest this.

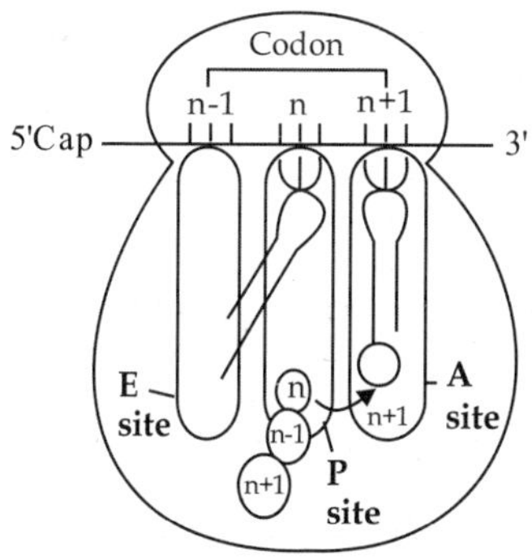

## Essential Components Required for 5 Steps of Protein Synthesis (in Prokaryotes)

**Activation of amino acids**
- 20 aminoacids
- 20 aminoacyl-tRNA synthetase (of 2 classes)
- ≥ 32 t RNAs
- **ATP**
- $Mg^{++}$

**Initiation**
- **mRNA (Shine-Dalgarno** sequence)
- **Initiation codon (AUG)** in mRNA
- **N-formylmethionyl tRNA** $^{fMet}$ (i.e. f-Met + tRNA $^{fMet}$)
- 30S subunit of ribosome
- 50 S subunit of ribosome
- **Initiation factors (IF-1, IF-2, IF-3)**
- **GTP**
- $Mg^{++}$

**Elongation**
- Functional 70S ribosome **(initiation complex)**
- Aminoacyl tRNAs (as specified by codon)
- **Elongation factors** (EF-Tu, EF-Ts, EF-G)
- GTP
- $Mg^{++}$

**Termination & Ribosome recycling**
- **Termination /Stop codons (UAA,UAG, UGA** in mRNA
- **Release /Termination factors** (RF-1, RF-2, RF-3, RRF)
- **EF – G**
- **IF - 3**

**Folding** & Post translational modification

Enzymes & cofactors required for
- Removal of initiating & signal sequences
- Addition of acetyl, methyl carboxyl, phosphoryl group etc or oligosaccharide or prosthetic groups to aminoacid residues
- Proteolytic cleavage & modification of terminal residues.

## Aminoacyl t- RNA Synthetase (AtRS)

- This family of enzyme is *required for attachment of amino* acids to their corresponding t RNAs. ***Each amino acyl tRNA synthetase recognizes one specific amino acid and one or more corresponding t RNAs (isoaccepting t RNAs)***[Q]. **For amino acids with 2 or more corresponding tRNAs**, the same enzyme usually aminoacylates all of them. The *extreme specificity of synthetase* in recognizing both A.A & t-RNA is ***responsible for high fidelity of tranlation of genetic message***[Q]. So, it *implement genetic code by acting as molecular dictionaries*[Q] that can read both 3 letter code of nucleic acid and 20 letter code of aminoacid.
- Based on substantial differences in primary & tertiary structures and in reaction mechanism AtRS has been divided into **2 classes.**

| Class I | Class II |
|---|---|
| Arg, Cys, Gln, Glu, Ile, Leu, Met, Trp, Tyr, Val – (add tRNA synthetase to each) | Ala, Asn, Asp, Gly, His, Lys, Phe, Pro, Ser, Thr (tRNa synthetase) |
| In 2[nd] step, the aminoacyl group is transferred **initially to 2[1](OH) group of 3′ terminal A** residue **then to 3′ (OH) group** by transesterification reaction | In 2[nd] step, aminoacyl group is **directly transferred to 3[1] hydroxyl group of terminal A adenylate** |

- It catalyzes **2 step reaction** that result in ***covalent attachment of carboxyl group of a specific aminoacid to the 3′ end of its corresponding / cognate / isoaccepting tRNA***[Q]. The overall reaction **requires ATP** which is *cleaved to AMP and inorganic pyro phosphate (PPi)*. Thus ***2 high energy phosphate bonds are expended for activation of each aminoacid molecule***[Q], making the over all reaction irreversible. In 1[st] step the enzyme bound intermediate – aminoacyl adenylate (aminoacyl - AMP) is formed and in 2[nd] step the aminoacyl group is transferred from **enzyme bound aminoacyl AMP intermediate to 3' (OH) of terminal A (adenylate)** of corresponding tRNA.
- Amino acyl tRNA synthetase, aminoacylates tRNA that accomplishes 2 ends: (1) **it activates an amino acid for peptide bond formation** and (2) **it ensures appropriate placement of aminoacids in growing polypeptide chain**. As the identity of amino acids attached to tRNA is not checked on ribosome, the attachment of correct amino acid to tRNA is ***essential for fidelity of protein synthesis***[Q].

$$\textbf{Aminoacid+t-RNA+ATP} \xrightarrow[\text{Aminoacyl tRNA Synthetase}]{Mg^{++}} \textbf{Aminoacyl tRNA+AMP+PPi}$$

- In addition to extreme specificity & high fidelity it has a ***proof reading or editing activity***[Q] that can remove mischarged aminoacid from the enzyme or tRNA molecule. *The effect of forcing the substrate specific binding through 2 sucessive steps (filters) is multiplicative in proof reading.*
- Incorrect aminoacids bind to **separate hydrolytic (proofreading)** site in few AtRS. The active site of some AtRS that activate aminoacids with no close structural relatives (**eg Cys-tRNA synthetase**) can sufficiently discriminate between the proper substrate and incorrect aminoacids, and demonstrate **little or no proof reading activity**. Overall error rate of protein synthesis (1 mistake in $10^{-4}$ aa incorporated) is higher than that of DNA relication.
- **Interaction between aminoacyl tRNA synthetase and tRNA is called the second genetic code** b/o its critical role in maintaining accuracy of protein synthesis. Conserved sequences of tRNA cannot be used for discrimination. Discriminatory sequences are mostly concentrated in aminoacid & anticodon arm of tRNA. For example primary determinant of tRNA recognition by Ala-tRNA synthetase is **single G = U base pair in the amino acid arm** of t RNA $^{Ala}$. So even a short synthetic RNA minihelix with **critical G=U basepairing** but lacking most of remaining tRNA structure is amino acetylated specifically with alanine almost as efficiently as the complete tRNA$^{Ala}$.

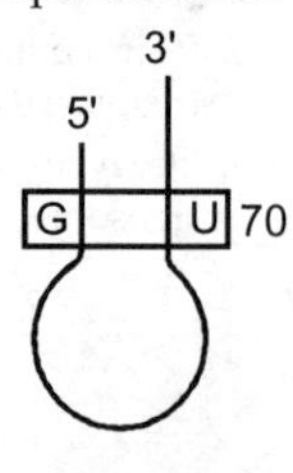

## Energy Requirements In Protein Synthesis

### Energy requirements

Total **4 ATP** and **5GTP** are used in protein synthesis in following steps

| | |
|---|---|
| - **Activation of aminoacid & formation of aminoacyl t- RNA complex** | **2 high energy $PO_4$ bonds** (ATP - → AMP) |
| - Formation of 43 S initiation complex when **e IF4A and eIF 4B bind and reduce** the complex secondary structure 5′ end of **m RNA** through ATPase and ATP dependent heticase activity | **1 ATP** (or high energy $PO_4$ bond) |
| - **Formation of 48 S initiation cmplex** by association of m-RNA with 43 S pre initiation complex. | **1 ATP ($PO_4$ bond)** |

| | |
|---|---|
| **Formation of 43 S pre initiation complex** involves binding of *GTP by eIF- 2*. This binary complex binds to *met t RNAi*, (methionine having anticodon *UAC*) specifically involved in binding to initiation codon. | 1 GTP |
| **Formation of 80 S initiation complex** (i.e. binding of 60 S subunit and 48 S initiation complex) involves hydrolysis of GTP bound to eIF- 2 by eIF- 5 | 1 GTP |
| **Binding of aminoacyl t RNA to 'A' site** requires elongation factor EF 1A and GTP | 1 GTP |
| For **translocation movment** of m-RNA forward by 1 codon and leaving the A site open for occupancy of another tRNA- EF1A- GTP- aminoacid complex requires EF2 and GTP | 1 GPT |
| **Releasing factor 3 (RF3)** with bound GTP is required for **termination** process | 1 GTP |

### Formation of peptide bond

- It is catalyzed by **peptidyl transferase**, a component of **28 S RNA** of **60S** (Harper) /**50 S** (Lippincott) ribosomal subunit. It is an example of ***ribozyme activity (i.e. r-RNA catalyzes the reaction)***[Q] and a *direct role of RBA in protein synthesis.*
- *α - amino (NH2) group of new aminoacyl t-RNA* in **'A' site** combines with carboxyl (COOH) group of peptidyl t- RNA occupying the ***'P' (peptidyl or polypeptide)*** *side*. At initiation, P site is occupied by ***aminoacyl - t RNA met[i]. Because the aminoacid on aminoacyl t RNA is already activated, no further energy source is required for this reaction***[Q].
- In eukaryotic cell, a single ribosome is capable of synthesizing 400 peptide bonds each minute.
- **Energy required for formation of one peptide bond** include the equivalent of hydrolysis of *2 ATP to ADP and 2GTP to GDP*, or the hydrolysis of **4 high energy phosphate bonds**

## Ribosomes

- Ribosome is a *cytoplasmic nucleoprotein* structure that acts as a ***machinery for protein synthesis*** from m RNA templates. Its role is to ***bring m-RNA and t-RNA together***[Q] to translate the information encoded in m-RNA (and transcribed from genes) into polypeptides.
- 1 ribosome can synthesize 5-6 peptide bonds /second. So many ribosomes, situated 80-100 nucleotides apart, work on same m-RNA simultaneously and these aggregates are called **polyribosomes** or **polysomes**. Ribosomes may be attached on walls of **endoplasmic reticulum (ER)** to form rough ER or may **exist free in cytoplasm.**
- **RER associated ribosomes** synthesize proteins that are exported from cell, are integrated into plasma, ER or golgi membranes or *lysosomes*. Free **cytosolic ribosomes** synthesize protein required in cytosol, nucleus, mitochondria & ***peroxisomes***[Q]. However mitochondria contain its own ribosome
- Ribosomes can be **free (cytoplasmic)** or **membrane (ER) bound**, contain about 65% of r-RNA and 35% of protein, are roughly spherical with a diameter of about 18nm - seen only on electron microscope and accounts for almost 25% of dry weight of cell.
- Ribosomes are large complexes of r-RNA and proteins with *one large and one small subunits*. The **small subunit** *binds m-RNA*, thus guiding *interaction b/w m-RNA codon and anticodon of t-RNA* to read the genetic information with exiquisite **fidelity**. Hence small subunit is **responsible** for accuracy, whereas the **large subunit**

## Energy Required in Protein Synthesis

- **4 high energy bonds** are required for addition of one aminoacid to growing polypeptide chain

| 2 from ATP in *aminoacyl t-RNA synthetase reaction*[Q]. | 2 from GTP<br>- *1 for binding of aminoacyl tRNA to A site*[Q]<br>- *1 - for translocation*[Q] |
|---|---|

- Additional ATP & GTP are required for **initiation** *in eukaryotes*. Whereas additional **GTP** is ***required for termination in both eukaryotes & prokaryotes***[Q].

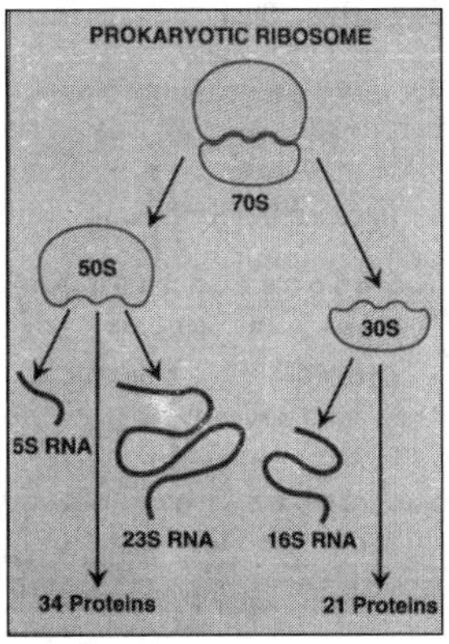


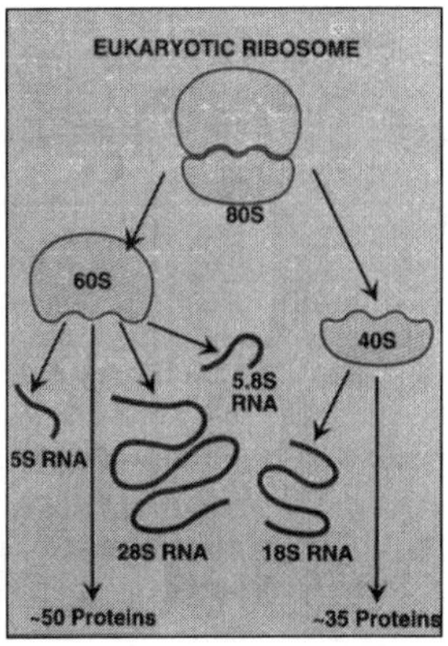

catalyzes the **formation of peptide bond.**

- Prokaryotic ribosome with sedimentation coefficient 70S (S=Svedberg units, a parameter sensitive to molecular size & shape) is composed of 2 unequal subunits with sedimentation coefficient of 30 S and 50S. Whereas eukaryotic 80S ribosome has 60S and 40S.

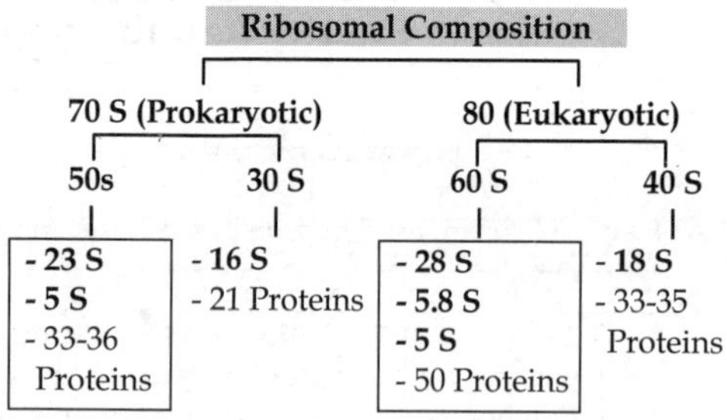


- Each *ribosome has 3 binding sites for t-RNA* – **A** *(for incoming aminoacyl t RNA),* **P** *(for peptidyl – t RNA)* and **E** (for empty t RNA about to exit), each of which **extend over both subunits**. Together they cover 3 neighbouring codes.
- Both ribosomal subunits *can be broken down into their RNA and protein components, then reconstituted* in vitro nearly identical in structure and activity to native subunit. Ribosomal subunits are *huge r-RNA molecules* that form the structural core. The *proteins are secondary elements* in complex *decorating the surface (forming Worm like structures)*. There is no protein within 18A° of active site for peptide bond formation. The large r-RNA component performs **peptidyl transferase** activity and thus ribosome is a **ribozyme.**
- *Ribosomal RNAs (28S + 16S)* constitute nearly 70% of total eukaryotic cellular RNA. All r-RNA molecules *except 5S r RNA*, which is independently transcribed are processed from a single 45S precursor RNA molecule in nucleolus. The highly methylated r-RNA are packaged in nucleolus with the specific ribosomal proteins. In cytoplasm, ribosomes remain quite stable and capable of *many translational cycles.*
- ***16s r-RNA of 30 subunit of prokaryotic ribosome identifies and binds shine – Dalgarno sequence***[Q].
- The r-RNA residues of large subunit of ribosomes that catalyze peptide bond formation (and have peptidyl tranferase activity) contain highly conserved nucleotide sequence[Q] – the ribonucleotide octet (5') AUAACAGG (3') in all cells.
- *Many negatively charged phosphoryl groups* in RNA backbone limit the stability of very large RNA molecules. So incorporation of *divalent cations or positively charged groups* and certain *peptides promote stability*. Ribozyme catalyzed synthesis of peptides could thus initially have evolved for structural maintenance of large RNA molecules but the greater catalytic potential of proteins marked the beginning of new era of protein dominated metabolic system.

## Protein Kinase & Protein Phosphorylation

| Eukaryotic Protein Kinase (PK) | Phosphorylate |
|---|---|
| Serine-Threonine PK | Serine (95%); also recognizes threonine (3%) |
| Tyrosine PK | Tyrosin (< 1%) only |
| Dual Function PK | Serine (Sr), threonine (Thr), tyrosine (Tyr) |

- **Attachment of phosphoryl groups** to specific aminoacid residue of a **protein is catalyzed by protein kinases; removal of phosphoryl groups** is **catalyzed by phospho protein phosphatases**.
- Phosphorylation is the *commonest type of regulatory post translational modification.* **The addition of phosphoryl group to a Ser, Thr,** or **Tyr** residue introduces a bulky charged group into a region that was only moderately polar. The oxygen atoms of a phosphoryl group can hydrogen bond with one or several groups in a protein, commonly the amide groups of peptide backbone at the start of an α-helix or the charged *guanidinium group of an Arg residiue*. The 2 negative charges on a phosphorylated side chain can also repel neighbouring negatively charged (Asp or Glu) residue. The interactions with **arginine, aspartic acid or glutamic acid, histidine & lysine** side chains is usually secondary to and after primary attachment with **serine (Sr) , threonine (Thr) or Tyrosine (Tyr)**
- When modifications caused by phosphorylation occur in a region of an enzyme critical to its three dimensional structure, phosphorylation can have dramatic effects on enzyme conformation and thus on substrate binding and catalysis. (either stimulating or inhibiting). For example phosphorylation **stimulates substrate binding & catalysis in glycogen phosphorylase** of muscle & liver, whereas it **inhibits isocitrate dehydrogenase.**
- Protein kinases catalyze the transfer of negatively charge phosphoryl (phosphate) group of ATP to hydroxyl moiety of only three aminoacids ie **serine (Sr, 95%), threonine (Thr, 3-4%) and tyrosine (Tyr** in < 1%) to form chemically stable phosphate ester **in eukaryotes**. Whereas **in prokaryotic** bacteria, fungi & plants phosphorylate **histidine and aspartate (or glutamate)** by **histidine** and aspartate protein kinases.

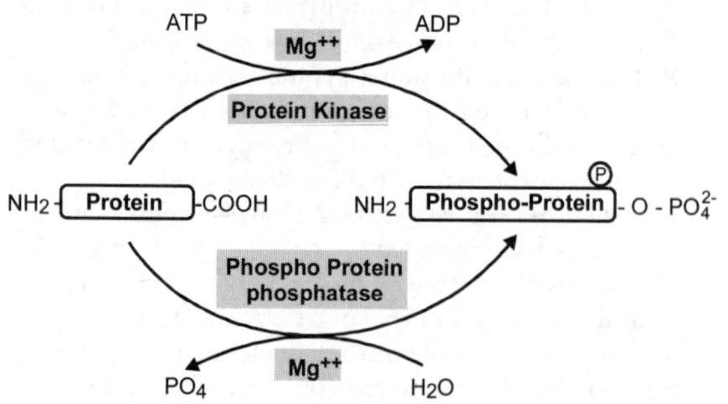

## Plasma Immunoglobulins (Antibodies)

- Antibodies are produed by **B** (or **plasma**) **cells** and provide **humoral immunity**. It destroyes target cells by following mechanisms.
  - **Activating classical complement pathway** i.e. complement fixation (by IgG & IgM)
  - **Antibody dependent cell mediated cytotoxicity (ADCC)** i.e. antibody coating will sensitize the target cells for killing by *killer (k) cells* (IgG)
  - **Agglutination** (by IgM > A > G)
  - **Opsonization** (IgG coating helps & makes phagocytosis easy as its Fc portion can fix with macrophage).
  - All immunoglobins contain a minimum of **2** identical **light (L) chains** (23 -kDa) and **2** identical **heavy (H)** chains (53 – 75 kDa) joined together by **disulfide bonds** forming a **Y shaped tetramer ($L_2 H_2$)**. Each chain has 2 ends – **amino ($NH_3^+$)** and ***carboxy ($COO^-$)*** and 2 regions.

### Constant (C) region

- It has *constant amino acid sequence,* and located *towards carboxy* (C) terminal.
- **Half (1/2) of light (L) chain** towards carboxy end (k/a $C_L$) and approximately three quarters **(3/4)** in IgG, A, D or 4/5 in Ig M,E of **heavy chain** towards carboxy terminal (k/a $C_H$) – constitute the constant region.
- Constant domain have a *characteristic, well conserved structural motif* – the **immunoglobulin fold** in all β-class of proteins. There are **3 to 4** of these constant domains in each heavy and 1 in each light chain.

#### $C_H$

- Constant region of heavy chain ($C_H$) is divided into **3** (in **IgG, IgA, Ig D**) or **4** (in **IgM, IgE**) **parts – $C_{H1}$, $C_{H2}$, $C_{H3}$, $C_{H4}$.**
- Distinguished by **differences in their CH regions**, humans have **5** different **types of heavy chains – determining 5 classes of immunoglobulin**. These are.

| Immuno-globulin | Heavy Chain | CH domains (number) |
|---|---|---|
| **IgG** | **Gamma (γ)** | 3 } **$C_H$1, $C_H$2, $C_H$3** |
| **IgA** | **Alpha (α)** | 3 |
| **IgD** | **Delta (δ)** | 3 |
| **IgM** | **Mu (μ)** | 4 } Also **$C_{H}4$** |
| **IgE** | **Epsilon (ε)** | 4 |

- **Hinge region between $CH_1$ and $CH_2$** domains is the area in which **papain** (proteolytic enzyme obtained from **papaya**) and pepsin cleave the immunoglobulin molecule. Papain cleaves distal disulfide bond to produce **2** antigne binding fragments (**Fab**) and 1 crystallizable fragment (**Fc**) whereas, pepsin digestion cleaves proximal S-S bond to generate 2 Fab fragments joined together by distal S-S bond and 1Fc.
- Hinge region allows both Fab arms to move independently thus confers **flexibility** to bind to antigen sites which may be at variable distance (on bacterial surface).
- **Constant regions** of immunoglobulin ***particularly basal crystalizable fragment (Fc)*** i.e. **CH2, CH3** (and **CH4 in IgM & IgE**) are responsible for **class specific effector functions** (like transplacental passage, complement fixation, opsonization, agglutination, binding to macrophage & mast cells, mediation of allergic response, presence in secretions, antigen receptors on B cells and polymeric forms containing J chains of immunoglobulins.
- 1 molecule of Ig has 2 Fab so it is termed **divalent**.

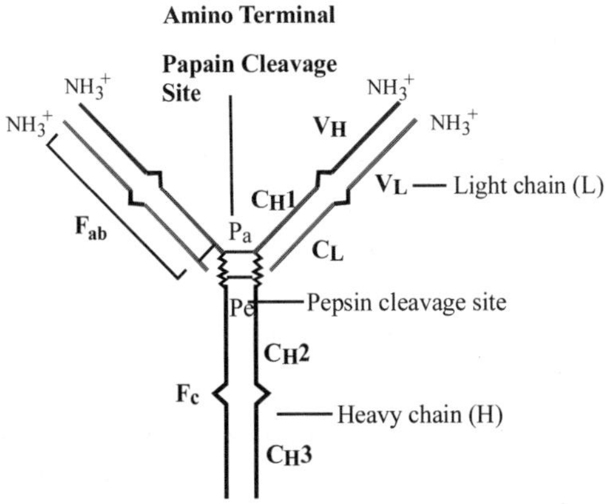


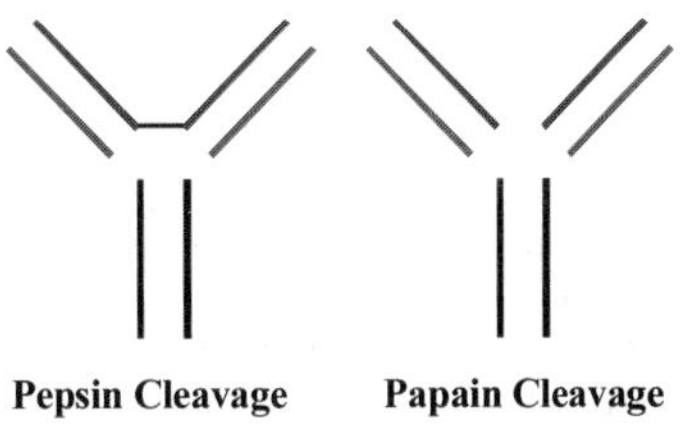


#### $C_L$

- Distinguished by **differences** in their **$C_L$** (constant region of light chain), humans have **2** different **types** of light chain – **kappa** (**κ**) and **lambda** (**λ**).
- Any immunoglobulin molecule always contains **either 2λ or 2k** but never a mixture of both.
- In human k chains are more frequent (60%).

### Variable (V) region

- It has *variable amio acid sequence* & located towards *amino terminal.*
- First 108 amino acids (out of 214) in light chain i.e. amino terminal half of light chain ($V_L$) and first 118 aa (out of 440) in heavy chain i.e. approximately **one quarter (1/4)** of **heavy chain** towards amino terminal **($V_H$)** constitute the variable region.
- Variable region are quite **heterogenous** and **no two** variable regions **have identical amino acid sequence**.
- Variable regions are comprised of relatively invariable regions and **hypervariable regions**.
- L chains have **3** and H chains have **4 complementarity determining regions (CDRs)** or **hyper variable regions** – which comprise the antigen binding site located on amino tips of Y and dictates amazing **specificity** of antibodies.
- Polypeptide zone b/w 2 hyper variable regions is k/a **frame work regions**.
- About 5 to 10 aminoacis in each hypervariable CD region contribute to antigen binding site, which is formed by CDRs of both $V_H$ & $V_L$
- **Epitope or antigenic determinant** is the site on antigen to which an antibody binds. Large antigen binds with all of CDRs whereas small antigen interact with only few (or one) CDR i.e. ----- a **mutual complementarity** b/w epitope & CDR surface. Binding involves **non covalent forces** and **bonds** (electrostatic, vander Walls, hydrogen and hydrophobic **bonds**)
- Various combinations of H & L chain CDRs can give rise to tremendous diversity of antibodies (specificity) k/a **combinatorial diversity**.
- **Antigen binding fragment (Fab)** has light chain ($V_L$ & $C_L$) and $V_H$ & $C_{H1}$ of heavy chain.

- Both light chain and heavy chain products of multiple genes like – variable region (**V**) gene, joining region (**J**) gene, constant region (**C**) gene and diversity region (**D**) genes. **V, J, & C** genes occur for both **L & H** chains – **$V_L/V_H$, J, $C_{L/H}$** genes whereas diversity region (**D**) **genes occur only for heavy (H) chains**. *J gene bears no relationship to J chain of IgA or IgM.*
- All normal classes & subclasses of immunoglobins are called **isotopes** if they contin **same light chain** and ***identical variable domains of both their light chains ($V_L$) and heavy chains ($V_H$)*** indicating **same antigen specificity**. This means different classes (isotopes) of immunoglobulins are differentiated by their **different $C_H$ regions** which are combined with the *same antigen specific $V_H$ region.*
- Human genome contains only ~ 29,000 coding genes but can produce $10^9$- $10^{10}$ different immunoglobin types b/o **gene rearrangements**, providing the immease diversity needed for recognition of enormous number of antigens. **Immense antibody diversity** depends on a number of factors including – **the existence of multiple gene segments** (30 λV, 300 kapa (κ) V; 1000 heavy chain V, 4J, 15D, 1C segments), ***their recombinations (somatic rearrangement of DNA or transposition of genes)***[Q], the **combinations of different light (L) & heavy (H) chains, junctional diversity** (i.e. addition or deletion of random number of nucleotides in joining certain gene segments l/t inaccuracies in V-J, V-D and D-J recombination), **N-region insertion** (nucleotides inserted b/w D and J by terminal transferase), combinatorial association, multispecificity, and a ***high frequency of somatic mutation***[Q].
- **C- terminal transmembrane domain** is present in membrane bound antibodies but absent in secreted (circulating) antibodies. The shift from membrane bound form to secreted form of immunoglobulins ***involves poly A-site choice (i.e. differential RNA processing)***[Q].

| | IgG | IgA | IgM | IgD | IgE |
|---|---|---|---|---|---|
| **Heavy (H) Chain** | γ | A (α) | μ | δ | ε |
| Heavy chain domains | 4 | 4 | 5 | 4 | 5 |
| Usual Structrue /Units | Monomer (1) | Monomer (1) Dimer (2) | Monomer (1), Pentamer (5) Hexamer (6) Dimmer (2) | Monomer (1) | Monomer (1) |
| **Antibody valence** | 2 | 2, 4 | 10, 12 | 2 | 2 |
| Additional Units in polymers | - | **S & J** | **J piece** | - | - |
| Subclasses (Isotypes) | G1, G2, G3, G4 | A1, A2 | - | - | - |
| % of total Ig in serum | 75 | 15 | 9 | 0.2 | 0.004 |
| Serum concentration (mg/dl) | 1000 | 200 | 120 | 3 | 0.05 |
| Serum half life (days) | 23 | 6 | 5/10 | 3 | 2.5 |
| **Rate of synthesis** (mg/kg/day) | 35 | 65 | 5 | 0.4 | 0.016 |
| **Sedimentation coefficient** (S) | 7 | 7 or 11★ | 19 | 7 | 8 |
| Molecular weight (X1000) | 150 | 170 or 400★ | 900 | 180 | 190 |
| **Complement Fixation-Classical** Alternative complement activation | + ($G_1$, $G_2$, $G_3$)<br>+($G_4$) | <br>+ | +<br>- | -<br>+ | -<br>- |
| **Natural antibodies, Primary response antibody Antigen recetors on B cells** | - | - | + | - | - |
| **Transplacental passage, Opsonization (produce opsonin $C_{3b}$), Antibody dependent cell mediated cytolysis (ADCC)** | + | - | - | - | - |
| Fixation to **mast cells Mediation of allergic responses** | - | - | - | - | + |
| **Found in secretions** | - | + | - | - | - |
| **Agglutination** | + | ++ | +++ | | |

★ Form is found in secretions (saliva, milk, tear etc) & fluids of respiratory, genital & intestinal tracts.

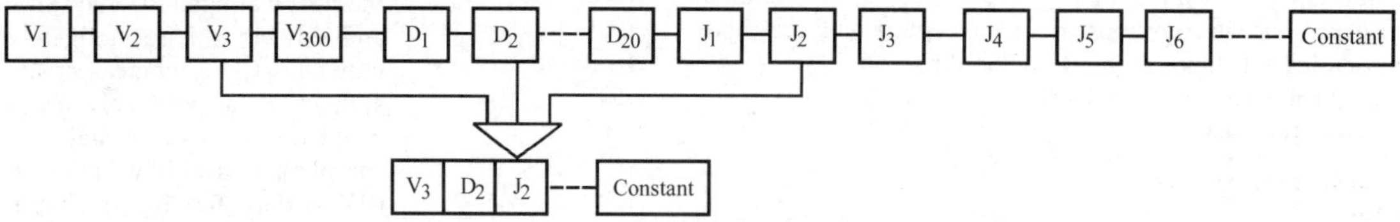


- A gene can give rise to multiple products by **differential RNA processing** i.e. – either by poly A site choice or alternative splicing or both. If there are ≥2 sites for cleavage and polyadenylation, use of one closest to 5′ end will remove more (& use of one closest to 3′ end will remove less) of primary transcript sequence-thus generating diversity in variable domain of Ig heavy chain. The mRNA site where cleavage occurs is marked by 2 sequences.

- Highly conserved (5′) **AAU AAA** (3′) sequences about 10 to 30 bases upstream on the 5′ side of cleavage site
- Less well defined **GU rich** sequence, 20 to 40 nucleotides downstream of the cleavage site.

**Cleavage generates free 3′-OH end of mRNA. Poly (80 - 250) A residues are immediately added by polyadenylate polymerase enzyme that does not require template but uses cleaved mRNA as primer. Poly A site choice generates diversity in variable domains and is responsible for *deciding whether an antibody will remain membrane bound or get secreted*[Q].** Alternative spling produce 3 different form of myosin heavy chains whereas, both mechanism come into play to produce 2 different hormones calcium regulating hormone clacitonin in thyroid and calcitonin gene regulated peptide (CGRP) in brain from single transcript.

## Protein Sorting (Localization /Targetting)

A major *sorting decision is made early when proteins are synthesized either on membrane bound polyribosomes (of RER) or on free polyribosomes of cytoplasm.* Protein synthesized on

### Cytosolic-Free Polyribosomes

- Protein synthesized on free ribosome **lack signal peptide** and are delivered into cytosol.
- They may be further directed to *mitochondria, nuclei,* and *peroxisomes* by specific signals or remain in cytosol if they lack a signal.

★ Proteins that contain targeting sequence that is subsequently removed are called **pre proteins.** Whereas in **pre-pro-proteins** a second peptide also has to be removed.

### Membrane bound (RER)- Polyribosomes

- Proteins synthesized in RER contain a **signal peptide** that mediate their attachment to membrane of endoplasmic reticulum.
- Proteins synthesized on RER may be destined to various membranes (eg ER membrane, golgi apparatus membrane and plasma membrane), to lysosome and for secretion.
- Golgi apparatus (all parts) is involved in **O-glycosylation** and *processing of oligosaccharide chains* of membrane & other N-linked glycoproteins and *sorting of various proteins* prior to their delivery to appropriate intracellular destination. (*trans golgi network* performs this role)

| **Secretory Proteins** destined for **regulated secretion** are carried in **secretory vesicles** | **Transport proteins** for various intracellular (eg lysosome, plasma membrane etc) destinations, and proteins that are **sereted in a constitutive manner** are carried in **transport vesicles.** |
|---|---|

## Intracellular Traffic & Sorting of Proteins

### Signal peptides & protein localization

- Signal peptide is an extension that is found in proteins ***synthesized on membrane bound polyribosomes***[Q]. But proteins whose entire synthesis occurs on free polyribosome lack this signal peptide (Blobel – Sabatini hypothesis)
- Signal peptide is also k/a ***leader or signal sequence, presequence or transient insertion singal.*** And it
  - Contain *12-35 amino acids with a central cluster of hydrophobic amino acids & at least one positively charged aminoacid near amino terminal.* Methionine is usually the amino terminal aminoacid
  - Is usually (not always) located at the amino terminal; and cleaved off at the carboxyl terminal end of an Ala residue by *signal peptidase*
- Signal peptide is *involved in process of protein insertion into ER membrane & lumen* in following manner
  - The m-RNA encodes an *amino terminal* **signal peptide**. It is recognized by **signal recognition particle (SRP)** that ***blocks translation after about 70 amino acids***[Q] have been polymerized (40 buried in large ribosomal subunit & 30 exposed).
  - SRP causing **elongation arrest** has 6 proteins & 7 S RNA (related to Alu family of highly repeated DNA sequences)
  - **SRP-R** (a receptor for SRP) is an integral **docking protein** on ER membrane, which has $\alpha$ and $\beta$ subunits. $\beta$ subunit spans the membrane & $\alpha$ is ***bound to GDP/GTP***[Q]
  - SRP imposed **elongation block is released** *as* the SRP-signal peptide-polyribosome complex binds to ***SRP-R***[Q]; thus *SRP guides the signal peptide to SRP-R & prevents premature folding and expulsion of proteins.*
  - **Translocation** consists of 3 membrane bound proteins (**Sec 61 complex**) that form a ***protein conducting channel***[Q] in ER. The *insertion of signal peptide into conducting channel, while the other end of parent protein is still attached to ribosome* is termed **cotranslational insertion**
  - Protein should be in *unfolded state* prior to entering conducting channel- otherwise it may not be able to gain access to the channel. When the process is complete the ribosome is dissociated into 2 subunits and signal peptide is hydrolysed by signal peptidase, located on luminal side of ER.
  - Amino acid sequence k/a **halt** or **stop transfer signal, retains proteins in membrane** as it prevents passage through membrane of ER, of proteins that are integral ER membrane proteins eg. cytochrome p 450
  - N- glycine chains are added (**cotranslational glycosylation**) occurs as proteins transverse the inner part of ER membrane.

### Chaperone (Folding) proteins

- **Chaperone** (literally meaning *older women incharge of young unmarried woman on certain social occasions*) are the proteins that have a role in *assembly and proper folding of newly synthesized proteins* so that they have biological activity. The exit of properly folded protein after synthesis from ER may be a rate limiting step.
- **Present** ***in a wide range*** **of species from bacteria to humans in various cellular compartments such as** ***cytosol, mitochondria, & lumen of endoplasmic reticulum*** **and many are so called** ***heat shock protein (hsp)***[Q]
- Bind mainly to *hydrophobic regions* of unfolded & aggregated proteins and act as ***a quality control or editing mechanism for detecting misfolded*** **or otherwise defective proteins.**
- Some are *induced by* conditions that cause unfolding of newly synthesized proteins eg. ***any stress to cell like radiation, heavy metals, free radicals, toxins, elevated temperature & chemicals***[Q]; and hence called **stress proteins. Heat shock proteins** were first identified in response to heat shock.
- Most exhibit **ATP ase activity** & bind ADP & ATP. The chaperon- ADP complex has high affinity for unfolded proteins, when bound ADP is replaced by ATP. Chaperon – ATP complex releases segments of proteins that has folded properly.
- Some **chaperone folding protein & enzyme located in rough endoplasmic reticulum are**
  - **Immunoglobin heavy chain binding protein (BiP, prewent in lumen)**
  - **Glucose regulated protein (GRP) 94**
  - **Calnexin** (calcium binding protein located in ER membrane that also binds to MHC antigen) & variety of other serum proteins, retaining them in ER until glycoprotein has folded properly.
  - **Calreticulin** (calcium binding protein)
  - **Protein disulfide isomerase (PDI),** an enzyme that promotes ***rapid reshuffling of disulfide bonds***[Q] until correct set is achieved.
  - **Peptidyl prolyl isomerase (PPI)** enzyme ***accelerates folding of proline containing proteins***[Q] by catalyzing the cis-trans isomerization aminoacid residue (x) – Pro bond

- Some sequences that direct proteins to specific organelle

| Targeting sequence (or compound) | Targeted organelle |
|---|---|
| Signal peptide sequence | Membrane of ER |
| Amino terminal KDEL sequence (Lys- Asp – Glu- Leu) in ER resident proteins in COPI vesicles | Luminal surface of ER |
| Di-acidic sequences (Asp-X-Glu) in membrane proteins in COP-II vesicles | Golgi membranes |
| Amino terminal sequence (20 – 80 residues) | Mitochondrial matrix |
| **Nuclear localization signal (NLS)** eg $Pro_2$ – $Lys_2$ – Arg – Lys- Val | Nucleus |
| **PTS** (peroxisomal matrix targeting sequence) eg Ser – Lys – Leu | Peroxisome |
| **Mannose 6 phosphate** | *Lysosome*[Q] |

- Misfolded proteins in ER are transported back to **proteasomes** present in cytosol by **retrograde transport** through *translocon* for ERAD. It may be powered by ATP ase present in proteasomes. Before entering proteasomes, most proteins are ubiquitinated.

★ About other options: **Proteases** are ***enzymes that hydrolyze proteins***[Q]. **Proteosomes** (eg 26 S component) ***help in degrading the proteins marked with ubiquitin***[Q]. **Template** is involved in the synthesis of nucleic acid.

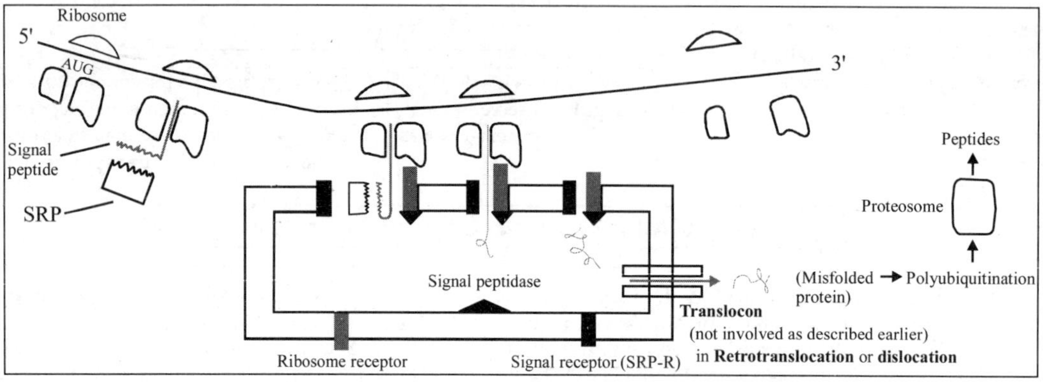


## Protein Degradation and Traffic

- Accumulation of misfolded proteins in endoplasmic reticulum (**ER stress**) can induce **unfolded protein response** (**UPR**). This results in increased folding capacity of ER (by increasing chaperones) and prevents a buildup of unproductive & potentially toxic protein products by inhibition of translation of misfolded proteins & induction of protein synthesis involved in degradation of misfolded proteins.
- **Retrotranslocation or dislocation** is the process by which misfolded proteins are transported back across ER to enter ***proteasomes*** in cytoplasm. **Chaperones** (of ER & cytosol) target misfolded proteins and ***polyubiquitin-binding proteins*** *escort* them to proteasomes. Energy for translocation is partly supplied by **p97** an **AAA-ATPase** (i.e. **A**TP **A**ssociated with various cellular Activities).
- **3** enzymes –**activating, conjugating** and **ligase** (latter confers substrate specificity) are involved in attaching ubiquitin to target protein. Minimum of 4 ubiquitin molecules must be attached to commit a target molecules for degradation. Ubiquitin can be **reused** after cleaving by **deubiquitinating** enzymes.
- Proteasome is *a large cylindrical structure composed of 50 subunits*. It has *1-2 regulatory caps containing ATPase* for unfolding target proteins and a *hollow core* for degrading it to small peptides. It has a important role in presenting small peptides (produced by degradation of viruses etc) to major histocompatibility *(MHC) class I molecules*, a key step in *antigen presentation to T-lymphocytes.*
- Vesicles involved in **endocytosis** and /or carrying cargo to *lysosomes* are **coated with clathrin.** Clathrin is involved in transport in post golgi apparatus locations including *endosomes, plasma membrane (PM) and trans golgi network (TGN).*
- Proteins synthesized on membrane bound polyribosomes (RER) is destined for golgi apparatus (GA) or PM. **COP II (Calthrin free) transport vesides** are involved in *antegrade (ER to GA) transport* and ***COPI (clathrin free) transport vesicles*** are involved in *retrograde (GA to ER) transport. Secretory* & transport **vesicles** carrying cargo from GA to PM are also clathrin free.
- *Key steps* and **molecular switches** in the life cycle of non clathrin coated vesicles are **budding** [*Sar 1* (GTPase); *Sec 12* (guanine nucleotide exchange factor = 'GERF), *coat proteins* (complet bud formation & contribute to curvature)] ; **pinching off** bud, **Uncoating/coat disassembly** (Sar1 has key role in both assembly & uncoating of coat proteins), vesicle **targeting** (*Rab proteins /* Ras related proteins / monomeric GTPases first observed in rabbit brain), **tetering** (or attachment) of vesicles to membrane (*Rab effector proteins*), **docking** (Vesicle or V- *SNAREs* pair with cognate target or t-*SNAREs*, forming 4 helix bundle; *SNAREs = SNAP* Receptors), **fusion** (interaction of SNAREs on same membrane forms eis – SNARE complex and on two different membranes forms trans SNARE complex or **SNARE pin**) and **dissociation** (require NSF or NEM sensitive ATPase and *α-SNAP* or soluble NSF attachment protein). ARF (a GTPase or ADP ribosylated factor) is involved in formation of both COP I & clathrin coated vesicles.

There are two major enzyme system responsible for degradation.

| Ubiquitin- Proteasome pathway or Endoplasmic reticulum associated degeneration (ERAD) | Lysosomes |
|---|---|
| • *Energy dependent,* requires ATP<br>• Mainly *degrade endogenous protein* (synthesized within cell)<br>• α- carboxyl glycine of ubiquitine becomes co- valently attached to lysine residue of protein ↓<br>Protein tagged with ubiquitine is *recognized by proteolytic proteasome*<br>↓<br>Protein degraded to Amino acid | • Non energy dependent<br>• Degrade extracellular protein:<br>- Plasma protein<br>- Cell surface membrane protein<br>• Extracellular proteins are taken into cell by endocytosis & then degraded by lysosomal enzyme |

## Diseases d/t

Conformational abnormalities in *intracellular transport of proteins and enzymes* (d/t mutation) resulting in **ER stress** and **protein misfolding**.

| **Disease** | **Affected protein** |
|---|---|
| **Alzheimer's disease** | ***β-amyloid***[Q] |
| **Prion diseases (like kuru, Creutzfeldt Jakob's disease, fatal familia insomnia)** | **Pr Psc** |
| **Cystic fibrosis** | CFTR |
| α-Antitrypsin deficiency with liver disease | α1-Antitrypsin |
| Chediak Higashi syndrome | Lysosomal trafficking regulator |
| Combined deficiency of factor 5 & 8 | Mannose binding lectin (ERGIC 53) |
| Diabetes mellitus (some) | Insulin receptor (α-subunit) |
| AD familial hypercholesterolemia | LDL receptor |
| Gaucher disease | β-glucosidase |
| Hemophilia A | Factors 8, 9 |
| Hereditary hemochromatosis | HFE |
| Hermansky-Pudlak syndrome | β-3A subunit of AP-3 adaptor complex |
| I-cell disease | N- acetyl glucosamie phospho transferase |
| Lowe oculocerebrorenal syndrome | PIP2- 5- phosphatase |
| Tay Sach's disease | β-hexosaminidase |
| Von Willebrand disease | Von Willebrand factor |

**Peroxisomal abnormalities**

1. **Hyper** oxaluria type 1
2. **Hyper** pipecolic academia
3. **Zellweger** and pseudo zell wager syndromes
4. **Adrenoleuko dystrophy** (ALD), neonatal ALD and psoudo neonatal ALD
5. Acatalasemia
6. Rizomelic chondrodysplasia punctuata
7. Infantile *Refsum* disease
8. Glutaryl CoA oxidase **deficiency**

Mn - "**Hyper ZAR-G deficiency**"

## Prion Proteins & Prion Disease

It is a protein that is highly resistant to proteolytic degradation. It exists in two isoforms

**Noninfectious normal cellular prion protein ($PrP^c$)**

- Human prion related protein is a *glycoprotein,* encoded on ***short arm of chromosome 20***[Q]
- It is monomeric, ***rich in*** $\alpha$ ***– helix***[Q] and does not cause disease
- It is precursor of $PrP^{sc}$.

**Pathological prion protein (PrPsc)**

- It ***rich in β-sheets***[Q] with many hydrophobic aminoacyl side chains exposed to solvents. $PrP^{sc}$ molecules therefore *associates strongly with one another forming insoluble protease resistant aggregates* of fibrils (similar to amyloid)
- One pathological prion or prion related protein can serve as template for conformational transformation of many $PrP^c$ molecules. So the prion disease ***can be transmitted by protein alone without involvement of DNA or RNA***[Q].
- It causes transmissible spongiform encephalopathies (TSE) or prion disease. These fatal neurodegenerative diseases are characterized by spongiform changes, astrocytic gliomas & neuronal loss resulting from insoluble aggregates in neural cells. These include ***mad cow disease (bovine spongiform encephalopathy) in cattles, scrapie in sheep, and Creutzfeldt- Jacob disease (most common), Gerstmann- Straussler – Sheinker disease, Kuru, & fatal familial insomnia in humans***[Q].

# Protein Misfolding

*Any alteration in protein folding causes wide variety of neurodegenerative disease in mammals,* perhaps the *most common of which is prions disease.* Prions diseases include:

- ***Fatal familial insomnia***[Q] → Humans
- Creutzfeldt – Jakob's disease → Humans
- ***Kuru***[Q] → Humans
- Scrapie → Sheep
- Bovine spongiform encephalopathy → Cow

Protein folding is a complex, trial and error process that can sometimes result in improperly folded molecules. Deposits of these misfolded proteins are associated with a number of neurological diseases.

**Prions diseases**

- Occur because of defect in the secondary – tertiary protein structure ***due to defect of folding of the peptide chain***[Q].
- Prions stands for ***proteinaceous infections particle devoid of nucleic acid***[Q].

**Alzheimer's disease**

- Occurs due to ***accumulation of misfolded protein called β- amyloid***[Q].
- The *A β amyloid* that is deposited in brain is *derived by proteolytic cleavages from larger amyloid precursor protein*
- A β peptide when aggregated in β-pleated sheet, is neurotoxic.
- **Apolipoprotein E** has been implicated as a potential mediator of this conformational transformation

## Gene Duplication

- **Gene duplication** is any duplication or amplification of segment of DNA (chromosome) that contains a gene.
- This **second copy of a whole gene** is introduced into chromosome as a result of *defective replication of the DNA (chromosome)* such as *inhomologus recombination, retrotransposition* or duplication of entire chromosome.
- The *second gene copy is superfluous (extra) and free from selective pressure (the process of natural selection) and mutation in this gene will not be deleterious.* So it becomes a means by which the **cell may evolve, by producing a new gene with a new function (protein/enzyme)** while retaining the original gene & gene function because (organism with) extra gene accumulate mutations faster than (organism with) single function gene.
- Freedom from pressure of natural selection and consequences of mutations in extra copy of gene allow them to acquire new capability (such as metabolism of new substrate) that may increase the fitness of organism for survival in new ecological niche (environment).

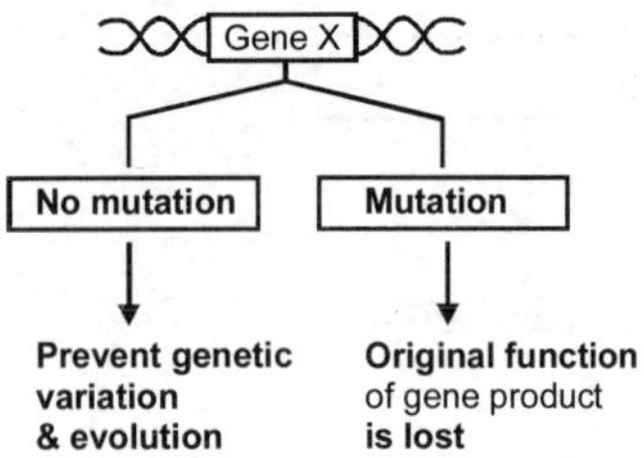


## Homologs, Paralogs & Orthologs

- When 2 genes share readily detectable sequence similarities (nucleotide sequence in DNA or aminoacid sequence in proteins they encode), their sequences are called **homologous** and proteins they encode are **homologs**.
- 2 homologous genes occurring **in the same species** are called **paralogous** and their protein products are **paralogs.** Paralogous genes are **derived from gene duplication** followed by gradual changes in the sequences of both copies. Paralog proteins are similar in sequence of aminoacid & three dimensional structure both, although they commonly acquire different functions during their evolution
- 2 homologous genes occurring **in different species** are called **orthologous** and their protein products are **orthologs**. Orthologs are commonly have **same functions in both organisms.**
- **Synteny is conserved order of genes on chromosome** over a large segment of genome of closely related species (eg human & mouse). It provides additional evidence for an **orthologous relationship between genes at identical location** within the related segment.
- Genes in segments of **human chromosome 9 & mouse chromosome 2** exhibit very high degree of homology **(orthology)** as well as **synteny (same gene order).**

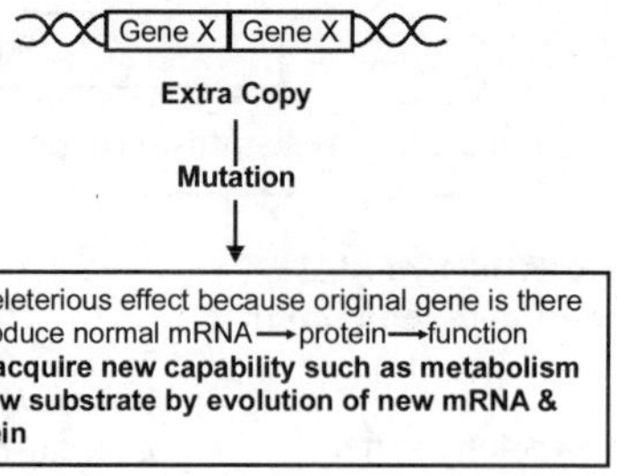


# Mutation

Mutation is defined as any *alteration in primary nucleotide sequence of DNA regardless of functional consequences*. It can involve (i) **Germ cells** to get transmitted to progeny or, (ii) **somatic cells**, which is *non hereditary* and may result in cancers etc. Types include.

### Base Substitution (or Point) Mutation

- It involves ***substitution (replacement or change) of one nucleotide base with another base***[Q] and can be of 2 types

| Transition | Transversion |
|---|---|
| *Purine base is replaced by another purine base or pyrimidine is replaced by another pytimidine base*[Q].<br>**Purine (A) ↔ purine (G)**<br>**Pyrimidine(T)↔Pyrimidine (C)** | It changes **purine to either of two pyrimidines or pyrimidines to either of 2 purines.**<br>**Purine** A/G ↔ **Pyrimidine** T/C |

- It may result in **disappearance** of already present restriction site **or creation** of a new **restriction site** by a particular restriction endonuclease (RE) l/t *generation of larger or smaller fragmens resectively* on digestion with that RE. In otherwords, **point mutation may l/t RFLP**[Q] (restriction fragment length polymorphism).

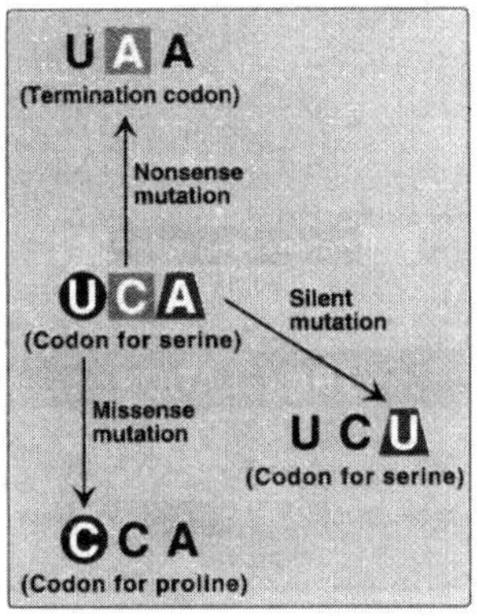


**Possible effect of changing a single nucleotide base in the coding region of an mRNA chain**

- The resulting **m-RNA will show a change only at a point complementary to a base change** at the corresponding locus. Point mutation or changing a single nucleotide base on mRNA chain may l/t any of these 3 effects. Effects of point mutation may be

#### Silent Mutation

- If mutation affects **non-essential DNA** or if it has a **negligible effect** on function of a gene, it is k/a silent mutation.
- The codon containing the changed base may **code for same amino acid.** This occurs **d/t redundancy /degeneracy** of genetic code.
- **No apparently detectable** effect usually occurs d/t **change in 3rd nucleotide of** genetic code. And because of **wobble phenomenon** translation of a gene is least sensitive to a change at 3rd position.
- **For example CUU, CUA, CUG,**

#### Missense Mutation

- Codon containing the changed base may **code for a different aminoacid.** The substitution of a **mistaken/ missense/** or **incorrect** amino acid is called a missense mutation.

#### Nonsense Mutation

- The codon containing the changed base may ***become a stop/termination codon***[Q]. This creation of stop codon at inappropriate site is called a non sense mutation.
- It would result in **premature termination** of peptide chain and **only a fragment of intended protein molecule** will be produced.

Mutations **altering the amount or structure of protein** produced by translation.

### 1. Frame Shift Mutation

**Insertion type** | **Deletion type**

- Insertion or deletion of **one or two** or **non multiples of 3 nucleotides** into the coding gene results in an m-RNA in which the **reading frame is distorted** upon translation. This **reading frame change /alteration/distortion** in an mRNA, all the way down to the mutant site is a **feature of frame shift mutation & is not seen in point mutations.**
- The machinery translating the mRNA can not recognize that a base is missing (deleted) or added (inserted), *since there is no punctuation in reading of codons* – is the reason of altered reading frame.
- This can result in production of **garbled protein** (i.e. protein with completely/radically different amino acid sequence) or **truncated/short /prematurely terminated** – proteins (d/t premature creation of termination codon) or perhaps reading through the normal termination codon until another nonsense codon is encountered. (d/t deletion/insertion just prior to or within non sense codon)
- Following an insertion in a gene, a deletion (or vice versa) can restore the proper reading frame. And the corresponding mRNA on translation would contain a garbeled amino acid sequence b/w insertion & deletion and a correct sequence after that.
- If **3 or multiples of 3 nucleotides** are deleted/inserted in a coding region, the *corresponding number of aminoacids is missing/added* in the protein. Loss of 3 bases *maintains the reading frame* but can result in serious pathology like *cystic fibrosis* (**CF**).
- In CF, deletion of one codon (i.e. 3 bases) result in loss of 1 aminoacid **phenyl-alanine at 508th position (ΔF508) in CFTR (cystic fibrosis trans membrane conductance regulator) protein.** CFTR protein normally is a **chloride channel** in epithelia cells & its loss l/t production of thick, sticky secretion in lungs & pancrease causing damage to both.

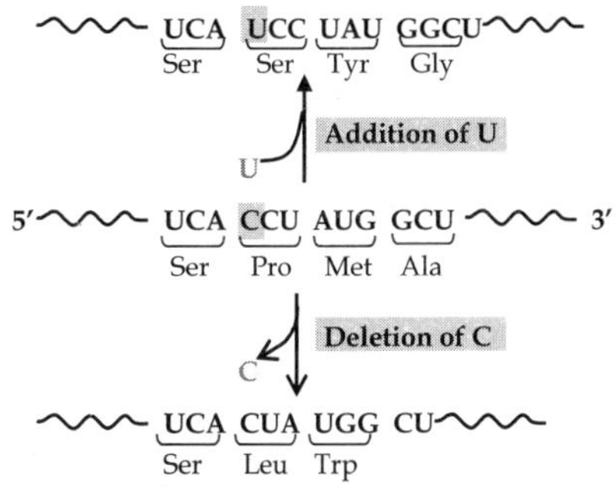


**Frame Shift mutation d/t insertion & deletion of 1 base l/t production of garbled protein**

### 2. Trinucleotide Repeat Expansion/Dynamic Mutation

- A sequence of 3 nucleotide bases that is repeated in tandem becomes amplified in number, so that too many copies of triplet occur.
- If this occurs in **coding region**, the protein will **contain many extra copies of one aminoacid** Eg CAG amplification in Hutington disease l/t insertion of many extra glutamine aa in

**and CUC̲ all code** leucine **and both UCU̲ & UCA̲ code serine**

- Example: **Homologous substitution** of **valine** at **67th** position of **β-chain-HbA** with another aminoacid has **no apparent effect** and result **in functionally normal hemoglobin** types.

| Hemoglobin type | Homologous substituted aminoacid at 67th position on β-chain of Hb-A |
|---|---|
| **Normal Hb A** | Valine |
| **Hb-Milwaukee** | *Glutamic acid*Q/*glutamate* |
| **Hb-Bristol** | *Aspartic acid*Q/aspartate |
| **Hb- Sydney** | *Alanine*Q |

- The incorporation of mistaken different aminoacid, depending upon its location in specific protein – might be *acceptable (mostly), partially acceptable or unacceptable*

- There is high probability that *prematurely terminated partially produced peptide or protein fragment will not function in its assigned role. Eg. β-thalassemia*
- If a *stop codon is changed into a coding codon*, this l/t elongation of protein to produce **run on polypeptide.** Eg Hb constant spring (α-thalassemia) .

| | Acceptable Mutations | Partially Acceptable | Unacceptable mutations |
|---|---|---|---|
| | - Change in aa has no functional consequence i.e. it **does not alter the normal function of protein**<br>- **Conserved mutation** means altered aa has the same properties of original aa eg **glutamic acid to aspartic acid**. Most point mutation would result in replacement of one aa by another with rather similar functional groups –a natural mechanism to avoid drastic changes. The resulting protein may not be distinguishable from the normal one. | - It will result in a protein molecule with **partial but abnormal function**<br>- **HbS** *hinders normal function* since it l/t sickle cell anemia when mutant gene is present in homozygous state and is considered *partially acceptable* because HbS does not bind & release $O_2$ abnormally. | - It results in **totally non functional protein,** that may be incompatible with normal life.<br>- For example **HbM** mutation generate molecules that oxidize $Fe^{2+}$ of heme to $Fe^{3+}$, producing **methemoglobin,** which cannot transport oxygen |
| **Protein** | **Hb-Hikari (β-chain)** | **Hb-S/Sickle Cell (β-chain)** | **Hb-M (Boston), α-Chain** |
| **Aminoacid change** | In HbA-**β-chain-61 position**, lysine is replaced by **asparagine**<br>**61 Lysine →Asparagine** | In HbA-**(β-chain)-6th position glutamate** is replaced by **valine**<br>**6,Glutamic acid→valine** | In HbA-**α-chain-58th position,** histidine is replace by **tyrosine**<br>**58Histidine →Tyrosine** |
| **Codon change** | **Transversion**<br>AAA or AAG<br>↓ ✕ ↓<br>AAU or AAC | **Transversion**<br>GAA or GAG<br>↓ ↓<br>GUA GUG | CAU or CAC<br>↓ ↓<br>UAU UAC |

★ **Null mutation** l/t no functional gain

Hutington protein making it unstable that accumulates causing neurodegenerative disorder.

- If amplification occurs in **non coding regions,** the result may be decrease in amount of protein produced, eg, **fragile X syndrome & myotonic dystrophy**. In fragile X syndrome the amplification results in gene silencing through **DNA hyper methylation** (as we know transcriptionally active **DNA is hypomethylated** whereas hypermethylation silences gene expression).

| Disease | Repeat | Gene product |
|---|---|---|
| **Hutington disease** | CAG | Hutington |
| **Spinocrebellar ataxia** 1, 2, 3 (Machado Joseph disease), 6, 7, 12 | CAG | Ataxin 1, Ataxin 2, SC3 (MJD1), Alpha 1A voltage dependent Ca++ channel, Ataxin 7, Protein phosphatase 2A |
| **Dentorubral pallidoluysiane atrophy (DRPLA)** | CAG | Atrophin |
| **X-chromosome spinobulbar muscular atrophy (DRPLA)** | CAG | Androgen receptor |
| **Friedreich ataxia** | GAA | Frataxin |
| **Fragile -X- syndrome** | CGG /GCC | FMR ½ protein |
| **Dystrophia myotonica** | CTG / CUG | Myotonin protein kinase |

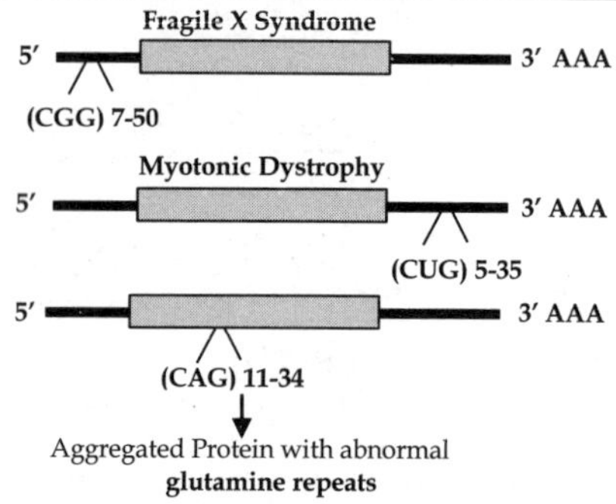


**3. Splice Site Mutation**

- Improper splicing can alter the way in which introns are removed from pre mRNA l/t production of aberrant proteins.
- Eg incorrect splicing of β-globin mRNA l/t **β-thalassemia** and in **myotonic dystrophy** gene silencing occurs d/t splicing alterations.

**Suppressor Mutations**

- Suppressor mutations can suppress/counteract some effects of missense, nonsense & frame shift mutations by producing abnormally functioning, mutated, **suppressor t-RNA molecules** with alterations in anticodon region. These are capable of binding to & decoding altered mutated codones, thereby suppressing the effects of mutations in distinct mutated mRNA encoding structure genes.
- Suppressor t RNA usually result in *decreased viability* as these are incapable of distinguishing b/w a normal & a mutated codon. Eg **nonsense S-tRNA** can suppress normal termination signals to allow a read through when it is not desirable and a **frameshift S-tRNA** may read a normal codon plus a component of a juxtaposed codon to provide a frame shift when it is not desirable.
- Since reading through of translation has on occasion been observed, S-tRNA may exist in mammalian cells.

## Sickle Cell Hemoglobin (HbS)

- A **point mutation** involving **T- to - A** *DNA substitution* (which inturn results in an **'A - to- U'** change in the *m-RNA*) corresponding to the 6th codon of β globin gene result in sickle cell disease

**Partially accecpted missense (Point) mutation involving (T) to (A) substitution in β globulin gene (DNA) at 6th position** → **(A) to (U) substitution in** corresponding positionof **m RNA** and so codon

| | Codes Amino acid | In protein |
|---|---|---|
| GAA / GAG | **Polar Negatively Charged Glutamate at β 6** | **HbA β chain** |
| ↓ becomes | | |
| GUA / GUG | **Non polar hydrophobic Valine at β 6** | **HbS - β chain** |

- The corresponding single nucleotide change within the codon would be **GAA or GAG of glutamic acid to GUA or GUG of valine**. This is a **partially accepted missense mutation**; partially accepted because HbS does bind & release $O_2$, albeit abnormally; missense because it hinders normal function & result in sickle cell anemia.
- Restriction fragment length polymorphism (RFLP) is an inherited difference in the pattern of restriction (endonuclease) enzyme digestion d/t presence or absence of an extra restriction site. This single base *change in sickle cell disease result in RFLP*[Q].
- The mutation results in **single amino acid substitution (GLu $^{6(\beta)}$ – Val):** i.e. ***a surface localized charged (polar, hydrophilic) aminoacid glutamate is replaced by hydrophobic (non polar) amino acid valine (without any charge)***[Q] ***at position 6 in two β-chains***. The R group of valine has no electric charge, whereas glutamate has a negative charge at pH 7.4. So HbS has 2 fewer negative charges than HbA (1 for each β-chain)
- This replacement creates a **'Sticky hydrophobic patch'** (contact point) on the outer surface at position 6 of β-chain of both oxy HbS and deoxy HbS (but not in Hb A)
- **Complementary sticky patch** is found in both **HbA and HbS**, but is exposed only in their **deoxygenated (T) state.**
- HbA remains a true solute at rather higher concentrations because of polar exterior surface that is compatable and non reactive with nearby Hb molecules. In contrast ***HbS when deoxygenated is less soluble***[Q].

  Thus at low $PO_2$, deoxy HbS can polymerize to form long , insoluble fibers. These twisted helical fibers ***distort the erythrocyte into characteristic sickle shape***[Q].

  Binding of **deoxy Hb A** *terminates fiber polymerization*, since HbA lacks the second sticky patch necessary to bind another Hb molecule.

**1° Hydrophobic sticky patch on oxy & deoxy HbS** — Produced **d/t replacement of polar glu → non polar valine**

**2° Complementary Sticky site on deoxy HbA and deoxy HbS** — Produced d/t **deoxygenation** — **Decreased solubility**

↓

**Polymerization & Sickling**

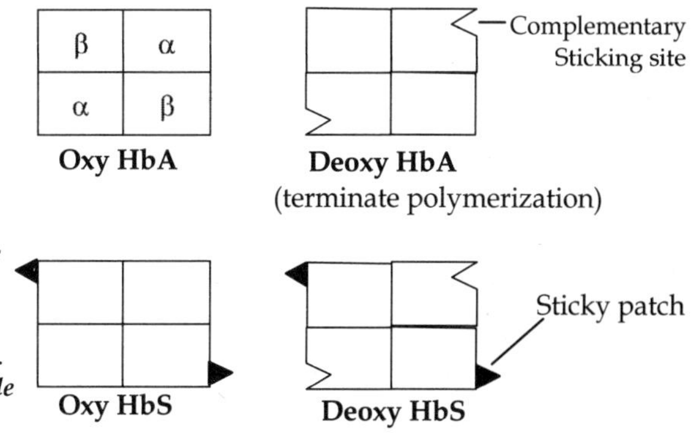


- In dilute solutions, HbS has interactions with $O_2$ ($P_{50}$, Hill coefficient) that are similar to those for HbA. However *Bohr effect on concentrated HbS is more pronounced* l/t greater release of $O_2$ in the capillaries & increased propensity for sickling. Sickled RBCs are less deformable less freely mobile through microvasculature & often block blood flow especially in *spleen & joints*. These cells lose water, become fragile, & have a considerable short life span l/t hemolysis & anemia.
- In **heterozygous (Hb A/ HbS, sickle cell trait)** individuals, sickling decreases by at least a factor of 1000, thereby accounting for the *asymptomatic natue except during extreme physical exertion*. For reasons that remain to be elucidated, ***hetrozygosity is associated with an increased resistance to malaria***[Q], specially for lethal forms like *plasmodium falciparum*. HbS trait causes parasites to grow poorly or die at low $O_2$ concentration b/o *low $K^+$ levels caused by potassium efflux* from RBC on heboglobin sickling.
- This is the selective advantage that HbA/HbS hetrozygotes exhibit over either normal HbA/HbA or homozygous HbS/ HbS and offer an explanation for persistence of HbS in gene pool d/t natural selection. Emerging t/t include *inducing HbF expression* to inhibit polymerization.

★ 90% of human genome variation occurs d/t **single base change in DNA** and is k/a **single nucleotide polymorphism** (**SNPs** or pronounced "**snips**"). This results in **disappearance** (of already present) or **creation** of a new **restriction site** by a particular restriction, endonuclease enzyme.

In either case, cleavage with that restriction endonuclease results in fragments of **lengths differing from normal** (i.e. **RFLP**=restriction fragment length polymorphism), which can be detected by *DNA - hybridization (southern bloting)*. In Hbs, point mutation abolishes the recognition site of **restriction endonuclease Mst II** that recognizes the nucleotide sequence **C C T N A G G** (N=any nucleotide). A to T mutation in $\beta^s$ globin gene codon *eliminates a cleavage site*, resulting in generation of **larger 1.35 kg fragments** (in place of *normal 1.15 kb fragments*) on DNA digestion with Mst II restriction endonuclease.

## Methods used for Detection of Mutation

| Common Techniques | Principle |
|---|---|
| Cytogenetic analysis | Unique visual appearance of various |
| Fluorescent in situ hybridization (FISH) | Hybridization to chromosomes with fluorescently labeled probes |
| Southern blot | Hybridization with genomic probe or cDNA probe after digestion of high molecular DNA |
| Polymerase chain reaction (PCR) | Amplification of DNA segment |
| Reverse transcriptase PCR (RT-PCR) | Reverse transcription, amplification of DNA segment - absence or reduction of mRNA transcription |
| DNA sequencing | Direct sequencing of PCR products<br>Sequencing of DNA segments cloned into plasmid vectors |
| Restriction fragment polymorphism (RFLP) | Detection of altered restriction pattern of genomic DNA (southern blot) or PCR products |

| Other Techniques | Principle |
|---|---|
| Single-strand conformational polymorphism (SSCP) | PCR of DNA segment: Mutations result in conformational change and altered mobility |
| Denaturing gradient gel electrophoresis (DGGE) | PCR of DNA segment: Mutations result in conformational change and altered mobility |
| RNAse cleavage | Cleavage of mismatch between mutated and wild type sequence |
| Oligonucleotide specific hybridization (OSH) | Hybridization of PCR products to wild -type or mutated oligonucleotides immobilized on chips or slides |
| Microarrays | Hybridization of PCR products to wild-type or mutated oligonucleotides |
| Protein truncation test (PTT) | Transcription/translation of cDNA isolated from tissue sample |
| Pyrosequencing | Clonal amplification of single DNA fragments on microparticles followed by massive parallel sequencing |
| Multiplex ligation-dependent probe amplification (MLPA) | Quantification of PCR-generated amplicons reflecting the number of copies of a specific DNA sequence |

# Chapter -4 CYTOGENETICS AND MOLECULAR GENETICS, RECOMBINANT DNA & GENOMIC TECHNOLOGY

## QUESTIONS

### Cytogenetics

**1. The long and short arms of chromosomes are designated respectively as:**
- A. p and q arms ☐
- B. m and q arms ☐
- C. q and p arms ☐
- D. 1 and s arms ☐

**2. Karyotyping under light microscopy is**
- A. L Banding ☐
- B. G banding ☐
- C. C Banding ☐
- D. FUdR banding ☐

**3. Rapid method of chromosome identification in intersex is:**
- A. FISH ☐
- B. PCR ☐
- C. SSCP ☐
- D. Karyotyping ☐

**4. Which of the following technique can be used for exact localization of a genetic locus?**
- A. Chromosome painting ☐
- B. Western blot ☐
- C. Comparative genomic hybridization ☐
- D. FISH ☐

**5. Subtelomeric rearrangement of genes is frequently associated wih mental retardation. All of the following techniques can be used to diagnose them except:**
- A. FISH ☐
- B. MAPH ☐
- C. cGH array ☐
- D. MALDI ☐

**6. Which of the following is used to detect the chromosomal differences between neoplastic cells and their normal counterparts?**
- A. PCR ☐
- B. Comparative genomic hybridization ☐
- C. Spectral karyotyping ☐
- D. Western blotting ☐

**7. Nanotechnology has found tremendous application in the diagnosis of cancers because of all of following advantages, except:**
- A. Nanocrystals exibit bright, photostable fluorescence ☐
- B. Nanocrystals have a narrow spectrum wavelength ☐
- C. Peak spectrum wavelength is tunable ☐
- D. Nanocrystals exhibit a narrow difference between their excitation and emission peak spectra ☐

**8. Transfer of genetic material in 1 meiotic division between 2 non-homologous chromosomes:**
- A. Translocation ☐
- B. Non- disjunction ☐
- C. Inversion ☐
- D. Isochromose ☐
- E. Deletion ☐

**9. Aneuploidy is due to:**
- A. Non-disjunction at meiosis ☐
- B. Mosaicism ☐
- C. Deletion ☐
- D. Translocation ☐

**10. Differential expression of same gene depending on parent of origin is referred to as:**
- A. Genomic imprinting ☐
- B. Mosaicism ☐
- C. Anticipation ☐
- D. Nonpenetrance ☐

**11. Normal parent with 2 siblings having osteogenesis imperfecta. Pattern of inheritance is**
- A. Mutation ☐
- B. Anticipation ☐
- C. Genomic imprinting ☐
- D. Germline mosacism ☐

**12. Prenatal diagnosis at 16 weeks of pregnancy can be performed using all of the following, except:**
- A. Amniotic fluid ☐
- B. Maternal blood ☐
- C. Chrionic villi ☐
- D. Fetal blood ☐

**13. Rich source of IgG is:**
- A. Stomach ☐
- B. Visceral peritoneum ☐
- C. Small intestine ☐
- D. Large intestine ☐

**14. Rh factor is**
- A. IgM antibody ☐
- B. Mucppolysaccharide ☐
- C. IgG antibody ☐
- D. Fatty acid ☐
- E. Glycoprotein ☐

**15. Barr body is found in the following phase of the cell cycle:**
- A. Interphase ☐
- B. Metaphase ☐
- C. GI phase ☐
- D. Telophase ☐

**16. Movement of protein from nucleus to cytoplasm can be seen by**
- A. FISH ☐
- B. FRAP ☐
- C. Confocal microscopy ☐
- D. Electron microscopy ☐

### Luminescence

**17. Fluorescence means**
- A. Spontaneous illumination in dark ☐
- B. Release of longer wavelength light on absorbing light of shorter wavelength ☐
- C. Release of shorter wavelength light on absorbing light of longer wavelength ☐
- D. Release of equal wavelength light at constant rate ☐

**18. Which statement is incorrect?**
- A. Chemiluminescence: excited electron in higher orbit comes to lower orbit by emitting energy in form of photon ☐
- B. Bioluminescence: is a form of chemiluminescence ☐
- C. Photoluminiscence: absorbed radiation emitted as light ☐
- D. Electrophotochemiluminescence: Light-emitting reaction which take place by the use of electrical current ☐

**19. Firefilies produce light due to:**
A. NADH ☐
B. GTP ☐
C. ATP ☐
D. Phosphocreatinine ☐

**20. Nephelometry is based on the principle of**
A. Light attenuated in intensity by scattering ☐
B. Refraction of light ☐
C. Reduced transmission of light ☐
D. Filtration of solutes by kidney ☐

**21. DNA estimation can be done by**
A. Spirometer ☐
B. Spectrophotometer ☐
C. pH meter ☐
D. Sphygmometer ☐

**22. Immunoflorescent probes are used in:**
A. FRET ☐
B. Microarray ☐
C. RIA ☐
D. Recombinant DNA ☐
E. ELISA ☐

## Restriction Endonuclease

**23. RFLP, True are:**
A. Endonuclease cuts DNA at nucleotide level: ☐
B. It acts at specific site ☐
C. Only cohesive ends are produced ☐
D. Only blunt ends are produced. ☐

**24. Restrinction Endonucleas function → true about:**
A. Cut both the strands of ds DNA ☐
B. The cut ends produced are sticky ☐
C. The cut ends produced are blunt. ☐
D. Cuts single strand of DNA ☐

**25. Restriction endonuclease is** :
A. Break single stranded DNA ☐
B. Break double stranded DNA ☐
C. Break peptide chain ☐
D. Break RNA ☐

**26. Correct statements regarding restriction endonuclease is/are**:
A. Restriction endouclease recognizes specific sites of DNA sequence ☐
B. Restriction endonuclease recognizes short sequence of DNA ☐
C. It acts at 5' – 3' direction ☐
D. It acts at 3' – 5' direction ☐

**27. DNA fragments formed by the action of Restriction Endonucleases, are separated by**:
A. Gel electrophoresis ☐
B. Agarose gel eletrophoresis ☐
C. Paper Chromatography ☐
D. High pressure liquid chromatography ☐

**28. DNA restriction is done by the following method**:
A. Paper chromatography ☐
B. Electrophoresis agargel method ☐
C. Spectrophotometer ☐
D. Spectrometry ☐

**29. After digestion by restriction endonucleases DNA strands can be joined again by**
A. DNA polymerase ☐
B. DNA ligase ☐
C. DNA topoisomerase ☐
D. DNA gyrase ☐

**30. True about Restriction enzymes:**
A. Palindromic ☐
B. Produce DNA sticky end ☐
C. Restrict replication of DNA ☐
D. Restriction sites are not specific ☐
E. Breaks at sugar-phosphate bond ☐

**31. True statement about Restriction endonuclease:**
A. Palindromic sequences observed ☐
B. Protects bacteria from infection by virus ☐
C. Present only in eukaryotes ☐
D. Restrict replication of DNA ☐

**32. Which of the following represents the most charachteristic function of Type II Restriction Enzyme**
A. Prevent folding of proteins ☐
B. Remove formed DNA ☐
C. Prevent supercoiling ☐
D. Cut DNA at palindromic sites ☐

**33. True about DNA methylation:**
A. Alters gene expression ☐
B. Genetic code remains intact ☐
C. Role in carcinogenesis ☐
D. Protective mechanism against cleavage by restriction endonuclease ☐

**34. Bacteria aquires restriction endonuclease by horizontal transfer. The result would be**
A. Bacteria can undergo mutation ☐
B. Bacteria causes death of host DNA ☐
C. Bacteria cannot survive because it lacks DNA methylase that protects the host DNA ☐
D. It helps in DNA proof reading in bacteria ☐

## Polymorphism and RFLP

**35. True about polymorphism is:**
A. Single locus → multiple normal alleles ☐
B. Single locus → multiple abnormal alleles ☐
C. Single phenotype:Single locus → multiple normal alleles ☐
D. Single phenotype: Single locus → multiple abnormal alleles ☐

**36. Correct statement about Restriction fragment gene**
A. Detected by Southern blot ☐
B. Detected by Northern blot ☐
C. Used for identification of gene for genomic mapping ☐
D. RFLP is a DNA variation sequence ☐

**37. Restriction fragment length polymorphism is used for**:
A. Analysis of chromosome structures ☐
B. DNA estimation ☐
C. Synthesis of nucleic acid ☐
D. Detecting proteins in a cell ☐

**38. For measurement of long DNA molecules (50-100 KB) following is used**
A. Chromosome walking ☐
B. Nitch ☐
C. RFLP ☐
D. SSLP ☐

**39. RFLP, true is /are:**
A. Detects mutation ☐
B. Recognizes triuncleotide repeates ☐
C. Detects deletion ☐
D. Blunt ends are produced ☐
E. Always short ends are produced ☐

**40. Microsatellite sequence is**:
A. Small satellite ☐
B. Extra chromosomal DNA ☐
C. Short sequence (2-5) repeat DNA ☐
D. Looped-DNA ☐

## DNA Fingerprinting

**41. DNA fingerprinting is based on possessing in DNA of:**
- A. Constant Tandem Repeat ☐
- B. Variable Number Tandem Repeats (VNTR) ☐
- C. Non- repeatative sequence ☐
- D. Exon ☐
- E. Intron in eukaryotes ☐

**42. DNA fingerprinting was founded by:**
- A. Watson ☐
- B. Galton ☐
- C. Jeffrey ☐

**43. DNA finger printing is done by:**
- A. Splitting DNA ☐
- B. DNA of WBC ☐
- C. DNA from nucleated cells ☐
- D. All of the above ☐

## PCR

**44. True about polymerase chain reaction (PCR):**
- A. Carried out by thermostable DNA polymerase ☐
- B. Exponential ☐
- C. Additive ☐
- D. Specific ☐
- E. Single-stranded DNA is required ☐

**45. In PCR:**
- A. Thermostable enzyme is needed ☐
- B. 211 copies formed after 'n' numbers of multiple ☐
- C. Non specific ☐
- D. Thermolabile enzyme ☐
- E. Primer is needed. ☐

**46. True about polymerase chain reaction is:**
- A. Enzymatic DNA amplification ☐
- B. Recombinent DNA amplification ☐
- C. Seperation of protein fragments is serum ☐
- D. None ☐

**47. Which of the following is not true about PCR:**
- A. Thermostable enzyme is used ☐
- B. Annealing is done after DNA denaturation ☐
- C. Specific primers re required ☐
- D. Required atleast 1 week time for synthesis ☐
- E. DNA polymerase has to be added on each cycle ☐

**48. The enzyme used in polymerase chain reaction (PCR) is:**
- A. Thermostable enzyme ☐
- B. Enzyme stabiliser ☐
- C. Inorganic ion ☐
- D. Inorganic metal ☐

**49. True statements about PCR:**
- A. Protein amplification ☐
- B. DNA amplification ☐
- C. Same as western blot test ☐
- D. Detection of infecting organisms ☐

**50. True about PCR:**
- A. Primers required ☐
- B. DNA dependent RNA polymerase ☐
- C. DNA polymerase ☐
- D. RNA dependent DNA polymerase ☐

**51. Enzyme(s) used in polymerase chain reaction is/are:**
- A. Restriction endonuclease ☐
- B. DNA polymerase ☐
- C. Alkaline phosphate ☐
- D. RNA polymerase ☐
- E. Reverse transcriptase ☐

**52. Which of the following is/are features of polymerase used in recombinant synthesis:**
- A. Thermostable ☐
- B. Doesn't require primer ☐
- C. Unusually active ☐
- D. Replicates double stranded DNA ☐

**53. In PCR Acquaticus thermophilus is preferred over E.coli. because:**
- A. Thermostable at temperature at which DNA liquefies. ☐
- B. Proof reading done. ☐
- C. Done in more precisely. ☐
- D. Does not require primer. ☐
- E. Better DNA replication. ☐

**54. True about DNA polymerase used in PCR:**
- A. Obtained from virus ☐
- B. Obtained from bacteria ☐
- C. Used for joining the two strands ☐
- D. It is heat stable ☐
- E. Add nucleotide ☐

**55. Which of the following is used in PCR?**
- A. Ca++ ☐
- B. Mg++ ☐
- C. Li+ ☐
- D. Na+ ☐

**56. For PCR which of the following is not required:**
- A. Taq polymerase ☐
- B. d-NTP ☐
- C. Primer ☐
- D. Radiolabelled DNA probe ☐

**57. For PCR which of the following is not required:**
- A. Taq polymerase ☐
- B. d-NTP ☐
- C. Dideoxynucleotides ☐
- D. Magneswium ☐

**58. SYBR Green Dye is used for:**
- A. HPLC ☐
- B. Immunofluorescence ☐
- C. PCR ☐
- D. ELISA ☐

**59. Real time PCR is used for:**
- A. Multiplication of RNA ☐
- B. Multiplication of proteins ☐
- C. Multiplication of specific segments of DNA ☐
- D. To know how much amplification of DNA has occurred ☐

**60. Prenatal diagnosis of Hemophilia is best done by:**
- A. PCR ☐
- B. Linkage analysis ☐
- C. Cytometry ☐
- D. Microarray ☐

## Ligase Chain Reaction

**61. DNA Amplification is done in:**
- A. PCR ☐
- B. NASBA (Nucleic acid sequential based amplification) ☐
- C. Ligase chain reactions ☐
- D. DNA sequencing ☐

## Cloning

**62. In molecular cloning, Blue-white screening is used for:**
- A. To screen for recombinant vectors ☐
- B. To detect gene mutations ☐
- C. To identify desired chromosomal DNA insert in plasmid vectors ☐
- D. To detect host DNA in situ ☐

**63. True about Monoclonal antibody:**
- A. Produced by hybridoma technology ☐
- B. Non-specific ☐
- C. Requires in small quantity ☐
- D. Used for blood grouping ☐

**64. True about Hybridoma:**
- A. Immortalise myeloma cell ☐
- B. Hybridoma cell produced by fusion of T-cell & myeloma ☐
- C. Cell is of human origin ☐
- D. Prior immunization is done ☐
- E. Produce monospecific & monoclonal Ab ☐

**65. Methods of producing fusion of cells are A/E**
- A. Attaching inactive viral particles on cell membrane ☐
- B. Adding polyethylene glycol ☐
- C. Applying a small electric current ☐
- D. Reducing surface tension ☐

**66. In gene cloning, largest fragment can be incorporated in:**
- A. Plasmid ☐
- B. Bacteriophage ☐
- C. Cosmid ☐
- D. Retrovirus ☐

**67. In DNA transfer the vectors used from smallest to largest is:**
- A. Cosmids, Plasmids, Bacteriophage ☐
- B. Plasmids, Bacteriophage, Cosmids ☐
- C. Bacteriophage, Cosmides, Plasmids ☐
- D. Cosmids, Bacteriophage, Plasmids ☐
- E. Plasmids, Cosmids, Bacteriophage ☐

**68. Which is true about phage DNA**
- A. Antibiotic susceptibility ☐
- B. Restriction enzyme sites ☐
- C. Hexagonal DNA ☐
- D. Carries short segment of DNA ☐

## Site Directed Mutagenesis

**69. Which test uses oligomer with single base pair substitution as primer**
- A. PCR ☐
- B. RFLP ☐
- C. Error coded mutation analysis with PCR ☐
- D. Site directed mutagenesis ☐

## Site Specific Recombination

**70. Site specific recombination is**
- A. Palindromic ☐
- B. Ser-form Holliday intermediate ☐
- C. RE + ligase ☐
- D. Inversion in same orientation / Non precise ☐

## Linkage Analysis

**71. Which of the following statement is true about Linkage analysis?**
- A. Detection of Characteristic DNA polymorphism in a family is associated with disorders ☐
- B. Useful to make pedigree chart to show affected and non-affected family members ☐
- C. Used to make a pedigree chart to show non-paternity ☐
- D. Non-Gene maping method of genetic study ☐

## Analyzing Technique

**72. True about western blot:**
- A. Separation of proteins are based on mass ☐
- B. SDS-PAGE electrophesis is used for separation ☐
- C. Enzyme linked antibodies are used ☐
- D. Confirmatory in AIDS ☐

**73. Antigen antiboey reaction is detected by:**
- A. ELISA ☐
- B. Southern blot ☐
- C. Northern blot ☐
- D. Western blot ☐
- E. Eastern blot ☐

**74. Western blot technique is done for**
- A. Mitochondrial RNA ☐
- B. Double strand DNA ☐
- C. r- RNA ☐
- D. Protein ☐

**75. Nothern blot is used for the separation of:**
- A. mRNA ☐
- B. DNA ☐
- C. Protein ☐
- D. Protein DNA interaction ☐

**76. Northern blot test is used for:**
- A. DNA analysis ☐
- B. RNA analysis ☐
- C. Analysis of proteins ☐
- D. Enzyme analysis ☐

**77. Probe used in western blot:**
- A. Antibody ☐
- B. M-RNA ☐
- C. DNA ☐
- D. t-RNA ☐
- E. PCR ☐

**78. The following methods can be used to detect the point mutation in the beta (β)-globin gene that causes sickle cell anemia, *except*:**
- A. Polymerase chain reaction with allele-specific oligonucleotide hybridization ☐
- B. Southern blot analysis ☐
- C. DNA sequencing ☐
- D. Northern blot analysis ☐

**79. Which of following techniques is used for detection of variations in DNA sequence and Gene expression:**
- A. Northern Blot ☐
- B. Southern Blot ☐
- C. Western Blot ☐
- D. Microarray ☐

**80. Which of the following tests is not used for detection of specific aneuploidy:**
- A. FISH ☐
- B. RT-PCR ☐
- C. QF-PCR ☐
- D. Microarray ☐

**81. Gene expression can be detected by all except:**
- A. RT-PCR ☐
- B. cDNA microarray ☐
- C. Southern blot ☐
- D. Northern blot ☐
- E. Immunohistochemistry ☐

## Gene Library

**82. True about gene library:**
- A. Also known as chromosome ☐
- B. Library that contains books on gene ☐
- C. Computer base with all gene knowledge ☐
- D. DNA Nucleotide or fragment ☐
- E. Complete collection of gene copies of one organism ☐

## Recombinant DNA Technology or Genetic Engineering

**83. Biotechnology is/are used for**
A. Viral vaccine production ☐
B. To cure genetic disorder ☐
C. Genetic crop ☐
D. Gene production ☐
E. Production of genetic products ☐

**84. Starting material for production of insulin from bacteria is:**
A. Genomic DNA from beta pancreatic cells of human ☐
B. Genomic DNA from lymphocytes of human ☐
C. mRNA from beta pancreatic cells of human ☐
D. mRNA from lymphocytes of human ☐

**85. Reverse transcriptase is:**
A. DNA dependent RNA polymerase ☐
B. RNA dependent DNA polymerase ☐
C. DNA dependent DNA polymerase ☐
D. RNA dependent RNA polymerase ☐
E. RNA polymerase ☐

**86. True about DNA reconstruction technology:**
A. Restriction endonucleases involved ☐
B. DNA ligase is used ☐
C. Acid phosphatase is used ☐
D. Reverse transcriptase needed ☐

**87. Enzymes used in DNA research programme are except:**
A. Polymerase ☐
B. Exonuclease ☐
C. Nuclease ☐
D. Alkaline phosphatase ☐
E. None ☐

**88. Which of the following is a strategy used to increase the yield of protein produced in recombinant protein synthesis?**
A. Promoter induction ☐
B. Genes for protease inhibitors ☐
C. Translation initiation ☐
D. Translation and transcription termination ☐

**89. Study of structure and products of gene is:**
A. Genomics ☐
B. Protenomics ☐
C. Bioinformatics ☐
D. Cytogenetics ☐
E. Pharmacogenomics ☐

**90. Study of multiplication of proteins in disease process is called:**
A. Proteomics ☐
B. Genomics ☐
C. Glycomics ☐
D. Nucleomics ☐

**91. Techniques used for protein expression proteomics study include(s):**
A. Gene Array Chips ☐
B. Mass Spectroscopy ☐
C. PolyAcrylamide Gel Electrophoresis (PAGE) ☐
D. RT-PCR ☐
E. Two-Dimensional Electrophoresis ☐

## Transgenic Organism

**92. Mutation that completely disrupt the function of the gene used in which of the following technique:**
A. Knock-out ☐
B. Non-sense mutation ☐
C. Restrictin fragment length polymorphism ☐
D. Targeted gene disruption ☐
E. Knock -in ☐

**93. True statement about transgenic mice:**
A. Developed from DNA insertion into fertilized egg ☐
B. Have same genome as parents except one or more genes ☐
C. Identical genome to parent mice ☐
D. Produced by breeding over several generations ☐
E. Homozygous are selected ☐

**94. Which of the following methods is most suited to assess function of a gene:**
A. Southern blot ☐
B. Northern blot ☐
C. Gene knockout animals ☐
D. Transgenic animals ☐

**95. Nude mouse is used in genetics because of the following properties:**
A. Absence of thymus ☐
B. Xenograft can be sustained for weeks ☐
C. Severe combined immunodeficiency mice is same as nude mice ☐

**96. Two transgenic plants are grown. One plant has a gene encoding a fluorescent pigment incorporated in its genome. The other plant has a fire fly luciferase gene incorporated in its genome. Which of the two plants will glow in the dark?**
A. Both plants will glow ☐
B. Neither will glow ☐
C. First one will glow ☐
D. Second one will glow ☐

## Gene Therapy

**97. Purpose of Gene therapy:**
A. Replacement of abnormal gene by normal gene ☐
B. Replacement of normal gene by abnormal gene ☐
C. Knock out of abnormal gene ☐
D. Introduction of viral gene ☐

**98. Gene therapy methods are:**
A. Electroporation ☐
B. Intranuclear injection ☐
C. Site directed mutagenesis ☐
D. Retrovirus ☐

**99. The first gene therapy (somatic enzyme) was successfully done in:**
A. SCID ☐
B. Phenylketonuria ☐
C. Thalassemia ☐
D. Cystic fibrosis ☐
E. Alkaptonuria ☐

## Genetic Disorder

**100. True abut 'X' Chromosome inactivation:**
A. X gene ☐
B. RNA interference ☐
C. Seen in Male ☐
D. Seen in Female ☐

**101. Which of the following are X- linked recessive disorders:**
A. Marfan Syndrome ☐
B. Phenylketonuria ☐
C. Neurofibromatosis ☐
D. Duchenne muscular dystrophy ☐
E. G-6-P dehydrogenase deficiency ☐

**102. Father to son inheritance is never seen in case of:**
A. Autosomal dominant inheritance ☐
B. Autosomal recessive inheritance ☐
C. X- linked recessive inheritance ☐
D. Multifactorial inheritance

**103. An affected male infant born to normal parents could be an example of all of the following, *except:***
A. An Autosomal dominant disorder ☐
B. An Autosomal recessive disorder ☐
C. A polygenic disorder ☐
D. A vertically transmitted disorder ☐

**104. Autosomal recessive disease are:**
A. Tuberous sclerosis ☐
B. Duchenne muscular dystrophy ☐
C. Cystic fibrosis ☐
D. Ataxia telangiectasia ☐
E. Factor VIII deficiency ☐

**105. A child with a small head, minor anomalies of the face including a thin upper lip, growth delay, and developmental disability can have all of the following, *except:***
A. A chromosomal syndrome ☐
B. A teratogenic syndrome ☐
C. A mendelian syndrome ☐
D. A polygenic syndrome ☐

**106. In a family, the father has widely spaced eyes, increased facial hair and deafness. One of the three children has deafness with similar facial features. The mother is normal. Which one of the following is most likely pattern of inheritance in this case?**
A. Autosomal dominant ☐
B. Autosomal recessive ☐
C. X-linked dominant ☐
D. X-linked recessive ☐

**107. Gene for major histocompatibility complex and HLA gene is located on:**
A. Long arm of chromosome 8. ☐
B. Short arm of chromosome 8 ☐
C. Long arm of chromosome 6 ☐
D. Short arm of chromosome 6 ☐

**108. True about MHC:**
A. Transplantation reaction ☐
B. Autoimmune disease ☐
C. Immunosupression ☐
D. Involved in T-cell function ☐
E. Situated at long arm of chromosome ☐

**109. MHC class II antigens are located on which of the following cells:**
A. Platelets ☐
B. Dendritic cell ☐
C. RBC ☐
D. T-cell ☐
E. G-cell ☐
F. B-cell ☐

**110. MHC II is/are presented by:**
A. Macrophage ☐
B. Dendritic cells ☐
C. Lymphocyte ☐
D. Epithelial cells ☐
E. Platelets ☐

**111. Which of the follwoing molecular phenomenon in $I_g$ genes is responsible for affinity maturation of antibody response**
A. Chain shuffling ☐
B. Junctional diverity ☐
C. Somatic hypermutation ☐
D. Altered RAA splicing ☐

## Answers:

### Cytogenetics

1. **C i.e. q and p arms** *[Ref: Robbins 7th/170-73; http://www.ring-chromosome-20.org/what_are_chromosomes.aspx]*
2. **B i.e. G banding** *[Ref: Nagesh Rao: Human genetics (1988) 78. 21-26]*
3. **A i.e. FISH** *[Ref: Robbin's 7/e p. 171- 73; http://members.aol.com/chrominfo/fishinfo.htm]*
4. **D i.e. FISH** *[Ref: Harper 29/e p. 442]*
5. **D i.e. MALDI** *[Ref: Teitz 6/e p 1225-28; Harrison 18/e p 510-12 665; Harper 29/e p-442]*
6. **B i.e. Comparative genomic hybridization**
7. **B i.e. Nanocrystals have a narrow spectrum wavelength**
8. **A i.e. Translocation** *[Ref: Robbins 7/e p-173 –75; Harrison 16/e p. 384- 85]*
9. **A i.e. Non disjunction at meiosis**
10. **A i.e. Genomic Imprinting** *[Ref: Robbins 7/e p 186; Harrison 16/e p. 375]*
11. **D i.e. Germline mosacism**
12. **D i.e. Fetal blood** *[Ref: Dutta 6th/108; www.americanpregnancy.org/prenatal testing]*
13. **C i.e. Small intestine** (Most probably) Most abundant immunoglobin in blood → IgG.
14. **A i.e. IgM antibody >> E i.e. Glycoprotein** *[Ref: Harrison 17/e p. 2155; Chakraborty Microbiology 1/e p. 141; Davidson 20/e p. 1074]*
15. **A i.e. Interphase** *[Ref: Tortora Principles of Anatomy & Physiology 10/e P-1098; Robbins 7/e P-178; Chandrasoma Taylor 3/e P- 227]*
16. **B i.e. FRAP** *[Ref: Lehninger 5/e p 383, 434-36, 760]*

### Luminescence

17. **B i.e. Release of longer wavelength light on absorbing light of shorter wavelength**
18. **None** *[Ref: Lehninger 5th/e p. 435, 509; Teitz 6th/ed pg- 63, 79-80, 167-68, 179]*
19. **C i.e. ATP** *[Ref: Lehninger 5th/ed pg- 509, 332; Teitz 6th/ed pg -79]*
20. **A i.e. Light attenuated in intensity by scattering** *[Ref: Tietz 6/e p. 80-179]*
21. **B i.e. Spectrophotometer** *[Ref: Lehninger 5/e p. 78; Teitz 5/e p 152]*
22. **A i.e. FRET; B i.e. Microarray; C i.e. RIA; E i.e. ELISA** *[Ref: Chatterjea 8/e p. 834; Lippincott 6/e p. 472]*

### Restriction Endonuclease

23. **B i.e. It acts at specific site**
24. **A i.e. Cut both strands of ds DNA; B i.e. Cut ends produced are sticky; C i.e. Cut end produced are blunt**
25. **B i.e. Break double stranded DNA**
26. **A i.e. Restriction endonuclease recognizes specific sites of DNA; B i.e. Restriction endonuclease reconises short sequence of DNA**
27. **B i.e. Agarose gel electrophoresis**
28. **B i.e. Electrophoresis agar gel method**
29. **B i.e. DNA ligase**
30. **A, B, C, E i.e. Palindromic, Produce DNA sticky end, Restrict replication of DNA, Breaks at sugar-phosphate bond**
31. **A, B, D i.e. Palindromic sequences observed; Protects bacteria from infection by virus; Restrict replication of DNA**
32. **D i.e. Cut DNA at palindromic sites**

*[Ref: Harper 29/e p 434-36; Chatterjea 7/e 261-63; Vassudevan 6/e 513-15; Lippincott 5/e 465-66; Lehninger 5/304-7,1052-55; Satyanaraan 3/579-80]*

33. **A i.e. Alters gene expression; B i.e. Genetic code remains intact; C i.e. Role in carcinogenesis; D i.e. Protective mechanism against cleavage by restriction endonuclease** *[Ref: Lehninger 5/e 994-96, 292, 223, 233; Wikipedia]*
34. **C i.e. Bacteria cannot survive because it lacks DNA methylase that protects the host DNA**

### Polymorphism and RFLP

35. **C i.e., Single phenotype, single locus, multiple normal allele**
*[Ref: Harper's 27/e p. 413-16; Lippincott's 4/e p. 473-79; Robbins 7/e p. 189-91, 146, 150]*
36. **A i.e. Detected by southern blot; C i.e. Used for identification of gene for genomic mapping; D i.e. RFLP is a DNA variation sequence**
37. **A i.e. Analysis of Chromosal structure**
38. **C i.e. RFLP**
39. **A i.e. Detects Mutation B i.e., Recognizes trinucleotide repeats C i.e., Detects deletion D i.e., Blunt end produced**
*[Ref: Lehninger 5/e p 319; Lippincot 5/e p 474-76]*
40. **C i.e. Short sequence (2-5) repeat DNA** *[Ref: Robbins 7th/307; Harrisons 16th/449; http://oneweb.utc.edu/~Margaret-Kovach/microsat.html]*

## DNA Fingerprinting

41. **B i.e. Variable Number Tandem Repeats (VNTR)**
42. **C i.e. Jeffrey** 43. **D i.e. All of the above** *[Ref: Lehninger 5/e p. 319-21; Lippincott's 5/e p. 83, 475; Harper 28/e p. 404]*

## PCR

44. **A, B, D i.e. Carried out by thermostable DNA polymerase; Exponential; Specific**
45. **A & E i.e. Thermostable enzyme is needed & Primer is needed.** 46. **A i.e. Enzymatic DNA amplification**
47. **D i.e. Required atleast 1 week time for synthesis; E i.e. DNA polymerase has to be added on each cycle** 48. **A i.e. Thermostable enzyme**
49. **B i.e. DNA amplification; D i.e. Detection of infecting organism** 50. **A i.e. Primers required, C i.e. DNA polymerase**
51. **B i.e. DNA Polymerase**
52. **A i.e. Thermostable, D i.e. Replicates double stranded DNA** 53. **A i.e. Thermostable at temperature at which DNA liquifies**
54. **B i.e. Obtained from bacteria; D i.e. It is heat stable; E i.e. Add nucleotide**
55. **B i.e. $Mg^{++}$** 56. **D i.e. Radiolabelled DNA probe**
57. **C i.e. Dideoxynucleotides** 58. **C i.e. PCR**
*[Ref: Vassudevan 6th/e p. 616-18; Lehninger 5th/e p. 317-18; Chattarjea 7th/e p. 267-72; Harper 28th/e p. 395, 319; Lippincott 5th/e p. 479-82; Harrison 17th /1764; Harrison's 18th/2312]*
59. **D i.e. To know how much amplification of DNA has occurred**
60. **A i.e. PCR** *[Ref: Hall – Advances in genetics (1995) vol 32 p-121; Chen. Atlas of genetic diagnosis & counciling (2006) p-478]*

## Ligase Chain Reaction

61. **A i.e. PCR > B i.e. NASBA; C i.e. Ligase chain reaction** *[Ref: Lippincott]s 4/e p. 479-83; Chatterjea 7/e p. 267- 71; Robbins 7/e p- 361]*

## Cloning

62. **C i.e. To identify desired chromosomal DNA insert in plasmid vectors.**
*[Ref: Lippincott's 4/e p. 467- 70; Harper's 27/e p. 406 – 9, 419; Wikipedia]*
63. **A i.e. Produced by hybridoma technology; C i.e Requires in small quantity; D i.e. Used for blood grouping**
64. **A, D, & E i.e. Immortalise myeloma cell, Prior immunization is done & myeloma & Produce monospecific & monoclonal Ab** *[Ref: Harper 29/e p 647-48; Vasudevan 6/e p 617]*
65. **D i.e. Reducing surface tension** *[Ref: Harper 28/e 580]*
66. **C i.e. Cosmid** *[Ref: Harper's 27/e P-406-08]*
67. **B i.e. Plasmid, bacteriophage, cosmid** *[Ref: Chattergea 7/e p. 262]*
68. **B i.e. Restriction enzyme sites** *[Ref: Harper's 27/e P- 407; Anantha Narayan 6/e p. 426- 28]*

## Site Directed Mutagenesis, Site Specific Recombination, Linkage Analysis & Analyzing (Hybridization) Techniques

69. **D i.e. Site directed mutagenesis** *[Ref: Lehninger 5/e p. 312-13]*
70. **C i.e. RE + ligase** *[Ref: Lehninger 5/e 1010-12]*
71. **A i.e. Detection of characteristic DNA polymorphism in a family is associated with disorder**
*[Ref: Robbins 7/e p-189-91; Human genetics 2000, 8:738-43, Harper's 28/e p. 396-99]*
72. **A i.e. Separation of proteins are based on mass; B i.e. SDS-PAGE electrophesis is used for separation; C i.e. Enzyme linked antibodies are used; D i.e. Confirmatory in AIDS**
73. **A, D i.e. ELISA, Western blot** *[Ref: Harper 29/e p 439-40; Vasudevan 6/e p 612-14; Lippincott's 5/e p. 485; Lehninger 5/e p. 174]*
74. **D i.e. Protein** 75. **A i.e. m- RNA** 76. **B i.e. RNA analysis**
77. **A i.e. Antibody** *[Ref: Lippincott's 4/e p. 470- 74, 483-84; Harper's 27/e p. 409-12, 313-14]*
78. **D i.e. Northern blot analysis** *[Ref: Harrisons 16th/365, 378, 595]*
79. **D i.e. Microarray** *[Ref: Lippincott 5/e 483-85; Vassudeven 6/e 614; Lehninger 5/e p. 325-28]*
80. **D i.e. Microarray** *[Ref: Harrison 17/e p 406, 390; Robbin's 7/e p 171-73]*
81. **E i.e. Immuno histochemistry >> C i.e. Southern Blot** *[Ref: Harrison 18/e p 508; Lippincott 5/e p 465-85]*

## Gene Library

82. **D, E i.e. DNA Nucleotide or fragment, Complete collection of gene copies of one organism** *[Ref: Lehninger 5/e 315; Lippincott 5/e 469-70; Chatterjea 7/e p-265; Vassudeven 6/e p 516; Satyanarayan 3/e p 596-97]*

## Recombination DNA Technology or Genetic Engineering

83. **A, B, C, D, E i.e. Viral vaccine production; To cure genetic disorder; Genetic crop; Gene production, Production of genetic products** *[Ref: Lehninger 5/e 337; Vasudevan 6/e 512-14; Chattarjea 7/e-275, 279]*
84. **C i.e. mRNA from beta pancreatic cells of human:** *[Ref: Harper 28/e p388; Lehninger 5/e p 334-37, 316]*
85. **B i.e. RNA dependent DNA polymerase**
86. **A, B & D i.e. Restriction endonucleases involved, DNA ligase is used, Reverse transcriptase needed**
87. **E i.e. None** *[Ref: Harper's 29/436; Cjhatterjea 7th/e p. 261-63; Lehninger 5/e p. 305]*
88. **B i.e. Genes for protease inhibitors** *[Ref: Herper 28/e 392]*
89. **A i.e. Genomics**
90. **A i.e. Protenonomics**
91. **A, E > B, C i.e. (Gene Array Chips, Two-Dimensional Electrophoresis >Mass Spectroscopy; PolyAcrylamide Gel Electrophoresis (PAGE)** *[Ref: Lippincott's 4/e p. 484-85; Harper 29/e p 28-33; Stedman's dictionary 27/e p-739]*

## Transgenic Organism

92. **A, D i.e. Knock-out, Targeted gene disruption**
93. **A i.e. Developed from DNA insertion into fertilized egg; B i.e. Have same genome as parents except one or more genes; E i.e. Homozygous are selected:** *[Ref: Harrison 18/e p 490-94; Harper 29/e p 447; Lippincott 5/e p 486; Leheninger 5/e p 334; Vasudevan 6/e p 621]*
94. **D i.e. Transgenic animals**
95. **A i.e. Absence of thymus; B i.e. Xenograft can be sustained for weeks** *[Ref: Harrison 18/e p 2699-2701, 490-93; Harper 29/e p 447; www.genetic-nude mouse-1768]*
96. **A i.e. Both plants will glow** *[Ref: Lehninger 5/e 316, 434, 332]*

## Gene Therapy

97. **A i.e. Replacement of abnormal gene by normal gene.**
98. **A i.e. Electroporation, B i.e. Intranuclear infection, C i.e. Site directed mutagenesis, D i.e. Retrovirus**
99. **A i.e. SCID** *[Ref: Harper's 28/e P-380, 400, 504, 625; Lippincott's 5/e P- 485-56; Vasudevan 6/e p. 517-18; Lehninger 5/e p. 331-35, 312, 1004; Chatterjea 7th/e p. 278-87]*

## Genetic Disorder

100. **A i.e. X-gene; D i.e. Seen in females** *[Ref: Kumar & Clark 6/e p. 172-73; Harrison 16/e p. 375]*
101. **D & E i.e. Duchenne muscular dystrophy & G-6-P dehydrogenase deficiency**
102. **C i.e. X– linked recessive inheritance** *[Ref.: Chandrasoma Taylor 3rd/e P-234, 235, 236; Robbins 6th/e P-146]*
103. **A i.e. Autosomal dominant disorder** *[Ref: Harrison 16/e P- 374]*
104. **C & D i.e. Cystic fibrosis & Ataxia telangiectasia** *[Ref: Harrison 17/ed pg- 398-401, 494; Robbins 7th/ed pg- 151-52]*
105. **D i.e. A polygenic syndrome** *[Ref: www.som.tulane.edu/departments/peds_respcare/genetic.htm]*

106. **A i.e. Autosomal dominant (most likely)** *[Ref: http://www.babyhearing.org/HearingAamplification/ Causes/BasicGenetics.pdf; http://www.emedicine.com/ped/topic2422.htm]*
107. **D i.e. Short arm of chromosome 6** *[Ref: Harrison 18/e p.497, 2680, 2685-94; Ganong 22/e P- 526; Robbins 7/e P 203]*
108. **A i.e. Transplantation reaction; B i.e. Autommune disease; D i.e. Involved in T –Cell function**
109. **B i.e. Dendritic cells; F i.e. B-cell**
110. **A, B i.e. Macrophage; Dendritic cells; C i.e. Lymphocytes**
111. **C i.e. Somatic Hypermutation** *[Ref: Principles of Cellular & Molecular Immunology by Austin and Wood 1993/408, 449, 450]*

# CYTOGENETICS AND MOLECULAR GENETICS, RECOMBINANT DNA & GENOMIC TECHNOLOGY: REVIEW NOTES

## Normal Karyotype & Chromosomal Nomenclature

- The study of chromosomes – Karyotyping – is the basic tool of cytogenetics. Chromosome spread is produced by use of mitotic spindle inhibitors (eg. colcemid) to arrest mitosis in dividing cells in metaphase, and then to stain the chromosome. In **metaphase spread** every chromosome takes the form of two chromatids connected at the centromere. A Karyotype is a photograph (image) of stained chromosome pairs arranged in order of decreasing length (in metaphase spread stage). Idiogram is details of banding of chromosome.

- Chromosomes have characteristic banding patterns created by *trypsin and Giemsa stain;* hence called **G banding**. The chromosomes need to be stained in order to see them with a microscope. When stained the chromosomes look like strings with light and dark 'bands'. Each chromosome arm is defined further by numbering the bands, ***the higher the number, the further that area is from the centromere.***

- Every cell of the human body has 46 chromosomes occurring in 23 pairs. Chromosomes are laid out in pairs, from largest (#1) to smallest (#22). The last pair are called the sex chromosomes labeled X or Y. Female have two X chromosomes (XX), and males have an X and a Y chromosome (XY).

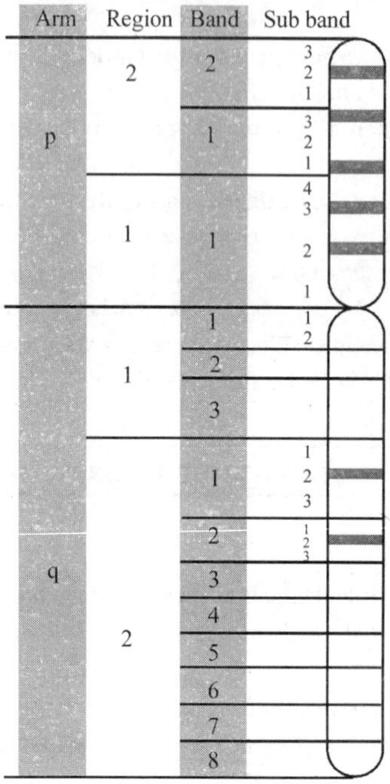


**X-Chromosome**

- Each chromosomes has a p and q arm; ***P (petit) is the short arm and q (next latter in the alphabet) is the long arm***[Q]. When a karyotype is made the q arm is always put on the bottom and the p on the top. The arms are separated by a region known as the centromere. So Xp 21.2 means segment located on short arm of X-chromosome, in region 2, band 1 and subband 2.

## Conventional Cytogenetic Analysis

- Theoritically, chromosomal preparations for analysis can be obtained *from any actively dividing tissue* by causing the cells to arrest **in metaphase** (the stage of cell cycle when chromosomes are maximally condensed). However, in practice only **amniocytes or chorionic villi** (for prenatal testing) and **blood, bone marrow or skin fibroblasts** (for post natal studies) are used.
- Analysis of *blood, bone marrow & chorionic villi* involve **short term culture** technique that yield result in **1-3 days**; whereas other tissues require **long term culture (1-3 weeks of processing)**.
- Cells are isolated at metaphase or prometaphase and treated chemically or enzymatically to reveal chromosome bands. Analysis of number of chromosomes and distribution of bands on individual chromosome allow the identification of numerical or major structural abnormalities.
- Each human chromosome has a ***centromere /primary constriction (that divides chromosome into short (p) and long (q) arms***[Q] and is responsible for segregation during cell division) and **telomeres or chromosomal ends** capping the p & q arms. Each chromosome consists of **single chromatid** copy of double helix DNA *prior to DNA replication* and **2 identical sister chromatids** after DNA replication (until cell division including metaphase)

| p | Short arm |
|---|---|
| Q | Long arm |
| + | additional chromosome |
| - | missing chromosome |
| T | translocation |
| del | deletion |
| dup | duplication |
| inv | inversion |
| der | derivative |
| r | ring chromosome |
| I | isochromosome |

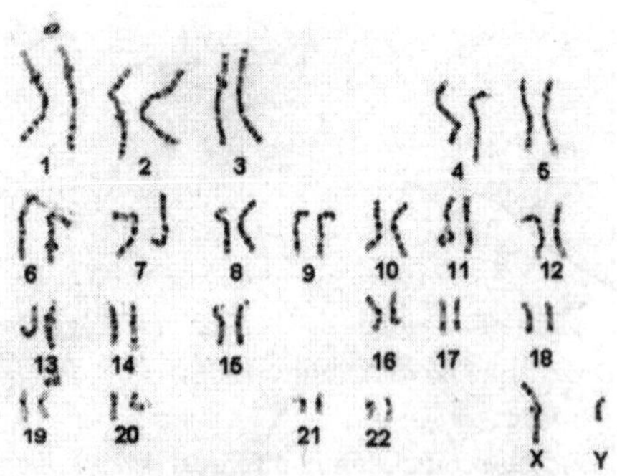


**Karyotype**

## Different Types of Banding

**G- Banding**

- It is a technique used in cyto genetics to produce visible karyotype by staining *condensed chromosomes* in cells *blocked in mitosis.*
- The metaphase chromosomes are *treated with trypsin* (to partially digest the protein) & stained *with giemsa*. The acid-saline- giemsa protocol utilizes acetic acid fixation, air drying, denaturing chromosomes mildly with proteolytic enzymes, salts, heats, detergents or urea , and finally giemsa stain.
- It yields a series of lightly & darkly stained bands. The **dark regions** tend to be *hetrochromatin, late replicating, AT rich and the light bands are euchromatic, early replicating GC rich.*

**FUdR (Fluro- deoxy- uridine Banding)**

- FUdR is used to induce fragile sites in chromosomes. Fragile sites on chromosome undergo breakage at an increased frequency under certain culture conditions
- Common or constitutive fragile sites (c- fra) can be induced by low folate levels. Chemicals such as FUdR, aphidicolin and caffeine also enhance c- fra.
- **Rare** or **heritable fragile sites (h-fra)** are located on autosomes (16), and the 17$^{th}$ is on x- chromosome.

**R - Banding**

- It is **reverse G banding** i.e. the dark regions are euchromatic, guanine - cytosine rich regions and the bright bands are hetrochromatic adenine - thymine rich regions.

**T- Banding**

Visualize *telomeres*

**C- Banding**

Giemsa specifically stain the centromere and other *regions* containing constitutive hetrochromatin i.e. 2° constrictions of human chromosomes 1, 9, 16, & distal segment of Y chromosome long arm.

**Q- Banding**

- Metaphase chromosomes ae stained with a **fluorescent quinacrine mustard** stain to produce temporary Q bands on chromosome. The pattern of bands is similar to that seen in G banding
- It is useful in identifying *Y chromosome, Y bodies in interphase nuclei and various DNA polymorphisms* involving satellites and centromeres.

## Molecular Cytogenetics: Fluorescence in Situ Hybridization (FISH)

***Conventional cytogenetic karyotyping*** *is applicable only to cells that are dividing or can be induced to divide in vitro.* This limitation can be overcome with *DNA probes labelled with fluorescent dyes* that recognizes chromosome specific sequences - a technique k/a FISH. ***The primary advantage of interphase FISH is that it can be performed very rapidly (usually <24 hours) because cell growth is not required***[Q].

**Method**

- In principle, FISH is similar to other **DNA-DNA hybridization method** in which fluorescent labeled DNA probe is hybridized with target DNA to counterstain it & allow its detection under fluorescene microscope
- Sample DNA (**interphase nuclei**, or **metaphase spread chromosome**) is denatured into complimentary strands and *fluorescent labelled DNA probe* is added. *Probe hybridizes with sample DNA* at the target site as the sample DNA reanneals (reforms) back into double helix.
- Then the probe signals are *visualized under fluorescent microscope* & sample *DNA is scored for presence or absence of the signals.*

**Types of FISH & Array Technology & their Utilty**

- FISH can be utilized to **identity specific chromosomes, characterize de novo duplications or deletions and clarify subtle chromosomal rearrangements**. However, its greatest utilization in constitutional analysis is in *detection of microdeletions* and in cancer cytogenetics for analysis of *structural rearrangements.* Though conventional cytogenetic studies can detect some microdeletions, initial detection &/or **confirmation with FISH, is essential**.
- It **can demonstrate *subtle microdeletions, complex translocations, telomere alterations, & specific rearrangements* in metaphase cell that are not readily detectable by routine karyotyping**
- To physically map (localize) a newly isolated gene & to identify extra material of unknown origin.
- It diagnose microdeletion syndromes such as Cri-du-chat / Miller - Dieker / Smith-Magenis/Kallman / Williams / Wolf-Hirschhorn/Prader-Willi-Angelman/Di-George/Velo cardial- facial / CATCH-22 / Shprintzen - syndromes.
- In addition to **metaphase FISH, other types include**

**1. Interphase FISH**

- It can be used **to make a rapid diagnosis** in instances when metaphase chromosome preparations are not yet available; also *increases number of cells available for examination* , allows for investigation of nuclear organization, and provides results when cell do not progress to metaphase.
- When there is strong clinical indication of any trisomy, the **aneuploid screen test (uncultured amniotic fluid interphase FISH study)** is performed on *amniotic fluid cells, using DNA probes for chromosomes 13, 18, 21 X and Y.* The results are obtained usually within 24 -48 hours and will ascertain ~60% abnormalities detected prenatally.
- *Interphase FISH* is used to *enumerate* one or more *chromosomes in interphase nuclei,* as well as to detect specific chromosomal rearrangements characteristic of certain cancers However, its application is not only limited to interphase nuclei. Many site specific translocations a/w specific types of malignancies (cancer

**Types of FISH Probes**

1. **Chromosome libraries (chromosome specific paints)** are probes that *hybridize to sequence that span the entirety of chromosome* from which they are derived and as a result they can used to **paint individual chromosomes**
2. **Repetitive probes** recognize **amplified DNA sequences** present in chromosomes. Eg **alpha- satellite DNA probes** are complementary to DNA sequences found at the **centromeric regions of all human chromosomes**.
3. **Single copy probes**, available d/t human genomic project, can be as small as 1kb (though normally are much larger) and are **packaged into fosmids** (40 kb) or **bacterial artificial chromosomes** (BACs) (100-200kb).

★ The *mobility of ds DNA* in gel electrophoresis depends on strand size & length but *is relatively independent of nucleotide sequence*. However, *mobility of single stranded DNA is highly affected by a small change in nucleotide* sequence because relatively unstable SS DNA forms intrastrand base pairing, loop & folds that give the single strand a unique 3rd structure, regardless of its length. **Single stranded conformation polymorphism (SSCP)** is electrophoretic seperation of single stranded nucleic acids based on their differences in nucleotide sequence (often a single base pair) that results in a different secondary structure & a measurable difference in its mobility through gel. So the SSCP *can detect point mutations.*

cytogenetics) can be identified. For example, probes for both **Abelson (Abl) onchogene** and **break point cluster region (bcr)** involved in **CML** are labeled in red and green respectively; so the fusion of both genes in CML combines the fluorescence and appears as a yellow hybridization signal.

- **Oncogene activation by DNA sequence amplification** (& overexpression of gene product) leads to increase *in DNA copy number* causing cytogenetically recognizable chromosome alteration k/a **homogenous staining regions (HSRs)** if *integrated within chromosome or* ***double minutes (d mins)*** *if extrachromosomal*. It can be *identified through comparative geneomic hybridization, FISH* which allow visualization of chromosomal aberrations. Microarray based, non cytogenetic approaches identify changes in copy number and short tag based sequencing approaches are used to evaluate amplification. With both microarrays & sequencing technologies, the entire genome can be surveyed for gains and losses of DNA sequences, thus pinpointing chromosomal region likely to contain gene important in development or progression of cancer

• In addition to standard metaphase & interphase FISH, several **enhanced techniques** include.

**2. Spectral Karyotyping (SKY) and multicolor FISH (mFISH)**

- In, **chromosomal painting** whole chromosomes can be labeled with a series of fluorescent DNA probes that binds to a particular chromosome at multiple sites. Chromosomal painting has limited ability *to visualize all 46 human chromosomes simultaneously*. This hurdle has been overcome by **spectral karyotyping** (or **spectacular Karyotyping = SKY**) which uses a combination of 5 fluorochromes & computer generated signals to visualize entire human genome.
- SKY and m-FISH use combinatorially labeled probes that *create a unique color for individual chromosomes*. It is *useful in identification of unknown chromosome material* (eg accessory marker chromosomes containing additional material) and most commonly *in complex rearrangements* seen in cancer specimen

**3. Fiber FISH**

- Chromosomes are mechanically stretched which provides a higher **resolution of analysis than conventional FISH**

**4. FISH - Comparative Genomic Hybridization (CGH)**

- ***Comparative genomic hybridization (FISH-CGH)*** *can be* ***used to detect chromosomal differences between neoplastic cells and their counterparts***[Q]. *It can quickly and efficiently analyse copy number variations (CNVs) in relation to ploidy level* in a test sample DNA compared to another reference sample (which is mostly related). It detects amplification or deletions of smaller DNA region or whole chromosome by comparing DNA of a patient (target) with a normal person.
- It can be used only when DNA in available from a specimen of interest (eg cancer). The entire DNA specimen from the sample of interest is labeled in one color (eg green) and the normal control DNA specimen is labeled by another (eg red) color. These are mixed in equal amounts and hybridized to normal metaphase chromosomes. Computerized analysis of (red to green) color ratio determines where the DNA of interest may have gains or losses of material.

**5. Array - CGH (a-CGH, Chromosomal Microarray Analysis / CMA, Virtual Karyotyping)**

- Similar to FISH - CGH, except that the test DNA is hybridized to DNAs that are **spread on arrays, rather than hybridized to normal chromosomes.**
- ***Comparitive genomic hybridization (CGH)*** *directly compares the DNA, content of differentially labelled normal & tumor cells* by their co- hybridization to normal metaphase chromosome spread or to series of genomic DNA clones aligned on glass slides **(array CGH)**. In this way tumor specific alterations in gene copy number can be ascertained.
- It provides a *higher resolution* (upto 50kb). **CGH arrays** utilize either BACs or **oligonucleotides**, whereas **genotyping arrays** utilize *single nucleotide polymorphisms* **(SNP arrays).** It is used in prenatal diagnosis & study of ***cryptic chromosomal imbalances in patients with mental retardation and multiple congenital anomalies.*** It is also used to ***detect microdeletions and micro duplications in cancer and previously unidentified genomic disorder***[Q]. This technology is still in development, but it will ultimately be the **initial method of study for constitutional abnormalities**.

★ Both **MAPH (multiplex amplification & probe hybridization)** and **MLAP (multiplex ligation dependent probe amplification)** techniques for detection of small scale copy number changes & gene deletions rely on sequence specific probe hybridization to genomic DNA followed by PCR amplification of hybridized probe and semiquantitative analysis of resultant PCR product. The relative peak heights / band intensities indicate initial concentration of each target.

## Cytogenetic Disorders (Chromosomal Mutations)

### Due to abnormal number of chromosomes

- **Euploid** means any exact multiple of haploid number (23) and **aneuploidy** means chromosomes *not in exact multiple of 23.*
- The usual cause of aneuploidy are

#### Non disjunction

Occurs when a ***homologous pair of chromosome fails to disjoin at 1st meiotic division***[Q], or two chromatids fail to seperate either at 2nd meiotic division or in somatic cell divisions resulting in 2 aneuploid cells. If this occurs in gametogenesis, gametes formed have either *an extra (n+1) or one less (n-1) chromosome.* Fertilization of such gametes by normal gametes result in – **trisomic (2n+1)** or **monosomic (2n-1)** zygotes

#### Anaphase lag

- ***One homologous chromosome in meiosis or one chromatid in mitosis lags behind***[Q] & is left out of cell nucleus. The result is one normal cell and one with monosomy
- All autosomal monosomies are fatal d/t loss of too much genetic information
- Monosomies & trisomies of sex chromosomes & trisomy of 21 autosomal chromosome are compatabile with life.

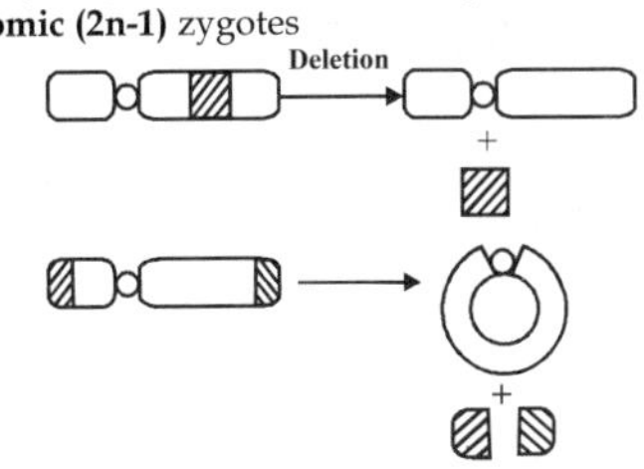


### D/t alteration in structure of chromosomes

- **Deletion** means *loss of portion of chromosome* & may be of 2 types
- **Terminal deletion** at ends
- **Interstitial deletion** refers to 2 breaks within chromosome arms f/b loss of material b/w the breaks & fusion of broken ends (most common type)
- **Ring chromosome** is special form of deletion, produced when break occurs at both ends of chromosomes with fusion of damaged ends.
- **Inversion** refers to rearrangement that involves two breaks within single chromosome with *inverted reincorporation of segment.*
- **Paracentric** inversion involves only one arm of chromosome
- **Pericentric inversion** has breaks on opposite side of centromere

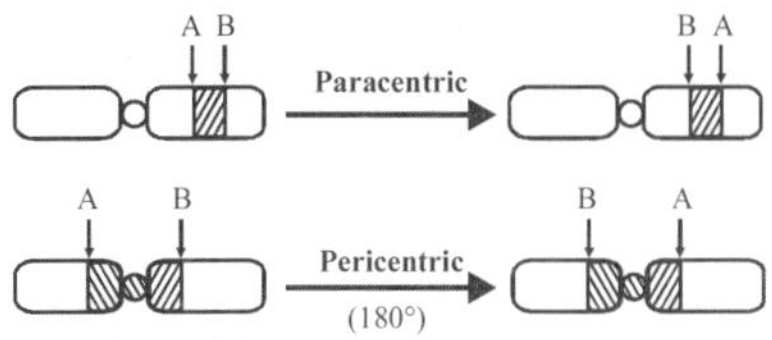


- **Isochromosome** results when one arm of chromosome is lost and the other is duplicated resulting in a chromosome containing *2 short arms or 2 long arms only*. Most common isochromosome (in live birth) involves long arm of X [i (x) (q 10)]. & is associated with monosomy for genes on short arm of X and trisomy for genes on long arm of X
- **Translocation** l/t ***transfer of a segment of chromosome to another nonhomologous chromosome***[Q]
- **Reciprocal translocation** is ***mutual swapping of ends between any two non homologous chromosomes***[Q]. It may be balanced or unbalanced (eg during meiosis).

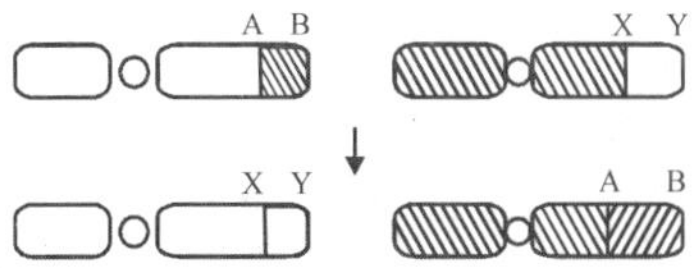


- **Robertsonian translocation (or centric fusion)** is *tanslocation b/w two acrocentric chromosomes (13, 14, 15, 21, & 22).* The *break occurs close to centromere* of each chromosome and transfer of segments l/t one very long & one extremely small chromosome. 14-21 fusion may cause Down syndrome.

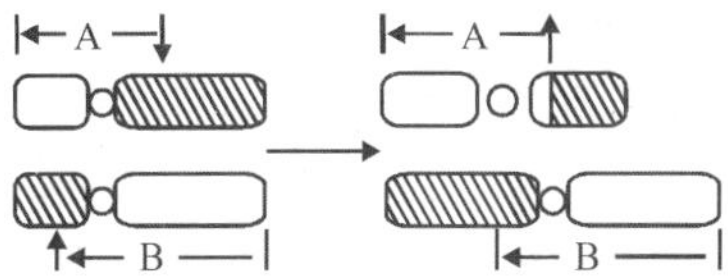


## Genomic Imprinting

It is selective ***inactivation of a gene or set of genes on either the maternal or paternal chromosome***[Q]. It occurs in ovum or sperm before fertilization & then is stabily transmitted to all somatic cells through mitosis and so can be of two types

### Maternal genomic imprinting

- It is ***inactivation of maternal allele (genes or chromosome)*** [Q]
- Paternal allele are functional
- Example is ***Angleman syndrome***[Q]

### Paternal genomic impringing

- It is *inactivation of paternal allele* (gene or chromosome)
- Functional allele are provided by only maternal chromosomes
- Example is ***Prader Willi Syndrome***[Q]

## Barr Body

- When two X chromosomes are present in a cell (as in a normal female) one of them becomes inactivated and condensed on the nuclear membrane and is called the **'Barr body'**. This process is termed as X chromosome lyonization (inactivation)
- Presence or absence of Barr bodies helps in *ascertaining the sex of an individuals*
  - ***Absence of Barr body indicates that the patient has only one X chromosome (eg. Normal male XY or Turner's syndrome(XO))***
  - Nuclei of cells in females (XX) contain a darkly staining Barr body that is not present in the nuclei of cells in males.
- Barr bodies are most easily seen in a smear of squamous epithelial cells obtained by **scraping the buccal mucosa** [Q]
- Barr bodies react differently to histological stains and are best seen as dark staining bodies with in ***the nucleus*** of ***non dividing interphase cells.***

## Fluorescence Recovery After Photobleaching (FRAP)

Lateral diffusion can be shown experimentally by attaching **fluorescent probes** to the head groups of lipids/proteins and using the **fluorescence microscopy** to follow the probes over time. Two techniques involve

| Fluorescence Tagging of Membrane Surface | Single Particle Tracking |
|---|---|
| • Lipids (protein etc) on the outer leaflet (layer) of membrane are **labeled by** reaction with a membrane -impermanent **fluorescent probe, so the surface is uniformly labeled when viewed with fluorescence microscope**. A small area (5μm²) of a cell surface with fluorescent tagged lipids is **photobleached by intense laser radiation** so that the irradiated patch **no longer fluoresces** (emit fluorescent light) when viewed with less intense (non bleaching) light in the florescence microscope.<br>• However, the photo bleached membrane region **recovers its fluorescence within milliseconds** as unbleached lipid molecules diffused into the bleached patch and bleached lipid molecules diffuse away from it by rapid lateral diffusion.<br>• The **rate of fluorescence recovery after photo bleaching or FRAP is a measure of rate of lateral diffusion** of the lipids<br>• FRAP can be used to *assess structure of membranes* (biological & artificial both), *define fluid mosaic model* and investigate ***diffusion (motion) of biological macromolecules including lateral diffusion movements with in the plane of membranes and movements into & out of nucleus***[Q]. | • The *motion (movement) of a single fluorescently labeled lipid (protein / etc) molecule* in the cell membrane is *recorded on video by fluorescence microscopy on a much shorter time scale* (eg 50 ms = 2250 frames with time resolution of 25μs=40000 frames/s).<br>• The pattern of movement confirms **rapid lateral diffusion within a confined (small discrete) region with occasional hops** into an adjoining region. It suggests that lipids are corralled by molecular fences that they can occasionally jump by **hop diffusion.** Membrane *proteins (like glycophorin & $Cl^-$ - $HCO_3^-$ exchanger in RBC) immobilized by their association with spectrin* (a filamentous cytoskeleton protein) form the fences that define the regions of relatively unrestricted lipid motion.<br>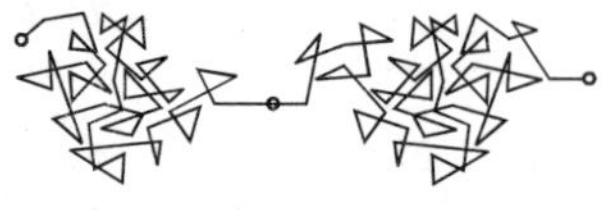<br>**Hop Diffusion of Single Lipid Molecule** |

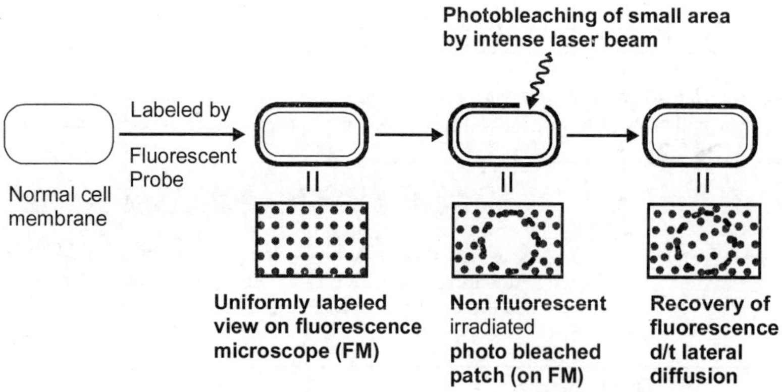


## Fluorescence Resonance Energy Tranfer (FRET)

- **Fluorescent probes** derived from naturally occurring fluorescent protein, the **green fluorescent protein (GFP)** of jelly fish Aequorea victoria or other variants like **BFP (blue), YFP (yellow), CFP (cyan)** along with **fluorescence microscopy** are used to visualize biochemistry of living cells by means of **FRET (fluorescence resonance energy transfer)**. FRET can be used **to measure cAMP and activity of PKA (pyruvate kinase A).**
- When two molecules are **very close (within 1 to 50A°)**, the energy of excited donor molecule passes directly to near by acceptor molecule without emission of a photon, exciting the acceptor (the efficiency of FRET is **inversely proportional to 6th power of distance between donor & acceptor)**. The acceptor now decays to its ground state by **fluorescence** (which can be located to specific regions of single living cell); ***the emitted photon has lower energy (longer wave length) than both exciting light and the fluorescence emission of donor***[Q].

## Atomic Force Microscopy (AFM)

In AFM, the **sharp tip of a microscope probe** attached to a (flexible) cantilever **is moved across an uneven surface eg membrane. Electrostatic & vander Walls interactions** between the tip and sample produce a force that moves the probe or sample up and down (in z dimension) as the probe encounters hills (up) and valleys (downs) in the sample. A laser beam reflected from the cantilever detects motion of 1A°. A series of scans in plane of membrane (x & y dimensions) yields a **three dimensional contour map of the surface** with resolution near the atomic scale - 0.1 nm in vertical and 0.5 to 1 nm in lateral dimensions. When several images of individual units are superimposed with compute, **a high resolution image of protein** is yielded. So AFM is **used to visualize membrane proteins** such as **membrane (microdomains) rafts** (enriched in sphingolipids, cholesterol & GPI linked proteins) or **single membrane protein** such as bacteriorhodopsin, aquaporin & Fo (proton driven rotor of chloroplast ATP synthase) etc.

## Movements of Lipid in Membrane Bilayer

### Uncatalyzed Lateral Diffusion

Lipid and protein molecules **diffuse laterally (or undergo Brownian movement within the bilayer)** by changing places with neighbouring molecules at very fast rate (1μm/s). This *rapid uncatalyzed lateral diffusion in the plane of membrane bilayer* tends to randomize the position of individual molecules in a few seconds.

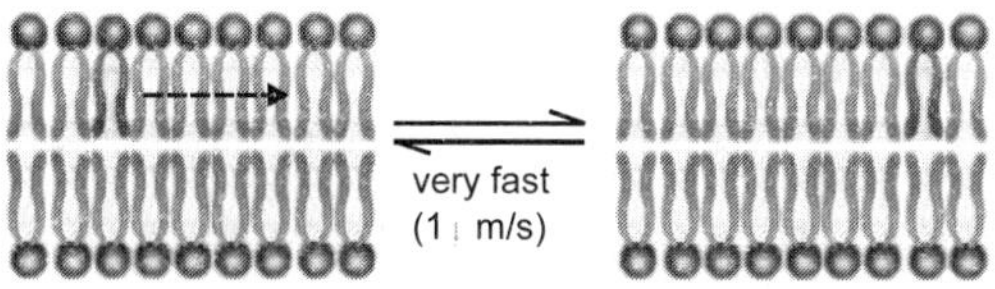


### Uncatalyzed Transbilayer (Flip-Flop) Diffusion

Transbilayer (flip-flop) diffusion of a lipid molecule from one leaflet of membrane to other occurs **very slowly** ($t_{1/2}$ in days) because it requires polar (charged) head group to leave its aqueous environment and move into hydrophobic interior of membrane, a process with large, positive free energy change. However, in the *endoplasmic reticulum* this movement is essential for lipids to get from their site of synthesis to their eventual point of deposition as *membrane glycerophospholipids are synthesized on cytosolic surface whereas sphingolipids are synthesized/ modified on luminal surface of ER membrane.*

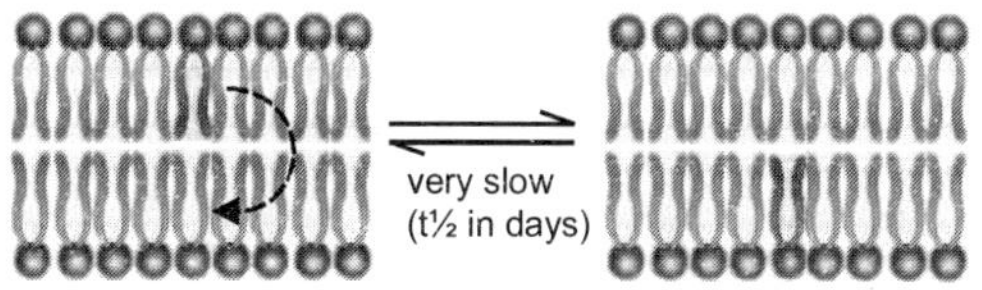


### Catalyzed Transbilayer Translocations

- **Use translocaters (flippases, floppases & scramblases)** to facilitate transbilayer movement of lipid by a path that is much **faster and more energetically favourable**.
- The combination of asymmetric biosynthesis of membrane lipids (ie different lipids on different sides), slow flip flop diffusion and presence of selective energy dependent translocaters is responsible for transbilayer asymmetry in lipid composition, *creating a larger surface on one side of membrane and generating curvature essential in budding of vesicles.*
- **3-types of translocater's include**

#### Flippase

- Structurally & functionally related to **P type ATPase** (active transporters); move **PE** (phosphatidylethanolamine) & **PS** (phosphatidyl serine) **from outer (extracellular) to cytosolic (lumenal) leaflet (side) of plasma membrane.** They consume about 1 ATP per molecule of phospholipid translocated
- Keeping PS out of extracellular surface *protects cells from apoptosis (programmed cell death)* by protecting against macrophages that carry PS receptors.

#### Floppase

- Are members of **ABC transporter family**; all of which actively *transport hydrophobic substrates outward across the* plasma membrane.
- Flippase transport plasma membrane phospholipids **from cytosolic (inner) to extracellular (outer) leaflet and use ATP**

#### Scramblase

- Are proteins that move any **membrane phospholipid** across the membrane **down its concentration gradient** (from leaflet where it is in higher concentration to leaflet where it has a lower concentration), ie in **either direction towards equilibrium**.
- They **do not require ATP but are activated by increase in cytosolic calcium ($Ca^{++}$)**, which may result from cell *activation, cell injury or apoptosis.*

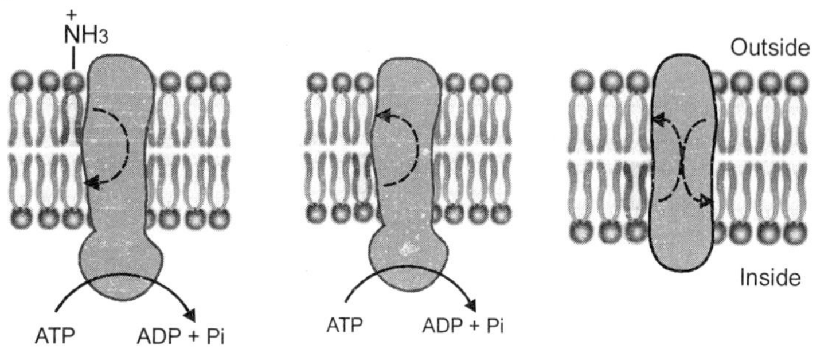


## Luminescence

***It is the emission of light or radiant energy when an electron returns from an excited or higher energy level to a lower energy level***[Q]. It can be **caused by chemical or biochemical reactions, electrochemical reaction, electro magnetic radiation (photons)**, subatomic movements or stress on crystal. It is a **cold body radiation** as the emission of light by a substance is not resulting from heating, which differentiates it from **incandescence** (ie light emitted by a substance after heating). It can be of various types.

### Chemi /Bio / Electrochemiluminescence & Luminometry

- These are types of luminescence in which the ***excitation event is caused by a chemical, biochemical or electrochemical reaction and not by photo illumination (or photoluminescence)***[Q] as seen in fluorescence.
- Physical event for light emission in chemi / bio / electro-chemiluminescence is similar to fluorescence in that it occurs from an excited singlet state, & the light is emitted when the electron returns to the ground state

### Photoluminescence

It is a kind of luminescence where energy is supplied by **photons (electromagnetic radiation)**. It can be of 2 types

#### I. Phosphorescence & Phosphometry

- It is a type of luminescence ***produced by certain substances after absorbing radiant energy or other type of energy***[Q]
- It is distinguished from fluorescence in that

- This type of light emission is measured by **luminometry**

**Chemiluminescence**

- It is emission of light when *an electron returns from an excited or an higher energy level to a lower energy level*
- Excitation event is caused by **chemical reaction** & involves oxidation of an organic compound such as luminol, isoluminol, acridinum ester, or luciferin by an oxidant such as $H_2O_2$, hypochlorite, or $O_2$
- Light is emited from the excited product formed in oxidation. These reactions occur in presence catalyst such as enzymes (eg alkaline phosphatase, horseradish peroxidase, & microperoxidase), metal ion and metal complexes ($Cu^{++}$ & $Fe^{+3}$ phthalocyanine complex) & hemin

**Bioluminescence**

- It is ***special form of chemiluminescence found in biological systems***[Q]
- In it an enzyme or photoprotein or **biological catalyst (eg luciferase & acquorin)** increase the efficiency of luminescence reaction
- The quantum yield is ~ 0.1 – 10% for chemiluminescence and 10-30% for bioluminescence

**Electrochemiluminescence (ECL)**

- It differs from chemiluminescence in that the reactive species that produce electro chemiluminescent reaction are ***electro chemically generated from stable precursors at the surface of an electrode***[Q]
- Ruthenium (Ru+2), tris (bipyridyl) chelate is the M.C. used ECL label & ECL is generated at an electrode via oxidation reduction type of reaction with tripropylamine.
- This chelate is relatively small, very stable & has been used to label haptens or large molecules (eg protein or oligonucleotides)
- ECL is used both in immunoassays and nucleic acid assays. It has the advantage of improved reagent stability, simple reagent preparation and enhanced sensitivity.

1. It continues even after radiation causing it has ceased
2. The decay time of emission of phosphorescence light is longer ($10^{-4}$ to $10^{-2}$ S)
3. Phosphorescence shows a larger shift in emitted light wavelength than fluorescence.

- Phosphometry measures phosphorescence

**Fluorescence & Flurometry**

- Fluorescence is emission of electromagnetic radiation by a substance after the absorption of energy in some form (eg the emission of light of one color / wave length when a substance is excited by irradiation with light of a different wavelength. In other words fluorescence ***occurs when a molecule absorbs light at one wave length and reemits light at a longer wave length (or lower energy)***[Q]
- It is differentiated from phosphorescence in that its life time is < 10 mili seconds after excitation ceases. Eg. fluorescent paint stops glowing as soon as UV lamp is turned off but phosphorescent paint keeps glowing for a while.
- An excited fluorescent molecules such as **green fluorescent protein (GFP) or YFP or CFP** etc can dispose of the energy from absorbed photon by either

1. **Fluorescence** ie ***emitting a photon of slightly longer wave length (lower energy)***[Q] or
2. **Non radiative** fluorescence resonance energy transfer **(FRET)**, where energy of excited donor passes directly to a nearby (within 1 to 50 A°) acceptor molecule without emission of a photon, exciting the acceptor. The acceptor ow decays to ground state by fluorescene; emitted photon has **longer wave length (lower energy)** than both original exciting light & donor emission.

- An atom / molecule that fluoresces is termed **fluorophore**
- **Fluorometry** is measurement of emitted fluorescence light.

## Bioluminescence Cycle

- **Bioluminescence** is a *special form of chemiluminescence found in biological system*[Q].
- Bioluminescence requires considerable amount of energy. In firefly, ATP is used in a set of reactions that ***convert chemical energy into light energy***[Q]

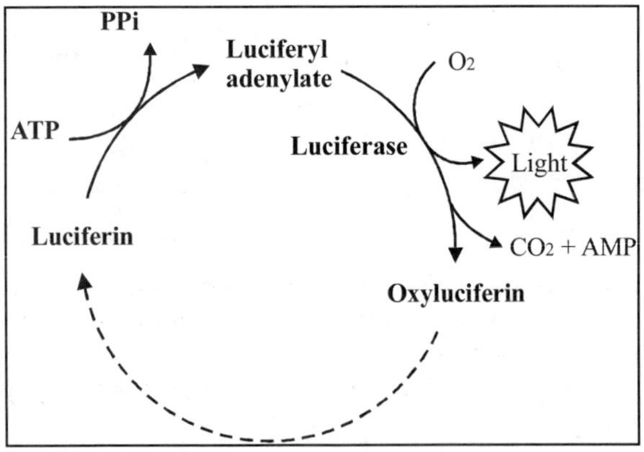


- The light is produced through a chemical reaction involving **luciferin,** (a heat resistant complex carboxylic acid substrate), **luciferase** (enzyme), **ATP** and $O_2$
- The generation of light flashes requires activation of luciferin by pyrophosphate cleavage of ATP to form **luciferyl adenylate**. In the presence of molecular oxygen (O2) and luciferase, the luciferin (adenylate) undergoes a multistep oxidative decarboxylation to oxyluciferin This process is accompanied by emission of light.
- Colour of flashes differ in different firefly species and seems to be determined by *difference in the structure of luciferase*. Luciferin is regenerated from oxyluciferin in a subsequent series of reactions.
- It has the highest quantum efficiency (Qc= 88%). The quantum yield (total photons emitted per total molecule reacting) is ~ 0.1– 10% for chemiluminescence and 10-30% for bioluminescence
- Since the light producing reaction is **dependent on ATP**. It allows researchers to determine the presence of ATP and hence the **presence of life**.
- In lab, pure firefly luciferin and luciferase are used to measure minute quantities of ATP by the intensity of light flash produced. As little as a few picomoles ($10^{-12}$ mol) of ATP can be measured in this way
- This method is used by NASA **to find life on other planets**. It is also used for **antibiotic susceptibility testing.** If light is produce on mixing above mixture to cultured sample of TB bacteria and antibiotic, it indicates the failure of drug and presence of growing and thriving bacteria.
- In **gene activation therapy**, if light is visible on ultraviolet cameras, this means that genes treated with luciferase are active.

## Spectrophotometer : Lambert Beer Law & Absorption of Light by Molecule

- Biomolecules absorb light at characteristic wave lengths, just as **tryptophan, tyrosine** and to a much lesser extent phenylalanine absorb ***ultraviolet light near a wavelength of 280 nm***Q.

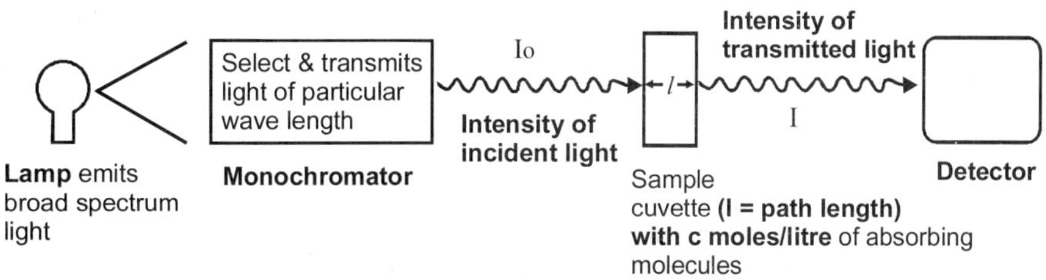


**Components of Sphectrophotometer**

- The fraction of incident light absorbed by solution at given wavelength depends on thickness of absorbing layer (pathlength) and concentration of the absorbing species. So Lambart Beer Law is **Absorbance** $= \log \frac{I^\circ}{I} = \varepsilon Cl$

  where ε is molar extinction coefficient and it has been assumed that incident light is parallel, mono chromatic (of single wave length) and solvent & solute are randomaly oriented. So *each successive millimeter path of absorbing solution absorbs not a constant amount but a constant fraction of light*. However, ***with fixed path length absorbing layer, absorbance is directly proportional to the concentration of absorbing solute***Q. ***So it can be used in quatitative estimation of DNA, RNA or aminoacids***Q.

## Restriction Enzyme / Restriction Endonucleases (RE)

- These are originally called **restriction enzymes** because their presence in a given bacteria ***restricted the growth of certain bacterial viruses (i.e. bacteriophages)***Q. This **defensive enzyme** protects the host bacterial DNA from the DNA genome of foreign organisms (particularly infective bacteriophages) by specifically ***inactivating the invading phage DNA by digestion***Q.
- *Werner Arber* discovered that their biological function is to recognize an *cleave foreign DNA* (eg the DNA of infecting virus) and ***such DNA is said to be restricted. RE restrict DNA replication (viral-replication).***Q
- However, REs are found only in cells that also contain **site specific DNA methylase enzyme-** ***which methylates the host DNA, rendering it an unsuitable substrate for digestion by restriction enzymes (and thus protecting it from RE)***Q. So restriction enzymes and site specific DNA methylase are *companion enzymes* an always exists in pairs in a bacterium – and sometimes called as **restriction modification system**.
- Immense size of DNA was the main obstacle in its molecular analysis, which was over come by a group of bacterial enzyme called restriction endonucleases (restriction enzymes). RE ***cleaves double stranded (d s) DNA into smaller, more manageable & precisely defined DNA segments***Q called **restriction fragments**. RE used as **molecular scissors or chemical knife** is the *key enzyme in recombinant DNA technology or genetic engineering*. There are 3 types of Res

| Features | Type I RE | Type III RE | Type II RE |
|---|---|---|---|
| Structure, components & activities | **Single large, multisubunit, multifunctional** enzyme containing both **endonuclease (nuclease) & methylase activities in one enzyme** | **Single large, multisubunit, multifunctional** enzyme containing both **endonuclease (nuclease) & methylase activities in one enzyme** | Simple **homodimers** (2 identical proteins linked together) with **separate nuclease & methylase** activities (ie both not in one enzyme). |
| **Nuclease subunit structure & Requirements for cleavage** | - **Hetero – trimer**<br>- **Require ATP** for cleavage<br>- Cofactors **ATP, $Mg^{++}$, SAM**<br>- **2** recognizition sites in **any orientation** | - **Hetero-dimer**<br>- **ATP not required** for cleavage<br>- Cofactors **$Mg^{++}$, SAM**<br>- **2** recognizition sites in **head to head orientation** | - **Homodimer**<br>- ATP not required for cleavage<br>- Cofactors **$Mg^{++}$**<br>- **Single** recognizition site |
| **Site of DNA cleavage and methylation** | - Cleaves at **random sites that can be > 1000 base pairs** (bp) away from recognition sequence (RS)<br>- Methylates at RS | - Cleaves DNA, 25 bp (24-26) from recognition site (towards 3' end)<br>- Methylates at RS | - Cleaves DNA within recognized sequence itself (ie at or near RS)<br>- Methylates at RS |
| **DNA translocation** | - Present<br>- **Require ATP for moving along DNA** | - Absent<br>- Require ATP for moving along DNA | - Absent<br>- **Require no ATP** |
| **Restriction modification** | By single multifunctional enzyme | By separate enzymes sharing a common subunit | Separate restriction (nuclease) & modification (methylase) |
| **Enzyme turnover** | Absent | Absent | Present |

★ Type II RE is first isolated by Hamilton Smith (Beta Hind 1) and Daniel Nathans first used them to cut DNA for mapping & analyzing genes & genome.

- Restriction endonucleases *recognize and cleave (cut or splice) double stranded DNA in a predictable manner at specific sequences*[Q] k/a (**recognition sequences or restriction sites**) that are typically **4-6** (Lehinger) /**4-7** (Harper) bp long, to generate a set of smaller fragments. Restriction enzymes are endonucleases ie they break nucleic acid chains somewhere within the DNA rather than at the ends of molecule.
- To cut DNA, a RE makes *2 incisions through each sugar – phosphate backbone (i.e. phospho-diester bond of each strand) of double stranded DNA*[Q]. The **average size of DNA fragments** produced by cleaving genomic DNA with RE depends on the frequency with which a specific restriction site occurs in DNA; which inturn depends on their size. In a DNA in which all 4 nucleotides are equally abundant [i.e. (C=G) = (A = T) =50%] and randomly distributed, a RE tht recognizes a 6 bp sequence cuts once every 4096 ($4^6$), whereas another RE that recognizes a 4 bp sequence cuts once every 256 bp ($4^4$) and so produces smaller DNA fragments. The fragment size produced by RE cleavage can be increased by simply terminating the reaction before completion – **partial digest** – or by using special class of endonuclease called **homing endonuclease** (by group I introns) which cleave *14-20 bp DNA sequence*. However, in natural DNA the recognition sequence tend to occur less frequently because neucleotides are neither random nor equally abundant.
- If a piece of DNA from a species is made to react with a specific RE, a characteristic array of cut DNA fragments will be produced, this is k/a **restriction map**. The ends of all fragments have same DNA sequence. These restriction fragments of known size are isolated (enriched) by *electrophoresis on agarose or polyacrylamide gel*[Q] or **HPLC**. Restriction map serves as DNA fingerprint because the fragments of DNA from one organism will have a characteristic pattern.

**Specificity**

- Restriction endonucleases have specific recognition sites with **palindrome arrangement** where they cut *ds DNA (at specific DNA sequence )*[Q] with in the molecule producing short fragments (other enzymes cut DNA randomly)
- RE recognizes short stretches of DNA **about *4 to 7 base pairs long*** (usually having 4 or 6 base pairs)
- These sequences differ for each RE and are **palindromes**, i.e., they show *two fold rotational symmetry*. **Palindrome** (meaning to **run backwards**) are also known as **inverted repeat sequences**. It is similar to a *word that reads backwards or forwards similarly* eg madam. Which means with in a short region of double helix, the nucleotide sequence on one strand, read *$5^1 \rightarrow 3^1$, is identical* to that of the *$2^{nd}$ strand,* also read in *$5^1 \rightarrow 3^1$ direction*. So, if rolated 180 degrees around the axis of symmetry – the structure remains same.

Palindrome cut by Eco R1 endonuclease

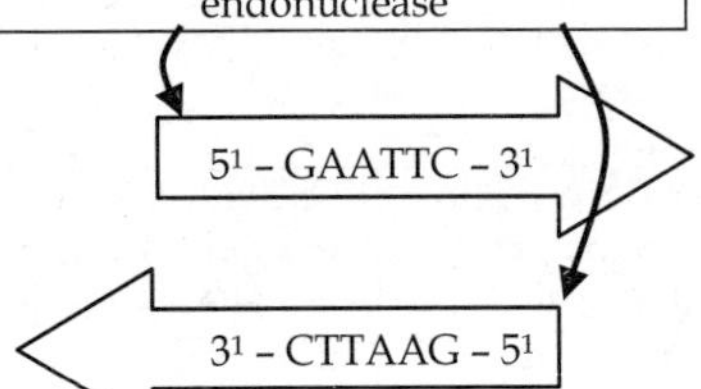


**Sticky & Blunt ends**

RE cleaves DNA so as to produce a 3' – OH group on one end & $5^1$ – $PO_4$ group on other end. DNA cut results in

**Sticky /Cohesive/ Overlapping/ Staggered ends**

- Produced due to **staggered cut** (by *Taq1, Bam HI*), resulting in DNA fragments having *single stranded (SS) sequences that are complementary to each other.*
- This leaves 2-4 nucleotides of one strand unpaired at each resulting end. These unpaired strands are called **sticky-ends** because these can base pair with each other or with complementary sticky ends of other DNA fragments.
- **DNA ligase** joins sticky ends produced by same RE
- **Terminal transferase** enzyme add new ends & change it into blunt end.

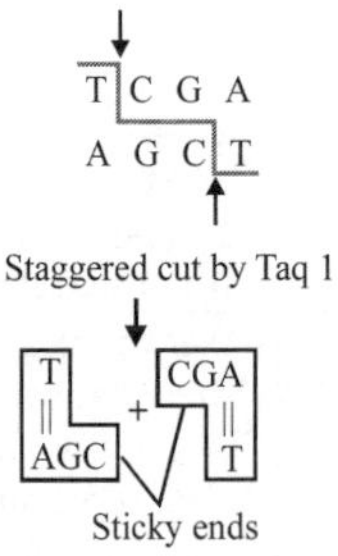


**Blunt ends**

- Cleaves both strands of DNA at the opposing ***phosphodiester bonds***[Q], leaving no unpaired bases on the ends.
- Produced d/t straight cut, (by HpaI, Hae III) that are double stranded & therefore donot form hydrogen bonds with each other.
- **Bacteriophage $T_4$ ligase** can covalently joint blunt ended fragments.

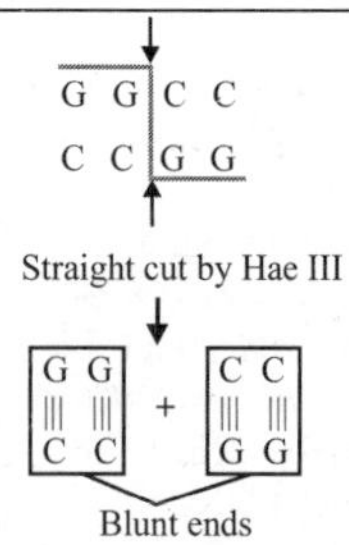


**Restriction site & nomenclature**

- A DNA sequence recognized by RE is called restriction site. RE that *recognizes 4 base* pair sequences produces *more cuts and shorter segments* than the RE requiring sequence of 6 base pairs.
- The $1^{st}$ letter of name of RE is from the *genus of bacterium* from which it is isolated (E). Next two letters are from *name of species (Co).* The additional subscript letter indicates the *type or strain (R)* and a *final roman number* indicate the *order in which the enzyme was discovered* in that particular organism (I) eg. ECoRI.

- After isolating target DNA (restriction) fragment, it is joined to similarly digested cloning vector (i.e. vector digested by some RE) by ***DNA ligase***[Q] (*which catalyzes formation of new phosphodiester bonds by using ATP*). Fragments produced by 2 RE (eg EcoRI & Bam HI) will not link. New DNA sequences can be created by inserting synthetic DNA fragments (**linkers**) b/w the ends that are being ligated. **Poly linkers** are inserted DNA fragments with multiple recognition sequences for RE (often useful later as points for inserting DNA by cleavage & ligation). So it has an *important role in recombinant DNA technology* and preparing *chimeric DNA molecules.*
- Ligating sticky ends is technically easy but is a/w the problems like sticky ends may reconnect with themselves, without net gain of DNA, forming heterogeneous tandom inserts or sticky end sites may not be available in a required (convenient) position. To escape these problems blunt ends can be generated. Blunt ends can be ligated directly (however not directional) by **bacteriophage $T_4$ ligase** – a technique though less efficient than sticky end ligation, has advantage of ligation of any pairs of ends. 2 alternatives to circumvent problems listed above include

1. **Homopolymer tailing** by **terminal transferase** i.e. if poly d (G) is added to vector and poly d (C) is added to 3' end of foreign DNA, the two molecules can ony link to each other.
2. Adding synthetic sticky ends (**linkers**)

- Some pro /eu-karyotic **recombinases** (like *CRE recombinase* identifying bacterial lox P sites or *Flp recombinase* identifying yeast FRT sites) are used as an adjunct to RE to catalyze DNA in corporation.

## Polymorphism

Any two nonrelated individuals share 99.9% of their DNA sequences. So the remarkable diversity of humans is encoded in only 0.1% of DNA (~ 3 million base pairs). Genomic variations are differences in sequence of DNA among individuals. And genomes of non-related people differ at *about 1 of 1200 to 1,500 DNA bases* (or *0.1% of genome*). These variations are due to.

**Polymorphism**

- It is ***normal, clinically harmless variations of DNA sequence, that does not affect the phenotype***[Q]
- Traditionally defined as **sequence variation at a given locus (allele) in >1% population.**
- It occurs ~ *once in every 500 nucleotides or about $10^7$ times per genome due to deletion, insertion or single base substitution occuring in non-coding region like introns & intergenic region* or at sites that cause no change in function of encoded protein.
- So ***polymorphism is single phenotype single locus and multiple normal allele***[Q].

**Mutations**

- It is **infrequent (<1%) but potentially harmful genome variation that is associated with specific human disease**
- Single mutation may l/t many end effects (**pleiotropism**) or mutations at several genetic loci may produce the several genetic loci may produce the same trait **(genetic heterogeneity).**
- Structural alterations of β-globin

| Alteration | Disease | Function affected |
|---|---|---|
| Point mutation | Sickel cell disease | Protein folding |
| | β-Thalassemia | Transcription control, Frame shift & non sense mutation RNA processing. |
| Deletion | β°- Thalassemia<br>Hemoglobin lepore | MRNA production |
| Rearragnement | β-Thalassemia type III | MRNA production |

## Restriction Fragment Length Polymorphism (RFLP)

- Human genome contains **sequence variations at a given locus (allele) that do not affect phenotype in >1% population**. This property of the molecule to exist in >1 form is k/a **polymorphism**. So polymorphism is **presence of single normal phenotype, single locus (site) and multiple allele (sequence variations)** in >1% of population. Polymorphism is a normal variation and is clinically harmless. Whereas mutation is *infrequent, (seen in <1%), abnormal, and potentially deleterious genetic variation that may lead to pleiotropism (one mutation – many effects) or genetic heterogeneity (many mutation – one effect).*
- **Restriction fragment length polymorphism (RFLP)** is a **genetic variation that can be observed by cleaving the DNA into fragments (restriction fragments) with a restriction endonuclease**. The existence of two or more types of restriction fragment patterns is called RFLP. The length of restriction fragment is altered if the genetic variation (polymorphism, mutation etc) alters the DNA so as to create or abolish a site of restriction endonuclease cleavage (a restriction site). Differences in DNA sequence (**polymorphism or mutation**) can *create or abolish a site of restriction endonuclease cleavage* (a **restriction site**) and thus *result in variation in length of restriction fragments*. If DNA of an individual has **gained a restriction site**, then restriction enzyme cleavage *yields at least one additional fragement*. And if mutation cause a **loss of restriction site** *fewer fragments are produced*. Two types of DNA variation that result in RFLP are.

**Single nucleotide polymorphism (SNPs, pronounced Snips) or site polymorphism**

- It is DNA variation that just *involves single base*. SNPs are *responsible for 90% of human genome* variation.
- Typically the SNPs are *biallelic* (i.e., only two choices exist at a given site) and can occur anywhere in genome – within intron, exon or intergenic regions. However, *<1% of SNPs occur in coding region.*
- Serve both as physical landmark within the genome & as a genetic marker whose transmission can be followed from – parent to child. It *is genetic marker of choice for* study of complex genetic traits.

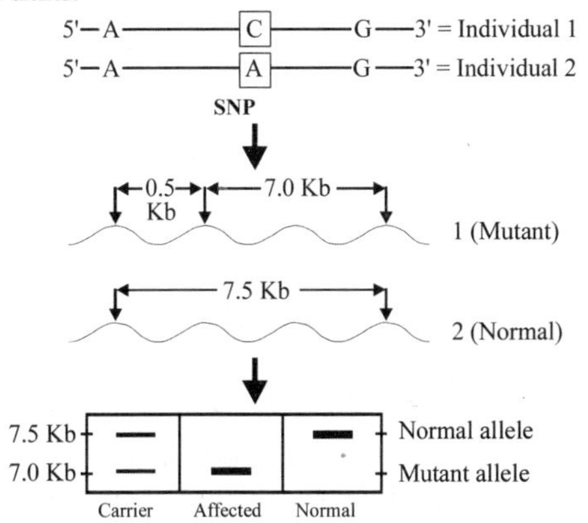


**Southern blot analysis**

**Length polymorphism / Tandem repeats**

- Human DNA contains short repetitive sequence of non coding DNA. This ***variable number of tandem (one after another) repeats* (VNTR), is unique for any individual & therefore serve as a molecular finger print**
- It may be of two types

**Microsatellite DNA polymorphism**

- ***Short (2-6 base pairs) inherited tandem repeats of usually < 1kb***[Q]
- Occurs ~ 50,000-1 lac times in human

**Minisatellite repeats**

- Larger *(1-3 kb)*, & repeat motifs is usually *15-70 base pairs.*

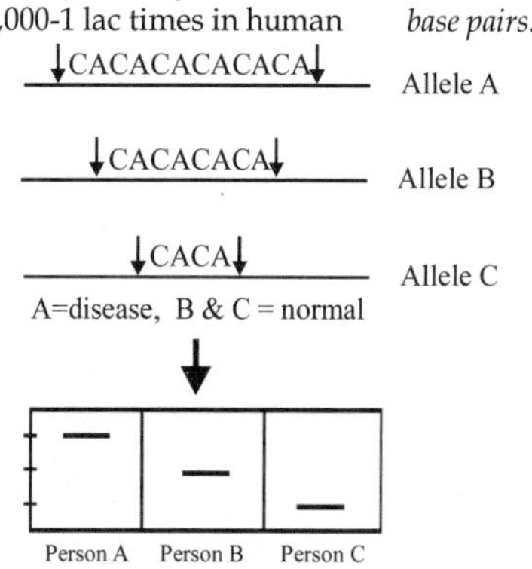


**Southern blot analysis**

- **Procedure**

DNA sample is treated with **restriction endonuclease enzymes** which cleaves DNA in restriction fragments of defined length. These fragments are **separated by agarose gel electrophoresis on the basis of size. Detection** of RFLP relies **on southern blotting hybridization** procedure. DNA is denatured by soaking agarose get in alkali, and then blotted on to nylon (nitrocellulose) paper

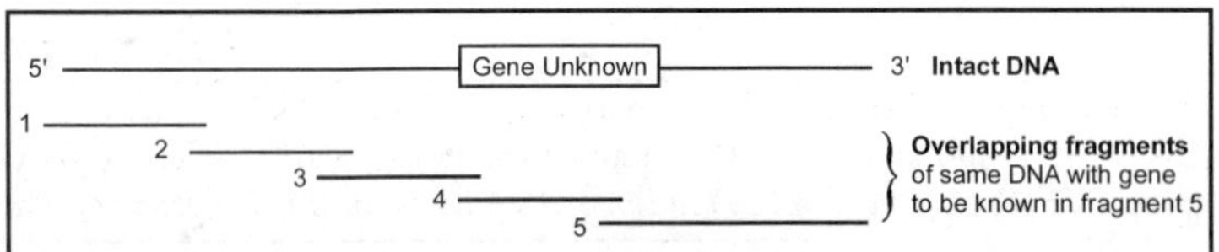


**Chromosomal Walking**

to reproduce the distribution RFs in gel. This *nitrocellulose membrane is immersed in radioactively labeled DNA probe* (southern-blotting). Autoradiography (x-ray exposure to film) reveals the fragments to which the probe hybridizes. The method is *very accurate*: However, it *requires large samples of undergraded DNA* (>25ng) that is often not available at crime scene.

- **Clinical Applications of RFLP**

- **Tracing chromosome from parent to offspring:** An individual who is heterozygous for a polymorphism has a sequence variation in the DNA of one chromosome and not in the DNA of companion (homolgous) chromosome. In such cases each chromosome can be traced from parent to offspring by determining the absence or presence of polymorphism. This is useful in **disputed parenthood.**
- **Prenatal diagnosis of genetic disease:** Disease will produce alteration in size & distribution of RE fragments of DNA obtained from fetus (blood, amniotic fluid or chorionic villi). Examples include

1. *Sickel cell anemia* can be directly diagnosed by RFLP, as the point ( $A \rightarrow T$ ) mutation *abolishes recognition site of restriction endonuclease mst II* that recognizes nucleotide sequence CCTNAGG (N = any nucleotide). Normal DNA digested with Mst II yields a 1.15 kb fragment whereas a 1.35 kb fragment is generated from $\beta^S$gene.
2. *Phenyl ketonuria* can be indirectly diagnosed using RFLP. Mutation in phenylalanine hydroxylase (PAH) gene do not directly affect any RE site. To establish diagnosis one has *to analyze DNA of affected family member with a goal to identify genetic markers or variants (RFLP) that are tightly linked to the disease.* Once these polymorphism marker that are consistently / closely linked to a disease producing mutation gene – (ie they closely show close linkage and are coinherited) are identified. The RFLP analysis can be carried out for prenatal diagnosis.

- **RFLP results from single base changes /mutation (eg sickle cell disease)** or **from deletions or insertions (copy number variations = CNVs)** of DNA into a restriction fragment (eg thalssemias) and have proved to be **useful diagnostic tools**. Thy have been found at known gene loci and in sequence that have no known function; thus RFLPs may disrupt the function of gene or may have no apperent biological consequence.
- **RFLPs / SNPs are inherited in mendilian fashion**, so these can be used in *definition of inherited disease in which the functional deficit is unknown.* RFLPs / SNPs can be used to **establish linkage** groups, which in turn by the process of **chromosomal walking**, will eventually **define the disease locus**. Chromosomal walking involves *repeated cloning of overlapping DNA segments (of 100-200 kb) to isolate/determine any gene in unknown location of large piece of DNA. In chromosomal walking, a fragment representing one end of long piece of* DNA is used to isolate the next overlapping segment. The direction of extension is determined by restriction mapping and the procedure is repeated sequentially until the desired sequence is obtained. **X chromosome linked disorders** are particularly amenable to chromosomal walking since only a single allele is expressed and a complete **linkage map (& genomic sequence)** of this chromosome have been determined. The gene for X-linked disorder **Duchenne muscular dystrophy** was found using RFLPS (& chromosomal walking). Similarly, defect was localized (linked) to terminal region of short arm of chromosome 4 in **Huntington disease** and to alpha-globin locus on chromosome 16 in **polycystic disease**.
- Comparison of **genetic makeup** of humans & related species **(genetic maping)**
- **For DNA finger printing (DNA typing or DNA profiling):** Alee Jaffreys described this technique in 1985. It is based on **sequence polymorphisms** (slight sequence differences) between individuals. It is a potent weapon of crime detection (forensic medicine).

1. *Some sequence changes affects restriction site and result in RFLPs*. It is very accurate method but requires larg sample of undergraded DNA (>25ng). That amount of DNA is often not available at a crime scene.
2. More sensitive DNA typing method use PCR and focus on **short tandem repeats (STRs)**. An STR locus is a short DNA sequence, repeated many times in tandem at a particular location in a chromosome; mostly & 4bp long. The DNA sequences flanking STR are unique to each type of STR & identical (except for very rare mutations) in all humans. PCR primers are added to this flanking DNA & designed to amplify the DNA across the STR. Since each human inherits one chromosome from each parent, the STR lengths on two chromosomes are often different generating 2 signals from 1 individuals. If multiple STR loci are analyzed, *a profile can be generated that is essentially unique to a particular individual*. PCR amplification allows DNA fingerprints to be obtained from **< 1ng of partially degraded DNA**, an amount that can be obtained from a single hair follicle, a drop of blood, a small semen sample that might be months or years old. Combined DNA Index System **(CODIS)** uses **13 STR loci** for DNA typing in USA. The **amelogenin gene** present on human sex chromosome, has slightly different flanking DNA on X and Y chromosomes. It is used as a marker for sex determination of DNA donor. **Multiplex STR kits** include 13 CODIS loci, amelogenin and 2 additional loci (total 16) . The chances of accidental match between two individuals in human population is < 1 in $10^8$ (quintillion).

## Microsatellites

- Microsatellites" are defined as loci (or regions within DNA sequences) where short sequences of DNA (nucleotides; adenine- A, thiamine- T, guanine- G, cytosine- C) are repeated in tandem arrays. This means that the sequences are repeated one right after the other. The lengths of sequences used most often are di-, tri-, or tetra-nucleotides.
- They can be used for DNA fingerprinting, in forensic and paternity/parentage work. At the same location within the genomic DNA the number of times the sequence (eg.AC) is repeated often varies between individuals, within population, and/or between species.

So one population may commonly have 13 AC's (dinucleotide repeat sequence) repeated in a row while another population has 18 AC's repeated at the same location within the genomic DNA.

- Predicting the progression of disease: Microsatellites are acutely prone to replication errors that result in expansions and contractions of repeat unit (repeat length variability) because of misalignment of the template and daughter strands. Variability of microsatellite repeat lengths leads to genomic instability and, plays a role in the progression of disease, presumably by gene inactivation. DNA mismatch repair (MMR) enzymes maintain genomic stability by removing replication errors from DNA.
- Defective DNA mismatch repair (MMR) enzymes in association with microsatellite instability (MSI) are thus implicated in the progression of several diseases and cancers. Examples includes : Fragile syndrome, Huntington's chorea, Myotonic dystroply, Spinobulbar muscular atrophy, Kennedy's disease, Hereditary non polyposis colon cancer
- Provides clue to genetic bases of disease: The association of a specific polymorphism in affected family members and the lack of this association in unaffected members may be the first clue about genetic bases of a disease.

## DNA Fingerprinting (DNA Typing or Profiling)

- *Alec J. Jeffrey*[Q] of Leicester University (U.K), in 1984 serendipitously discovered *fundamentals of genetic finger printing*.
- Because every person's DNA sequence is different, the fragment in DNA specimen from one individual to another are different in number & length. DNA finger printing uses restriction fragment length polymorphism (RFLP) or repeat sequence DNA to establish a unique pattern of DNA fragments for an individual. The DNA markers analyzed for such finger printing are most commonly ***short tandem repeat polymorphisms.*** VNTR (variable number of tandem repeats) are short sequences of DNA at scattered locations in genome, repeated in tandem (one after another) that give rise to polymorphism in chromosome. Short tandem repeats are similar to VNTR but smaller in size.
- **DNA fingerprinting (by PCR)** has revolutinized the analysis of evidence from crime scenes in determining whether the ***sample comes from specific individual and varification of paternity***[Q]. DNA fingerprinting is ***done by nucleated cells***[Q] eg ***blood***[Q] (WBC & RBC), semen, vaginal epithelial cells, tooth pulp, bone marrow, hair roots, muscle, skin, mucous membrane.

## Polymerase Chain Reaction (PCR)

- PCR, invented by **Karry Mullis**, is an **in vitro (test tube) enzymatic method of amplifying** a **selected (target) sequence of DNA**. It is like *Xerox machine for gene copying*. It is **sensitive, selective (specific) and extremely rapid means of amplifying any desired DNA sequence** which can be as short as 50-100 bp and as long as 10kb.
- It is so sensitive that it allows the DNA in a single cell, sperm or hair follicle; from any source – virus, bacteria, plant, animal or, human even when the targetedsequence makes up less than one part in a million of the total initial sample to be amplified. PCR has allowed successful **enzymatic cloning** of DNA from > 40,000 years old sample.
- **Specificity** is based on the use of ***2 oligonucleotide primers that hybridize to complementary sequences on opposite strands of separated ds (double standed) DNA***[Q]. (So ds DNA is required not SS DNA).
- Each newly synthesized strand can act as a template for the successive cycles thus each cycle of amplification **doubles the amount of DNA** in sample resulting in an **exponential increase** in target DNA, hence the name **polymerase chain reaction**. Typically *20-30 cycles* run during PCR amplify the DNA by a *million to billion folds in a few hours*. 20 cycles provide amplification of $2^{20}$ (i.e. $10^6$) and 30 cycles $2^{30}$ (i.e. $10^9$).
- Major **advantages of PCR over traditional cloning methods** (using recombinant DNA techniques), as a mechanism for amplifying specific DNA sequence are *sensitivity, speed and less technical difficulty*. It is an **in vitro (test tube)** method not requiring living cell. The cycles are generally repeated by automated **Tempcycler**.
- The **double stranded (ds) DNA** is first heated to separate (melt) the 2 strands of template DNA containing the target sequence (**denaturation**); Vast excess of **2 primers** (one for each flanking sequence) is added and allowed to bind DNA (**annealing** or **priming**); each DNA strand is copied by **thermostable DNA (Taq) polymerase enzyme** obtained from Thermus aquaticus, starting from the primer sites **(chain extension)** in presence of **all 4 dXTPs / dNTPs (deoxyribo nucleoside triphosphate)**. So it is **enzymatic (non-recombinant) DNA amplification**. The cycles of denaturation, annealing & chain extension are repeated.
- **Clinical applications of PCR** *utilize its ability to amplifly (increase) the minimal (or almost negligable) amount of DNA*, which is then detected by southern blot technique. So it is used in detecting low abundance nucleic acid sequence (DNA). For example.

**Detection of infectious disease**

- To detect bacterial, viral etc infectious disease agents in early and latent phase (when the agent load is very less). So PCR offers rapid & sensitive method of detecting viruses that have long latency such as HIV.
- Can detect even one virus or bacteria present in sample
- To detect viral load by reality-PCR

★ PCR uses cells obtained from amniocentesis or chorionic villus sampling for prenatal diagnosis; somatic cells for postnatal dignosis and nucleated cells for finger printing.

**Detection of variations & mutations in genes**

- To ***detect allelic polymorphism, specific aneuploidy***[Q]; to compare normal cloned gene with an uncloned mutant gene and to study evolution using DNA from archeological samples.
- PCR (f/b electrophoresis & southern blot) is used for detection of **direct mutational analysis to prenatally or postnatally diagnose** the presence or absence of inherited disorders like ***Cystic fibrosis, hemophilia, β-thalassemia & sickle cell anemia etc***[Q]. It also detects carriers.
- Detects DNA abnormalities characteristic to cancer and establish precise tissue types for transplantation.
- For quantitative RNA analysis after RNA copying & m-RNA quantitation by RT-PCR (using retroviral reverse transcriptase).
- To score in vivo protein – DNA occupancy using chromatin immunoprecipitation assay.

**PCR in Law**

- **DNA fingerprinting** by means of PCR has revolutionized *forensic analysis of crime scene and paternity verification*. The DNA markers analyzed for such fingerprinting are most commonly *short tandem repeat polymorphism*.
- Sex determination

## Steps of a PCR

- **Each *cycle doubles the amount of DNA*** in the sample, leading to an *exponential (logarithmic) increase in DNA* with repeated cycles. Steps in each cycle are.

1. **Primer construction:- Flanking sequence** is nucleotide sequence of short segment on each side of *target DNA*. It brackets the DNA *sequence of interest*. In PCR ***it is not necessary to know the nucleotide sequence of target DNA but it is necessary to know the flanking sequence***[Q]**.**

- Two *synthetic single stranded oligonucleotides* (usually 20-35 nucleotides long) which are ***complementary to respective flanking sequence***[Q] are constructed. These serve as primers. ***The 3'- OH end of each primer points towards the target sequence***[Q]**.** Primer is added in vast excess.

2. **Denaturation of DNA duplex (94-98°C).** The DNA to be amplified is heated to seperated double stranded DNA (ds DNA) into single strands. (SSDNA)

3. **Annealing of primers to SSDNA (37-60°C).** Separated strands are cooled & allowed to ***bind (anneal) to the 2 primers (one for each strand) at flanking sequence***[Q]. Primer is added in vast excess.

4. **Chain extension of primer (~72°C)**

- ***DNA polymerase & deoxyribo nucleoside triphosphate (d-NTP)***[Q] are **added in excess** to initiate synthesis of two new chains complementary to original DNA chains, *starting at primer site*. ***DNA polymease adds nucleotides to 3¹- OH end of primer***[Q] and strand grows across the target DNA making complementary copies of target.

- ***Magnesium concentration is critical***[Q] as it affects DNA polymerase activity and fidelity, denaturation temperature , primer annealing & dimer formation and PCR specificity. 0.5-5mM is usually used $Mg^{++}$ concentration. Excess results in *accumulation of nonspecific amplification products seen as multiple bands on agarose gel, whereas, insufficient $Mg^{++}$ result in reduced* yield of desired PCR products.

- Cycles of heat denaturation (seperation), annealing (binding) of primers to flanking sequence and extension of annealed primer with DNA polymerase are repeated. Initially, *E.coli DNA polymerase* was used in PCR, that was destroyed & so has to be added by each heat denaturation cycle. The advantage of using thermostable DNA polymerase (such as ***Taq polymerase from a thermophilic bacteria Thermus aquaticus***[Q]) ***is that the enzyme itself is not denatured and therefore does not have to be added at each successive cycle***[Q]**.**

- The amplified DNA sequences can be analyzed by *gel electrophoresis & ethidium bromide staining, southern hybridization (blotting), direct sequence determination, RFLP / sequencing and incorporation of biotin / digoxigenin labeled dUTP during amplification and detection by colorimetric / luminescent techniques.*

## Types of PCR

1. Conventional DNA based PCR
2. **Reverse transcriptase PCR (RT-PCR)**

- In this mRNA or rRNA is starting material which is converted to *complementary DNA (c-DNA) by reverse transcriptase.* So it is a normal PCR preceded by reverse transcription
- **Tth polymerase** (instead of Taq polymerase) from *Thermus thermophilus* is used which has both reverse transcriptase & DNA polymerase activity.
- In normal PCR, DNA is detected which could be from living or non living organism but in RT-PCR, mRNA is detected indicating its origin from living organism (only living cells chang DNA to mRNA). So it is used in *expression mapping* i.e. determining when & where certain genes are expressed.

3. **Asymmetrical PCR** is used to generate single strands by adjusting primer concentrations to favor one strand. After 10-15 cycles the second primer is used up and only one strand complementary to first strand continues to be copied up.
4. **Inverse PCR** amplifies the sequences on either side of known stretch by circularizing a piece of DNA & hybridizing primers in an opposite orientation.
5. **Nested PCR,** improves *sensitivity & specificity by using 2 sets of primers in 2 successive PCR runs*. This means a fragment is amplified by using a set of primers (eg genus specific) and second amplification of some internal sequence is done by using another set of primers in first run product.

- This reduces contamination in products d/t amplification of unexpected primer binding sites but requires more detailed knowledge of sequence and proves hybridization may not be necessary.

6. **Anchored (one sided) PCR or RACE** (rapid amplification of (cDNA ends)

- It is used to amplify the ends of m-RNA transcripts when one end of sequence is known using a specialized *reverse transcription – (RT) PCR*
- To unknown end a segment of *guanine is covalently* attached which serves as template with polycytosine primer. It is used to obtain (amplify) unknown 5' end (5' RACE-PCR) or 3' end (3' RACE-PCR).

7. **PCR using other DNA polymerases**

- ***DNA ligase in ligation amplification reactions***[Q]
- **T7 RNA polymerase** in transcription based systems
- **Q β replicase** from bacteriophage

8. **In situ** (paraffin embedded or cytospin coated glass slides) **PCR amplification** (by protease + DNA polymerase) **and product detection** (by hybridization or direct incorporation of biotin / digoxigenin labeled nucleotides)
9. **Real Time PCR (RT- PCR)** has many advantages over conventional RT-PCR

- **RT-PCR or quantitative (q)PCR, combines PCR (DNA) amplification and detection into a single step** by eliminating gel electrophoresis for detection. *It is a software driven automated easy to perform procedure that can be easily standardized. It has higher sensitivity, specificity, reproducibility and sample output (~ 200 samples / day)*
- Allows for *quantitative measurement* and rapidity d/t reduced cycle times & removal of post PCR detection procedure. The amplicon could be visualized as amplification progressed. It is **used to know *how much amplification of DNA has occurred***[Q]**.**
- ***All real time PCR rely upon fluorescent reporter (probes) such as SYBER – green, Taq man, and molecular Beacons***[Q] for detection & quantitation. The signal of which increases in ***direct proportion to the amount of PCR product in reaction*** **[Quantitative Real time PCR (RQ-PCR)].**
- It can detect viral load *(no. of viruses present in sample) so help planning treatment.*

10. **Quantitative (Q-) PCR** (preferably real time) is used to quantify PCR product i.e. determining whether a sequence is present or not and if it is present the number of copies in sample.
11. **Multiplex PCR** uses multiple – unique primer sets within a single PCR targeting multiple genes in a single test run that would otherwise reuire several repeated PCR runs.

**Heat - Denaturation (seperation)**

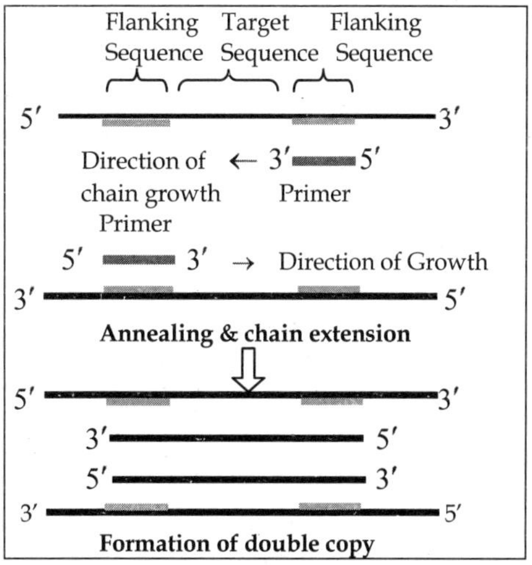


**Detection of pre or post natal disease with known mutation eg cystic fibrosis, sickle cell anemia, β-thallasemia & hemophila**

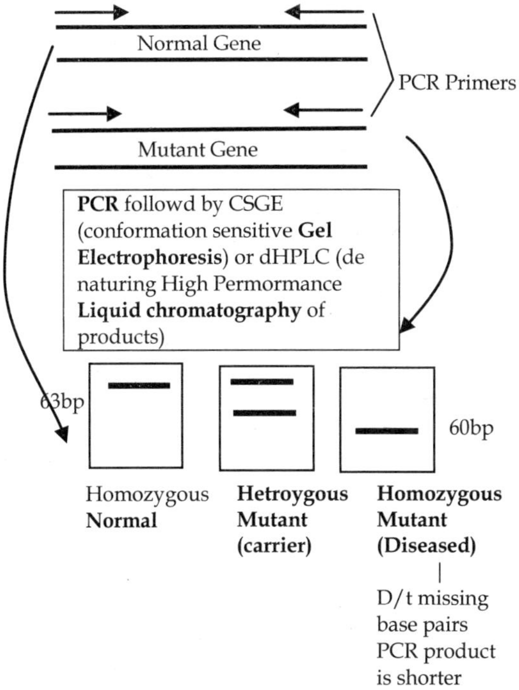


| Direct Mutation Analysis (eg by **PCR**) | Indirect linkage Analysis |
|---|---|
| Involves *identification of specific base pair change or mutation responsible for disease* | Involves *segregation of genetic markers known to be linked to a gene* responsible for disease. And it is determined that wheres an individual inherited a chromose present in family that carries the abnormal gene |
| As it is a direct method, not based on segregation of genetic markers in family members, it does not require DNA analysis of multiple family members. | DNA analysis of multiple family members is required to identify the markers that segregate with abnormal chromosome in each affected pedigree |
| Involves physical isolation and sequencing of gene | Dose not involve physical isolation & sequencing of gene |
| Determines unequivocally whether suspect has inherited the disease or not. So has become **gold standard** | Being less specific it's use is restricted to genetic diseases if mutation sequence is not known. |

### Ligase Chain Reaction (LCR)

- LCR, is amplification of target DNA after multiple rounds of denaturation, annealing & ligation of two pairs of synthetic nucleotide (which hybridize to complementary strands of a target DNA) with a thermostable ligase
- **Gap- LCR** reduces the background generated by target independent blunt end ligation. In this DNA polymerase fills in a gap b/w annealed probes which are sub sequently joined by DNA ligase.

### Nucleic Acid Sequence Based Amplification

- NASBA is a *continuous, isothermal, enzyme based* method of nucleic acid *amplification. It amplifies RNA (especially or DNA* from a pool of total nucleic acid.
- It uses a mixture of *reverse transcriptase, RNA polymerase, ribonuclease- H, and 2 transcript specific DNA primers*
- $5^1$ extension of *forward primer* contain promoter sequence for bacteriophage T7 DNA dependent RNA polymerase and $5^1$ extension of *reverse primer* has complementary binding sequence for an electro chemiluminescent (ECL) tag.

★ **DNA sequencing** is the process of determining the exact order of 3 billion bases (A,T, C & G) that make up the DNA of 24 different human chromosomes.

## Gene / DNA / Molecular Cloning

- It is a technique by which large number of identical DNA molecules can be produced. In this technique a DNA fragment to be cloned (amplified) is inserted into the DNA strands of cloning vector eg. plasmid, phages or cosmids to make a new recombinant or chimeric DNA. When the DNA strand of vector multiplies, it also multiplies the inserted DNA fragment. Clones produced is later removed by using restriction enzymes.

- Cloning of DNA fragment involves 4 steps
  - **Fragmentation** by *restriction endonuclease* involves isolation of DNA of intrest (that is to be cloned) and linearization of circular vector DNA that contain same sticky ends
  - **Ligation** is gluing together of DNA of interest with vector DNA to make a new recombinant or chimeric DNA molecules, by DNA ligase enzyme.
  - **Transfection** is inserting newly formed pieces into cells. And finally the cells are cultured. In this way the chimeric DNA (so the DNA of interest) is amplified.
  - **Screening or selection** ***for selecting or identifying the cells that have been successfully transfected with the vector DNA containing the desired insertional DNA sequence in the required orientation***[Q]. This can be done by.

| **Antibiotic resistance markers** | **Colour selection markers which provide blue white screening ($\alpha$ -factor complementation) on X- gal (a colourless galactose sugar) medium** | **PCR, restriction fragment analysis & or DNA sequencing** |
|---|---|---|
| Allow only cells in which the vector has been transfected, to grow | It is based on *lac operon*. The hydrolysis of x-gal by $\beta$ glactosidase cause blue colour in colonies & indicate that colonies contain unligated vector. Whereas, white colonies indicate insertion of foreign DNA & loss of cells ability to hydrolyse marker. | Congirmatory method |

## Hybridoma Cells and Monoclonal Antibodies

- Generally when an antigen is injected into an animal it results in formation of *polyclonal (not monospecific)* antibodies by mixture of B cells. These antibodies are directed against a number of different sites (epitomes or determinants on antigen).
- By **Kohler- Milstein** method, limitless amounts of **monoclonal - monospecific** (specific for one epitope)antibodies can be obtained, by producing **hybridoma cell**. The method involves **cell fusion** & resulting permanent cell line is called a **hybridoma**.
- **B cells** previously ***treated with an antigen***[Q] or mixture of antigens & obtained from mouse spleen are mixed with **mouse myeloma** cells in presence of PEG (polyethylene glycol). PEG causes cell fusion and formation of **hybridoma cell**, which when cloned produce **monoclonal monospecific** antibodies.
- Hybridoma cells can be *frozen & stored and subsequently thawed* when more of antibody is required; this ensures its long term supply. It can also be grown in the abdomen of mice, providing relatively large supplies of antibodies. Attempts to produce human monoclonal antibodies are under-way.
- **Monoclonal antibodies** are produced by **hybridoma technology (in vitro)** or by one clone secreting specific type of antibody in **multiple myeloma (in vivo)**. In **monoclonal antibody preparation** all molecules ***are specific against a particular antigen***[Q] and have **increased avidity** for attaching with antigen. So in a reaction where polyclonal antibodies require 1ml the **monoclonals require very little (only 1 microliter) quantity**. So the initial cost of production may be high but it decreases gradually in long run.
- Monoclonal antibodies are now useful in detection of **1) serum proteins, 2) enzymes, 3) hormones, 4) drugs 5) bacterial & viral antigens, 6) cell surface receptors, 7) HLA antigen, and 8) Cancer cells etc**
- **Monoclonal monospecific antibodies** are used in
  - To measure the amounts of many individual proteins
  - To determine nature of infectious agent
  - To subclassify both normal (eg lymphocytes) & tumor cells (eg leukemia)
  - To direct therapeutic agents to tumor cells
  - To accelerate removal of drug (eg digoxin) from circulation in toxicities
  - ***Nephelometric assays of blood components*** *and* ***blood grouping***[Q]
  - As **immunosuppressants** in clinical conditions like autoimmune disease (Rheumatoid disease)
  - To do ELISA tests
  - Monoclonal antibodies made in mice can be **humanized** (used in humans) by attaching the *complementarity determining regions [CDRs)* (i.e. the sites that binds antigen) onto appropriate sites in a human immunoglobin molecule. This produces an antibody that is very similar to human antibody, thus markedly decreasing immunogenecity & chances of anaphylactic reactions
  - **Quantitative preparation of specific cells and pure antigens**

| **Myeloma cell** | **B Cell** |
|---|---|
| - Do not produce antibody<br>- Immortal<br>- HGPRT-ve rendering salvage path of purine | - Produce specific antibody<br>- Not immortal<br>- HGPRT +ve |

M + B → Fused in presence of **polyethylene glycol (PEG)**

**Hybridoma - cells**

- Immortalized (like parental myeloma cell)
- Produce antibody & are HGPRT +ve (gained from parental B- cells

↓

Grown in presence of **HAT (Hypoxanthine - aminopterinthymidine)** containing medium

| | | |
|---|---|---|
| **B Cell** will die in medium as they are not immortal | **Myeloma** cell will also die in presence of HAT, since the aminopterine in HAT suppress purine synthesis by denovo pathway by inhibiting reutilization of tetrahydrofolate | **Hybridoma cell** will **survive & grow** because they are hypoxanthine - guanine-phosphoribosyl-transferase (HGPRT) +<br>If cloned produce **monoclonal monospecific antibodies** |

## Cloning Vectors

**Plasmid**
- Accept DNA pieces about *6- 10 kb long*
- *Small, circular,* duplex DNA molecules
- Confer *antibiotic resistance to host cell*
- Its complete DNA sequence is known hence precise location of restriction cleavage site for inserting the foreign DNA is available

**Phages**
- Accept *DNA fragment 10-20 kb long*
- *Linear DNA molecule* into which foreign DNA can be inserted at several restriction enzyme sites.

**Cosmids**
- ***Accept larger fragment of DNA, 35-50 kb long***[Q].
- Are plasmids that contain DNA sequence, called *cos sites*, required for packaging lambda DNA into phage particle.

### Cloning Capacities.

| Vector | DNA insert size |
|---|---|
| Plasmid, PBR322 | 0.01- 10kb (kilobases) |
| Phage | 10- 20kb |
| **Cosmid** | ***35- 50kb***[Q] |
| BAC (bacterial artificial chromosome), PAC (E. Coli bacteriophage P1 based) vectors | 50- 250kb |
| YAC (Yeast artificial chromosome) | 500- 3000kb |

## Site Directed Mutagenesis: Alternation in cloned genes produce modified proteins

Cloning can be used not only to overproduce proteins but to produce protein products with *subtle alteration in native* forms. Specific aminoacids may be replaced by **site directed mutagenesis** in two ways

If the appropriate (known) restriction sites flank the sequence to be altered, researchers can simply remove a DNA segment & replace it with a synthetic one that is identical to original except for the desired change

- When known restriction sites are not present, **oligonucleotide - directed mutagenesis** can create a specific DNA sequence change
- A short synthetic DNA strand with a specific base change is annealed to single stranded copy o cloned gene. The mismatch of a single base pair in 15-20 bp does not prevent annealing at appropriate temperatures.
- This annealed strand acts as a primer for synthesis of a duplex DNA (with one mismatch), which is then used to transform cells.
- Cellular DNA repair systems will remove and replace the altered base and restore the gene to its original sequence in 50% cases whereas, ***the other half will remove and replace the normal base , retaining the desired mutation***[Q]
- Changes can also be introduced that involve more than 1 basepair. Or even the parts of 2 genes can be ligated to create **fused gene** and **fusion protein**.

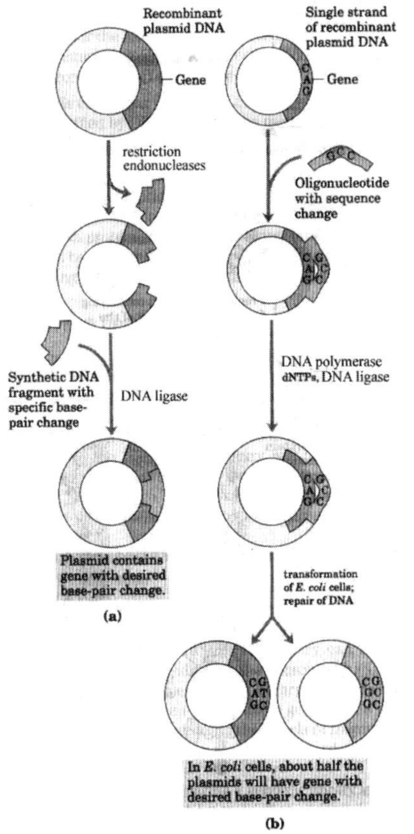


Two approaches to site-directed mutagenesis

## Site Specific Recombination (Exchange) / SSR

- SSR occurs only at a particular short (20-200 bp), unique DNA sequence – the **recombination site (RS)**, where the recombinase enzyme acts. Recombination sites recognized by site specific recombinase are **non palindromic *(partially asymmetrical)*** [Q] and 2 sites align in same orientation during reaction . The outcome depends on location & orientation of recombination sites. If 2 sites are on
  - Same DNA molecule with
    - Same orientation → **Deletion** of intervening DNA
    - Opposite orientation → **Inversion**
  - Two different DNA molecules → If one or both DNAs are circular the result is **insertion**
- ***Recombinase is a site specific endonuclease and ligase in one package***[Q]. Auxillary proteins may regulate timing or outcome of reaction.
- 2 classes of SSR system, with rely on either **Tyr** or **Ser** residues in the active site. A separate recombinase recognize and bind to each RS on same or two different DNA molecules. One DNA strand in each site is cleaved at a specific point & recombinase becomes covalently linked to DNA at cleavage site through phospho tyrosine bond. This transient protein DNA linkage preserves phosphodiester bond that is lost in cleaving the DNA so ATP is unnecessary in subsequent steps. The cleaved DNA strands are rejoined to new parteners to form **Holliday intermediates**, with new phosphodiester bonds created at the expense of protein DNA linkage. The reaction is completed by repeating the process at a 2$^{nd}$ point within each of 2 RS.
- SRS system that employ an **Ser residue active site** , ***both strands of each RS are cut concurrently & rejoined to new partners without the Holliday intemediates***[Q]. In both systems, ***exchange is precise and reciprocal***[Q], regenerating RS when the reaction is complete.

## Linkage Analysis : Indirect DNA Diagnosis

- Direct gene diagnosis is only possible if nucleotide sequence of mutant gene is known, which is not the case in most genetic disorders. Therefore ***mutant gene is indirectly tracked on the basis of its linkage to detectable genetic markers such as naturally occuring variations or polymorphism***[Q]; SNPs, RFLP, STRs (short tandem repals or micro satellites)
- In essence, one has to determine whether a given fetus or family member has inherited the same relevent chromosomal region as a previously affected family member.
- **Linkage analysis** is a statistical technique used to identify location on a chromosome of a given gene involved in a trait or disease relative to a known location of chromosomal marker, in terms of recombination frequency rather than as a specific physical distance. The greater the frequency of recombintion (segregation) between two genetic markers, the farther apart they are assumed to be.
- With linkage analysis all members of family are genotyped for polymorphic markers and then compared to determine which markers are present in family members affected by the disorder. So the primary aim is to determine whether there exist pieces of genome that are passed down through families (with multiple patients) in a pattern that is consistent with a particular inheritance model and that is unlikely to occur by chance alone. Since linkage analysis does not detect mutations in gene directly, further investigation is required once genome of interest is identified.
- **Pedigree** is a diagram of family relationship that uses symbols to represent people (square = male, circle = female) and lines to represent genetic relationship (horizontal line = mating, vertical line extending downward from a couple represent their children). It is often analyzed to *determine the mode of inheritance (dominant or recessive)*. All the individuals that possess the trait / disease are shaded.

## Blotting & Hybridization Techniques

- **Visualization (or detection) of a specific DNA segment (Southern) or RNA fragment (Northern) or particular antigen/protein (Western)** *in a complex mixture of thousands of containinating molecules* requires convergence of a number of techniques (like *restriction enzymes, Agarose / SDS-PAGE electrophoresis, denaturing, blotting renaturing, fixing, probe hybridization* which are collectively termed **blot transfer**.
- Blot technique was developed by EM Southern in 1975, to detect a specific segment of DNA in the whole genome. Southern blotting is named after its inventor, *Edward Southern* and others (northern, western) began as laboratory jargon.

### Procedure

- **Electrophoresis:** For blot transfer, the sample (DNA or RNA or protein) is isolated from cell line or tissue and this complex mixture is pipetted into a well in an agarose or ***sodium dodecyl sulfate (SDS) - polyacrylamide gel for electrophoresis. Electrophoresis seperates sample (DNA / RNA / Protein) according to molecular size (mass)***[Q]; the smaller fragments more most rapidly. In southern blotting, sample DNA is *digested with one or more restriction enzymes* before pipetting and ***exposed to direct electrical current during electrophoresis. DNA being negatively changed move towards anode***[Q].
- **Blotting (Adsorption / Transfer) to Nitrocellulose (Nylon) membrane:** DNA / RNA / Protein within the gel is transferred **(blotted or adsorbed) over to nitrocellulose or nylon paper (membrane)** by covering the gel with paper, resulting in an exact replica of the pattern on the gel. In Southern blotting, *DNA is denatured by exposure to mild alkali (like NaOH) to make it single stranded* before adsorption. During the transfer the SDS is largely removed from some proteins, and there is enough refolding & restoration of conformation so that the antibody probe can react with protein on membrane.
- **Adding Probe & Hybridization:** Before adding probe, DNA is bound (fixed) on the nitrocellulose membrane by exposure to *heat (temp at 80°c) and or UV*. Then paper is **exposed to labeled probe**. The probe is **complementary DNA strand** (c-DNA) labeled with radioisotope or nonradioactive fluorescent label in Southern (DNA) and Northern (RNA) blot tests. *The nucleotide sequence of cDNA is complementary to DNA or RNA*. There will be many DNA/RNA fragments on membrane but only few pieces that contain the target DNA / RNA, hybridize with cDNA probe to make a **DNA-cDNA hybrid in Southern blot or RNA-cDNA hybrid in Northern blot.** Similarly a **labeled antibody probe forms complex with protein (antigen)** in **Western (immuno) blot test** and **labeled nucleic acid probe forms complex with protein in south-Western blot test**.
- **Washing & Autoradiography:** After thorough washing to remove excess probes, the x-ray plate or imaging screen is placed over the nitrocellulose paper in dark for few days. The radiation from fixed probe will produce its *marks in form of several specific bands corresponding to the DNA/RNA/ protein fragment that recognized the probe.*

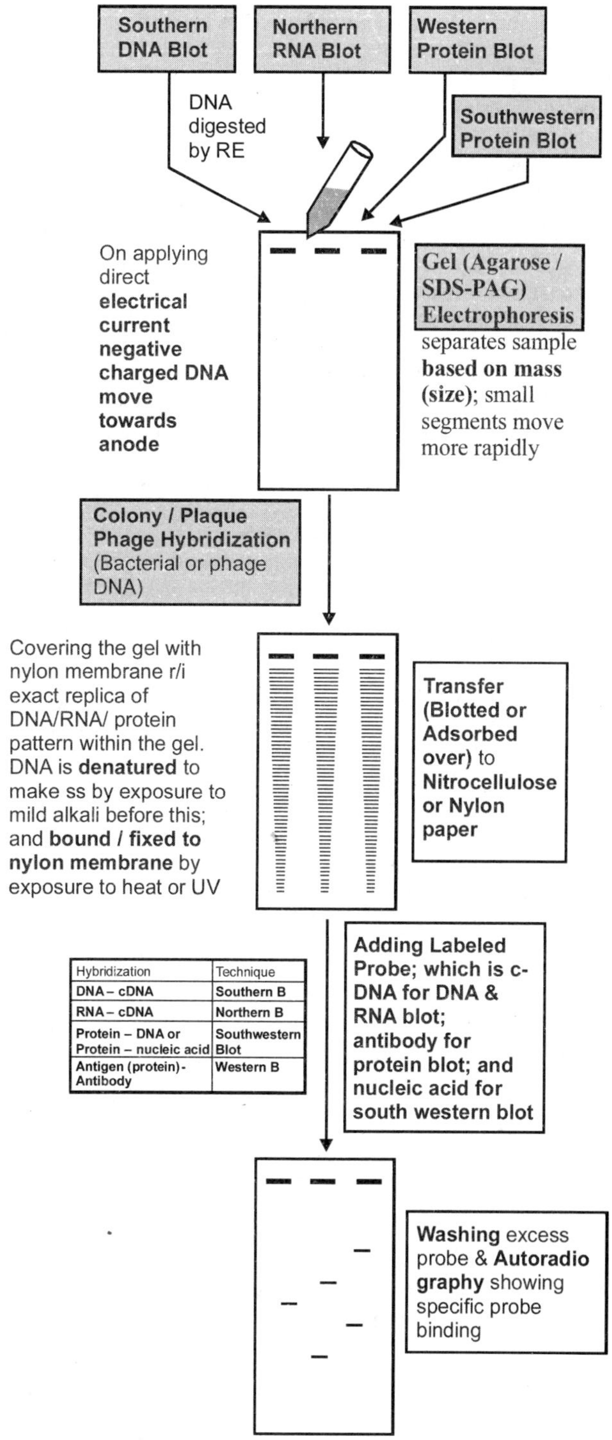


| Hybridization | Technique |
|---|---|
| DNA – cDNA | Southern B |
| RNA – cDNA | Northern B |
| Protein – DNA or Protein – nucleic acid | Southwestern Blot |
| Antigen (protein) - Antibody | Western B |

### Variants

- In **Southwestern hybridization blot technique**, proteins are separated by electrophoresis, blotted to a membrane, renatured, and analyzed for an **protein-DNA (nucleic acid) interaction** by incubation with a specific labeled nucleic acid probe.
- **Colony or Plaque or Phage Hybridization** is a method by which **specific clones of bacteria or phage** grown as colonies on agar plate are **identified and purified**. Nitrocellulose paper is overlaid over agar plate sticking clones from each colony which are fixed permanently by heat (UV and denatured or lysed with NaOH so that its DNA is available to hybridize with cDNA probe. It results in a **clonal isolate (bacterial colony) or individual phage plaque** containing a unique DNA insert.

### Use

- Blotting procedure are **useful in determining amount of gene (DNA)/RNA/ protein** in a given tissue / sample. If a specific base is changed and a restriction site is altered these procedures **can detect point mutations and gene alterations (deletion, insertion or rearrangements)** because the required electrophoresis step sepeates the molecules on the basis of size. Therefore Southern, Northern & Western blot transfer techniques are used to **size, identify and quantitate specific gene (DNA), RNA and protein – respectively**. Mutant genes like HbS, DMD, PKU & cystic fibrosis as well as presence of viral DNA (HBV, HBC) can be identified by Southern blot method. Similarly ***Western blot method confirms diagnosis of AIDS***[Q] (in ELISA positive or HIV positive patients) by demonstrating presence of antibodies in patients serum to a specific HIV protein.
- All hybridization procedures depend on specific base pairing of complementary nucleic acid strands. **Perfect matches hybridize readily & withstand stringent conditions (high temperatures and low salt concentrations).** In the hybridization & washing reactions, less than perfect matches do not tolerate such stringent conditions; thus hybridization either never occur or is disrupted during washing steps. **Gene homology detection and cross species comparison of a gene can be done by varying stringency**.

### Analysis of Gene (DNA) and Products of Gene Expression (mRNA and Proteins)

| Technique | Sample analyzed | Gel used | Probe | Purpose |
|---|---|---|---|---|
| **Southern blot** | *DNA*[Q] | Yes | Radioactive DNA probes | Detects DNA changes & mutation |
| **Allele specific oligonucleotide (ASO)** | DNA | No | Allele specific oligo nucleotide probe | Detects DNA mutation |
| **Microarray** | M-RNA or C-DNA | No | DNA probe | - ***Genotyping* (i.e., gene variation or mutation) by using DNA sample.**<br>- ***Gene expression analysis*** (i.e., patterns of m-RNA production) by using m-RNA & converting it to c-DNA by reverse transcriptase.<br>- Analyze thousands of gene & mRNA at same time<br>- **Tumor fingerprint or transcriptional profile** used to determine the differing (global) pattern of gene expression in two different cells types eg normal & cancer cells (in order to develop most appropriate form of chemotherapy). |
| **Northern blot** | *RNA*[Q] | Yes | DNA probe | Measures ***mRNA***[Q] amounts & sizes |
| **Western (immuno) blot** | *Protein*[Q] | Yes | ***Labeled antibody***[Q] | Measure protein amounts |
| **South Western blot** | Protein, DNA (?) | Yes | **Labelled nucleic acid (DNA) probe** | Examines **protein – DNA (protein-nucleic acid) interactions** |
| **ELISA** | Protein or antibodies | No | ***Antibody***[Q] (specific for protein to be measured) | Detects proteins (antigens) or antibodies |
| **Proteomics** | *Protein*[Q] | Yes | - | Measures abundance, distribution, post translational modifications, function & interactions of cellular proteins |

★ The base sequence of DNA that have been cloned & purified can be determined in the laboratory by – **Sanger dideoxy enzymatic (manual) method** and **Maxam & Gilbert chemical (manual) method**.

## Probes

### DNA probe

- Probe is a *short single stranded piece of DNA*, labelled with a *radioisotope (eg* $P^{32}$*)* or a *non-radioactive probe (eg. biotin)*, and can pick a specific gene or DNA sequence out of the mixture of thousands or millions of irrelevant DNA fragments cleaved by restriction endonucleases. The nucleotide sequence of a probe is *complementary* to the DNA of interest, called the **target DNA.**
- Utility of probes depends on *phenomenon of hybridization (or annealing)* in which a single stranded sequence of a target DNA binds to a probe containing a complementary nucleotide sequence.

### Synthetic oligonucleotide probe

- If sequence of all or part of target DNA is known, single stranded oligonucleotide probes of 20-30 nucleotides can be synthesized that are complementary to gene of interest
- **Allele specific oligonucleotide (ASO)** probe is used to detect the presence of *sickel cell mutation in β-globin gene*

### Biotinylated probes

- Disposal of radioactive probes is expansive, so *now vitamin biotin* coupled nucleotide are used to synthesize probes
- Biotin binds to egg white protein avidin. Avidin can be attached to fluorescent dye detectable optically with great sensitivity. Thus a DNA fragment that hybridizes with biotinylated probe can be made visible by immersing the gel in a solution of dye coupled avidin.

### Antibodies

- When no information is available to guide the synthesis of a probe for direct detection of DNA of interest.
- In this case ***antibody labeled probe directed against the protein of interest***[Q] is used to identify which bacterial colony produces the protein & therefore contains CDNA of interest.

## DNA-Microarray / DNA – Chips

- DNA microarrays *contain thousands* (500-5000) *of immobilized DNA probes /sequences* (few dozen to hundreds of nucleotide long) from known genes organized in an area no longer than a microscope slide. DNA segments (from DNA libraries) are *amplified by PCR* and placed on small wells in a solid polystyrene plates, using robotic devices. Upto million such spots are deposited in a predesigned array on a surface area of just few $cm^2$. An alternate way is to synthesize DNA directly on the solid surface using *photolithography*.
- C-DNA (obtained directly or from mRNA of patients particular cell type or stage) is added to each well, hybridize and fluorescence is assessed to assess genes being expressed in those cells/stage.
- This is based on principles of nucleic acid hybridization like Southern or Northern blot tests but allows simultaneous study of multiple genes or entire genome rather than single gene. Hybridization means binding of complementary strands of nucleic acid a/t Watson-Crick rules (i.e. A = T and G=C binding). *Southern blot for DNA & Northern blot for RNA allows the study /detection of single gene whereas microarray technique (for DNA & RNA) allows detection of multiple genes or entire genome.* So it can be considered as multiple Southern or Northern blot analysis running in parallel.

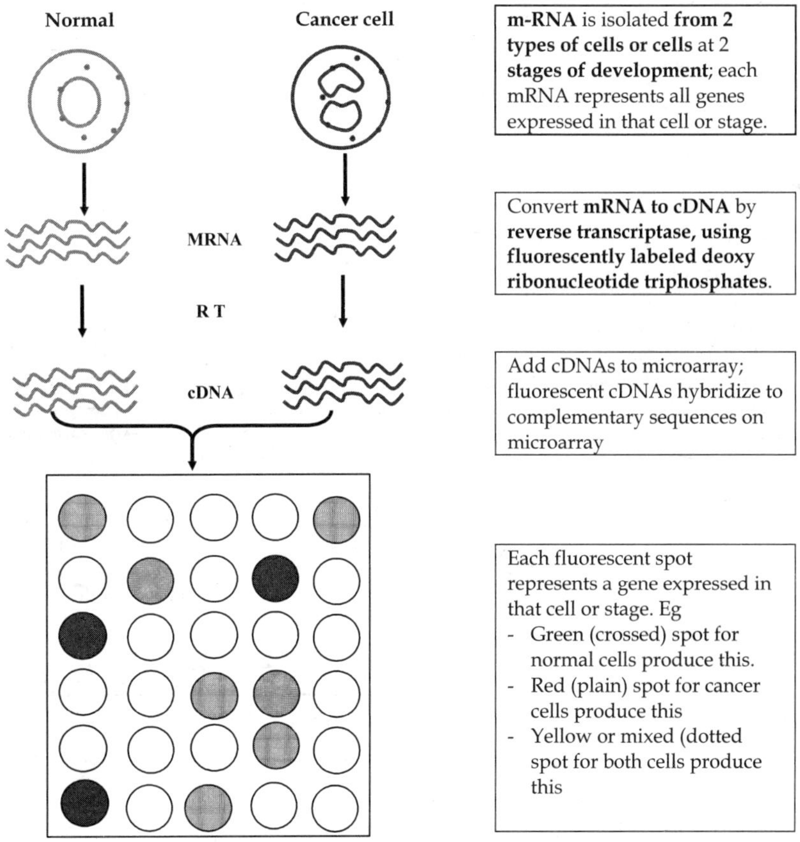


**DNA Microarray Analysis of gene expression**

- Microarrays are used to analyze a sample for presence of **mutation / gene variation (genotyping)** or to determine the patterns of mRNA production (**gene expression analysis**).
  - **For genotyping and mutational analysis**, the cellular sample is genomic DNA. **Microarray based CGH (comparative genomic hybridization)** test can be used as high resolution whole genome scan for the detection or screening of unknown (non specific) abnormalities, mutation or genomic imbalance including deletions, duplication and aneuploidies. Microarray based CGH cannot detect balanced translocations or inversions
  - Microarray is the **most powerful tool for screening gene expression profile** of biological samples. It allows researcher to explore, *expression patterns of thousand of genes (or entire genome)* in a single analysis thus permitting **comprehensive analysis of gene expression profile**. For expression analysis the mRNA from a particular cell type (eg normal and cancer cells) or from same cell type in different stags of development is converted to cDNA & labeled with fluorescent tag. This mixture is then exposed to microarray chip. The amount of fluorescence bound to each spot is a measure of the amount of that particular mRNA in the sample. This tells which genes are expressed in which stage of development or in which cells. The spots that fluoresce provide a **snapshot of all genes being expressed** in the cells at the moment they were harvested - gene expression on genome wide scale.
  - For a gene of unknown function, the time & circumstances of its expression can provide important *clues about its role in the cells.*
  - **Tumor finger print or transcriptional profile** of cancers to tailor treatment regimens.
  - *Genetic fingerprint* of different diseases / malignancies - classifying them, understanding genetic pathophysiology and identifying diagnostic or prognostic markers.

# Methods for Analysis of Gene (DNA, Mutation) & Products Gene Expression (RNA and Protein)

## Methods used for Detection of Mutation (& Analysis of Gene or DNA)

1. Cytogenic analysis
2. Fluorescent in situ hybridization (FISH)
3. *Southern blot*[Q]
4. *Polymerase chain reaction (PCR)*[Q]
5. *Reverse transcriptase PCR (RT PCR)*[Q]
6. *DNA sequencing and DNA cloning*[Q]
7. *Restriction fragment polymorphism (RFLP)*[Q]
8. *Single stranded conformational polymorphism (SSCP)*[Q].
9. *Denaturating gradient gel electrophoresis (DGGE)*[Q]
10. RNAse cleavage
11. Oligonucleotid specific hybridization
12. **Microarrays (c DNA microarrays or DNA chips)**
13. Protein truncation test (PTT).
14. **Pyrosequencing**
15. **Multiplex ligation dependent probe amplification (MLPA)**

## Analysis of Gene Expression Product

### Determination of mRNA levels

1. *Northern blot*[Q]
2. **Microarrays**: In this mRNA from a particular cell is **converted to cDNA** and amplified by **RT-PCR or rererse transcriptase PCR**

### Analysis of Proteins

- *Amount of protein in cells donot always directly correspond to amounts of mRNA* as some mRNAs are translated more efficiently & some proteins undergo post translational modifications.
- For detecting **one or limited number of proteins, antigen (protein) labeled antibody binding is used eg in**
  1. **ELISA (Enzyme linked immuo sorbent assay)**
  2. **Western (Immuno) blots**
- When **analyzing abundance & interactions of large number of proteins** (called **proteomics**), automated methods are employed such as.
  1. *Two dimensional (2D) gel electrophoresis*[Q]
  2. *Mass spectroscopy*[Q]
  3. *Multidimensional liquid chromatography*[Q]
  4. **Bioinformatics**

# DNA (Gene) Library

DNA or gene library is *collection of cloned restriction fragments of DNA of an organism*. It can be of 2 types

## Genomic - DNA library

- It is the *largest type* of DNA library, created when the *complete genome of a particular organism is cleaved into thousands of fragments by restriction endonuclease* and all the fragments are cloned by insertion into a *cloning vector*.
- This (amplified DNA fragments) represent the entire genome of an organism including introns and control regions. It is prepared by RE & cloning in following way
  - 1[st] step **is partial digestion of DNA** (of an organism) by restriction endonucleases (RE) in which either the amount or the time of action of enzyme is limited.
  - RE that cut very frequently (recognize 4bp) are generally used. Complete digestion is not done as it would fragment the gene of interest (i.e. it is not contained in any one clone) as most genes contain > 1 restriction sites. Whereas partial digestion provides gene of interet in DNA fragments of range of sizes (~ 20 kb)
  - *Too small or too large fragments* (inadequate for cloning) *are removed* by electrophoresis or centrifugation. Clonic vector (BAC or YAC) plasmid is cleaved with the same RE and ligated to partially digested genomic DNA fragments.
  - Now each transformed yeast or bacterium cell grows into a colony or clone of identical cells, each bearing the same plasmid containing one of many genes represented in overall library.
- *Hybridization* methods can order individual clones in sequence by identifying clones with overlapping sequences. **Sequence tagged site (STS)** can provide landmarks for genomic sequencing projects. A set of over lapping clones represents a catalog for a long contiguous segment of a genome, often referred to as a **contig**.

## Complementary (c) DNA library

- It is a *specialized library* designed to *study gene function* – so it includes only those *genes that are expressed i.e. are transcribed into mRNA*. So cDNA libraries lack introns & control regions.
- **It is prepared by *using m-RNA as a template to make a complementary DNA (cDNA) catalyzed by enzyme reverse transcriptase (RNA dependent DNA polymerase)***[Q]. (The mRNA is isolated from tRNA and r-RNA by the presence of its poly tail)
- The resulting double stranded c-DNA can be amplified by PCR or cloning (i.e. inserting into a suitable vector and creating a population of clones) resulting in c-DNA libraries.
- To aid mapping of large genomes, cDNAs can be partially sequenced to produce a useful type of STS called **expressed sequence tag (EST)**.
- cDNA libraries are made more specialized by cloning cDNAs into a vector that fuses cDNA sequence with the sequence for **marker** or **reporter gene**-thus forming reporter construct. 2 useful markers include
  - **Green fluorescent protein (GFP)** gene which generates fusion protein which is highly fluorescent protein that literally lights up.
  - **Epitope tag** protein that bounds mono clonal antibody & precipitates.
- Because cDNA has no intervening (intron & control regions etc) sequences, it can be cloned into an **expression vector** for synthesis of eukaryotic proteins (like human insulin) by bacteria. These (plasmid of) expression vector contain bacterial promoter (for transcription) and *Shine Dalgarno sequence* /SDS (to initiate translation).

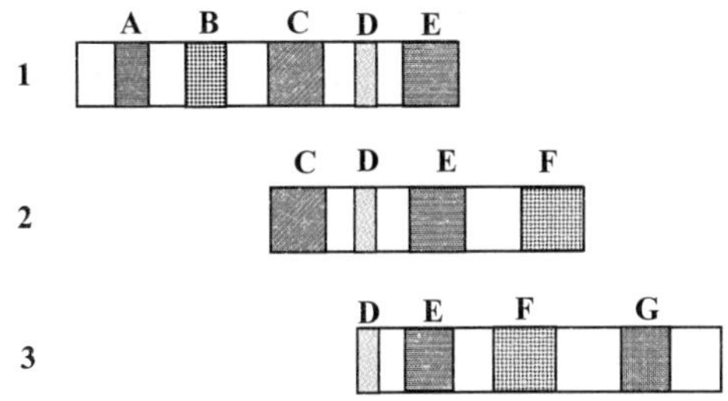


So the sequence of partially digested & cloned fragments is 1 → 2 → 3

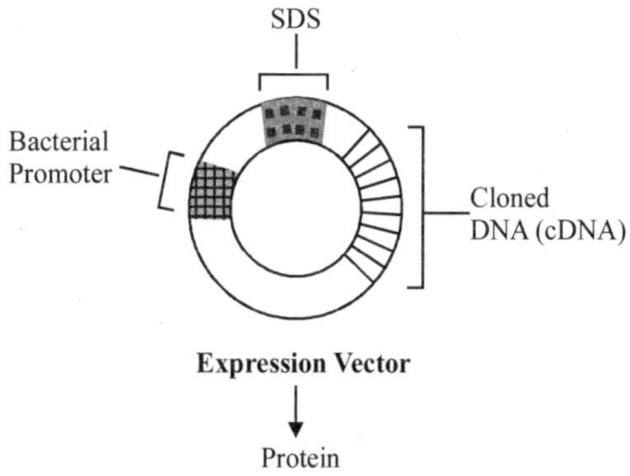


## Biotechnology / Recombinant DNA technology / Genetic Engineering

It is a method by which a living organism or its parts (i.e. DNA/genes) are used *to change / incorporate* a particular character to another living organism.
It involves use of *restriction endonuclease* (to cut a particular gene) and PCR or cloning (to amplify it). It can be used for

- **Quantitative production of human biomolecules, genetic products by bacteria eg**
  - Human insulin
  - Erythropoietins, anticoagulants
  - Plasminogen activators
  - Cell growth factos, GF, Colony stimulating factor
  - ***Interferons, interleukins***[Q]
  - *Recombinant vaccines* eg rabies vaccine, hepatitis B vaccine
  - Monoclonal antibodies
  - Superoxide dismutase

  This method produces biological substances without any risk of contamination (like hepatitis B virus)
- **Creation of gene library**

**Somatic Gene Therapy**

- It is intracellular delivery of desired genes to ***cure a genetic disorder***[Q] by correcting an existing abnormality.
- It is tried in SCID, cystic fibrosis, Duchene MD, familial hyper cholesterolemia etc.

**Gene production**

New genes can be produced to be incorporated in
- ***Genetic crops***[Q]
- **Transgenic animals**

Production of specific **DNA probes** for diagnosis/identification of
- Antenatal genetic disease
- Mutation / onchogenesis
- Sex, parent or criminal etc.

## Production of Human Insulin by Genetic Engineering

- Because obtaining a human DNA with specific insulin gene is a laborious process, it is easier to ***begin the process by obtaining insulin mRNA from beta cells of pancreas***[Q], where insulin is produced in abundance (and obtaining specific mRNA is easier).
- **Complementary (c) DNA containing the insulin gene** is prepared by using human insulin mRNA (from pancreatic beta cells) as a template and **reverse transcriptase enzyme**.
- This **c-DNA containing insulin gene to be cloned is inserted into plasmid vector**. Bacterial plasmids are small, circular, duplex DNA molecules whose natural function is to confer antibiotic resistance to host cell. They exist as single or multiple copies within bacterium and replicate independtly from the bacterial DNA while using primarily the host replication machinery. The complete DNA sequence of many plasmids are known; so the precise location of RE cleavage sites for inserting foreign DNA (for cloning) is available. Plasmids are easily separated from host chromosome because of smaller size and the desired plasmid - inserted DNA can be easily removed by cutting plasmid with enzyme specific for restriction site into which the original piece of cloned DNA was inserted. **Plasmids produce millions of clones containing same insulin gene.**
- Bacteria (E.coli) containing insulin gene are grown in optimal conditions; insulin produced is isolated, collected & purified.

**Insulin mRNA of human pancrease beta cells**
↓
**c-DNA by reverse transcriptase**
↓
**Cloned into plasmid vector** to produce many copies of same gene
↓
Bacteria (E.coli) grown in optimal production conditions
↓
Produced insulin is collected isolated & purified

## Recombination DNA Technology (Research) & Enzymes Used in it

- It is a *genetic engineering which effects artificial modification* of genetic constitution of a living cell by introduction of foreign DNA experimental techniques. It involves.
  - *Splicing the DNA by restriction endonuclease,*
  - *Preparation of chimeric DNA molecule* followed by
  - *Cloning* for production of large number of target DNA molecules
- The biological tools required are – **enzymes, vector (vehicle) DNA** (i.e. bacterial plasmids, cosmids & bacteriophage), and **passenger (foreign) DNA** (i.e. complementary DNA, synthetic or random DNA to be introduced into the vector). Enzymes used are

**Enzymes used in Recombinant DNA Technology / Genetic Engineering**

| Enzyme | Function | Primary Use |
|---|---|---|
| **Restriction Endonuclease (Type II)** | - Cleave DNAs at a specific base sequences k/a **recognition sequences** or **restriction sites**.<br>- **Cut (splice or cleave)** DNA of any source into short pieces in a **sequence specific manner** in contrast to other methods. eg enzymatic, physical or chemical that break DNA in random fashion. | **Key enzyme** used as **chemical knife**, in recombinant DNA technology<br>Originally called **restriction enzymes** because their presence in a given bacteria restricted the growth of certain viruses (bacterio phages) |
| **Example** | **Cleaved Sequence** | **Bacterial Source** |
| Eco RI | G AATT C<br>C TTAA G | E. Coli Ry 13 |
| H Pa I | GTT AAC<br>CAA TTG | Haemophilus parainfluenzae |
| Bam HI | G GATC C<br>C CTAG G | Bacillus amylliquifaciens H |
| Eco RII | CCTGG<br>GGACC | E. Coli R 245 |
| Pst I | CTGCA G<br>G ACGTC | Providencia stuartii 164 |
| **DNA ligase** | Catalyzes the formation of new photodiester bonds in a reaction that uses ATP (or similar cofactor) between DNA molecules | ***Joining DNA molecules eg after digestion by RE. DNA strands can be joined again by DNA ligase***[Q]. |
| **Bacteriophage λ Exonuclease** | ***Removes nucleotides from 5′ ends of dsDNA to expose single stranded 3′ end***[Q] | DNA sequencing |
| **Exonuclease III** | ***Removes nucleotides from 3′ ends of DNA***[Q] | DNA sequencing; mapping protein-DNA interactions |
| **BAL 31 Nuclease** | Degrades both the 3′ and 5′ ends of DNA | Progressive shortening of DNA molecules |
| **S1 Nuclease** | ***Degrades single-stranded DNA***[Q] | Removal of "hairpin" in synthesis of cDNA; RNA mapping studies (both 5′ and 3′ ends) |
| **DNase I** | Under appropriate conditions, produces single-stranded nicks in DNA | Nick translation; mapping of hypersensitive sites; mapping protein-DNA interactions. |
| **Alkaline phosphatase** | - Dephosphorylates 5′ ends of RNA and DNA<br>- Removes terminal phosphate from either 5′ or 3′ ends (or both) - Lehninger | Removal of 5′-PO4 groups prior to kinase labeling to prevent self-ligation. |
| **Thermostable DNA polymerase I (E. coli)** | - ***Synthesizes double-stranded DNA from single-stranded DNA***[Q]<br>- ***Fills gap in duplex by stepwise addition of nucleotides to 3′ end*** | Synthesis of double-stranded cDNA; nick translation; generation of blunt ends from sticky ends. |
| **Reverse transcriptase *(RNA dependent DNA polymerase)***[Q] | ***Synthesizes DNA from RNA template***[Q] (i.e. makes DNA copy of an RNA molecule) | Synthesis of cDNA from mRNA; RNA (5′ end) mapping studies. |
| **Polynucleotide kinase** | - Adds a phosphate to 5′-OH end of polynucleotide to label it or permit ligation.<br>- Transfers terminal phosphate (γ position) from ATP to 5′-OH groups of DNA or RNA | $^{32}P$ labeling of DNA or RNA |
| **Terminal transferase** | Adds nucleotides (**homopolymer tails**) to 3′-OH ends of DNA (linear duplex). | **Homopolymer tailing** |

## Genomics

- ***Study of organism's entire genome (i.e. set of genes)***[Q]
- **Genome** is set of all genes expressed by an organism
- *Genome of an organism is constant, so it's less complicated* process and involves study of structure of genome including maping & sequencing and ***enables primary sequence of protein to be identified easily***[Q] from small amounts of sequence data. All that remains is to aquire open reading frame (ORF) that encodes protein.
- Picture provided is both *static & incomplete* and *represents the begining* of the task of undarstanding the dynamics of growth, aging & diseases process.

## Glycomics

Deals with the ***structure & function of chains of sugar (oligosaccharides)***[Q]. Glycome refers to the identity of the entirely of carbohydrates in an organism

## Bioinformatics

A scientific discipline that combines the tools and techniques of mathematics, computer science and biology with the aim of understanding the biologic significance of variety of data.

## Cytogenetics

Branch of genetics concern with structure and function of cell, especially the chromosome.

## Pharmacogenomics

The study of genetically determined variations in responses to drugs in human or in laboratory organisms.

## Proteomics

- ***Quantitative & qualitative study of entire proteome (all expressed protein)***[Q]. **Preteome** is the set of all proteins expressed by a cell at particularly time. It is *more complicated* as it involves the ***study of all protein expressed by a genome, including their relative abundance, distribution, post translational modifications, functions, & interactions with other macro molecules***[Q].
- It aims to identify the entire complement of proteins expressed by a cell *under diverse condition*. So it provides *more complete, dynamic & advanced picture* of growth, aging & disease. Example includes **identification of proteins whose levels of expression correlate with medically significant events**, like whose appearance or disappearance is associated with a specific physiological condition or disease.
- Basic steps include **sample preparation, protein separation, protein imaging and identification**. It can be done by

1. **Gene Array (DNA Chips)** in which the expression of m RNA that encodes protein is detected. It is more sensitive the 2 D gels, particularly with respect to low abundance proteins. However, changes in expression of mRNA encoding a protein do not necessarily reflect comparable changes in level of corresponding protein.
2. **Multidimensional protein identification technology (Mud PIT)** employs *successive rounds of chromatography* to resolve the peptides produced from digestion of complex biological sample into many simpler fractions that can be analyzed by **mass spectroscopy**.
3. **2-Dimensional electrophoresis: Isoelectric focusing (IEF) is used in conjunction with SDS-PAGE** for 2D (two dimensional) electrophoresis, which *seperates polypeptides based on PI on one dimension and molecular mass (Mr) in second*. 2D electrophoresis is particularly used for separating the components of complex mixtures of proteins. Individual polypeptides are then extracted and analyzed by **Edman sequencing** or **mass spectroscopy**.

★ Proteins & peptides must be **purified** prior to analysis by various **chromatography techniques**. Then protein **purity is assessed by SDS-PAGE** (sodium dodecyl sulfate polyacrylamide gel electrophoresis). **Edman reaction** enables peptide & proteins to be sequenced. **Mass spectroscopy** is more sensitive method for determining sequences of peptides and proteins. MS determines mass of molecules and can be used to *analyze metabolites, carbohydrates and post translational modification* such as phosphorylation or hydroxylation that add *readily identified increaments of mass to a protein*.

## Human Genome Project

### Principle Methods Used

| Procedure | Comments |
|---|---|
| Detection of specific cytogenic abnormalities | For instance, a small deletion of band Xp21.2 was important in cloning the gene involved in Duchenne muscular dystrophy |
| Extensive linkage studies | Large families with defined pedigrees are desirable. Dominant genes are easier to recognize than recessives |
| Use of probes to define marker loci | Probes identify STSs, RFLPs, SNPs etc; thousands, covering all the chromosomes, are now available. It is desirable to flank the gene on both sides, clearly delineating it. |
| **Radiation hybrid mapping** | Now the *most rapid method of localizing a gene or DNA fragment to a subregion of a human chromosome* and constructing a physical map. |
| Use of rodent of human somatic cell hybrids | Permits assignment of a gene to one specific chromosome but not to a subregion. |
| Fluorescence in situ hybridization | Permits localization of a gene to one chromosomal band. |

### Major Findings

- More than 90% of the genome has been sequenced; gaps, large and small, remain to be filled in.
- Estimated number of protein – coding genes ranges from 30,000 to 40,000.
- Only 1.1-1.5% of the genome codes for proteins.
- There are wide variations in feature of individual chromosomes (eg in gene number per Mb, SNP density, GC content, numbers of transposable elements and CpG islands, recombination rate).
- Human genes do more work

| Use of pulsed-field gel electrophoresis (PFGE) to separate large DNA fragments | Permits isolation of a large DNA fragments obtained by use of restriction endonucleases (rare cutters) that result in very limited cutting of DNA. |
|---|---|
| **Chromosome walking** | *Involves repeated cloning of overlapping DNA segments*; the procedure is laborious and can usually cover only *100-200 kb.* |
| **Chromosome jumping** | By cutting DNA into relatively large fragments and circularizing it, one can *move more quickly and cover greater lengths of DNA than with chromosomal walking.* |
| Cloning via YACs, BACs, cosmids, phages, plasmids | Permits isolation of fragments of varying lengths |
| Detection of expression of mRNAs in tissues by Northern blotting using one or more fragments of the gene as a probe | The mRNA should be expressed in affected tissues |
| **PCR** | Can be used to *amplify fragments of the gene;* |
| **DNA sequencing** | Establishes the highest resolution physical map. Identifies open reading frame. Facilities with many high throughput instruments could sequence millions of base pairs per day. |
| Databases | Comparison of DNA and protein sequences obtained from unknown gene with known sequence in databases can facilitte gene identification |

than those of the roundworm or fruit fly (eg alternative splicing is used more frequently).
- The human proteome is more complex than that found in invertebrates.
- Repeat sequences probably constitute more than 50% of the genome.
- Approximately 100 coding regions have been copied and moved by RNA-based transposons.
- Approximately 200 genes may be derived from bacteria by lateral transfer.
- More than 3 million SNPs have been identified

## Nude (Nu) Mouse / Nude Defect

- Nude defect is characterized by **absence of both hair and thymus**. A profound T cell defect can result from faulty thymus development (eg **Di George syndrome** d/t detection in long arm of chromosome 22 and **CHARGE** – coloboma of eye, heart anamoly, choanal atresia, retardation, genital and ear anomalies syndrome d/t CHD 7 deficiency) leading to virtually no T cells. However, expansion of oligo clonal T cells can occur; these cases require thymic graft.
- **Nude mouse** is a laboratory mouse *mutant with disruption of FOX N1 gene* ***(an autosomal recessive mutation on chromosome 11 nu locus), causing lack of body hair and absent/deteriorated thymus (=thymus aplasia)***Q. Because of lack of thymus, nude mice can not produce mature T cell lymphocytes resulting in **deficiency / greatly reduced number of T cells**. Nude mouse **do not generate cytotoxic effector cells, CD 8/4 T cells and are insusceptible to graft versus host disease.** Therefore these **can receive various types of Xenograft and allograft transplants**, in form of tissue and tumor grafts and ***sustain them for weeks***Q (used in research to test new methods of imaging & treating tumors).
- Nude mouse are unable to mount most immune responses such as
  1. **Lack graft rejection** (d/t lack of CD4+ and CD8+ T cells)
  2. Lack **cell mediated immune response** (which requires CD4 + and/or CD8+ Tcells)
  3. Lack **delayed type hypersensitivity response** (requires CD4 + T cells) and some **antibody formation** that require CD4 + helper T cells.
  4. Lack **killing of malignant / virus infected cells** (which requires CD8+ cytotoxic cells)
- Most nude mice are **leaky** (more so on aging) and **have few T cells**. Therefore, now these are less popular in research and **knock out** (eg RAG1 & RAG2 **knock out**) mice with more complete defects in immune system are preferred.

## Genetically Modified Animals

**Genetically modified animals** are produced by *transgenic* pronuclear injection, forward genetics (i.e. mutations created randomly by ENU=N-ethyl-N-nitrourea), *targeted knock in and knock out*, congenic strains (mating of inbred donor, diseased phenotype with inbred recipient strain to identify genome responsible for disorder) and *cloning.*

### Transgenic Expression (Animals)

- Transgenic animals are produced by pronuclear injection of transgene (genomic DNA or cDNA construct) into the nuclei of fertilized ovum. There is *no way to control where that gene eventually resides (ie random integration of transgene).* Transgene has variable copy number and variable expression in each individual founder. Transgenic (animals)

### Targeted (Directed or Conditional) Approaches; Knock out & Knock In

Creation of gene knock in and knock out (targeted) take advantage of the fact that *a segment of DNA (gene) can be substituted by another homologous (identical) or nearly identical DNA segment* by recombination. This allow integration of deletions that disrupt gene function (**targeted knock out**) or integration of selected mutations into **targeted gene** (i.e. targeted knock in).

expression can be

1. **Loss of function models** using **antisense** and **dominant negative transgenes**
2. **Gain of function models** d/t **over expression** using tissue specific promoter
3. Inducible expression (tetracycline, ecdysone)

- It can be produced by ***microinjecting one or few cloned genes into the nuclei of fertilized egg (ovum) of experimental animal (eg mouse)***Q. The successful introduction of recombinant DNA into an animal can be illustrated by an experiment that permanently altered an easily observable inheritable physical trait. Microinjection of DNA into the nuclei of fertilized mouse eggs can produce efficient transformation (chromosomal integration). When the injected eggs are introduced into a female mouse & allowed to develop, the new gene is often expressed in some of new born mice.
- Unlike, somatic cell gene replacement therapy (or gene therapy) which *would not be passed on to offspring, this process of generating transgenic animal would alter germ cell lines and be passed on to offsprings*.
- If gene becomes successfully integrated into a chromosome, it will be present in both somatic cells and germline of resulting animal & is *passed along from generation to generation*.
- So transgenic animals ***have same genome as parents except few (1 or more) genes***Q that have been integrated or inactivated. Those in which the germline has been altered can be identified by testing their offspring. By careful breeding of these mice, **transgenic line** in which all the mice are homozygous for new gene or genes can be established.
- Hundrends of transgenic animals are established and these are useful for *analysis of tissue specific effect on gene expression and effects of over production of gene products (eg those from the growth hormone gene or onchogenes*) and in discovering genes involved in development.
- A *giant super mouse* is produced by injecting the gene for rat growth hormone into fertilized mouse egg or transgenic cows or goats can be designed to produce human proteins like *clotting factor in* their *milk*.
- Similarly genetic hypogonadism in mice can be treated (in offsprings) by injecting DNA with coding sequence for GnRH (gonadotropin releasing hormone) precursor.
- Transgenic stratigies can be divided into 2 main approches

1) Expression of a gene by random insertion into genome (pronuclear injection of trransgene)
2) Deletion or targeted mutagenesis of a gene by homologous recombination with the native endogenous gene (knock out, knock in).

- Transgenic expression of gene can be useful for studying **disorders that are sensitive to gene dosage**. Eg over expression of PMP 22 gene l/t high level of peripheral myelin protein 22 (type I Charcot-Marie tooth disease); SRY gene in females induce formation of testis. ***Transgenic introduction of CAG trinucleotide repeat causes Hutingtons disease, whereas targeted delition (knock out) of Hutington's disease gene does not induce neurological disorder***Q. (ie gain of function for CAG encoded polyglutamine containing protein)
- Transgenic strategies can be **used as precursors to gene therapy**. Eg expression of dystrophin corrects Duchenne's muscular dystrophy in mouse

| Targeted Knock In Animals | Targeted Knock Out (Gene Disruption) Animals |
|---|---|
| • *Introduction of a subtle mutation* (s) into a gene by substitution of a normal endogenous gene with a mutant gene (carrying a specific mutation) by homologous recombination in embryonic stem cell is called **(targeted) knock in**. It occurs d/t substitution of endogenous gene with gene carrying a subtle mutation (i.e. adding few genes).<br>• These are predominantly used in mice and can accurately model human disease<br>• Targeted expression of onchogene is used to study mechanism of neoplasia & to generate immortalized cell lines. Eg expression of simian virus (SV) 40 large T antigen under direction of insulin promoter induces formation of islet cell tumors. | • It is substitution of functional gene with inactive gene by homologous recombination in embryonic stem cell.<br>• It is *selective removal of a gene from genome*. Gene knockout animals are *made by creating a mutation that totally disrupts the function of a gene*. In other words, rather than introducing a functional gene into animal, a non functional version is inserted.<br>• It is a way of *establishing the function of inactivated gene* or to study corresponding human disease.<br>• Both Mi RNAs and DNA recombinases inactivate gene expression.<br>• Techniques disrupting targeted genes take advantage of particular promoter enhancer combinations driving expression of *DNA recombinases or mi RNAs, both of which inactivate gene expression (targeted knock out)*.<br>• It is predominantly used in mice. Tissue specific knock out is possible (Cre / Iox). ***Absence of phenotype may occur d/t gene redundancy***Q or subtle phenotype. For eg **deletion of HPRT gene (Hprt) does not cause characteristic features of Lesch Nyhan syndrome in mice** b/o their reliance on adenine phosphoribosyl transferase (APRT) in purine salvage. **Deletion of retinoblastoma gene (Rb) encoding p 105 does not l/t retinoblastoma** or other human syndromes in mice. However, mice with combinatorial deletion of several Rb related proteins exhibit features similar to human disorder. |

This replacement of one gene in embryonic stem cell creates a *heterozygous transgenic animals*. The mating in 2 such animals will result in *25% of homozygous offsprings* (a/t mendelian law). Careful breeding will establish **transgenic (animal) line** ***in which all animals are homozygous for new gene / genes***Q.

**Forward Genetics**

- Mutations created randomly by ENU (N-ethyl-N-nitrourea)
- Selection of phenotype followed by genetic characterization
- Useful for identifying novel genes

**Congenic strains**

- Mating of an inbred donor strain with a disease phenotype with an inbred recipient strain in order to define the genomic region responsible for the disorder
- Useful for mapping disease-causing genes

**Cloning**

- Introduction of nucleus into enucleated eggs (nuclar transfer)
- Successful in several mammalian species including sheep (Dolly), mice, cows, monkeys
- Cloning of genetically identical individuals
- May effect lifespan
- Ethical concerns

## Gene Therapy

- It implies to *correct the basic genetic abnormality*. The principle is to *insert the normal, cloned DNA for defective gene* into somatic cells.
- **Gene therapy** is a procedure involving *inserting (or sometimes deleting portions of gene* in diseased patients for the purpose of cure. In *somatic gene therapy*, the recipient's genome is changed but the change is not passed along the next generation. Whereas, in germ line gene therapy, change is passed to next generation.
- **Antisense gene therapy** or **gene silencing** selectively inactivate (or turn off) a mutated gene by RNA interference using short synthetic double stranded **siRNA (small interfacing RNA)**

- Procedure involves
- ***Replacement***[Q]: Mutant gene removed & replaced with normal gene.
- **Correction** : Only mutated area of affected gene would be corrected & the remainder will be unchanged.
- ***Augmentation:*** Introduction of foreign genetic material into a cell to compensate for the defective product of mutant gene.
- Gene of interest is usually administered via a **viral** (retro, adeno, adenoassociated, lenti viruses etc) **vector** or **non viral plasmid liposome (cationic lipid) complex**, used as gene transfer vehicle.
- **Gene therapy is used in**

- **SCID (severe combined immunodeficiency disease)** or **bubble bay syndrome,** which occurs d/t mutation in either *adenosine deaminase gene* or a X-linked gene coding for an *interleukin receptor subunit*, is the *first disease that was successfully treated by gene therapy.*
- ***Cystic fibrosis***[Q]
- Familial hypercholesterolemia
- Duchene muscular dystrophy, Hemophilia, Leber's hereditary optic neuropathy.
- *Lesh – Nyhan syndrome, phenylketonuria (PKU)* are most likely candidates for future gene therapy. Single gene disorders are best candidates for gene therapy. However, unfortunately most prevalent disorders such as heart disease, high BP, Alzheimer's disease, diabetes and arthritis are multigene disorders.

**Techniques to transfer genes (foreign material) into cells**

- ***Sites directed recombnation***[Q]
- Soil bacterium Agrobacterium tumefaciens (containing Ti plasmid) and Agrobacterium E. coli are used for plants
- ***Intranuclear microinjection***[Q]
- **Transduction** using viral vectors like *retrovirus, adenovirus, adeno associated virus, herpes simplex virus and lenti viruses.* Adenovirus lacks a mechanism for integrating DNA into chromosome. Therefore adenoviral vector is expressed for only a short time and then destroyed. This is useful if the objective is **transient expression of gene**. Adenovirus are used for introduction of cystic fibrosis gene in respiratory tract cells. Other possible vectors are- Epstein Barr viruses, herpes, simian virus 40, papilloma, non human lentiviruses, and hepatitis viruses.
- **Transfection** using non-viral methods like plasmid liposome complex using calcium phosphate precipitated DNA. Liposomes (cationic lipids) are small vesicles consisting of lipid bilayer that encloses an aquous compartment.
- **Electroporation :** It employs *pulsed electric field* using small electric current, which *transiently increase the permeability of plasma* membrane thus allowing intake of extracellular macromolecules including DNA.

Mn-"**SITE**"

## Inheritance of X-linked Recessive Disease

**X linked recessive inheritance** is a sex linked disorders i.e. they are transmitted by sex chromosomes. Remember that all sex linked diseases are linked to X chromosome so it is quiet obvious that none of the sex linked disease (whether X-linked recessive or X-linked dominant) will be transmitted from father to son, as **father transmits only 'Y' chromosome to the son.** Other characteristic of this disorder is that it is mostly seen in males. Where as the diseases transmitted through non sex chromosomes (autosomes) have equal male and female incidence.

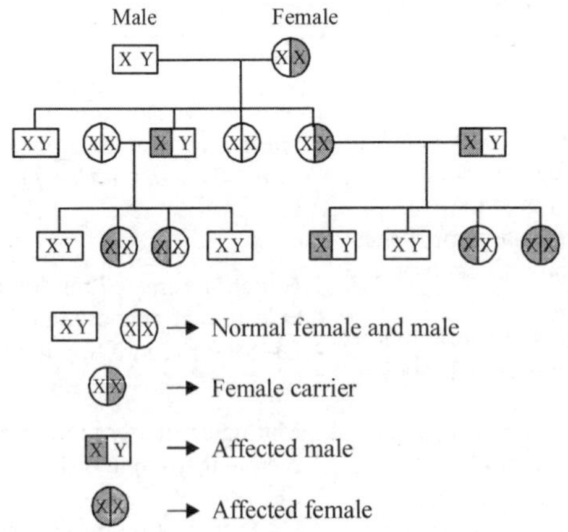


- *An affected male does not transmit the disorder to his sons, but all daughters are carriers*
- *Sons of heterozygous woman have 50% chance of receiving the abnormal gene*
- *It usually affects males because of the presence of Y chromosome which is not homologous to X chromosome and therefore the mutant genes on the X is not paired with alleles on the Y*
- *It is rare in females only possible when mother is carrier and father has overt disease.*

Most of the X linked disorders are X linked recessive. There are only **few X-linked dominant conditions**. These are

- Pseudohypoparathyoidism
- Hypophosphetemic rickets.
- Vit D resistant rickets
- Incontinentia pigmenti

**X-linked Recessive Disorders**

(1) ***Duchenne & Becker muscular dystrophy***[Q]
(2) ***Hemophilia A and B***[Q]
(3) *Chronic granulomatous disease (70% XLR, 30% AR)*
(4) ***Glucose 6-$PO_4$ dehydrogenase deficiency***[Q]
(5) *Agammaglobulinemia*
(6) *Wiskott Aldrich syndrome*
(7) *Diabetes insipidus*
(8) *Fragile X syndrome*
(9) *Lesch Nyhan syndrome*
(10) *Fabry disease*
(11) *Hunter's disease*
(12) *Colour blindness*
(13) *Ocular albinism*
(14) *Sideroblastic anemia*

## Autosomal Recessive (AR) Disorders

### Metabolic

| | |
|---|---|
| **All** | **Al**binism[Q] |
| **Anti** | α1 **Anti**trypsin deficiency[Q] |
| **Ha** | **Ha**rtnup disease[Q] |
| **He** | **He**mochromatosis[Q] |
| **Ho** | **Ho**mocystinuria[Q] |
| **Gla** | **Gala**ctosemia[Q] |
| **Gly** | **Glyco**gen storage disease[Q] |
| **La** | **La**urence Moon Biedl Syndrome[Q] |
| **Ly** | **Ly**sosomal storage disease[Q] |
| **Will** | **Wil**son's disease[Q] |
| **Use** | **Us**her's syndrome[Q] |
| **Cystic** | **Cystic** Fibrosis[Q] |
| **Urea** | Phenylketon**uria**[Q] |

Mn – **"All Anti Ha He Ho Gla Gly, La Ly will Use Cystic Urea"**

### Hematopoetic

| | |
|---|---|
| **See** | **S**ickle cell anemia[Q]<br>Thala**semia** - α & β[Q] |
| **And** | Leucocyte **adhesion** deficiency |
| **Check** | **Chediak** – Higashi syndrome[Q] |
| **My** | **Mye**loperoxidase deficiency |
| **Fan** | **Fan**coni syndrome |

Mn – **"See And Check My Fan"**

### Endocrine

- Congenital adrenal hyperplasia
- Pendred syndrome

### Nervous

- *Friedrich ataxia*[Q]
- Neurogenic muscular atrophy
- Spinal muscular atrophy

### Skeletal

| | |
|---|---|
| All | **Al**kaptonuria |
| Pets | Osteo**petr**osis |
| Fail | Klippel **Feil** syndrome |
| Don's | **Dan**los **Ehl**er syndrome |
| Exam | |

### Urinary

- *Barter syndrome*[Q]
- *Gitelman syndrome*[Q]
- Nephronophthisis
- Nephrogenic diabetes insipidus (also XL)
- *AR polycystic kidney diseasse*[Q]

### Gastrointestinal

- Familial Mediterranean fever

### Other

- Bloom syndrome

## Genetically Transmitted Disorders

Normal parents means parents who are 'clinically normal' with no manifestation of any 'disease' during any part of their life time. But these may still be 'abnormal' (1) genetically i.e. carrying single allele of recessive disease that needs 2 recessive alleles to be manifested or (2) non genetically carrying silent or infective agents.

### Autosomal dominant (AD)

For a child with an autosomal dominant disorder to be affected at least one parent needs to have the affected allele

*Because the allele is dominant it will always express phenotipiclly and hence both parents can not be normal*

Genotype of Affected Child with autosomal dominant disorder

Tt (phenotypically abnormal parent 1) + Tt (phenotypically normal parent 2)

T ↓ t

Tt (affected offspring in AD disorder)

### Autosomal recessive (AR)

For a child with an autosomal recessive disorder to be affected he needs to have atleast two recessive alleles, one from each parent.

***Because the allele is recessive, it might not express in either parents and both parents can be phenotypically normal.***

Genotype of Affected Child with autosomal recessive disorder

Tt (phenotypically normal parent 1) + Tt (phenotypically normal parent 2)

T ↓ t

TT (affected offspring in AR disorder)

### Polygenic disorder

- A trait is called 'polygenic' if multiple genes on thought to contribute to the phenotype.
- Polygenic disorders include Hypertension Diabetes, Asthma
- ***A male infant with asthma or diabetes may will be born to normal parents***

### Vertically transmitted disorder

- Passage of disease causing agent (pathogen) 'vertically' from mother to baby during the perinatal period is called 'vertical transmission'.
- ***A vertically transmitted agent night lie dormant in the mother and not manifest in her clinically (normal mother) but may manifest in the child.***

## Types of Defects

**Genetic**

**Single gene defect (Mendelian disorder)**
- Autosomal dominant disorders
- Autosomal recessive disorders
- X linked dominant disorders
- X linked recessive disorders

**Polygenic (Multifactorial)**
- Diabetes
- Hypertension
- Coronary / ischemic heart disease
- Congenital heart disease
- Neural tube defect
- Pyloric stenosis
- Hirschspning disease
- Cleft lip or cleft palate
- Gout
- Schizophrenia

**Chromosomal**
- Abnormal number of chromosomes (Trisomy, Monosomy etc) Polyploidy
- Abnormal shape/Structural abnormalities

**Congenital Malformations (eg Teratogenic)**

Abnormal development unrelated to genes or chromosomes.
(eg Teratogenic event)

## Wadenburg Syndrome Type -1

*Waardenburg's Syndrome (WS) is a rare* ***autosomal dominant syndrome*** *characterized by pigmentary disturbances (skin,* ***hair****, iris),* ***sensorineural hearing loss****, and other developmental anomalies such as* ***dystopia canthorum (widely spaced eyes)*** *and blepharophimosis.*

| Type | I (Waardenburg) |
|---|---|
| **Distinguishing Features** | Dystopia canthorum (Widely spaced eyes)<br>Hearing loss (25%) |
| **Inheritance** | Autosomal Dominant (AD) |
| **Gene Defect/ Function** | P AX3/transactivates promotor for MITF |

**Facial features**
- Broad high nasal root
- Synophrys or medial flaring, or both, of the eyebrows
- Hypoplastic alae nasi
- **Dystopia canthorum (lateral displacement of inner canthi or widely spaced eyes or hypertelorism)**

**Hair features**
- White forelock (present at birth or developing later; also may disappear later) White body hair, eyebrows, eyelashes
- Dark tufts of hair or black forelock
- Premature graying (i.e. <30 y)

**Aural features**
- **Sensineural hearing loss (SNHL) (deafness)**

**Eye features**
- Complete or segmental heterochromia
- Brilliant sapphire blue eyes

**Skin features**
- Hypopigmentation, possibly on the face, trunk, or limbs with or without an associated white forelock
- Patches ofhyperpigmentation in some families with WS

**Less commonly associated findings**
- Neural tube defects
- Sprengel shoulder (ie, congenital upward scapular displacement)
- Cleft lip or palate
- Hirschsprung disease (primarily in cases of WS4 but reported in families with WS1 and WS2) Contractures and limb muscle hypoplasia (in patients with WS3)

## Major Histocompatibility Complex (MHC)/ Human Leukocyte Antigen (HLA) Complex

- In humans the gene encoding MHC or HLA complex are clustered on ***a small segment (4 megabase region) of chromosome 6 short arm***[Q] ***(6p 21.3)***[Q]. HLA class I and class II genes whose products are critical for ***immunological specificity and transplantation histocompatibility***[Q] and they play a major role in **susceptibility to a number of autoimmune diseases.**
- **Function:** Binds peptide fragments of foreign protein for presentation to appropriate *antigen specific T- Cells. Thus involved in*: 1) ***Transplantation reaction***[Q] ***2)*** Immune response & tolerance 3) Disease susceptibility ***(autoimmune ds***[Q], infectious & Inflammatory disease) 4) Complement component.
- They are classified into **3 categories**

| Feature | Class I Antigen (MHCI) | Class II Antigen (MHC II) | Class III (MHC III) |
|---|---|---|---|
| **Expressed on (presented by)** | ***All nucleated cells & platelets***[Q] | ***Antigen presenting cells including Dendritic cells***[Q] in lymphnode & spleen, ***Langerhans cells***[Q], Macrophages, ***B cells***[Q] ***& activated T cells***[Q] | Class III is present in between I & II |
| **Encoded by (component loci)** | 3 closely linked loci designated HLA-**A**, HLA-**B** and HLA-**C** | ***HLA-D*** *(HLA* ***DP, D***[Q], **DR**) | C4B, BF, C2 TNF α & β |
| **Encoding molecule** | **Cell surface glycoprotein involved in antigen presentation** | **Cell surface glycoprotein involved in antigen presentation** | **Components of complement system** |
| **Recognized by** | ***CD8+ Tcells***[Q], NK cell recognizition | ***CD4+ helper Tcells***[Q] | |
| Function | - Immune response against intracellular infection, tumors, allografts<br>- Graft rejection<br>- Cell mediated cytolysis<br>- Component of hormone receptor | - Graft versus host response<br>- Mixed leucocyte reaction (MLR)<br>- Influence functional capacity of mature peripheral T cells. | |

# Chapter -5 STRUCTURE & FUNCTIONS OF PROTEINS AND ENZYMES

## QUESTIONS

### Structure of Protein

1. **The primary structure of a protein refers to:**
   A. Linear structure and order of the amino acids present ☐
   B. Regular confirmational forms of a protein ☐
   C. Complete three-dimensional structure of the polypeptide units of a given protein ☐
   D. Subunit structure of the protein ☐
2. **Alpha helix and Beta pleated sheet are examples of:**
   A. Primary structure ☐
   B. Secondary structure ☐
   C. Tertiary structure ☐
   D. Quaternary structure ☐
3. **Which one of the following is not true for an α-helix:**
   A. It is one of the most important secondary structure ☐
   B. It has a net dipole moment ☐
   C. All hydrogen bonds are aligned in the same direction ☐
   D. Long stretches of left handed α-helices occur in proteins ☐
4. **An amino acid which does not participate by αhelix formation is:**
   A. Leucine ☐
   B. Glycine ☐
   C. Proline ☐
   D. Lysine ☐
5. **An alfa helix of a protein is most likely to be disrupted if a missense mutation introdues the following amino acid with in the alpha helical structure:**
   A. Alanine ☐
   B. Aspartic acid ☐
   C. Tyrosine ☐
   D. Glycine ☐
6. **Folding of protein chain is due to :**
   A. Amide bond ☐
   B. Hydrogen bonds ☐
   C. Phosphodiesterase bonds ☐
   D. Disulphide bond ☐
7. **The 3 dimensional shape of a protein is maintained mainly by:**
   A. Strong covalent interactions ☐
   B. Interactions with other proteins ☐
   C. Multiple weak interactions ☐
   D. Interactions with prosthetic groups ☐
8. **Proteins are linear polymers of amino acids. They fold into compact structures. Sometimes, these folded structures associate to form homo-or hetero-dimers. Which one of the following refers to this associated form?**
   A. Denatured state ☐
   B. Molecular aggregation ☐
   C. Precipitation ☐
   D. Quaternary structure ☐
9. **An Immunoglobulin molecule represents the following level of organized protein structure:**
   A. Primary structure ☐
   B. Secondary structure ☐
   C. Tertiary structure ☐
   D. Quartenary structure ☐
10. **True about Isopeptide bond:**
   A. It makes protein resistant ☐
   B. Bond is formed b/w carboxyl terminus of one protein and the amino group of a lysine residue on another ☐
   C. Involves in post-transcriptional modification of protein ☐
   D. Enzyme acts as catalyst for the bond formation ☐
11. **Stability of the toxoid in snake's venom is due to:**
   A. Disulfide bonds ☐
   B. Hydrogen bonds ☐
   C. Ionic bonds ☐
   D. Van Der Wall's bond. ☐
12. **Keratin in skin is softer than keratin in nail because keratin in skin has:**
   A. Less number of disulphide bonds ☐
   B. Less number of salt bridges ☐
   C. High sodium content ☐
   D. Different affinity for water ☐
13. **Biomineralization is seen in:**
   A. Pinna ☐
   B. Molluscs shell ☐
   C. Hooves of cattle ☐
   D. Nails ☐
14. **Different sequence of amino acids having similar structure of proteins is an example of**
   A. Divergence ☐
   B. Convergence ☐
   C. Opportunistic ☐
   D. Incidental ☐
15. **There are more than 300 variants of human hemoglobin gene. Among these only a few are fatal. Hence, the most important factor to be conserved in a protein for its function is the:**
   A. Amino acid sequence ☐
   B. Ligand binding residues ☐
   C. Structure ☐
   D. Environment ☐
16. **Which of the following is not true in relation to glycoproteins:**
   A. Are proteins to which oligosaccharide are covalently attached ☐
   B. The carbohydrate units of glycoprotein have several repeats ☐
   C. Carbohydrate content is same but proteins are different ☐
   D. Carbohydrate chain is often linear ☐
17. **Which of the following is a component of polysaccharide-**
   A. Synovium ☐
   B. Glucosamine ☐
   C. Glucoronic acid ☐
   D. Ascorbic acid ☐
18. **Regarding proteoglycans, false is:**
   A. Chondroitin sulfate is a Proteoglycan ☐
   B. They hold less amount of water ☐
   C. They are made up of sugar and aminoacids ☐
   D. They carry charge ☐
19. **Compounds with large amount of carbohydrate & small amount of protein**
   A. Glycoprotein ☐
   B. Glycosaminoglycan ☐
   C. Proteoglycan ☐
   D. Glycocalyx ☐

**20. Which of the following aminoacids in a protein commonly acts as a potential O-Glycosylation site for attachment of an oligosaccharide unit:**
A. Glutamine ☐
B. Cysteine ☐
C. Serine ☐
D. Asparginine ☐

**21. All steps of N- glycosylation occur in ER except**
A. Dolichol synthesis ☐
B. Glycosyl transferase ☐
C. Protein- oligosacharide transferase ☐
D. Final trimming ☐

**22. Glycosyl transferase of O-glycosylation is found in**
A. RER ☐
B. SER ☐
C. Golgi ☐
D. Lysosome ☐

**23. Difference between High mannose & complex glycoprotein**
A. Core pentasacharide ☐
B. Protein chain ☐
C. Asparagine ☐
D. Presence of GlC – NAc – Gal – NANA in complex glycoprotein ☐

**24. Following organelles are involved in the formation of N-glycosylated product:**
A. Golgi apparatus ☐
B. Nucleolus ☐
C. SER ☐
D. RER ☐
E. Peroxisomes ☐

**25. Characteristics of glycoprotein:**
A. Protein linked with glycosidic bond ☐
B. Core protein ☐
C. Sugar residues are long in carbohydrate portion of glycoprotein. ☐
D. Participate in cell surface recognition. ☐

**26. All are true about denatured proteins except:**
A. Amino acid sequence remains intact ☐
B. The biological function remains intact ☐
C. The isoelectric pH changes ☐
D. Recovery after denaturation is not possible ☐

**27. True about denaturation of proteins is all except:**
A. Unfolding occurs ☐
B. Disruption of secondary structure occurs ☐
C. Sequence of amino acids remain the same ☐
D. Biological activity is retained ☐

**28. Random arrangement of molecule results in**
A. Crystallization ☐
B. Precipitation ☐
C. Denaturation ☐
D. High Solubility ☐

**29. Protein that precipitates on heating to 45° C and redissolves on boiling is:**
A. Bence Jones Protein ☐
B. Gamma globulin ☐
C. Albumin ☐
D. Myosin ☐

**30. Optical transmission through a solution depends on:**
A. Time ☐
B. Concentration ☐
C. Scale ☐
D. Path length ☐
E. Spectrophotometer

**31. Cytochrome C of the bacteria has 50% identity of amino acid sequence with that of human. Which of the following is the most conserved parameter in these two proteins?**
A. Quarternary structure ☐
B. Tertiary structure ☐
C. Amino acid sequence ☐
D. Loop and turn segments ☐

**32. Which of the following is a denaturing substance?**
A. Guanosine ☐
B. Guanidine ☐
C. Glutamate ☐
D. Glycine ☐

**33. Which of these is a denaturating substance:**
A. Guanosine ☐
B. Guanidine ☐
C. Glutamate ☐
D. Glycine ☐

**34. The structural proteins are involved in maintaining the shape of a cell or in the formation of matrices in the body. The shape of these proteins is:**
A. Globular ☐
B. Fibrous ☐
C. Stretch of beads ☐
D. Planar ☐

**35. Structural proteins are:**
A. Fibrous ☐
B. Globular ☐
C. Branched ☐
D. Compound ☐

**36. In a centrifugal distribution, protein that is precipitated first is:**
A. Fibrous ☐
B. Globular ☐
C. Completely disorganized ☐
D. None of the above ☐

**37. True about Collagen:**
A. Triple helix ☐
B. Beta- pleated structure ☐
C. Vit C is necessary for post-translational modification ☐
D. Glycine residue at every third position ☐

**38. Which of the following are intracellular events occurring in fibroblast during synthesis of collagen:**
A. Hydrolysis of procollagen to collagen ☐
B. Glycosylation of proline ☐
C. Formation of triple helix ☐
D. Formation of covalent cross link b/w fibrils ☐
E. Self assembly of tropocollagen molecules into fibrils ☐

**39. The 40 nm gap in between the tropocollagen molecule in collagen which serve as the site of bone formation is occupied by which of the following-**
A. Carbohydrate ☐
B. Ligand moiety ☐
C. $Ca^{++}$ ☐
D. $Fe^{+++}$ ☐

**40. Albumin and globulin are classified as:**
A. Conjugated proteins ☐
B. Simple globular proteins ☐
C. Unconjugated proteins ☐
D. Derived proteins ☐

**41. Which is /are not transport protein (s):**
A. Transferrin ☐
B. Collagen ☐
C. Ceruloplasmin ☐
D. Hemoglobin ☐
E. Albumin ☐

**42. Which of the following is/are storage protein :**
A. Myoglobin ☐
B. Ovalbumin ☐
C. Ricin/Hepcidin ☐
D. Ferritin ☐
E. Glutelin ☐

**43. A Protein estimation test is confused with:**
A. Phosphates ☐
B. Nitrates ☐
C. Sulphates ☐
D. Bile salts ☐

**44. Intact peptide bond is necessary for which test:**
A. UV diffraction ☐
B. Ninhydrin ☐
C. Diazo reaction ☐
D. All ☐

**45. All of the following assays are used for estimation of total serum protein, except**
A. Biuret ☐
B. Bradford ☐
C. Lowry's ☐
D. Bromocresol green ☐

**46. Which of the following estimates blood creatinine level most accurately**
A. Jaffe method ☐
B. Kinetic jaffe method ☐
C. Technicon method ☐
D. Enzyme assay ☐

**47. False positive test of protein in dipstick test seen in:**
A. Chlorpropamide ☐
B. IV contrast agent ☐
C. Viral infection ☐
D. IV administration of drugs ☐

## Methods of Protein Separation (Purification)

**48. Protein separation based on mass / molecular weight (size) is /are done in all except:**
A. Ultrafiltration ☐
B. Native gel electrophoresis ☐
C. 2D gel electrophoresis ☐
D. Gel Filtration chromatography ☐
E. Ultracentrifugation ☐

**49. Protein fragments separation is /are done by:**
A. Western blot ☐
B. Chromatography ☐
C. Centrifugation ☐
D. Ultrafiltration ☐
E. Electrophoresis ☐

**50. In SDS-PAGE (Sodium Dodecyl Sulfate-Polyacrylamide Gel Electrophoresis) proteins are separated on basis of:**
A. Mass ☐
B. Charge ☐
C. Density ☐
D. Molecular weight ☐
E. Solubility ☐

**51. Proteins are separated on the basis of size by:**
A. SDS-PAGE ☐
B. HPLC ☐
C. Affinity Chromatography ☐
D. Ion-exchange Chromatography ☐

**52. Separation of proteins based on size is done by:**
A. Affinity chromatography depending on charge ☐
B. SDS-Polyacrylamide gel electrophoresis ☐
C. Ion exchange chromatography ☐
D. High performance liquid chromatography ☐
E. Electrophoresis ☐

**53. Protein purification and separation can be done by all except:**
A. Chromatography ☐
B. Centrifugation ☐
C. Electrophoresis ☐
D. Densitometry ☐

## Ammonium Sulfate Fractionation

**54. Protein is purified using ammonium sulfate by:**
A. Salting out ☐
B. Ion exchange chromatography ☐
C. Mass chromatography ☐
D. Molecular size exclusion ☐

## Chromatography

**55. The following separation technique depends on the molecular size of the protein :**
A. Chromatography on a carboxymethyl (CM) cellulose column ☐
B. Iso-electric focussing ☐
C. Gel filtration chromatography ☐
D. Chromatography on a diethylaminoethyl (DEAE) cellulose column ☐

**56. Molecular separation of two proteins with same charge can be done by:**
A. Ion exchange chromatography ☐
B. Dialysis ☐
C. Gel diffusion chromatography ☐
D. Electrophoresis ☐

**57. The best method to differentiate proteins is by:**
A. Gel chromatography ☐
B. Affinity chromatography ☐
C. Ion exchange electrophoresis ☐
D. None of the above ☐

**58. In chromatography mass movements of the substances is due to:**
A. Diffusion ☐
B. Electrophoresis ☐
C. Paper chromatography ☐
D. Osmosis ☐

**59. In which type of chromatography, the proteins are bound to another substance:**
A. Hydrophobic chromatography ☐
B. Affinity chromatography ☐
C. Paper chromatography ☐
D. Gel chromatography ☐

**60. Method of chromatography in which molecules that are negatively charged are selectively released from stationary phase into the positively charged molecules in mobile phase is termed as:**
A. Affinity chromatography ☐
B. Ion-Exchange chromatography ☐
C. Adsorbtion chromatography ☐
D. Size-Exclusion chromatography ☐

**61. Fastest moving amino acid in methanol- chloroform electrophoresis is**
A. Glycine ☐
B. Aspartic Acid ☐
C. Valine ☐
D. Leucine ☐

**62. Which amino acid migrates fastest on chromatography on carboxy methylcellulose medium?**

A. Aspartic acid ☐
B. Valine ☐
C. Lysine ☐
D. Glycine ☐

## Electrophoresis

**63. True regarding electrophoresis are all except**
A. Isoelectric focusing use ampholytes & pI ☐
B. Adversly affect structure & function ☐
C. Depends on size not on shape ☐
D. Commonest method of purifying protein ☐
E. Use electric field & quickly estimate no. of proteins ☐

**64. Supercoiled DNA is separated by relaxed DNA by:**
A. ELISA ☐
B. Gel electrophoresis ☐
C. DNA footprinting ☐
D. DNA fingerprinting ☐
E. Microarray assay ☐

**65. Which process separates the fragments of DNA** :
A. Gel centrifugation ☐
B. Paper chromatography ☐
C. High speed centrifugation ☐
D. Thin layer chromatography ☐

**66. The two fragments of DNA are separated by**:
A. High speed centrifugation ☐
B. Thin layer chromatography ☐
C. Paper chromatography ☐
D. Gel chromatography ☐

**67. The molecular weight of a protein can be determined by -**
A. Native Poly Acrylamide Gel Electrophoresis (PAGE) ☐
B. Sodium Dodecyl Sulphate PAGE ☐
C. Isoelectric focussing ☐
D. Ion Exchange Chromatography ☐

**68. A protein with molecular weight of 100 kD is subjected to SDS PAGE electrophoresis. The SDS PAGE electrophoresis pattern show two widely separated bands of 20kD and 30kD after addition of Mercaptoethanol. The true statement regarding this will be.**
A. The protein has undergone complete lysis ☐
B. The protein is a monomer of 20 kD and 30kD protein ☐
C. The protein is a dimmer of two 20kD and 30kD proteins ☐
D. The protein is a tetramer of 20kd and 30kD proteins ☐

**69. Hemoglobin electrophoresis is based on**
A. Molecular weight ☐
B. Charge ☐
C. Solubility ☐
D. Calorimetric properties ☐

## Detection of Protein Structure

**70. Method (s) to determine protein structure is /are:**
A. X-RAY Crystallography ☐
B. NMR Spectroscopy ☐
C. Electrophoresis ☐
D. Infra red spectroscopy ☐

**71. All of the following can determine the protein structure, Except:**
A. High performance liquid chromatography ☐
B. Mass spectrometry ☐
C. X- ray crystallography ☐
D. NMR spectrometry ☐

**72. Sequence in a long chain of protein is identified by-**
A. Restriction fragment length polymorphism (RFLP) ☐
B. Chromosome walking ☐
C. Leucine Zipper ☐
D. SSOP ☐

**73. The tertiary structure of protein is detected by**:
A. X- ray diffraction / crystallographs. ☐
B. Spectrophotometry ☐
C. Electrophoresis. ☐
D. Chromatography. ☐

**74. Trypsin cleaves :**
A. Arginine ☐
B. Glutamate ☐
C. Lysine ☐
D. Proline ☐

**75. All is true about fragment cleavage in 1° structure determination Except**
A. Trypsin cleaves lysine residue (C) ☐
B. Trypsin cleaves arginine next to proline ☐
C. Trypsin & lysyl endoproteinase cleave C terminal of lysine ☐
D. Cysteine reduced by 2 mercapto ethanol ☐
E. Performic acid break disulfide bond

**76. Chymotrypsin cleaves carbonyl terminal of:**
A. Phenylalanine ☐
B. Arginine ☐
C. Lysine ☐
D. Tryptophan ☐
E. Tyrosine ☐

**77. Molecular size is assesed by** :
A. Sedimentation ☐
B. Absorption mass spectroscopy ☐
C. Liophilization ☐
D. Salting out ☐

**78. The substance present in the gall bladder stones or the kidney stones can be best identified by the following techniques**:
A. Fluorescence spectroscopy ☐
B. Electron microscopy ☐
C. Nuclear magnetic resonance ☐
D. X-ray diffraction ☐

## Enzyme: Kinetics

**79. In competitive inhibition-**
A. Vmax unchanged ☐
B. Apparent Km unchanged ☐
C. Apparent Km decreased ☐
D. Vmax decreased ☐
E. Rate independent of substrate concentration ☐

**80. Disopropyl phosphofluoridate (DFP) reacts with serine proteases irreversibly and therefore is :**
A. Allosteric inhibitor ☐
B. Competitive inhibitor ☐
C. Non competitive inhibitor ☐
D. A repressor ☐

**81. The type of enzyme inhibition (in which succinate dehydrogenase reaction is inhibited by malonate) is an example of**:
A. Non competitive ☐
B. Uncompetitive ☐
C. Competitive ☐
D. Allosteric ☐

**82. True about reversible non-competetive inhibitors:**
A. Lower Vmax ☐
B. Lower Km ☐
C. Not affect Km ☐
D. Not affect Vmax ☐
E. Affect both V max & Km ☐

**83. True about competitive inhibition of enzyme:**
- A. ↑ Km ☐
- B. ↓ Km ☐
- C. ↑ Vmax ☐
- D. No change in Km and Vmax ☐
- E. V max remain same ☐

**84. In noncompetitive antagonism the true statement is:**
- A. Km value decrease; V max normal ☐
- B. Km value decreased; V max decreased ☐
- C. Km value normal; V max decreased ☐
- D. Km value decreased; V max increased ☐

**85. Km increased but Vmax same enzyme is:**
- A. Competitive ☐
- B. Non competitive ☐
- C. Irreversible ☐
- D. Uncompetitive ☐

**86. Km value is defined as:**
- A. Substrate concentration at Vmax/2 ☐
- B. Substrate concentration of twice Vmax ☐
- C. Substrate concentration of thrice Vmax ☐
- D. Substrate concentration of one third Vmax ☐

**87. True about Km**
- A. Half the substrate concentration at which velocity is maximum ☐
- B. Substrate concentration at which reaction rate is half the maximum ☐
- C. Michaelis constant ☐
- D. Dissociation constant of enzyme-substrate complex ☐
- E. Dissication constant of enzyme-product complex ☐

**88. Hormone substrate concentration affects the velocity of enzymatic action, this is known as -**
- A. Zimmerman reaction ☐
- B. Salkowski reaction ☐
- C. Michales Menton reaction ☐
- D. Lieberman-Burchard reaction ☐

**89. Michaelis-Menten hypothesis states that -**
- A. Rate of enzymatic reaction is independent of substrate concentration ☐
- B. Rate of non enzymatic reaction is proportinal to substrate concentrate ☐
- C. Km is the enzyme-substrate complex association constant ☐
- D. Enzyme-substrate complex formation is essential in enzymatic reaction ☐

**90. Which of the following enzymes are activated in dephosphorylated state:**
- A. HMG Co A reductase ☐
- B. Glycogen phosphorylase ☐
- C. Glycogen phosphorylase kinase ☐
- D. Citrate lyase ☐
- E. Glycogen synthase ☐

**91. Enzyme regulated by phosphorylation:**
- A. Glucokinase ☐
- B. Glycogen synthetase ☐
- C. Pyruvate dehydrogenase ☐
- D. Isocitrate ☐
- E. Citrate lyase ☐

**92. All of the following enzymes are regulated by calcium or calmodulin, except:**
- A. Adenylate cyclase ☐
- B. Glycogen synthase ☐
- C. Guanylyl cyclase ☐
- D. Hexokinase ☐

**93. "All enzymes are not proteins." This statement is justified by:**
- A. All enzymes do not follow the Michaelis Menton hypothesis ☐
- B. RNAs act as ribozymes ☐
- C. Antibodies take part in the catalysis of many reactions ☐
- D. Metals are involved in attachment to enzymes and catalysts. ☐

**94. Definition of Ribozyme:**
- A. RNA molecular that acts catalytically to change it self or another RNA molecule ☐
- B. t-RNA ☐
- C. m–RNA ☐
- D. Ribosome ☐
- E. Ribonucleoprotein ☐

**95. One of the following enzyme is not a protein:**
- A. DNAase ☐
- B. Abzyme ☐
- C. Eco RI ☐
- D. Ribozyme ☐

**96. Ribozymes is/are :**
- A. Splicing of heterogenous RNA (hnRNA) to form mRNA ☐
- B. Splicing of polypeptide chain and mRNA ☐
- C. Transcription of mRNA ☐
- D. Recognition of codons in introns ☐
- E. RNA polymerase ☐

**97. Enzyme activity is expressed as:**
- A. Millimoles /lit? ☐
- B. Milli gm/lit? ☐
- C. Mg/dl ☐
- D. Micromoles/min ☐

**98. True about enzyme specificity:**
- A. Amount of enzyme required per second, per mole or product formation ☐
- B. Number of sites per substrate ☐
- C. Amount of enzyme binding with various substrates ☐
- D. Number of enzyme units per milligram of enzyme protein ☐
- E. Amount of enzyme causing transformation of 1 μmol of substrate per minute under standard conditions ☐

**99. Enzymes Ea,Eb and Ec are under allosteric control of S2 and P1 and P2 respectively. If Ec is defective what would occur -**

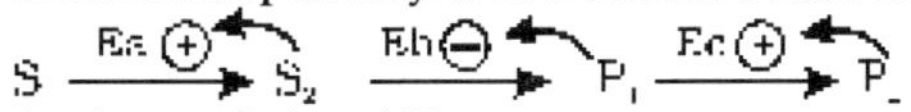


- A. Accumulation of S1 ☐
- B. Accumulation of P1 ☐
- C. Accumulation of S2 ☐
- D. Decrease of S2 ☐

**100. Non- functional enzymes are all except:**
- A. Alkaline phosphatase ☐
- B. Acid phosphatase ☐
- C. Lipoprotein lipase ☐
- D. Gamma glutamyl transpeptidase ☐

**101. True about isoenzymes is:**
- A. Same quaternary structure ☐
- B. Same distribution in different organs ☐
- C. Same enzyme classification with same umbers ☐
- D. Catalyze the same reaction ☐

**102. True about isoenzymes is/are:**
- A. Different km value ☐
- B. Act on different substrate ☐
- C. Consist of multimeric complex ☐
- D. Same electrophoretic mobility ☐
- E. Have different physical properties ☐

**103. The predominant isozyme of LDH in cardiac muscle is:**
- A. LD-1. ☐

B. LD-2. ☐
C. LD-3. ☐
D. LD-5. ☐

**104.In which of the following conditions the level of creatinine kinase-1 increases?**
A. Myocardial Ischemia ☐
B. Brain Ischemia ☐
C. Kidney damage ☐
D. Electrical cardioversion ☐

**105.Force not acting in an enzyme substrate complex :**
A. Electrostatic ☐
B. Covalent ☐
C. Van der waals ☐
D. Hydrogen ☐

**106.The serine proteases do not include**
A. Pepsin ☐
B. Trypsin ☐
C. Elastase ☐
D. Chymotrypsin ☐

**107.Active sites of serine protease contain:**
A. Histidine ☐
B. Lysine or threonine ☐
C. Arginine ☐
D. Serine ☐

**108.If chymotrypsin molecule undergoes a ser-195-ala mutation then :**
A. Chymotrypsin will not bind the substrate ☐
B. Chymotrypsin will bind the substrate as well as cause cleavage ☐
C. Chymotrypsin will bind the substrate but will not cause cleavage ☐
D. No affect will be observed ☐

**109.Tyrosinase is -**
A. Oxidase ☐
B. Transferase ☐
C. Lyase ☐
D. Isomerase ☐

**110.Hexokinase is a:**
A. Transferase ☐
B. Reductase ☐
C. Oxidoreductase ☐
D. Oxidase ☐

**111.Fumarase is a:**
A. Oxidoreductase ☐
B. Transferase ☐
C. Oxidase ☐
D. Lyases ☐

**112.Enzymes mediating transfer of one molecule to another are:**
A. Transferases ☐
B. Oxidases ☐
C. Lysases ☐
D. Peptidases ☐

**113.Enzymes that move a molecular group from one molecule to another are known as:**
A. Ligases. ☐
B. Oxido-reductases. ☐
C. Transferases. ☐
D. Dipeptidases. ☐

**114.Addition of water in C-C bond is by the enzyme:**
A. Hydroxylase ☐
B. Dehydrogenase ☐
C. Hydrolase ☐
D. Hydratase ☐

**115.Which of the following enzymes does not participate in oxidation-reduction reactions?**
A. Oxygenases ☐
B. Peroxidases ☐
C. Hydroperoxidases ☐
D. Dehydrogenases ☐

**116.All of the following enzymes are involved in oxidation – reduction reactions, Except**
A. Dehydrogenases ☐
B. Hydrolases ☐
C. Oxygenases ☐
D. Peroxidases ☐

**117.Detoxification of drugs is controlled by:**
A. Cytochrome ☐
B. Cytochrome P450 ☐
C. Cytochrome C ☐
D. Cytochrome A ☐

**118.All of the following are true regarding oxygenases except :**
A. Incorporate 2 atoms of oxygen ☐
B. Incorporate 1 atom of oxygen ☐
C. Required for hydroxylation of steroids ☐
D. Required for carboxylation of drugs. ☐

**119.Which of the following is not a rate limiting enzyme:**
A. HMG CoA Reductase ☐
B. Phosphofructokinase ☐
C. Acetyl CoA carboxylase ☐
D. Malanoate dehydrogenase ☐

**120.In which of the following reactions is Magnesium required:**
A. ATPase ☐
B. Dismutase ☐
C. Phosphatase ☐
D. Aldolase ☐

**121.Coenzymes are .........organic compounds :-**
A. Lipoprotein ☐
B. Proteinaceous ☐
C. Non-protein ☐
D. Any of the above ☐

**122.The combination of main supporting enzyme is called:**
A. Apoenzyme ☐
B. Coenzyme ☐
C. Holoenzyme ☐
D. Constitutive enzyme ☐

**123.Which of the following acts as co-enzymes and not as co-factors:**
A. Pyridoxine ☐
B. Biotin ☐
C. Thiamine ☐
D. Folic acid ☐
E. Co-balamin ☐

**124.Coenzyme, in an enzymatic reaction usually functions to :**
A. Activate the substrate ☐
B. Increase the active sites of apoenzyme ☐
C. Enhance the specificity of aponzyme ☐
D. Accept one of the cleavage products ☐

**125.Thiamine deficiency decreases cellular metabolism because:**
A. Thiamine is a coenzyme for pyruvate dehydrogenase and alfa-ketoglutarate dehydrogenases ☐
B. Activity of transketolase is inhibited ☐
C. It is required for the process of transamination ☐
D. It is a cofactor in oxidative reduction ☐

**126.Vitamin K is required for:**
A. Carboxylation ☐
B. Hydroxylation ☐
C. Oxidation ☐
D. Reduaction ☐

**127.Which coenzyme is responsible for carboxylation reaction?**
A. Biotin ☐
B. FAD ☐
C. NADH ☐
D. Thiamine pyrophosphate ☐

**128.Treatment of Multiple Carboxylase Deficiency is:**
A. Biotin ☐
B. Pyridoxine ☐
C. Thiamine ☐
D. Folic acid ☐

**129.Which of the following acts as cofactor after it's modification:**
A. Vit-C ☐
B. Pantothenic acid ☐
C. Biotin ☐
D. Zinc ☐
E. Copper ☐

**130.Zinc is cofactor for:**
A. Alcohol dehydrogenase ☐
B. Pyruvate Carboxylase ☐
C. Pyrvate Carboxylase ☐
D. Alpha- KG dehydrogenase ☐

**131.Zinc acts as co-factor in:**
A. Lactate dehydrogenase ☐
B. Carbonic anhydrase ☐
C. Glutathione peroxidae ☐
D. Alkaline phosphatase ☐
E. Superoxide dismutase ☐

**132.Selenium deficiency causes:**
A. Dermatitis ☐
B. Cardiomyopathy ☐
C. Diarrhoea ☐
D. Alopecia ☐
E. Gonadal atrophy ☐

**133.Selenium is co-factor for :**
A. Glutathione peroxidase ☐
B. Glutathione reductase ☐
C. Glutathione synthetase ☐
D. Glutathione dehydrogenase ☐

**134.Cofactor associated with the enzyme Glutathione peroxidase is**
A. Zinc ☐
B. Cadmium ☐
C. Molybdenum ☐
D. Selenium ☐

**135.Abzyme is a/an**
A. Isoenzyme ☐
B. Allosteric enzyme ☐
C. Abnormal enzyme ☐
D. Antibody with a catalytic activity ☐

**136.Copper containing enzymes is/are:**
A. Superoxide dismutase ☐
B. Cytochrome oxidase ☐
C. Myeloperoxidase ☐
D. Tyrosinase ☐
E. Amine oxidase ☐

**137.Biological role of metallothioneins is to sequester harmful metal ions. These bind**
A. $Cd^{++}$, $Cu^{++}$ & $Zn^{++}$ ☐
B. $Al^{+++}$, $Hg^{++}$ & $NH_4^+$ ☐
C. $Pt^{++}$, $As^{+++}$ & $PO_4^-$ ☐
D. $Fe^{+++}$, $Na^+$ & $K^+$ ☐

**138.Increased copper excretion in urine is seen in all except**
A. Primary sclerosing cholangitis ☐
B. Wilson's disease ☐
C. Primary biliary cirrhosis ☐
D. Hepatocellular carcinoma ☐

## Answers:

### Structure & Functions of Proteins

1. **A i.e. Linear structure and order of amino acids present**
2. **B i.e. Secondary structure**
3. **D i.e. Long stretches of left handed α- helices occur in proteins**
4. **C i.e. Proline**
5. **B i.e. Aspartic acid**
6. **B i.e. Hydrogen bond**
7. **C i.e. Multiple weak interaction**
8. **D i.e. Quaternary structure**
9. **D i.e. Quartenary structure** *[Ref: Lehninger 5/e p 140-117, 92; Lippincott 5/e p 16-17; Vasudevan 6/e p 32-33; Harper 29/e p 36-40; Chattarje 8/e p 89-91]*
10. **All i.e. (It makes protein resistant, Bond is formed b/w carboxyl terminus of one protein and the amino group of a lysine residue on another, Involves in post-transcriptional modification of protein, Enzyme acts as catalyst for the bond formation)**
11. **A i.e. Disulfide bond** *[Ref: Lippincott's 3/e P-19; Harper's 27/e P-33-35]*
12. **A i.e. Less number of disulphide bonds:** *[Ref: Vasudevan 6/e p 584; Harper 29/e p 626-27, 43-44; Lehninger 5/e p 71, 123]*
13. **B i.e. Molluscus shell** *[Ref: Internet]*
14. **B i.e. Convergence** *[Ref: Convergent evolution among immunoglobins F : M Frick;]*
15. **B i.e. Ligand binding residues** *[Ref: Lehninger 4th/160; Harper's 27/e P-369]*
16. **C i.e. Carbohydrate content is same but proteins are different D i.e. Carbohydrate chain is often linear**
17. **B i.e. Glucosaminoglycan**
18. **B i.e. They hold less amount of water**
19. **C i.e. Proteoglycan**
20. **C i.e. Serine**
21. **D i.e. Final trimming**
22. **C i.e. Golgi**
23. **D i.e. Presence of GlC – NAc – Gal – NANA in complex glycoprotein**
24. **D i.e. RER > A i.e. Golgi apparatus**
    *[Ref: Lippincott 5/e p 444; 166-70; Vasudevan 6/e p 124]*
25. **A i.e. Protein linked with glycosidic bond; D i.e. Participate in cell surface recognition**
26. **B i.e. Biological function remains intact**
27. **D i.e. Biological activity is retained**
28. **C i.e. Denaturation>B i.e. Precipitation**
29. **A i.e. Bence Jones proteins** *[Ref: Harper's 27/e P-45-46; Leninger 2/e P- 141, 160, 63, 66- 61; Lippincott's 4/e p. 20, 171; Ananthanarayan 7/e p. 90; Harrison 16/e p. 251]*
30. **B i.e. Concentration; D i.e. Path Length** *[Ref: Lehninger 3/e P- 121; 2/e 314, 207]*
31. **B i.e. Tertiary structure** *[Ref: Homology of pseudomonas cytochrome C-551 with eukaryotic Ctyochrome C by northwest university school of medicine]*
32. **B i.e. Guanidine**
33. **B i.e. Guanidine** *[Ref: Lippincott's 3/e P-21, 23, Lehninger 3/e P 192]*
34. **B i.e. Fibrous proteins**
35. **A i.e. Fibrous**
36. **A i.e. Fibrous**
    *[Ref: Harper's 27/e P-38; 26/e P-30; Chatterjea 6/e P-78; Lehninger 5/e p. 125]*
37. **A i.e. Triple helix**
38. **C i.e. Formation of triple helix** *[Ref: Harper 28th/ed pg-528-30; Lippincott 4th/ed pg- 43-49]*
39. **C i.e. Calcium**
40. **B i.e. Simple globular protein** *[Ref: Chatterjea 7/e p. 81-82; Lehninger 5/e p. 85]*
41. **B i.e. Collagen:** *[Ref: Harper's 29/e p 48, 632; Chattarjae 8/e p 105-06]*
42. **B, D, E > A i.e. Ovalbumin, Ferritin, Glutelin > Myoglobin** *[Ref: Chatterjaea 8/e p 617, 83-85; Satyanarayan 3/e p 163; Harper 29/e p 635]*
43. **A i.e. Phosphates** *[Ref: Chatterjea 6/e P- 657]*
44. **B i.e. Ninhydrin** *[Ref: Lippincott's 3/e P- 14- 15]*
45. **D i.e. Bromocresol green** *[Ref: Teitz 6/e p 687, 80-179]*
46. **D i.e. Enzyme assay** *[Ref: Reliability of plasma creatinine method in infants & children marie Jose clermont – Clinical pediatrics, vol. 25, No 11, 569- 572 (1986); Recommendations for improving serum creatinine methods- Gary L. Myers, Clinical chemistry 52 : 5 – 18 – 2006; Measurement of serum creatinine – Micheal whiting].*
47. **B i.e. IV Contrast agent; A i.e. Chlorpropamide** *[Ref: Schnier: Manual of nephrolgy 6/e p- 116- 17]*

### Methods of Protein Separation (Purification)

48. **B, C i.e. Native gel electrophoresis; 2D gel electrophoresis**
49. **B, C, D, E i.e. Chromatography, Centrifugation, Ultrafiltration, Electrophoresis**
50. **A, D i.e. Mass; Molecular weight**
51. **A i.e. SDS- PAGE**
52. **B i.e. SDS- Polyacrylamide gel electrophoresis**
53. **D i.e. Densitometry**
    *[Ref: Chatterjea 6/e P-749- 50, NMS 4/e P 19- 23; Harper's 27/e p. 21-24]*

## Ammonium Sulfate Fractionation

54. **A i.e. Salting out** *[Ref: Lehninger 5th/ed pg-85-92; John Baynes Mechanical Biochemistry 3rd/ed pg- 14-15; Harper 28th/ed pg-21]*

## Chromatography

55. **C i.e. Gel filtration Chromatography** 56. **C i.e. Gel diffusion Chomatography** 57. **A i.e. Gel Chromotography**
58. **A i.e. Diffusion** 59. **B i.e. Affinity chromatography**
*[Ref: Chatterjea: 7/e p. 769-72; Harper's 28/e p. 21-23; Vasudevan 6/e p. 601-4]*
60. **B i.e. Ion-Exchange chromatography** 61. **B i.e. Aspartic acid** 62. **Ai.e. Aspartic acid**
*[Ref:Lehninger 5th/e p. 85-88, 173, 364-65; John Baynes Mechanical Biochemistry 3rd/e p. 16; Harper 28th/e p.22; Vasudevan 6/e p. 601-4]*

## Electrophoresis

63. **C & D i.e. Depends on size not on shape & Commonest method of purifying protein**
64. **B i.e. Gel electrophoresis** 65. **A i.e. Gel centrifugation** 66. **D i.e. Gel chromatography**
*[Ref: Lehninger 5th/ed pg- 958-56; Teitz 6th/ed pg- 278; Micklos: DNA science 2/ed pg-438-39; Pierce: Genetics 2/e p-515; John Baynes Mechanical Biochemistry 3rd/ed pg- 467-66]*
67. **B i.e. Sodium Dodecyl Sulphate PAGE** 68. **C i.e. The protein is a dimmer of two 20kD and 30kD proteins**
*[Ref: Lehninger 5th/ed pg- 88-91; Harper 28th/ed pg-23-24; John Baynes Mechanical Biochemistry 3rd/ed pg-16-17]*
69. **B i.e. Charge** *[Ref Cahill, Mathew. Handbook of Diagnostic Tests. Springhouse, 1995. ;Jacobs, David S., et al. Laboratory Test Handbook. 4th ed.; Pagana, Kathleen Deska. Mosby's Manual of Diagnostic and Laboratory Tests. St. Louis1998]*

## Detection of Protein Structure

70. **A, B, E i.e. X-RAY Crystallography, NMR Spectroscopy, Electrophoresis** *[Ref: Vasudeven 6/e 34; Harper 28/e 23-27-37-39; Lehninger 5/e 75-90; Lippincott 5/e 21; John Baynes 3/e p 15-17, 55]*
71. **A i.e. High performance liquid chromatography**
72. **B i.e. Chromosome walking** 73. **A i.e. X-ray diffraction / Crystallography**
74. **A i.e. Arginine; C i.e. Lysine** 75. **B i.e. Trypsin cleaves arginine next to praline** 76. **A,D,E i.e. Phenylalanine; Tryptophan; Tyrosine**
*[Ref: Harrison 17th /1764; Harrison's 18th/2312Lehninger 5th/ed pg-95-96; Vasudevan 6/e p. 33; Harper 28/e p. 462; John Baynes Mechanical Biochemistry 3rd/ed pg- 18-19]*
77. **B i.e. Absorption mass spectroscopy**
78. **D i.e. X-ray diffraction** *[Ref: Harper's 28/e P-26-27; Campbells Urology 8/e P- 3274]*

## Enzymes

79. **A i.e. $V_{max}$ unchanged** 80. **C i.e. Non competitive inhibitor** 81. **C i.e. Competitive**
*[Ref: Chattarjea 7/e p 121-24; Harper 28/e 70-74-77-79; Lippincott 5/e 62-64; KDT 6/e p 40]*
82. **A, C i.e. Lower Vmax, Not affect Km** 83. **A, E i.e. ↑ Km, V max remain same**
84. **C i.e. Km value normal; $V_{max}$ decreased** 85. **A i.e. Competitive** 86. **A i.e. Substrate concentration at $V_{max}/2$**
*[Ref: Chattarjea 7/e p 121-24; Harper 28/e 70-74-77-79; Lippincott 5/e 62-64; KDT 6/e p 40]*
87. **B, C i.e. Substrate concentration at which reaction rate is half the maximum; Michaelis constant**
88. **C i.e. Michales – Menton reaction** 89. **D i.e. Enzymes substrate complex formation is essential in enzymatic reaction**
90. **A, E i.e. HMG CoA reductase; Glycogen synthase** 91. **B, C & E i.e. Glycogen synthetase, Pyruvate dehydrogenase & Citrate lyase**
*Ref: Lippincott 4th/e p.63, 110; Lehninger 5th/e p. 220-27, 571-77; Harper 28th/e p.81; Chattarjea & Shinde 7/e p. 118- 19]*
92. **D i.e. Hexokinase** *[Ref: Harper's 28/e p. 450; Vasudevan 6/e p. 412, 587; Lehninger 5/e p. 436-37]*
93. **B i.e. RNAs act as ribozymes** *[Ref: Harper's 27/e P-315, 318, 364]*
94. **A i.e., RNA molecular that acts catalytically to change itself or another RNA molecule** 95. **D i.e. Ribozyme**
96. **A i.e. Splicing of heterogenous RNA to form mRNA; D i.e. Recognition of codons in intron**
*[Ref: Harper's 27/e P-315, 318, 364; 26/e P-308, 356; Lippincott's 3/e P-436]*

97. **D i.e. Micromoles / Minute** *[Ref: Lippincott's 3/e P- 54, NMS. Biochemistry 4/e P-59-60; Vasudevan 4/e p- 44]*

98. **E i.e. Amount of enzyme causing transformation of 1 μ mol of substrate per minute under standard condition**

99. **C i.e. Accumulation of $S_2$** *[Ref: Harper's 27/e P-75-77; 26/e P- 74]*

100. **C i.e. Lipoprotein lipase** *[Ref: Harper 28th/ed pg- 59]*

101. **D i.e. Catalyze the same reaction:**

102. **A i.e. Different Km value; C i.e. Consist of multimeric complex; E i.e. Have different physical properties**

103. **A i.e. LD-1** 104. **B i.e. Brain Ischemia**

*[Ref: Chatterjea 8/e p 123, 644-647, 522; Lippincott 5/e p 65-66; Das 8/e p 94; Harper's 29/e P-63-65; Harsh Mohan 4/e 296; Debajyoti Das 8/e P 94]*

105. **C i.e. Vander Waals** *[Ref: Textbook of Biochemistry Thomas M.Devlin 4/e P 156]*

106. **A i.e. Pepsin** 107. **D i.e. Serine** *[Ref: Harper's 27/e P-53-55]*

108. **C i.e. Chymotrypsin will bind the substrate but will not cause cleavage**

109. **A i.e. Oxidase** 110. **A i.e. Transferase** 111. **D i.e. Lyases**

112. **A i.e. Transferase** 113. **C i.e. Transferase** 114. **C i.e. Hydrolase**

*[Ref: Chattergea & Shinde 7/e p. 469, 116; Harper's 28/e p. 52; Lippincott's 5/e p. 53-54]*

115. **None >>> B i.e. Peroxidase**

116. **B i.e. Hydrolases** *[Ref: Harper 28th/ed pg- 98-102; Lippicott's 4th/ed pg – 53; Lehninger 5th/ed pg- 816, 518-20]*

117. **B i.e. Cytochrome P 450** 118. **D i.e. Required for carboxylation of drugs**

*[Ref: Harper 28/e p. 98-102; Lehninger 5/e p. 816]*

119. **D i.e. Malonate dehydrogenase** 120. **C i.e. Phosphatase** *[Ref: Harper's 27/e P-78-79; Chatterjea 6/e P-559]*

121. **C i.e. Non protein** 122. **C i.e. Holoenzyme**

123. **A i.e. Pyridoxine; B i.e. Biotin; C i.e. Thiamine; D i.e. Folic acid** 124. **D i.e. Accept one of the cleavage products**

125. **A i.e. Thiamine is a coenzyme for pyruvate dehydrogenase & $\alpha$ ketoglutarate dehyderogenase** 126. **A i.e. Carboxylation**

*[Ref: Lippincott's 4/e p. 54- 55, 101, 110, Harper's 27/e p. 50-51,490; Chattergea & Shinde 7/e p. 114- 16 ; Vasudevan 4/e p. 37- 39]*

127. **A i.e. Biotin** 128. **A i.e. Biotin** *[Ref: Nelson 17/e p. 412]*

129. **B i.e. Pantothenic acid** *[Ref: Harper's 27/e P-503]*

130. **A i.e. Alcohol dehydrogenase**

131. **A i.e. Lactate Dehydrogenase; B i.e Carbonic anhydrase; D i.e. Alkaline phosphatase; E i.e. Superoxide dismutase.**

132. **B i.e. Cardiomyopathy**

133. **A i.e. Glutathione Peroxidase** 134. **D i.e. Selenium**

*[Ref: Harper 29/e p 118, 201, 270, 541; Harrison 18/e p 604; Chattrjea 8/e p 211, 630-31, 560, 801; Indian Journal of Medial Science 1190; 44(7): p. 173-7]*

135. **D i.e. Antibody with catalytic activity** *[Ref: NMS Biochemistry 4/e P- 109]*

136. **A, B, D, E i.e. Superoxide dismutase; Cytochrome oxidase; Tyrosinase; Amine oxidase:**

137. **A i.e. $Cd^{++}$, $Cu^{++}$ & $Zn^{++}$** *[Ref: Harper 29/e p 640]*

138. **D i.e. Hepatocellular carcinoma** *[Ref: Robbins 7/e p. 910; Harper's 27/e p. 595-97; Chattergea 7/e p. 584-86]*

# STRUCTURE & FUNCTIONS OF PROTEINS AND ENZYMES: REVIEW NOTES

## Structural Organization of Protein

### Primary Structure

- Primary structure is **linear sequence of aminoacids held together by covalent bonds (mainly peptide and disulfide bonds).** It is **insufficient to perform chemical /physical task.**
- The aminoacids are numbered from N terminal end (free $NH_2$/amino group of terminal amino acid) as no 1 towards the C (free carboxy) terminal.
- **Peptide bonds form the backbone** and side chains of aminoacid residues project out side the peptide back bone
- α-carbons of adjacent aminoacid residues are separated by three covalent bonds $C_\alpha - C - N - C_\alpha$. **The peptide (C-N) bond has a partial double bond character** that keeps the entire 6 atom peptide group in a **rigid planar configuration.** Peptide C-N bond cannot rotate freely; **rotation is permitted about N-$C_\alpha$ and $C_\alpha$ - C bonds**. So backbone of polypeptide chain can be pictured as a series of rigid planes sharing a **common point of rotation at $C_\alpha$.**
- Peptide conformation is defined by 3 **dihedral angles** (or **torsion angles**) called **ϕ (phi)** with rotation occurring about **N-$C_\alpha$ bond; ψ(Psi)** with rotation occurring about **$C_\alpha$-C bond** ; and **ω (omega)** with central peptide (C-N) bond, where rotation is constrained and mostly (99.6% times) peptide bond is in trans configuration (omega = ± 180°) or very rare in cis configuration (ω=0°). Theoritically values of ϕ & ψ can be between – 180° and + 180° but many values (eg both O°) are prohibited d/t steric interferences. Allowed values are obtained by **Ramchandran plot**.

### Tertiary Structure

- **Tertiary structure** refers to **over all three dimensional arrangement of all atoms in a protein**. It indicates the **3-D confirmation of a single polypeptide chain** ie in 3D space how secondary structure features helices, sheets, loops and bends assemble to form domains and how these domains relate spatially to one another.
- Tertiary structure refers to ***spatial arrangement of long range aspects of aminoacids***[Q] (in comparison to secondary structure that includes adjacent aminoacids). Proteins with tertiary structure are sufficient to perform a particular task.
- On the basis of tertiary structure, proteins can be divided into **structural fibrous proteins** (having simple repeating elements of secondary structure) and **globular proteins** (often containing several types of secondary structure in same polypeptide chain).
- Complex structures of globular proteins can be analyzed by examining folding patterns called **motifs (super secondary structures or folds).** A motif is a recognizable folding pattern involving 2 or more elements of

### Secondary Structure

- **Secondary structure of protein** refers to **description of steric relationship (spatial arrangement) between aminoacids located relatively near each other in a selected segment of main polypeptide chain**, without regard to the conformation of its side chains or its relationship to other segments.
- **A regular secondary structure** occurs when each dihedral angle (ϕ & ψ) remains the same or nearly the same throughout segment. Where a regular pattern is not found, the secondary structure is called **undefined** or **random coil** (misnomer as polypeptide back bone in any protein is not random).
- The secondary structure of a polypeptide segment can be completely defined if ϕ & ψ angles are known for all aminoacids.
- **Circular dichroism (CD) spectroscopy**, based on principle that structural asymmetry in a molecule gives rise to differences in absorption of left handed versus right handed plane polarized light, is a method for **assessing secondary structure and moniter folding in proteins**. It can determine whether proteins are properly folded, estimate the fraction of protein that is properly folded in either of common secondary structures, an moniter transition b/w folded & unfolded states. For proteins spectra are obtained in **far UV region (190 to 250nm).**
- **Three dimensional secondary structure** is produced by folding or coiling of short (3-30) contiguous segments of polypeptides (peptide chain primary structure) and production of cross linkages or bonds mainly hydrogen bonds. It is *insufficient to perform a particular physical or chemical task*. Organization may result in formation of **geometrically ordered units** such as α helix, β sheets, loops and bends-

#### α- Helix

- Are *regular- helical coils* of peptide chain
- Formed by ***intra chain hydrogen bonds***[Q] b/w carbonyl O of 1[st] amino acid and amide N of 4[th] amino acid residue.
- α- helix may be left handed or right handed
- ***Left handed α helix is less stable***[Q] than right handed α- helix because of steric interference b/w the C=O and the side chains
- Only right handed α- helix has been found in protein structure
- *In one complete turn* of α- helix there are *3.6 amino acid residue.*
- ***Proline is never found in α- helix***[Q].
- Small or uncharged amino acids as *alanine, phenylalanine & leucine* are often found; whereas more polar a.a. such as *arginine, glutamate & serine* may repel & destabilize *α- helix*.

#### β- Pleated Sheets

- β- pleated structure is formed by ***inter chain hydrogen bonds***[Q].
- They are produced when *hydrogen bonds* are formed *between carbonyl oxygen and amide hydrogen of two adjacent chains.*
- The adjacent chains may be either parallel or antiparallel.
- Most common a.a to form β- pleated sheet - *Glycine, Alanine, Serine*
- ***Proline occurs although it tends to disrupts β- sheet by producing kinks***[Q]
- ***Silk fibroins a protein of silk worm is rich in β- pleated sheets***[Q].

#### Alpha (α) Helix (Pauley & Corey)

- This *spiral structure* is the *most common and stable* secondary conformation (structure) for a polypeptide chain. The polypeptide bond forms secondary structure and the connection (s) between them. It can be very simple as **β -α - β loop** or very elaborate such as **β barrel**. Motif is not a hierarchial structural element falling between secondary & tertiary structure; it is a folding pattern that can describe a small part of protein or an entire polypeptide chain. A motif segment may or may not be independently stable. A **domain** ***is a part of polypeptide chain that can fold stably and independently***Q or could undergo **movements as a** single entity with respect to the entire protein. Multiple domains of large proteins may have different functions and may retain their native 3D structure even when separated. Thousands of known protein structures are assembled from a repertoire of few hundred motifs.

## Quaternary Structure

- ***Quarternary structure results from interactions between the subunits of multi subunit (multimeric) proteins***Q. So quaternary structure is **3D arrangement of multiple polypeptide chain proteins**
- Some multimeric proteins have a repeated structural unit, consisting of a single subunit or a group of subunits known as promoter. Promoters are usually related by **rotational or helical symmetry** (ie individual subunit can be super imposed on other). Examples of rotational symmetry include **cyclic symmetry, dihedral symmetry and icosahedral symmetry** (in order of complexity).
- A multimeric protein with few subunits is called **oligomer. Dimer** contains 2 polypeptide chains.

| Homodimers | Heterodimers |
|---|---|
| Contain two copies of same polypeptide chain | Contain different polypeptide subunits |
| Represented as $X_2$ | Represented as α β |

- Examples: **Creatinine kinase (dimer), lactate dehydrogenase (tetramer), hemoglobulin (tetramer** of 2 alpha + 2 beta chains) and **immunoglobulin (tetramer** of 2 heavy + 2 light chain)

the back bone, side chain of aminoacids extend outward and the structure is **stabilized by hydrogen bond b/w N – H & C= O groups** of main chain

- In α-helix, the polypeptide backbone is *tightly wound (twisted) around an imaginary axis* (drawn longitudinally through the middle of helix) and *side chains (R-groups) protrude outwards* from helical back bone. The polypeptide backbone of α-helix is equally *twisted about each α-carbon atom* with a phi (ϕ) angle = -57° and psi (ψ) angle = -47°. Each complete turn of helix contains ~ **3.6** aminoacyl residues with **translation** (i.e. distance b/w each aminoacid) = 0.15 nm (1.5 A°) and **pitch** (i.e. distance per turn) = 0.54 nm (5.4 A°).
- Structure of α-helix is stabilized primarily by hydrogen bonds formed b/w
  - **Oxygen (O)** of peptide bond carbonyl and **hydrogen (H) atom** of peptide bond nitrogen of **4th** residue down the peptide chain (Harper)
  - Hydrogen (H) atom attached to electronegative nitrogen atom of peptide linkage and the electronegative carbonyl **oxygen (O) atom** of **4th** aminoacid on aminoterminal side of peptide bond (Lehninger).
- Every peptide bond (except those close to end of helix) participate in hydrogen bonding. So each turn is held to adjacent turn by 3-4 **hydrogen bonds** (supplemented by **Van der Walls** interactions), conferring significant stability.
- Experimentally, α-helix can form in polypeptides consisting of *either L or D stereoisomeric* aminoacids, with all residues of one type because *mixing of D & L aminoacids will disrupt the structure*. Theoretically, naturally occurring L aminoacids can form either right or left handed α-helices but extanded left handed α-helices are unstable and not observed.
- **Alanine** show the ***greatest tendency to form α-helix***Q. **Keratins** protein of hair, nail and skin and *hemoglobin / myoglobin* are rich in α-helical structure, whereas chymotrypsin virtually lack it. Not all aminoacids form α-helix, ***proline & glycine have least proclivity to form α-helixes***Q.

### Triple Helix

- ***Collagen rich in proline and hydroxy proline, can not form α- helix or β- pleated sheet. It forms triple helix***Q.
- Stabilized by interchain hydrogen bonds b/w different polypeptide chains.

### Reverse Turns or β- Bends

- β-bends reverse the direction of polypeptide chain, helping it form a compact globular chain.
- Usually occur on the surface of globular protein
- A.A frequently found in β- bends
  - Proline
  - Glycine

### Super Secondary Structures

- Greek key
- β-meander: consists of *5 β-pleated sheets connected by reverse turns*. It contains nearly as many hydrogen bonds as an α-helix.
- β- α- β unit

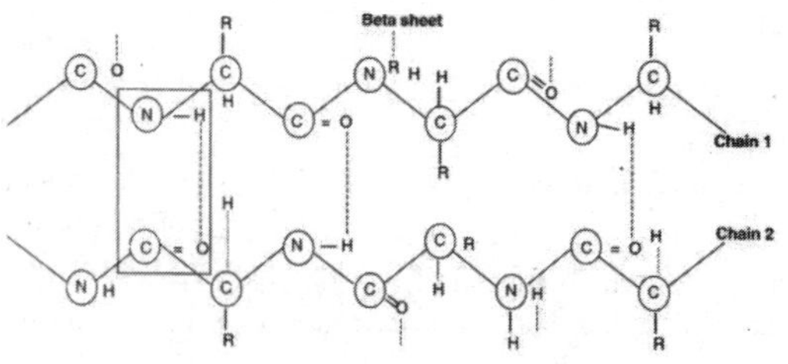

(H — O) HYDROGEN BOND—β-PLEATED SHEET

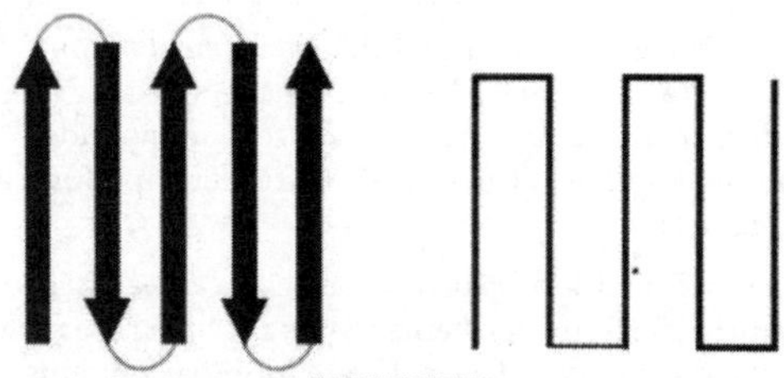
β-MEANDER

## Structural Organization of Protein

**Primary structure** is *linear sequence of amino acids held together by peptide bond*[Q].

↓ leads to

**Secondary structure is** regular arrangements of amino acids located near to each other in primary structure & is produced from folding or coiling of primary structure.

consists of
- *α- helix*[Q]
- *β- sheet*[Q]
- β- bends (reverse turns)
- Non- repetitive structure
- Supersecondary structures
  - β-α-β unit
  - β-meander
  - Greek-key

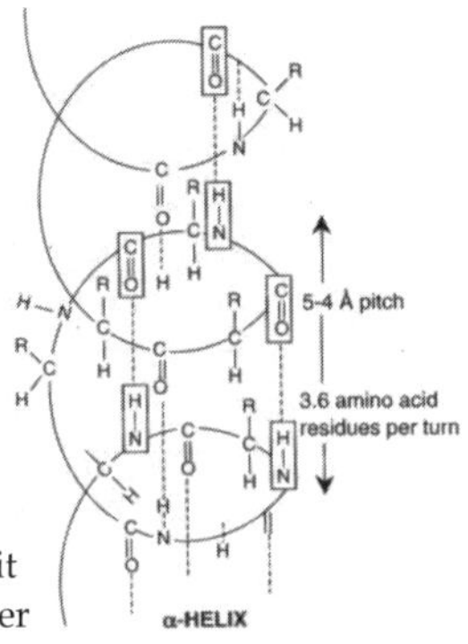


↓ leads to

**Tertiary structure** is is the three dimensional shape of the folded chain

Stabilized by
- Hydrophobic interaction
- Hydrogen bond
- Electrostatic interaction.
- Disulfide bonds

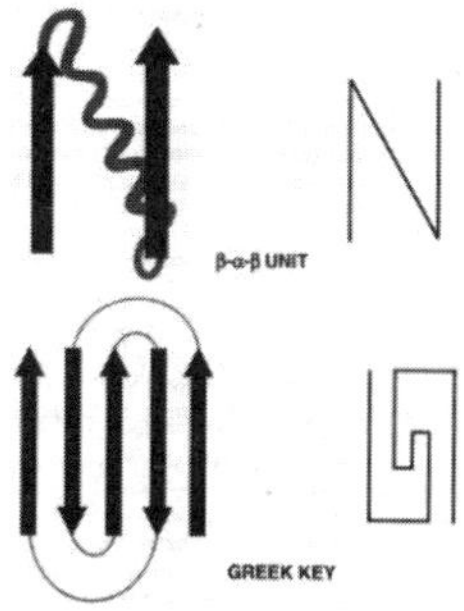


↓ may lead to

**Quaternary structure is** the arrangement of multiple polypeptide subunits in protien

Stabilized by
- Hydrophobic interaction
- Hydrogen bond
- Electrostatic interaction.

★ **Secondary and tertiary structure** of protein maintain the *3- dimensional shape of protein* and the main bonds involved are *weak non covalent bonds.* (Thus ***3-D shape is maintained by multiple weak interaction)***[Q].

### Aminoacids Affecting Stability or Disrupting α-Helices

**- Proline**
**- Hydroxy-proline**

- Since peptide bond nitrogen of proline *lacks a hydrogen atom to contribute to a hydrogen bond,* it can only be stably *accommodated within the first turn of α-helix.* When present else where, **proline disrupts α-helix.**
- Nitrogen atom of proline is a part of rigid imino ring & rotation about N-$C_{\alpha}$ bond is not possible. Hence proline **introduces a destabilizing** kink in α-helix.

**Glycine**

B/o small size, and more conformational flexibility, it induces bends.

**Charged aminoacids**

Disrupt α-helix by forming ionic bonds or electro statically repelling each other

| + | - |
|---|---|
| - Arginine<br>- Lysine<br>- Histidine | ***- Aspartate (aspartic acid)***[Q]<br>- Glutamate (glutamic acid) |

★ For stability +ve charged aa are found 3 residues away from –ve charge aa.

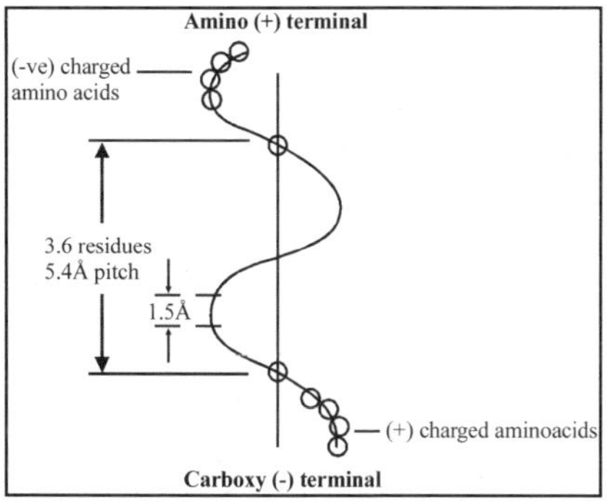


When present in large number or close together

**Bulky side chains**
- **Tryptopan**

**AA that branch at β carbon** (i.e. 1[st] C **in R group next to α-C)**
- **Valine**
- **Isoleucine**

**Bulk & Shape of AA**
- Asaparagine
- Serine
- Threonin

**Aminoacids at the end of helix**
- 4 aminoacids at each end do not fully participate in hydrogen bonding
- Electrical dipole of each peptide bond is aligned through hydrogen bonds of helix, resulting in a net dipole along the helical axis that increases with helix length
- For this reason negatively charged aminoacids are found near amino terminal and positively charged amino acids are found near carboxy terminal of α-helix; where they have stabilizing interaction

**Positive (+)** charged aminoacid at **amino (+) terminal)** and **negatively (-)** charged aminoacids **at carboxy (-) terminal** of α-helix is destabilizing.

## Various Types of Bonds

- **Hydrophobic (weak) interactions** are predominantly important for protein's stabilizing conformation (protein stability)
- Hydrophobic residues are largely buried in the protein interior, away from water and the number of **hydrogen bonds and ionic interactions with in protein is maximized**, thus reducing the number of hydrogen bonding & ionic group that are not paired with suitable partner. Because of favourable free energy change and cooperative bonding (i.e. one bond favours the formation of next bone), the **hydrogen bonds** often ***have an important role in guiding the protein folding process***[Q]. *(Langerhan's 115)*
- After folding into their native conformations, *some protein form interchain or intrachain disulfide bridges between Cys residues.* In eukaryotes, disulfide bonds are common in proteins to be exported from cells. The cross links formed in this way help to *protect the native conformation of protein from denaturation in extracellular environment*, which can differ greatly from intracellular conditions & is generally oxidizing, - *(Lehninger)*
- **Higher order of protein structure (tertiary & quaternary)** are stabilized primarily & often exclusively – by **non covalent** interactions, principle among these are ***hydrophobic interactionns***[Q] that drive most hydrophobic aminoacid side chains into the interior of protein shielding them from water. Other significant contributors include *hydrogen bonds and salt bridges between* carboxylates of aspartic and glutamic acid and the oppositely charged side chains of protonated lysyl, argininyl, and histidyl residue. Collectively these confer a high degree of stability to the biologically functional conformation of protein.
- Some (not all) peptides form **covalent disulfide (S – S) bonds** linking sulfhydryl group of cysteinyl residues by oxidation (requiring $O_2$). **Intrapolypeptide disulfide bonds** enhance the *stability of folded conformation* of a peptide, while ***interpolypeptide disulfide bond*** *stabilize quarternary structure* of certain oligomeric proteins.
- **Disulphide bonds:** are the S- S bonds between – SH group of two distant cysteine residues. A given cysteinyl residue can form many disulfide bond pairs, only one of which is appropriate for biologically folding. *The enzyme disulphide isomerase* facilitates shuffling of – S-S bonds by accelerating the rate at which disulphide undergo mutual exchange, thereby *accelerating process of protein folding and stabilizing proteins native conformation.*

**Bond Mainly Responsible For**

- **Primary structure**
  - *Peptide bonds*[Q]
- - **Secondary structure &**
  - **Folding**
  - *Hydrogen bond*[Q]
  - ★ **Chaperones** (i.e. Hsp 70 or 70 kDa **heat shock protein**) bind hydrophobic aa., shield them from solvent, prevent aggregation , thus ***providing opportunity for formation of appropriate 2° structure and folding***[Q]. Chaperonins (Hsp 60) act later in folding process by providing *sheltered environment* (d/t its donut shape) in which a polypeptide can fold until all hydrophobic regions are buried in its interior, eliminating aggregation.
  - ★ **Auxiliary proteins** assist folding
- - **Higher order (tertiary & quaternary) protein structure**
  - High degree of **stability to biologically functional** conformation of protein (**Protein stability**)
  - - ***Noncovalent Hydrophobic bonds***[Q] (main)
    - Hydrogen bond
    - Salt bridges
- Protection of native conformation of protein from denaturation
  - **Disulfide (Covalent) bond**
    - **Intrapolypeptide** disulfide bond
      - ***Enhance stability of folded conformation***[Q]
    - **Interpolypeptide** disulfide bond
      - Stabilize Quarternary structure of oligomeric proteins
- **Help in folding**
  - Auxiliary protein
  - Chaperones (Hsp-70)
  - Chaperonins (Hsp-60)
  - Disulfide isomerase
  - Disulfide bonds

## Isopeptide Bond

- **Isopeptide bond** is an amide bond formed **between the side (not main) chain carboxy terminal of one protein** (with either glutamate or aspartate) and **amino group of lysine** residue on side chain of another target protein.
- Bond formation is either **spontaneous** (in gram positive bacterial pilli & HK 97 bacteriophage capsid formation) or **enzyme (transglutaminase) catalyzed** (between lysine & glutamine). **Spontaneous proximity induced isopeptide bond formation** requires presence of glutamic acid, and is used in development of **isopeptag** (a new peptide tag) which can spontaneously & irreversibly react with its target through a covalent isopeptide bond. This molecular tool is used in development of new protein architectures – in vivo protein targeting and fluorescent microscopy imaging.
- Isopeptide bond formation is involved in **post translational modification of proteins**. Interchain isopeptide bonds **make proteins resistant** and produce stably linked protein dimmers, multimers & complexes like blood clots, as only few enzymes can hydrolyze this bond.
- A small peptide **Glutathione**, has isopeptide bond b/w side chain of glutamate & amino group of cysteine. Similary **ubiquitin protein**'s C terminal glycine residue gets attached to lysine side chain of other protein by isopeptide bond.

## Keratin: Fibrous – Intermediate Filament (IF) Protein

- **Keratin is a fibrous protein** and like all other fibrous proteins (such as **collagen & silk fibrion**) is adapted for **structural function. Keratins,** like all other **fibrous proteins (eg collagen & silk fibrion) are insoluble in water,** a property conferred by a **high concentration of hydrophobic amino acids both in interior of protein and onits surface**

**Right handed Alpha Helix and Left Handed Super Helix with Plenty of Hydrophobic Aminoacids.**

- α-keratin (helix) **secondary structure is right handed α helix.** *Two strands of α-keratin (right handed helix), oriented in parallel (with their amino terminals at the same end),* are wrapped about each other to form a **super twisted coiled coil with its helical axis twisted in a left handed super helix** (forming tertiary structure). The super twisting amplifies the strength of the overall structure, just as strands are twisted to make a strong rope. This super twisting to form a coiled coil is also responsible for discrepancy between the 5.4 A° per turn predicted for α helix by Pauling & Corey and 5.15 to 5.2 A° repeating structures observed in x-ray diffraction (of hair).
- The areas (surfaces) where 2–α helixes touch each other are made up of **hydrophobic aminoacid residues,** their R groups meshed together in a regular interlocking pattern – this **allows a close packing** of polypeptide chains with in left handed supertwist. That's why α keratins are ***rich in hydrophobic aminoacids Ala, Val, Leu, Ile, Met and Phe***[Q].

**Disulfide Bonds & Strength of Quaternary Structure**

- Intertwinging of 2-α helical polypeptides (coiled coils) forms **quaternary structure** of keratin. It is stabilized by **disulfide cross links** ***between pairs of cysteine (Cyst) residues of adjacent polypeptide chains***[Q] (enhancing the strength of fibrous proteins).
- **Protein α keratin,** formed by all **vertebrates,** is the **chief structural component of hair, nails, horns, hooves, wool, feathers, scales, claws, quills and much of the outer layer of skin.** So α- keratins form tough, insoluble protective structures of varying hardness and flexibility evolved for strength. ***In α-Keratins, the quaternary structure (formed by intertwinging of 2-α-helical polypeptide chains) is stabilized by disulfide bond cross links between pairs of cysteine (cyst) residues of adjacent polypeptide chains***[Q].
- The **extent of hardness, strength and flexibility** of α-keratins depends on the **number of disulfide bonds** (sulfur content / cysteine residues). ***The more the number of disulfide bonds between Cys residues of adjacent polypeptide chains, the more the hardness, toughness & strength and lesser the flexibility of the keratin is***[Q]. So decreasing order of disulfide bonds (or hardness) is ——————
- **Hair can be waved/curled** by moist heat and stretching out α-helix to fully extended β -conformation. **Reducing agent (thiol / or sulfhydryl group)** is applied with moist heat – the reducing agent cleaves disulfide cross link and moist heat breaks hydrogen bonds, thus causing α-helix to uncoil. After some time reducing agent is washed and oxidizing agent is applied to establish new disulfide bond pairs between Cys residues of adjacent polypeptide chains but not the same bond pairs as before the treatment. Similarly straightening of hair can also be done.

**IF Proteins**

Alpha -keatins are part of a broader family of proteins k/a intermediate filament (IF) proteins. IF is an intracellular fibrous system of filaments with an *axial periodicity of 21 nm and a diameter of 8-10 nm that is intermediate between that of microfilaments (6nm) and microtubules (23nm).*

| IF Proteins | Distribution |
|---|---|
| **Keratins<br>-Type I (Acidic)<br>-Type II (Basic)** | **Epithelial cells, hair, nails, horns, hooves, feathers etc** |
| **Lamins A, B and C** | **Nuclear lamina** |
| **Neurofilaments<br>- L (low),<br>- M (medium),<br>- H (high)** | **Neurons** |
| **Vimentin like<br>- Peripherin<br>- Glial fibrillary acid protein<br>- Desmin<br>- Vimentin** | **<br>- Neurons<br>- Glial cells<br><br>- Muscle<br>- Mesenchymal cells** |

They are all elongated, fibrous molecules with a central rod domain, an amino terminal head and a carboxy terminal tail. Mature filaments are composed of tetramers packed together in a helical manner forming a structure like rope. They are structural component of cells, and most are relatively stable components of cytoskeleton, not undergoing rapid assembly and disassembly and not disappearing during mitosis as do actin and microtubular filaments. **Lamins,** which form a *mesh work in apposition to inner nuclear membrane,* is an important exception – lamins subsequent to phosphorylation disassemble at mitosis and **reappear when it ends.**

**Skin** << **Hair** << **Nail** << **Rhinoceros Horn**

| Skin | Hair, Nail | Rhinoceros Horn |
|---|---|---|
| **Soft α keratin**<br>**Least number of disulfide bonds; more pliable (flexible) than hard keratins** | **Hard α-Keratins**<br>(Because of more disulfide bonds these are less flexible & much harder than soft keratins) | **Hardest & Toughest**<br>**(Upto 18% of residues are cysteines involved in disulfide bonds)** |

## Glycoprotein

- Are ***proteins that contain oligosaccharide (glycan) chains covalently attached to their polypeptide backbones***[Q]
- Carbohydrate chain is usually ***short (2- 10 units), branched & have several repeats***[Q]. Their carbohydrate content ranges from *1- 85%* by weight.
- Once a glycoprotein has been purified, the use of *mass spectrometry* and *high resolution NMR spectroscopy* can often identify the structures of its glycan chains. Analysis of glycoproteins can be complicated by the fact that they often exist as ***glycoforms***; i.e. ***proteins with identical aminoacid sequence but some what different oligosaccharide compositions***[Q].
- *Oligosacchride chains encodes biological information* and this depends upon their constituent sugars, their sequences and their linkages.
- Oligosacchride chain of glycoprotein is responsible for – *physiochemical properties* (eg solubility, viscosity, charge, conformation, denaturation & binding sites), *biological activity, protection against proteolysis, insertion into membranes, intracellular migration, sorting and secretion.* It affects embryonic development & differentiation and site of metastasis.
- Eight sugars predominate in glycoproteins and these are *mannose, fucose* (are GDP linked); *glucose, galactose, xylose, N- Acetyl galactosamine, N- Acetyl glucosamine* (are UDP linked) and *N- Acetyl neuraminic acid* (linked to CMP to form nucleotide sugar)
- *N- Acetyl neuraminic acid (Neu Ac)* is usually found at the *termini* of oligosaccharide chains attached to *subterminal galactose (Gal) or N- acetyl galactosamine (Gal Nac).* Other sugars are in internal positions. *Neuraminidase* is an *exoglycosidase* (i.e. act externally); endoglycosidase

F & H act internally; where as *galactosidase* is both *exo & end glycosidase*

- Based on their linkage between their polypeptide chains & oligosaccharide chains; glycoprotein can be of 3 types:
  i) **O- linked** i.e. containing O- glycosidic linkage, involving hydroxyl chain of serine/ threonine and sugar N- acetyl galactosamine ***(Gal Nac - Ser/Thr)***
  ii) **N- linked** i.e. containing N- glycosidic linkage, involving amide nitrogen of asparagine and N- Acetyl Glucosamine ***(Glc Nac - Asn)***
  iii) **GPI - linked/*Glycophosphatidyl inositol*-linked** i.e. glycan (oligosacchride) is linked to carboxyterminal of a.a. via phosphoryl ethanolamine.
- ***Glycophorin a RBC glycoprotein contain both O and N linked oligosacchrides***[Q]. Almost all plasma proteins except albumin are glycoproteins. *Selectins* (a glycoprotein) play a key role in *inflammation & lymphocyte homing*. Zona pellucida contain glycoproteins ZP 1- 3, that functions as a *receptor for sperm* (esp *ZP – 3*) & induce *acrosomal reaction*.
- *Asialoglycoprotein receptor* is involved in clearance of glycoprotein from plasma by hepatocytes.
- *Tunicamycin, deoxynojirimycin & swainsonine inhibit N but not O- glycosylation*. The extension of O- linked chains can be prevented by *Gal NAC – benzyl*.

Three inhibitors of enzymes involved in the glycosylation of glycoproteins and their sites of action

| Inhibitor | Site of Action |
|---|---|
| Tunicamycin | Inhibits GlcNAc-P transferase, the enzyme catalyzing addition of GlcNAc to dolichol-P, the first step in the biosynthesis of oligosaccharide-P-Pdolichol |
| Deoxynojirimycin | Inhibitor of glucosidases I and II |
| Swainsonine | Inhibitor of mannosidase II |

## Glycosaminoglycans (GAG)

- GAGs are ***large complexes of negatively charged, long, unbranched, hetropolysaccharide chains generally composed of a repeating disaccharide unit [acidic sugar – aminosugar]$_n$***[Q]
- They ***hold large amount of water***[Q] thereby producing the gel like matrix that forms the basis of body's ground substance, & lubricating other structures
- Because of their **strongly negative charges**, these hetropolysaccharide chains are extended in solution occupying space & repelling each other.
- They are *surrounded by a shell of water molecules* & when brought together, they slip past each other (like same poles of magnet) This l/t **slippery consistency** of synovial fluid & mucous secretions.
- When compressed, the water is squeezed out and GAGs occupy smaller volume. on release of compression the GAGs spring back to their original hydrated volume thus provides **cushioning**.
- Tend to attract polycations & positive ions such as Na+/K+ which result in their ability to attract water by osmotic pressure.

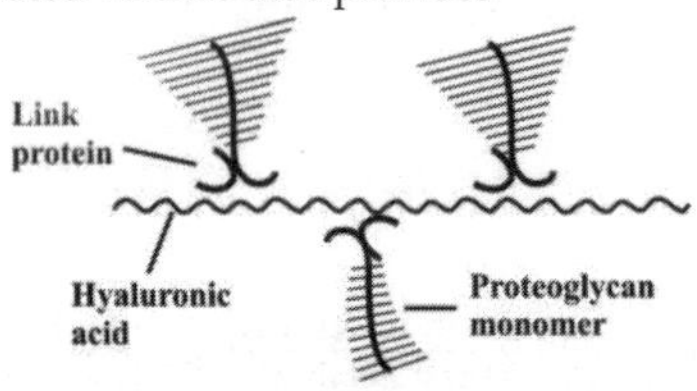


## Proteoglycan

- ***GAGs are generally associated with a small amount of protein forming proteoglycans which contain > 95% carbohydrate***[Q]. Whereas, glycoproteins contain primarily protein & a small amount of carbohydrate
- *All the GAGs, except hyaluronic acid, form proteoglycans*. It is also the only GAG which is *not sulfated* and also found in *bacterias.*
- Proteoglycan monomer resembles a *bottle brush* as it consists of a *core protein to which linear GAG chains* are covalently attached. Each chain may be composed of > *100 monosaccharide chains*, remain separated from each other b/o charge repulsion.

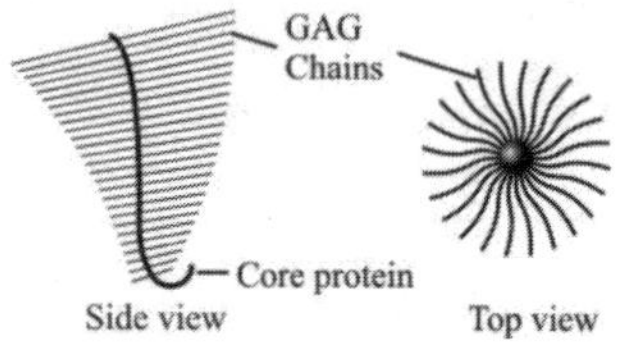


- Linkage b/w core protein & carbohydrate (GAG) chains is most commonly through *a serine residue & a trihexoside (galactose – galactose – xylose)* respectively. An O glycosidic bond is formed b/w hydroxyl group of serine & Xylose.

| Serine - OH | — Xylose– Galactose– Galactose — | [Acidic sugar / Amino sugar]$_n$ |
|---|---|---|
| **Serine side chain** | **Trihexoside** | **Repeating disaccharide unit** |

- Proteoglycan monomers associate with hyaluronic acid molecule to form proteoglycans aggregates *primarily through ionic interactions.* Association is stabilized by small link proteins.
- PGs can act as **sieves** restricting the passage of large molecules into ECM but allowing free diffusion of small molecules.
- Syndecan (membrane), versican & aggregan (extracellular matrix) and neurocan & cerebrocan (nervous system) are proteoglycans.

★ **So proteoglycan=GAGs+Protein (≤5%) =[Amino & Acidic sugar]$_n$ + proteins**

## Glycosylation: Glycosidic Linkages of Glycoproteins

Addition of carbohydrate (sugar or oligosaccharide) side chains to specific aminoacid residues of proteins forming glycoprotein is called **glycosylation**. There are **two types of glycosylation (& glycosides).**

### N-Glycosylation and N - Linked Glycosides

- In N-Glycosylation sugar chain is attached to ***amide ($NH_2$) group of asparagine***[Q] side chain (**Glc Nac – Asn**)
- N-linked oligosaccharide may be of complex or high-mannose variety both containing same **core pentasaccharide**. But additional sugars for complex oligosacchride are NANA (N-acetyl neuraminic acid), Fuc (L-fucose) & Glc NAc (N-acetyl glucosamine), whereas high mannose oligosaccharides contain primarily mannose (Man) only

### O- Glycosylation & O-Linked Glycosides

- In O-Glycosylation sugar chain is attached to hydroxy ***(OH) group of either serine or threonine***[Q] R group (**Gal Nac – Ser/Thr**)
- O – glycosylation begins with *transfer of an N-acetyl galactosamine (from UDP-Nac) onto a seryl or threonyl R group*. The **glycosyltransferases** responsible for stepwise synthesis of oligosaccharide are bound to ***membrane of golgi complex***[Q].
- **Tyrosine, hydroxylysine and hydroxyproline** aminoacids may also be involved in O-glycosylation.

- **Endo plasmic reticulum (synthesis) & golgi complex (final processing) are involved in N- glycosylation**[Q].

**ER**

- Protein & **dolichol** (80- 100 carbon ER membrane lipid) linked oligosaccharide are first synthesized.
- Sugars added to dolichol by membrane bound **glycosyl transferase** are first N- acetyl glucosamine f/b mannose & glucose
- Oligosaccharide is transferred from dolichol to asparagine side of protein by **protein – oligosaccharide transferase** present in ER
- **Trimming of carbohydrate chain begins** in ER by removal of mannosyl & glucosyl residues.

**Golgicomplex**

- **Final trimming & completion** of oligo saccharide chains by addition of variety of sugars (Nac glucosamine, Nac galactosamine, mannose, fucose, NANA) to produce **complex glycoprotein** or
- They are not processed, leaving branched, mannose containing chains in a **high-mannose glycoprotien.**

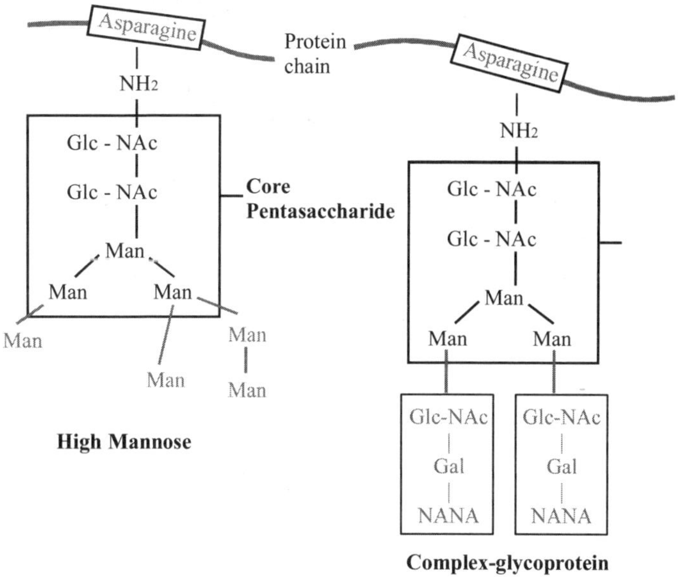


| Glycoproteins | Feature | Glycosaminoglycans |
|---|---|---|
| *Are* **proteins to which hetro oligosaccharides are covalently attached**[Q] | Composed of | **Protein including core & link protein + hetro polysacc haride chain**[Q] |
| - **Short hetrooligo saccharide chain**[Q]<br>- *Branched, may or may not be negatively charged.*<br>- *No repeating disaccharide units* | Chain | - *Long hetropolysaccharide chain*<br>- **Unbranched, Negatively charged**[Q].<br>- **Repeating disaccharide units**[Q] *[acidic sugar-amino sugar]$_n$*<br>- *Acidic sugar is* D- glucronic acid or L- iduronic acid *and aminosugar is D-glucosamine or* D- galacto-samine |
| - **Cell surface recognition**[Q]<br>- *Cell surface antigenicity*<br>- *Components of extracellular matrix & mucin*<br>- *Globular proteins in plasma* | **Function** | - *Chondroitin 4 & 6 sulfates, keratan, dermatan & heparan sulfate, heparin & hyaluronic acid are 6 major types*<br>- *Bind large amounts of water, producing gel like ground substance supporting cellular & fibrous component of tissues*<br>- *D/t viscosity also k/a mucopolysaccharides*<br>- *Mediate cell-cell signaling & adhesion* |
| - **N-glycosylation occurs in ER lumen & O-glycosylation in golgi complex**[Q]<br>- *In golgi complex proteins are sorted to their proper destination such as inclusion in cell membrane, lysosome or secretion from cell* | **Synthesis** | - **Glycosaminoglycans are synthesized in golgicomplex**[Q]<br>- *Sulfonation of amino sugar is last step. Source of sulfate is 3' – phophoadenosyl –5- phosphosulfate.*<br>- *All except hyaluronic acid form proteoglycan monomer, which consist of a core protein to which linear chains of glycosamino glycans are attached.* |

## Denaturation

- *Disruption of native structure* is termed denaturation. Physically denaturation may be viewed as ***randomizing the conformation of a polypeptide chain***[Q] with out affecting its primary structure.
- Since no covalent bonds in the back bone of the polypeptide chain are broken during this, the *primary structure remains intact*
- The comparatively weak forces responsible for maintaining secondary, tertiary and quaternary structure of protein are readily disrupted with resulting loss of biological activity.
- The biological activity of most proteins is destroyed by strong acids or bases, heat, ionic detergents (amphipaths), ***chaotropic agents (urea, guanidine)***[Q], heavy metals (Ag, Pb, Hg) or organic solvents.
- Denatured proteins are ***generally less soluble and they precipitate***[Q] (not always).
- Denaturation results in unfolding & disorganization of secondary & tertary structure of protein without hydrolysis of peptide bonds. ***Under ideal conditions it may be reversible, in which case the protein refolds into original native structure when denaturing agent is removed. However most proteins, once denatured remain permanently disordered***[Q].

## Collagen: Structure & Formation

- All collagens have a **triple helical** structure. **3 of these alpha chains** are then wound into **right handed superhelix**. A characteristic feature of collagen is occurrence of **glycine residue at every 3rd position** of triple helix of α- chin. This is necessary because glycine is the only amino acid small enough to be accommodated in the limited space available down the central core of triple helix.
- Repeating (Gly- X-Y)n structure is an absolute requirement for formation of triple helix while X & Y can be any other amino acids, about 100 of X are **proline** & 100 of Y are **hydroxyproline** both of which confer rigidity
- Biosynthesis of collagen involves.

### Intracellular events in fibroblast, osteoblast or chondroblast

1. **Cleavage of signal or leader peptide to form pro α chains** (from pre-pro α chains)

   Like most secreted proteins produced for export, collagen is synthesized on ribosomes in a precursor form preprocollagen, which contain a leader sequence that facilitates binding of ribosomes to RER & directs the polypeptide chain **into the lumen of endoplasmic reticulum.** The signal sequence is cleaved in ER to yield a precursor of collagen called **pro α chain**.
2. **Hydroxylation of prolyl & some lysyl residues**: proline & lysine residues found at Y position may be *post translationally modified (i.e. hydroxylated) to hydroxy proline & hydroxy lysine residues*, through the action of prolyl hydroxylase & lysyl hydroxylase enzymes. It requires *molecular oxygen ($O_2$),* ***reducing agent vitamin C (ascorbic acid)*** *and α ketoglutarate as cofactors.*

   So in scurvy collagen fibers cannot be cross linked greatly decreasing the tensile strength
3. **Glycosylation of some hydroxyl- lysyl residues** by addition of *galactose or galactosyl- glucose* through an **O-glycosidic linkage** (that is unique to collagen): Like hydroxylation, glycosylation also takes place in ER
4. **Formation of intrachain & interchain disulfide bonds in extension peptides:** Procollagen molecule contains polypeptide extension **(extension peptides)** of 20-35 kDa at both its amino & carboxy terminal. Both extension peptides have cysteine residues. While amino terminal propeptides form only intrachain disulfide (S – S) bonds, the carboxy terminal extension peptide forms both intra & interchain S-S bonds.
5. **Formation o triple helix**:

   Formation of these disulfide bonds assists in formation of triple helix, winding starts from carboxy terminal end. After formation of triple helix, no further hydroxylation or glycosylation can take place.

   Procollagen molecules are translocated to *golgi apparatus*, where they are packed in *secretory vesicles*. The vesicles fuse the *cell membrane* & release procollagen molecules into extracellular space.

### Extracellular events

6. **Cleavage of N and C terminal extension peptides of procollagen molecules.**

   Extracellular enzymes called **procollagen amino proteinase & procollagen carboxy proteinase** remove the extension peptides at amino and carboxy terminal ends, respectively.

   Cleavage may occur *within crypts or folds in the cell membrane*, releasing triple helical **tropocollagen** molecules which *spontaneously assemble* into collagen fibers.
7. **Self assembly of tropocollagen molecules into quarterly staggered collagen fibrils**

   Tropocollagen molecules spontaneously associate to form collagen fibrils. They form an ordered, parallel, overlapping array, with adjacent collagen molecules arranged in a **quarter staggered pattern** (such that each is displaced longitudinally from its neighbour by slightly less than a quarter of its length)
8. **Oxidtive demination of ε- amino groups of lysyl & hydroxylysyl residues to aldehydes and formation of intra and inter chain cross links**

   Lysyl oxidase, a copper containing enzyme that oxidatively deaminates the ε– amino group of lysine & hydrolysine residues, yielding reactive aldehydes

   The reactive aldehydes (allysine & hydroxy allysine) can condense with ε aminogroup of *unoxidized lysyl or hydroxylysyl residues* in neighbouring collagen molecules to form **collagen crosss links**, & thus, mature collagen fibers

   *Histidine* may also be involved in certain cross links.

## Tropocollagen or Collagen Molecule

It is a subunit of larger collagen aggregates such as fibrils & is approximately **300 nm long and 1.5 nm in diameter**, made up of ***three left-handed alpha* helix *polypeptides strands*** (its name is not to be confused with the commonly occurring alpha helix, a right-handed structure). These three left-handed helices are **twisted together into a *right-handed triple helix or "super helix"***, a quaternary structure stabilized by numerous *hydrogen bonds*. With type I collagen and possibly all fibrillar collagens if not all collagens, each triple-helix associates into *a right-handed super-super-coil* that is referred to as the collagen microfibril. Collagen fibrils are collagen molecules packed into an organized overlapping bundle. Collagen fibers are bundles of fibrils.

*A distinctive feature of collagen is the regular arrangement of amino acids in each of the three chains of these collagen subunits* - Gly-Pro-Y or Gly-X-Hyp, where X and Y may be any of various other amino acid residues. So ***Proline or hydroxyproline*** constitute about *1/6* &, ***Glycine*** accounting for the *1/3* of the sequence, this means that approximately half of the collagen sequence is not glycine or proline.

In the fibrillar collagens, the tropocollagen molecules are staggered from each other by about ***67nm*** (a **'D' unit** and changes depending upon the hydration state of the aggregate). Each *D-period contains 4 and a fraction collagen molecules*. This is because 300 nm divided by 67 nm does not give an integer (the length of the collagen molecule divided by the stagger distance D).

Collagen fibrils / aggregates are arranged in different combinations and concentrations in various tissues to provide varying tissue properties. **In bone**, entire collagen triple helices lie in a ***parallel, staggered array. 40 nm gaps between the ends of the tropocollagen subunits serve as nucleation sites for the deposition of long, hard, fine crystals of the mineral component, which is (approximately) hydroxyapatite, $Ca_{10}(PO_4)_6(OH)_2$with some phosphate***. It is in this way that certain kinds of cartilage turn into bone. Type I collagen gives bone its tensile strength.

## Simple & Conjugated Protein

Proteins can be divided *on the basis of their solubility and their physical properties*

**Simple proteins**

On complete hydrolysis yield only amino acids

Examples:
- *Albumin*[Q]
- *Globulin*[Q]
- Protamines
- Histones

**Conjugated protein**

Are simple proteins combined with a non- protein group called prosthelic group. Protein part is called **apoprotein** and entire molecule is called holoprotein.

| Class | Nucleo-protein | Muco-protein (mucoids) | Lipo protein | Glyco protein | Phospho protein | Chromoprotein | | | Metallo protein | | | | |
|---|---|---|---|---|---|---|---|---|---|---|---|---|---|
| | | | | | | Hemo-protein | Flavo protein | Visual purple | | | | | |
| Prosthetic group | DNA RNA | Hexo-samine | Lipids | Carbo hydrate | Phosphate | Heme (Fe-porphyrin) | Riboflavin (flavin) nucleotide | Carotenoid | Fe | Zn | Ca | Cu | Mo |
| Example | Chromatin | Mucin | $B_1$ lipo-protein | IgG | Casein Ovovitellin | Hb Mb Cytc, $P_{450}$ | Succinate dehydro-genase | | Ferritin | Alcohol dehydrogenase, carbonic anhydrase | Calmodulin | Plastocyanin, ceruloplasmin | Dinitrogenase |

## Transport or Binding Plasma Proteins

| Plasma Proteins | Function (Bind & Transport) |
|---|---|
| **Transthyretin (Prealbumin)** | **Thyroxine (T4) and retinol** (forms a complex with retinol binding protein) |
| **Albumin** | Osmotic protein binds & transports various ligands like **ions (Ca++), metals (Cu2+, Zn2+), bilirubin , free fatty** acids, metheme, steroids, other hormones & drugs |
| **Retinol binding protein** | Binds & transports **retinol** |
| **Ceruloplasmin** | Contains & transports **Cu++** (albumin is probably more important in physiological transport of Cu++); has **ferroxidase activity**. |
| **Corticosteroid binding globulin (Transcortin)** | Cortisol |
| **Thyroid binding globulin (TBG)** | **Thyroxine (T4, T3)** |

| Plasma Proteins | | Function (Bind & Transport) |
|---|---|---|
| **Haptoglobin** | | **Extracorpuscular (free) hemoglobin** (phenotype 1-1); **peroxidase activity** (phenotype 2-1) |
| **Sex hormone binding globulin** | | Testosterone , estradiol |
| **Hemopexin (HPX) = Beta-B-Globulin** | | **Heme** |
| **Transferrin (Siderophillin)** | | **Iron (Fe)** |
| **Trans cobalamine I, II, III ($\alpha_2\beta$ mobility)** | | **Vitamin $B_{12}$** |
| **Lipoproteins** | **$\alpha_1$ (HDL)** | Transport lipid, fat soluble vitamins, hormones and remove **cholesterol from tissue to liver (scavanger action)** |
| | **$\beta$ (LDL)** | Transport same but **carries cholesterol to tissues.** |

★ **Hemoglobin** is a tetrameric protein of RBC that **transport $O_2$ to tissues and return $CO_2$ & protons to lungs.**

## Storage Proteins

These are **biological reserves of metal ions and aminoacids** such as found in plant seeds, egg whites and milk. Examples includes

1. Plant albumins: **legumelin** in legumes and **leucosin** in cereals.
2. Animal albumins: **ovalbumin** in egg and **lactalbumin & casein** in milk
3. Globulins: ovoglobulin in egg and lactoglobulin in milk
4. **Gliadins (prolamines)** very rich in proline but poor in lysine: gliadin of wheat and **hordein** of barley
5. **Glutelins** (rich in glutamic acid): glutelin in wheat and **oryzenin** of rice
6. **Ferritin and hemosiderin** stores iron
7. **Myoglobin** , a monomeric protein of red muscles stores oxygen as a reserve against oxygen deprivation (Harper 29/48)*

## Heat Test for Protein

Take 2/3 of test tube full of urine sample. Hold the test tube from the bottom and heat the top portion of tube. Add a drop of 1% acetic acid. Do not mix.

**Normally (when Urine PH is Acidic)**

White turbidity or precipitates in the heated portion indicating the presence of albumin.

**If Urinary pH is Alkaline**

- Proteins may not be precipitated owing to formation of alkaline meta proteins, which are not precipitated on heating
- ***Phosphates may however be precipitate and give a false positive test***[Q].
- On acidification with 1% acetic acid, drop by drop, phosphate will disappear and precipitate of albumin will appear on acidification.

# Test Methods for Estimation of Substances

### Total Serum Protein Estimation

- **Calorimetric Assay (common methods)**

1. ***Biuret***[Q] protein assay
2. ***Lowry's (Folin-Ciocalteu)***[Q] protein assay
3. ***Smith (Bicinchoinic acidd)***[Q] protein assay
4. ***Bradford's (Coomassie G-250 dye) method***[Q]

- Nephelometric, Turbidimetric, Direct photometric, UV visible spectroscopy, Refractometric methods
- Kjeldahl method, Amido black protein assay, O-phthaldehyde & Nano orange methods.

### Blood Glucose Concentration

- Aztoor-king, Folin Wu & Nelson- Somogyi chemical methods.
- Glucokinase, Hexokinase & Glucose dehydrogenase enzymatic methods.

### Tests of Carbohydrate

- **Molisch's test**
- **Barfoed's, Benedict's and Fehling's tests** for detection of reducing sugar (ie with aldehyde & ketone group). **Seliwanoff's test** differentiate between aldose & ketone sugars.
- **Bial's Resorcinol test** detect presence of pentose (5C sugars)

### Tests for Lipids

- Brown paper (grease spot) test
- Sudan red test

### Uric Acid

- Phosphotungstic acid (PTA) chemical method
- Uricase enzymatic method

### Blood Urea

- Diacetyl monoxime (DAM) chemical method
- Urease & glutamate dehydrogenase enzymatic methods

## Clinical Laboratory Based Analytic Systems for Measuring Serum Creatinine to Assess GFR

### Alkaline picrate methods

- **Jaffe method** (1886) overestimates serum creatinine by as much as 15-25% d/t presence of interfering substance, particularly *proteins (albumin), acorbate, pyruvate, glucose, bilirubin, fetal hemoglobin & drugs*
- **Kinetic Jaffe assay** have improved specificity & minimized suceptibility to interfering substances.
- **Technicon continuous flow autoanalyzer** (Skeggs) provided the first opportunity to efficiently process increasing workloads & incorporated on line dialysis to remove protein & protein bound interfering substance such as bilirubin, but smaller molecules such as glucose, pyruvate, acetoacetate & cephalosporins were still able to cross the dialysis membrane & cause falsely increased results.

### Enzymatic criatinine method

- It uses these enzymes and this reaction

**Creatinine** —*Creatininase*→ Creatine —*Creatinase*→ Sarcosine —*Sarcosins oxidase*→ Formaldehyde + $H_2O_2$ + glycine

- The $H_2O_2$ generated can be measured by spectrophotometrically (Roche creatinine plus assay), using leuco dye (vitros dry chemistry system), or with blood gas analyzer electrodes (Radiometer dual electrode system)
- Bilirubin and creatinine interference is reduced by using more efficient $H_2O_2$ acceptor (triiodo- hydroxy benzoic acid), potassium ferocyanide& detergents. Ascorbate & dopamine are other interfering substances.

### High performance liquid chromatography (HPLC)

*Fairly sensitive & specific method* and include cation – exchange / normal-phase / reversed-phase and reversed phase ion-pair chromatography. Sample deprotinization improves specificity.

### GC- isotope dilution mass spectroscopy

Method of choice

# Method of Separation & Purification of Protein

(based on)

### Molecular size

| Technique | Property used |
|---|---|
| ***Denaturing gel/ SDS-PAGE (polyarcylamide gel) electrophoresis***[Q] | **Molecular weight (mass)** |
| ***Gel filtration (size exclusion) chromato-graphy***[Q] | Molecular weight (size) |
| **Dialysis/Ultra filtration** | Size |
| **Ultracentrifugation** | Mass/density |

★ **pI** is **pH** at which the net charge of molecule is zero. And electrophoresis in general is for separation of **charged molecules**.

### Charge & or Iso electric point (pI, pH) and combined

| Chromatography | Property used |
|---|---|
| *High performance liquid chromatography (HPLC)* | Charge, size, affinity |
| *Ion exchange chromatography* | Charge |
| *Chromato focusing chromatograpgy* | pI |
| **Electrophoresis** | **Property used** |
| *Isoelectric focusing (IEF) electrophoresis* | pI |
| *Native gel electrophoresis* | Mass/Charge |
| *2D gels electrophoresis* | Molecular weight & pI |

### Solubility

- **Ammonium sulfate precipitation (bulk method) i.e.**
  - **Salting in**
  - **Salting out**
- **Partition chromatography**

### Hydrophobicity

- **Reversed phase** chromatography
- **Hydrophobic interaction** chromatography

### Biological activity or affinity binding

- Affinity (absorption) chromatography
- Precipitation by antibodies

★ Ammonium sulphate, precipitation, centrifugation, and filtration are **bulk methods**

## Ammonium Sulfate / $(NH_4)_2SO_4$ = (Salt) Fractionation

Early purification (fractionation) utilize differences in **protein solubility** which depends on *pH, temperature, salt concentration etc.*

Salts of **divalent ion** such as ammonium sulfate / $(NH_4)_2SO_4$ and magnesium chloride ($MgCl_2$) are far more effective than salts of monovalent ions eg NaCl, KCl, and $NH_4Cl$. ***Ammonium sulfate is particularly effective and is often used to salt out protein*** [Q].

| Salting In | Salting out |
|---|---|
| In **low concentrations**, salt increase the solubility of many proteins, a phenomenon known as **salting in** | - The solubility of proteins is lowered at **high salt concentration**, an effect called salting out<br>- **Increasing the ionic strength (or salt concentration) gradually decrease the solubility of proteins.** So addition of certain salts eg ammonium sulfate can selectively precipitate some proteins, while others remain in solution<br>- At 33-40% saturated $(NH_4)_2SO_4$, human immunoglobins are precipitated (salted out) while albumin remains soluble. Most proteins will precipitate from an 80% saturated $(NH_4)_2SO_4$. Saturated ammonium sulfate is about 4.1 mmol/L |

## Chromatography

- This is a method of separation of molecules that involves passing (**diffusing**) a solution (the **mobile phase**) through a medium (**immobile or stationary phase**) that shows selective absorption for different solute components based on their size, charge, hydrophobicity & affinity etc. So chromatography separates or purifies proteins on the basis of *charge, size, hydrophobicity or affinity.*
- The stationary /immobile phase or matrix may be a *sheet of filter paper* (**paper chromatography**) or a thin layer of cellulose, silica or alumina (**thin layer chromatography** or **TLC**) or a column (cylinder container of glass, plastic or metal) containing small spherical beads of modified cellulose, acrylamide or silica whose surface has been coated with functional groups)– **Column chromatography**
- Either **ascending** or **descending chromatography** can be done based on the mobile phase being applied *from the bottom or at the top* respectively. Depending on methods of separation types of chromatography include-

### Size: Gel Filtration (Size Exclusion) Chromatography

- Separates protein on the basis of ***molecular size*** [Q] ***(stokes radius).***
- A number of gels (sephadex) when hydrated acts as molecular sieves. The pores on the surface of these gel allow smaller molecules to penetrate deeper whereas larger molecules are left outside, hence also called ***exclusion chromatography.***
- The **procedure is *extremely gentle*, permitting seperation of labile substances e.g. protein, nucleic acid like DNA fragments** [Q].
- The procedure is *highly reproducible with minimal losses.*
- Used to *determine molecular weight* of purified protein.

### Hydrophobicity: Hydrophobic Interaction Chromatography

- Seperates proteins based on their tendency to associate with a **stationary phase matrix coated with hydrophobic groups** (eg **phenyl Sepharose, octyl Sepharose**)
- *Proteins with exposed hydrophobic surfaces* adhere to the matrix via hydrophobic interactions, that are enhanced by *a mobile phase of high ionic strength*
- Nonadherent proteins are first washed away. The *polarity of mobile phase is then decreased to weaken hydrophobic interactions* by gradually *lowering salt concentration* f/b *adding glycerol or ethanol* (if interactions are very strong).

### Solubility: Partition Chromatography

- In this the components of mixture to be separated are partitioned b/w the two phases (eg solid – liquid, liquid-liquid, gas-liquid etc) depending on the **solubility (partition co-efficient)** of the particular substances. Stationary phase may be either solid or liquid over which a liquid or gaseous mobile phase moves
- Purifies proteins based on their relative affinity of different proteins for a given stationary or a mobile phase, which in turn depends on composition of both stationary & mobile phase.
- Proteins that interact more strongly with stationary phase are retained longer and provide a basis of partition (purification)
- Gas liquid chromatography (GLC), TLC or ascending / descending

### Biological Activity: Affinity Chromatography

- Affinity chromatography **separates proteins by their *binding specificities.* The *proteins retained on the column are those that bind specifically to a ligand*** [Q] (substance) that has an inherent ability to bind with the target molecule to be purified.
- It exploits the *high selectivity of most proteins for their ligands.* So **enzymes** can be purified by using coenymes or inhibitions as stationary phase. And so *antigen-antibody, hormone-receptor, enzyme-substrate, inhibitor-cofactor* can be sparated.
- After proteins that do not bind to ligand are washed through Bound proteins are eluted (washed out of column) either by competition with soluble free ligand or by *disrupting protein ligand interactions using urea, guanidine hydrochloride, mildly acidic pH or high salt concentration.*
- Stationary phase matrices available comercialy contain ligands such as *$NADP^+$ or ATP analogs and $Ni^{+2}$* (that bind protein with an attached polyhistidine tag & a glutathione matrix that binds a recombinant protein linked to glutathione – S- transferase

### Charge: Ion- Exchange Chromatography

- Separates proteins depending on the net electric ***charge of protein*** [Q].
- Chromatography ***on carboxymethyl cellulose or diethyl amino methyl cellulose column*** [Q] separates protein based on electrostatic attraction b/w charged molecules & oppositely charged groups on ion exchange resins.

### Size, affinity & charge; High Performance / Pressure Liquid Chromatograph (HPLC)

- The stationary phase used in classic column chromatography are spongy material whose compressibility limits flow of the mobile phase
- HPLC makes use of **high pressure pumps** that speed the movement of mobile phase (protein molecules) down the column, as well as higher quality chromatographic

paper chromatography is performed and some **location reagents** (eg ninhydrin for aminoacids & peptides; sulphuric acid for phospholipids; diphenylamine for sugars) is sprayed on paper to identify **RF (relative flow)** value. **RF (ratio of fronts) value** is the *ratio of distance traveled by the substance (solute) to the distance traveled by the solvent* in paper chromatography. The RF is constant for a particular solvent at a given temperature and the substance or aminoacid can be identified by their RF value.

**Adsorption coefficients** of molecules d/t van der waals interaction with stationary phase: **Absorption Chromatography**

- Protein mixture is applied to a column under conditions where **the protein of interest associates with the stationary phase** so tightly that its partition coefficient is essentially unity
- Non adhering first washed & then stabilizing forces are gradually disrupted by gradient of increasing salt concentration.

**incompressible** (sillica or alumina microbeads as) **stationary phase** that can withstand the crushing force of pressurized flow

- Reduced transit time **limits the diffusional spreading** of protein bands & *thus greatly improves resolution.*
- Used for high resolution separation of proteins peptides and aminoacids based on their charge, size & hydrophobicity. The eluates are monitored by *ultraviolet absorption, refractive index or fluorescence.* So it can give **high resolution separation** of mixtures of lipids or peptides whose property differ only slightly.
- **Reversed phase HPCL** uses a *hydrophobic stationary phase of aliphatic polymers* 3-18 carbon atoms in length. And peptide mixtures are eluted (separated) using a gradient of water miscible organic solvent such as *acetonitrile or methanol.*

## Ion Exchange Chromatogaphy (IEC)

- It separates (purifies) protein on the basis of differences in the **sign & magnitude of net electric** charge at a given pH.
- In IEC, the **stationary phase (column matrix)** is a synthetic polymer (resin) *containing bound (attached) charged groups* – **negatively charged** (carboxylic or sulfonic group) in **cation (+ ion) exchanger;** and **positively charged** (tertiary or quaternary amines) in **anion (- ion) exchanger**. The protein which has to be separated (purified) is percolated through the stationary phase in liquid form and it forms **mobile phase** of IEC. The proteins of mobilephase interact with resin of stationary phase by **charge - charge interaction (electro static attraction)**. Since the *net charge on a protein is determined by the pH*, this separation is also based on *ionic character of proteins & aminoacids* (**isoelectric point**).

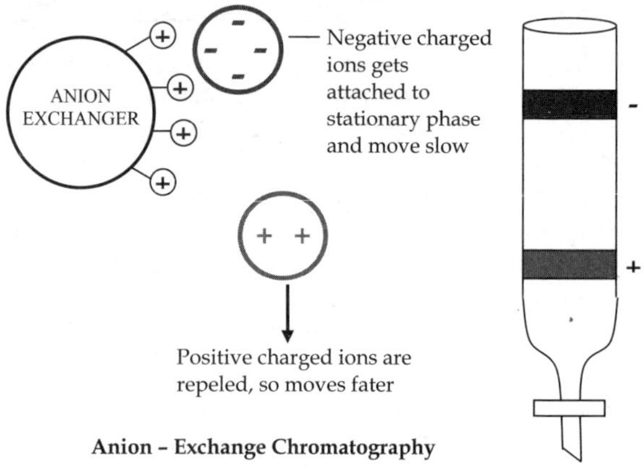


**Anion - Exchange Chromatography**

- Proteins, which are *polyvalent compete against monovalent ions* for binding to the stationary phase - thus the term ion exchange
- The affinity of each protein for charged group on column (stationary phase) is affected by the pH (which determines the ionization state & net charge of molecule) and **concentration of competing free salt ions**. Separation can be optimized by gradually changing the pH and or salt concentration of the mobile phase so as to create a **pH** or **salt gradient**.

- **On the basis of charge of stationary phase,** It is of 2 types

**Cation (Positive ion) Exchanger**

When a more positively charged ion (or molecule) is exchanged with another positively charged component bound to **negatively charged stationary phase**, the process is called cation exchanger. Cation exchange resins have **negatively** charged *sulphonic or carboxylic groups.*

| **Stationary phase (solid matrix) Resin** | **Charge** | **Negative** |
|---|---|---|
| | **Example** | - **Carboxymethyl cellulose** (O-$CH_2$-$COO^-$)<br>- Carboxylate (carboxylic) group.<br>- Sulfate (sulphonic) group |
| **Slowest moving amino acids** (in mobile phase) | | **Positively charged** aa. because they interact with stationary phase |
| **Fastest moving amino acids** (in mobile phase) | | **Negatively charged** |

**Anion (Negative ion) Exchanger**

When a more negatively charged ion (or molecule) is exchanged with another negatively charged component bound to **positively charged stationary phase** the process is called anion exchanger. Anion exchange resins have positively charged quaternary nitrogen ($N^+$)

| **Stationary phase (solid matrix) Resin** | **Charge** | **Positive** |
|---|---|---|
| | Example | - **Diethyl aminoethyl (DEAE) cellulose** (- O- $C_2H_4$ – $NH^+$ $[C_2H_5]_2$) = Strong anion<br>- Tertiary or quaternary amines (nitrogen)<br>- Dowex – 3 (weak anion)<br>- Amberlite IRC – 50 (weak cation) ?? (Vasudevan) |
| **Slowest moving amino acids** | | **Negative charged** |
| **Fastest moving amino acids** | | **Positively charged** |

★ At pH 7.5, albumin is negatively charged (pI = 4.8) and immunoglobin is positively charged (pI = ~ 8). So albumin **(anion) will move slowly in an anion exchanger** and immunoglobin **(cation) will move slowly in a cation exchanger.**

## Electrophoresis

- **Electrophoresis** is separation of proteins based on ***migration of charged proteins in an electric field***Q
- It is ***not geneally used to purify proteins in large amounts because it often adversely affects the structure & function of proteins***Q and simpler alternatives are available
- It is an *analytical method that quickly estimates number of different proteins in a mixture or the degree of purity* of a particular prtein preparation. Its advantage is that protein can be visualized as well as separated.
- *Polyacrylamide gel* acts as a molecular sieve slowing the migration of proteine ~ in proportion to **charge – to – mass ratio.** Migration is also affected by **size & shape**Q.
- The force moving the macromolecule is electrical potential (E)

### Isoelectric Focusing

- It determines isoelectric point (pI) of a protein and **separates protein according to their pI.**
- It is based on the fact that each protein has a different pH at which it is electrically neutral (pI)
- A **pH gradient** is generated within polyacrylamide matrix by allowing **ampholytes** or **ionic buffers** (i.e. low molecular weight organic acids & bases) to distribute themselves in an electric field generated across the gel.
- Applied protein migrate until it reaches the region where pH matches its **isoelectric point (pI), the pH at which the molecules net charge is zero.**

### Two dimensional Electrophoresis

- It is combining **isoelectric focusing and SDS electrophoresis** sequently
- It is *more sensitive* analytical method than either electrophoretic method alone
- It permits *fractionation of complex mixtures of proteins*
- It separates proteins of identical molecular weight that differ in pI, or protein with similar pI values but different molecular weight

$$\text{Electrophoretic mobility } (\mu) = \frac{\text{Velocity } (V)}{\text{E}} = \frac{\text{Net charge } (z)}{\text{Frictional Coffieicnt } (f)}$$

## Discrimination / Seperation of Nucleic Acid (DNA & RNA)

- Seperation by size through a gel matrix in presence of an electric field (i.e. gel electrophoresis) is the ***most common technique to discriminate different nucleic acids***Q
- Both *DNA & RNA are negatively charged* and will migrate towards a positively charged electrode.
- Seperation is primarily based on **molecular weight** with smaller molecules traveling faster than larger ones. **Physical conformation (or shape)** also affect & form the basis of separation. Because single stranded RNAgenerally hs a high degree of secondary structure. Electrophoresis of RNA is usually performed under denaturating conditions to abolish these structures. Electrophoresis of DNA is performed under non denaturing or denaturing conditions (to abolish hetroduplex, nicked or superhelical circular structures) depending on amplification. Under most gel conditions.

| Compact supercoiled (Form I) DNA | Floppy, relaxed or nicked circular DNA (Form II) | Linear (Form III) DNA |
|---|---|---|
| ***Fastest moving form***Q | ***Slowest migrating band***Q | Migrates at rate (form a band) intermediate b/w uncut supercoiled & nicked relaxed forms |

- When very large molecules (> 50kb) have to be separated, **pulsed electrical fields** are employed to help move these molecules through the polymer matrix **(Pulse- field gel electrophoresis, PFGE).** Conventional gel electrophoresis use current applied in single direction. Very large DNA fragments are thought to orient themselves with the voltage field. Once oriented, molecules of different lengths migrate at slow but similar rates. The trick to separating these large fragments is to make them change direction at regular intervals; longer DNAs take longer to orient correctly and so lag behnd shorter fragments. So in PFGE, an alternating current is applied to the gel, changing the direction of electrophoresis at intervals. That's why a normal agarase gel electrophoresis may take 1 – 4 hr, whereas PFEG often require 24 hrs to complete.
- **Polyacrylamide** gel is suited for *high resolution separation* (upto 0.1% size differences) of *short molecules* (upto 2kb), whereas *agarose gel* can separate nucleic acid fragments *from 20 bp to 10 mB (10,000 kb) but with limited resolution* (usually to a size difference 2-5%)

## SDS – PAGE

- A *denaturing anionic detergent, sodium dodecyl sulfate (SDS)* [dodecyl denoting 12 carbon chain = $CH_3 (CH_2)_{11}- SO_4 - Na^+$] is used in poly acrylamide gel electrophoresis (**PAGE**) system to separate, resolve & purify protein subunits according to **molecular weight.**
- Acrylamide is polymerized & cross linked to form porous matrix (stationary phase) which acts as a molecular sieve.
- SDS *denatures protein, & disrupts the hydrophobic interactions* of protein so that the protein is *partially unfolded and assumes a similar (rod like) shape.*
- SDS binds to protein at a **ratio of 1 molecule of SDS per 2 peptide bonds (or amino acid residues)** that is roughly *proportional to molecular weight of protein (or length of peptide chain).*
- The large number of bound anionic SDS contribute a **large net negative charge**, rendering the intrinsic charge of protein insignificant and *conferring on each protein a similar charge – to mass ratio.*
- Because SDS treated proteins have similar shape and charge to mass ratio; ***SDS – PAGE separates proteins almost exclusively on the basis of mass (molecular weight)***Q, with smaller polypeptides migrating more rapidly.
- A purified protein preparation can be readily **analyzed for homogeneity (purity)** on SDS-PAGE by staining with sensitive & specific dyes, such as **Coomassie blue**, or with a **silver staining** technique, which *binds to protein but not to gel itself.*
- Thus the researcher can moniter the progress of protein purification as the number of bands decreases after each new fractionation step. When *compared with positions of protein with known molecular weight*, the position of unidentified protein can provide a *good approximation of its molecular weight.*
- SDS- PAGE **separates the component polypeptides of multimeric proteins** when used with **2-merceptoethanol or dithiothreitol** to reduce and break disulfide bonds. **A separate band appears for each component.**

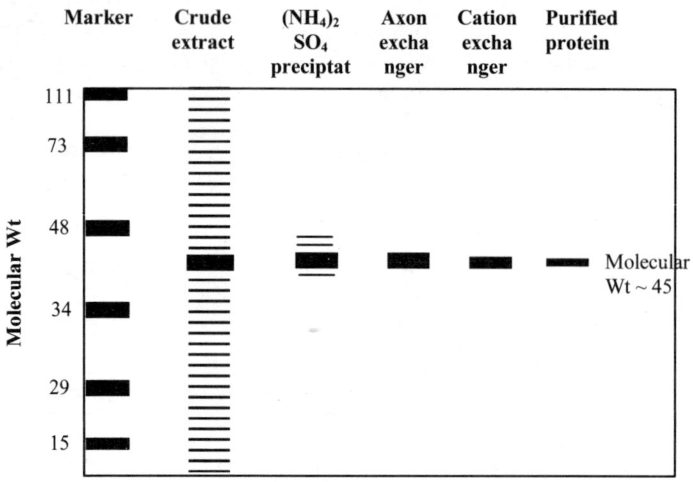

**SDS - PAGE**

So in above case 100 kD protein has 2 bands of 20 kD & 30 kD.

Hence Protein has 2 components of 20 kD & 30 kD (i.e. 50 kD). Since to be of 100 kD there must be 2 units of 50 kd (50× 2 = 100). So the 100 kD protein is a dimer of 20 kD & 30 kD component.

## Detection of Protein Structure

**Primary Structure detection**

- **Sanger's Reagent Method**
- Fragmenting polypeptide chain by endoproteases & chemical reagents.
- Automated protein sequencer **(sequenator)** using ***Edman's degradation technique***Q and **DNA sequencing.**
- **Mass spectrometry** to ***detect molecular mass, sequence of polypeptides & covalent modifications simultaneously***Q (more commonly used method)
- Protein sequencing, identification and molecular weight determination of intact protein can also be done by **matrix-assisted laser desorption ionization – time of flight (MALDI - TOF) mass spectrometry and Electrospray ionization mass spectrometry (ESI-MS)**
- Once partial aminoacid sequence is obtained, one can determine nucleotide sequence of DNA that encodes this polypeptide segment. Chemically synthesized oligonucleotide primers can be used to identify amplify (by PCR) and isolate gene containing appropriate sequence. **(Indirect hybrid technique)**

**Higher three dimensional (Secondary, tertiary and quaternary) structure detection**

- ***X ray crystallography (or diffraction)***Q
- **Polychromatic X-ray** crystallography (**Laue diffraction**)
- ***NMR (nuclear magnetic resonance) spectroscopy***Q
- ***Infra-red spectroscopy***Q
- Ultraviolet (UV) light spectroscopy
- Optical rotatory dispersion
- Circular dichromism

## Reagent & Cleavage Point

- *Trypsin cleaves peptide bonds on C- terminal side of arginine and lysine residues, provided the next residue is not proline*[Q]. **Chymotrypsin** cleaves peptide bond on ***carbonyl (C) terminal of phenylalanine, tryptophan and tyrosine***[Q]
- ***Lysyl endopeptidase cleaves c- terminal side of lysine***[Q] and cyanogens bromide cleaves C- terminal side of methionine.
- *Disulfide bonds interfere with sequencing procedure.* So before cleavage **proteins with cysteine** and **cystine** residue are either ***oxidized by performic acid***[Q] to ***cysteic acid or reduced by dithiothreitol (or β mercaptoethanol)***[Q] and idoacetate (to carboxymethylated cysteine) to **irreversibly break disulfide bonds.** This avoids spontaneous formation of inter or intra molecular disulfides during analysis.
- For **determination of structure of protein:** Purified protein (by process of salting out →dialysis → ion exchang & gel filtration chromatography →SDS PAGE) is cleaved by **protelytic degradation**. The cleaved peptides fragments are again purified by reverse phase HPLC and then sequenced on automated protein sequencer, using **Edman's degradation technique**, Now **Mass spectrometry, MALDI - TOF, ESI -MS** and indirect hybrid techniques are also used to determine 1° protein structure.

| **Reagent** (Biological source) | **Cleavage point** |
|---|---|
| **Trypsin** (bovine pancrease) | - ***Lysine, Arginine (C) provided next residue is not proline***[Q]<br>- Elastase esters of small neutral aliphatic aminoacids, chymotrypsin esters of aromatic aminoacids. |
| **Lysyl endoproteinase C** (bacterium Lysobacter enzymogenes) | Lysine (C) carboxy terminal |
| Submaxillarus protease (mouse submaxillary gland) | Arginine (C) terminal |
| Cyanogen bromide chemical | Methionine (C) |
| **V8 protease** (staphylococcus aureus) | Aspartate, Glutamate (C) |
| Asp - N- protease (Pseudomonas fragi) | Aspartate, Glutamate (N terminal) |
| **Chymotrypsin** (bovine pancreas) | Phenylalanine, Tryptophan, Tyrosine (C) or Leucine |
| **Pepsin** (Porcine stomach) | Leucine, phenyalanine (Phe), Tryptophan (Trp), Tyrosine (Tyr) - **N** amino side |

## Mass Spectrometry

- It determines the ***mass of molecules***[Q] (< 1000 Da by conventional spectrometers and larger mass by use of **flight spectrometers**)
- Initial difficulty of volatilizing large organic molecules has overcome by ***MALDI (matrix assisted laser desorption and ionization) and electrospray dispersion*** *(eg. Nanospray)* which permit the masses of even large polypeptides (>100000 Da) to be determined with *extraordinary accuracy (± 1Da)*
- Peptides inside the mass spectrometer are broken down in smaller units by collisions with *neutral helium atoms (collision induced dissociation)* and the masses of the individual fragments are determined.
- Since peptide bonds are much more labile than the carbon-carbon bonds, the most abundant fragments will differ from one another by units equivalent to one or two amino acids.
- Since with the *exception of leucine and isoleucine*- the molecular mass of each aminoacid is unique, the sequence of the peptide can be reconstructed from the masses of its fragments.
- It *detects covalent modification* i.e. is ideal for detecting the phosphate, hydroxyl and other groups on post translationally modified aminoacids. As each adds a specific and readily identified increment of mass to the modified amino acid
- **Tandem mass spectrometry** can *determine mass by analyzing complex peptide mixture with out prior purification*. It employs the equivalent of 2 mass spectrometers linked in series. It can detect metabolic abnormalities such as PKU, ethyl malonic encephalopathy, & glutaric academia type I.

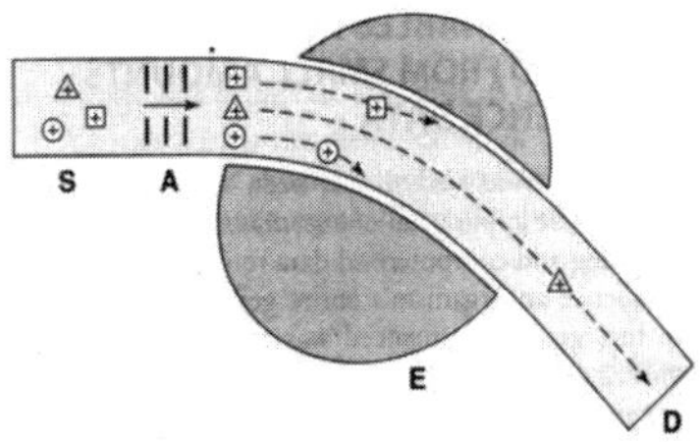


Basic components of a simple mass spectrometer. A mixture of molecules is vaporized in an ionized state in the sample chamber **S.** These molecules are then accelerated down the flight tube by an electrical potential applied to accelerator grid **A.** An adjustable electromagnet, **E,** applies a magnetic field that deflects the flight of the individual ions until they strike the detector, **D.** The greater the mass of the ion, the higher the magnetic field required to focus it onto the detector.

Mass increase resulting from common posttranslational modifications

| Modification | Mass Increase (Da) |
|---|---|
| Phosphorylation | 80 |
| Hydroxylation | 16 |
| Methylation | 14 |
| Acetylation | 42 |
| Myristylation | 210 |
| Palmitoylation | 238 |
| Glycosylation | 162 |

★ **Protein purity** is assessed by ***polyacrylamide gel electrophoresis (PAGE)***[Q]. The most widely used method is SDS- PAGE i.e. polyacrylamide gel electrophoresis in the presence of the anionic detergent sodium dodecyl sulfate (SDS).

★ **Sanger's reagent (1 fluoro,2, 4- dinitrobenzene)** was used to determine the polypeptide sequence of insulin. It als react with ε- amino group of lysine.

★ **Edman's reagent (phenyl- iso thiocynate)** selectively label the amino terminal residue of a peptide. It enables peptides and proteins to be sequenced.

## Enzyme Inhibition

Any substance that can *decrease the velocity of an enzyme catalyzed* reaction is k/a **inhibitor (I)**. The inhibition can be **reversible** or irreversible. **Reversible inhibitors** bind to enzymes through *non covalent bonds and can be dissociated (removed)* from its binding site (by dilution) without loosing its enzyme activity. Whereas, **irreversible inhibitors** bind to enzyme through *covalent bonds* and can be removed from its site of binding only at the loss of enzymatic activity (i.e. **irreversible inhibitors poison enzymes**). Two most common types of reversible inhibiton are competitive & non competitive. However the non- competitive can also be irreversible.

| | Competitive Inhibition | Non-Competitive - Inhibition |
|---|---|---|
| Direction | *Reversible*[Q] | *Reversible or irreversible*[Q] |
| Structure of inhibitor (I) | Resemble substrate (structure) and so are termed **substrate analogs.** | Bear **no** (or little) structure **resemblance** to substrate |
| Binding site | Inhibitor binds to **substrate binding portion of active site** (i.e. both inhibitor & substrate bind to **same site** and so inhibitor competes with the substrate (S) for that site) thereby blocking access by the substrate | Inhibitors bind enzymes at sites **distinct from substrate binding site** (i.e. substrate (S) and inhibitor (=I) bind enzyme (=E) at **different sites**) and so there is *no competition* between inhibitor & substrate for enzyme. |
| EIS complex | - Inhibitor can not bind to enzyme – substrate (ES) complex<br>- Either EI or ES complex is formed and EIS is not possible | - Inhibitor can bind to ES complex<br>- Both EI and **EIS complexes** can form; however EIS generates product at negligible rate. |
| Raising substrate concentration (i.e. dilution) | **Overcomes inhibiton** (i.e. at sufficiently high substrate concentration, **Vmax will be same** as observed in absence of inhibitor) | **Can not be overcome** (i.e. inhibitor **decreases Vmax**) |
| Substrate affinity to enzyme | - **Decreased** (i.e. once inhibitor binds to enzyme, the enzyme cannot bind to substrate)<br>- So more substrate is needed to achieve ½ Vmax (i.e. **Km↑**) | - **Does not change** (i.e. non competitive inhibitors donot interfere with binding of substrate to enzyme)<br>- Same amount of substrate is needed to achieve ½ Vmax (i.e. **Km is unaffected**) |
| V max<br>Km | *Same*[Q]<br>*Increased* **(↑)**[Q] | Lowered (↓)[Q]<br>Same[Q] |
| Michaelis - Menten equation | $V = \frac{V_{max}[S]}{Km\frac{1+(I)}{Ki}+S}$ | $V = \frac{V_{max}[S]}{Km\left[\frac{1+(I)}{Ki}\right][Km]+[S]}$ |
| Lineweaver - Burk plot | $\frac{1}{V} = \frac{Km}{V_{max}}[1+\frac{(I)}{Ki}]\times\frac{1}{[S]}+\frac{1}{V_{max}}$<br>For Non-Competitive - Inhibition<br>$\frac{1}{V} = \frac{Km}{V_{max}}\left[1+\frac{(I)}{Ki}\right]\times\frac{1}{[S]}+\frac{1}{V_{max}}+\left[1+\frac{(I)}{Ki}\right]$ | 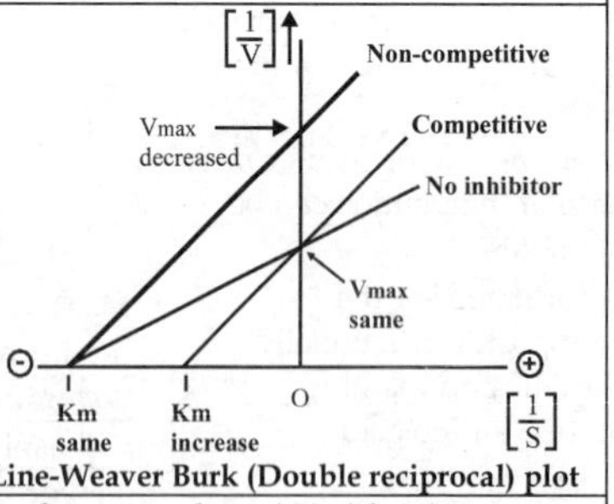<br><br>**Line-Weaver Burk (Double reciprocal) plot** |
| Eadic - Hofstee plot | No change in Y intercept (Vmax) but possesses steeper slope and smaller x intercept. | No change in slope (-Km) but Y intercept is lowered and x intercept declines in value |
| | 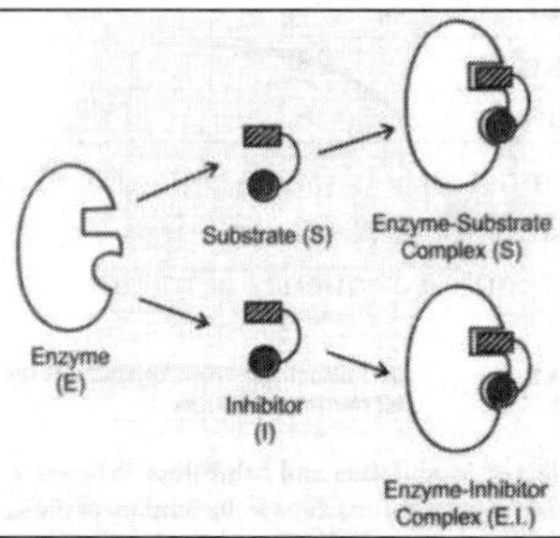<br> | 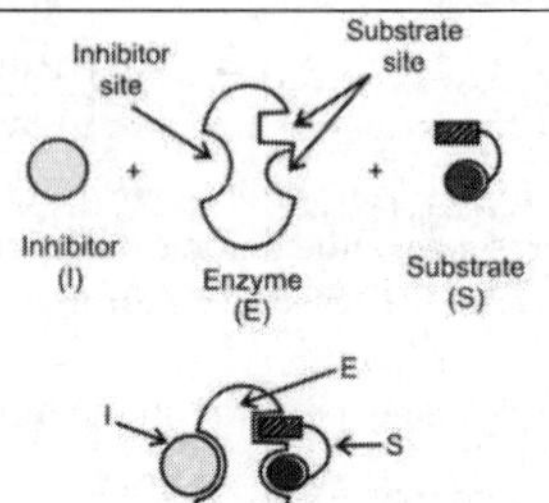<br> |

## Regulation of Enzyme Activity

### 1. Allosteric Inhibition

- Allosteric enzymes are regulated by molecules k/a **effector or modifiers** that bind **noncovalently at a site other than the active site** (k/a allosteric site) on a different region of enzyme molecule. Effector can *alter the affinity &/or the maximal catalytic activity of enzyme.*
- **Positive effectors** increase and **negative effectors** inhibit enzyme activity. When the substrate itself serves as an effector it is called **homotropic effector** but when both are different it is called **heterotropic effector**.
- Does *not follow Michaelis Menten hyperbolic kinetics*. Instead it gives a ***sigmoid curve & show cooperative binding.***[Q]
- Allosteric ***inhibitors*** shift the substrate saturation curve to the ***right*** & ***activators*** shift it to ***left***.
- Allosteric enzymes may be of *K & M series* according to their kinetics.
  - In **K- enzymes** eg *aspartate carbamoylase & phospho fructokinase,* allosteric inhibitor lowers substrate affinity to raise km, but ***Vmax is unchanged***
  - In **M-enzymes** eg *acetyl CoA carboxylase,* the allosteric inhibitor reduces the maximum velocity, but ***no change in km or substrate affinity.*** Allosteric activators produce a fall in K enzymes and a rise in Vmax
- When the final product allosterically inhibits the enzyme it is called feed back allosteric inhibition
  - ***Asparte transcarbamoylase (AT case)*** which catalyzes first reaction of pyrimidine synthesis is allosterically inhibited by *cytidine triposphate (CTP)*
  - *Threonine deaminase* first enz. of isoleucine synthesis is inhibited allosterically by *isoleucine*
- A metabolite may cause feed forward allosteric activation eg *F1. 6 Bi $PO_4$ activates pyruvate kinase*
- Allosteric effector oppositely influences two allosteric enzymes catalyzing reverse reations eg. *AMP activates phospho fructo kinase & inhibits F.D. pase*

| Enzyme/Drug | Competitive Inhibitor | Substrate |
|---|---|---|
| Lactate Dehydrogenase | Oxamate | Lactate |
| Aconitase | Transaconitate | Cis-aconitate |
| Succinate Dehydrogenase | Malonate | Succinate |
| HMG-CoA Reductase | HMG | HMG-CoA |
| Dihydrofolate Reductase | Amethopterin | 7,8 Dihydrofolate |
| **Allopurinol** | *Xanthine oxidase*, which produce uric acid from hypoxanthine | **Hypoxanthine** |
| **Sulfonamide** | Synthesis of folic acid (impermeable to bacterial wall) from PABA | **PABA** |
| **Methotrexate** | *Folate reductase* & prevent formation of $FH_4$ | **Folic acid** |
| **MAO Inhibitor eg Ephedrine & amphetamine** | *MAO (mono amine oxidase)* | **Cate -cholamines** |
| **Physos-tigmine** | Acetyl cholines terase (destroy ACH into choline &acetate) | *Ach* |
| **Dicoumarol** | Act as anticoagulant by inhibiting Vit K | *Vit K* |
| **Succinyl Choline** | Competitively fixes on post synapti c receptor. As it is not hydrolysed easily by the enzyme acetyl cholinesterase, it produces continued depolarization & muscle relaxation | *Ach* |

| *Enzyme* | *Allosteric activator* | *Allosteric inhibitor* |
|---|---|---|
| *Glutamate Dehydrogenase* | *ADP* | *ATP, NADH* |
| *Hexo kinase ICD* | *ADP* | *G-6-P, ATP* |
| *Protein Kinase* | *c-AMP* | - |
| *Pyruvate carboxylase* | *Acetyl CoA* | *ADP* |
| Phospho fructo kinase | - | *Citrate* |

2. By covalent modification eg **phosphorylation & dephosphorylation of enzyme.**

## Michaelis – Menten model & equation

- According to M-M- model, ***enzyme (E) reversibly combines with its substrate (S) to form enzyme – substrate (ES) complex that subsequently yields product (P), regenerating the free enzyme***[Q]

$$E + S \underset{K-1}{\overset{K}{\rightleftharpoons}} ES \xrightarrow{K_2} E + P$$

- M- M- equation describes how ***reaction velocity varies with substrate concentration***[Q].

$$Initial\ Velocity\ (V_0) = \frac{Maximum\ velocity\ (V_{max})[S]}{Michaelis\ constant\ (K_m) + [S]}$$

Where, [S] is substrate concentration & $K_m = (K-1+K_2)/K_1$. And it is assumed that concentration of substrate is much greater than enzyme, concentration of [ES] does not change with time and [ρ] is very small so rate of back reaction can be ignored. Conclusions extracted are

**Michaelis constant (Km)**

- It is characteristic of enzyme & its particular substrate and ***reflects the affinity of enzyme to that substrate***[Q]
- It is equal to substrate concentration at which ***reaction velocity is equal to 1/2 $V_{max}$***[Q]. It ***does not change with enzyme concentration***[Q].

| **Small (low) Km** | **Large (High) Km** |
|---|---|
| Reflects **high affinity** of enzyme for substrate, as low concentration of S is needed to half saturate E, i.e., to reach 1/2 $V_{max}$. | Reflects **low affinity** of E for S, because a high concentration of substrate is needed to half saturate enzyme |

- **Rate of reaction velocity is *directly proportional to enzyme concentration at all substrate concentrations***[Q]. Eg. when [E] is halved, $V_0$ & $V_{max}$ are reduced to half of original
- **Order of reaction**

| **When [S] << Km** | **When[S]>> Km** |
|---|---|
| - Velocity of reaction is approximately proportional to substrate concentration i.e., $V \alpha [S]$<br>- **1st order reaction** with respect to substrate. | - Velocity is constant and equal to $V_{max}$ (i.e., V = $V_{max}$)<br>- **Zero order** reaction, *independent of substrate concentration* |

★ **Line weaver – Burk (double – reciprocal) plot** is a straight line obtained by plotting $1/V_0$ versus $1/[S]$. It can be used to calculate Km & $V_{max}$, as well as to determine the mechanism of action of enzyme inhibitors.

## Catalytic Constant (Kcat) & Efficiency (Kcat/Km)

- Comparision of **relative catalytic activity** of different preparations of same enzyme or different enzymes can be done in
- Impure enzyme preparations by

$$\text{Specific activity} = \frac{V_{max}}{\text{Protein concentration}}$$

- Homogenous enzyme by

$$\text{Turnover number} = \frac{V_{max}}{\text{Moles of enzyme}}$$

- If number of active sites is known

$$\text{Catalytic constant } K_{cat} = \frac{V_{max}}{\text{Number of active sites } S_t}$$

It is best measure and unit is 1/time

- **Catalytic efficiency** is best expressed in terms of **ratio of Kcat/km**

## Inhibitory Potency

It is the concentration of inhibitor that produces 50% inhibition (**$IC_{50}$**)

## Calcium – Calmodulin

Calmodulin is calcium dependent (& binding) regulatory protein that is homologus to muscle protein troponin-C in structure & function. It can bind to **4 calcium ions**. Binding of Ca++ with calmodulin activates it (in a similar way of cAMP activates PKA). Enzymes & process activated by $Ca^{++}$ & mediated by calmodulin are

- **Adenylyl** *cyclase*[Q] (brain)
- C-AMP phosphodiesterase
- C-AMP gated olfactory channel
- Cyclic neucleotide **phosphodiesterase**
- ***Guanylate cyclase***[Q]
- C-GMP gated $Na^{+}$ & $Ca^{++}$ channels of rods & cones
- ***Glycogen synthase***[Q]
- Glycerol-3 phosphate dehydrogenase
- Glutamate decarboxylase

- $Ca^{++}$ dependent protein kinases (CaM kinase I-IV)
- $Ca^{++}$ - $Mg^{++}$ ATPase
- $Ca^{++}$ pump (plasma membrane calcium ATP ase)
- $Ca^{++}$ phospholipid dependent protein kinase
- Ca++ release channels of sarcoplasmic reticulum
- Ca++ dependent Na+ channel (paramecium)
- Calcineurin (phosphoprotein phosphatase 2B)
- L-type calcium channels
- Cytoskeletal protein

- Phosphorylase kinase
- phosphoprotein phosphatase 2B
- Phosphoinositide 3 kinase
- PhospholipaseC
- Phospholipase A2
- Pyruvate carboxylase
- Pyruvate dehydrogenase
- Pyruvate kinase

- RNA helicase
- Myosin light chain kinase
- NAD+ kinase
- Nitric oxide synthase
- NMDA type glutamate receptor

## Plasma Enzymes can be of Two Types

| Features | Functional Enzymes | Non Functional Enzymes |
|---|---|---|
| Function | Has physiological role | No known physiological role |
| Normal concentration in plasma in comparision to tissue | High | Low |
| Substrate in blood | Always present | Absent |
| Site of synthesis | Mostly in liver | In different tissues eg liver, heart, muscle |
| Cause of origin | Physiological need | Pathological process eg<br>- Cell damage & necrosis in viral hepatitis or MI<br>- Obstruction of normal path (bile duct = alkaline $PO_4$)<br>- Meastasis |
| Clinical importance | No | Diagnosis & prognosis of disease |
| Example | ***Lipoprotein lipase***[Q] etc | ***Acid & alkaline phosphatase , γ glutamyl trnspeptidase***[Q] etc. |

## Isozymes / Isoenzymes

Isozymes are the physically distinct forms of the same enzyme that catalyze the same reaction, and ***differ from each other structurally, electrophoretically and immunologically***[Q]. Isozymes arise through **gene duplication** in higher organisms. Isoenzymes may differ in their

1. **Quarternary structure** as many **isoenzyme multimeric complexes** contain ***different subunits in different (various) combinations***[Q] such as CPK1 has BB, CPK 2 has MB and CPK 3 has MM compositon.
2. **Physical properties** such as **heat resistance** because of genetically determined ***difference in aminoacid sequence***[Q]
3. **Electrophoretic mobility** (allowing them to be separated from each other by electrophoresis) because of **different electrical charges on the isoenzymes due to difference in contents of charged acidic & basic aminoacids**)
4. Properties such as **sensitivity to particular regulatory factors** or **substrate affinity** (eg glucokinase) **that adapt them to specific tissues or circumstances.**
5. **Tissue distribution: Different organs frequently contain characteristic proportions of different isoenzymes.** So pattern of isozyme in plasma may serve as *means of identifying the site of tissue damage.*
6. Although isoenzymes catalyze same reactions they differ in **rate of catalysis, pH optima, Kmax & Vmax** and even **enzyme classification.**

★ Each enzyme has a enzyme code number (EC No) of 4 digits

### Isoenzyme of Lactate Dehydrogenase (LDH)

- Lactate dehydrogenase is a tetrameric enzyme & consists of four subunits
- These subunits can occur in two isoform i.e.
  - H isoform (for heart)
  - M isoform (for muscle)
- All these isozymes though different physically they catalyze the same reaction of oxidation of LA to PA
- In normal serum, *LDH2 (H3M) is the most prominent isoenzyme.*

| LDH Isoenzymes | | | | |
|---|---|---|---|---|
| *Type* | *Polypeptide chains* | *Electrophorectic mobility* | *Tissue rich in isoenzyme type* | |
| LDH-1 | (H4) H H H H | Fastest moving d/t highest negative charge b/o higher Asp & glutamate content | found in *myocardium*[Q] | Heat resistance |
| LDH-2 | (H3M) H H H M | | | |
| LDH-3 | (H2M2) H H M M | | | |
| LDH-4 | (HM3) H M M M | | | Heat labile |
| LDH-5 | (M4) M M M M | slowest moving | found in *liver (Hepatic)*[Q] | |

separated by points; first being the main class, second indicating type of group involved in reaction (sub class), third denotes substrate on which group acts (sub sub class) and fourth digit is serial number of a particular enzyme.

| Serum **Non functional enzyme** | Diagnostic Use |
|---|---|
| Amylase,Lipase | Acute Pancreatitis |
| **Lactate dehydrogenase isoenzyme 5** | Liver diseases |
| Lactate dehydrogenase (isozyme) | Myocardial infarction |
| Aminotransferase<br>- Aspartae aminotransferase (AST, or SGOT)<br>- Alanine aminotransferase (ALT or SGPT) | <br>- Myocardial infarction<br>- Vitral Hepatitis |
| Ceruloplasmin | Hepatolenticular degeneration (Wilson's disease) |
| γ-Glutamyl transpeptidase | Liver disease |
| **Creatinine kinase (MB)** | Muscle disorder, MI |
| Acid phosphatase | Metastatic Ca of prostate |
| Alkaline phosphatase | Bone disorders, obstructive liver disease |

**Isoenzyme of CPK**

- **Creatinine phosphokinase exists as three isoenzymes in human tissue**:
  1. CPK- 1 or CPK – BB : Found in *Brain*
  2. CPK- 2 or CPK – MB : Found in *Myocardium and skeletal muscle.*
  3. CPK- 3 or CPK – MM: Found in *skeletal muscle*
- Thus creatinine phosphokinase *1 **is essentially found in brain & would be increased in brain ischaemia***[Q].

**Creatine phosphokinase (CPK) -2-CPKMB**

| Normally | Myocardial infarction |
|---|---|
| • *CPK -2 (MB isozyme)* occurs in very small quantity accounting for as less as *2% of total CK activity of plasma.*<br>• CKMB also exists in 2 form:<br>- $CKMB_1$ : Extracardiac form<br>- $CKMB_2$ : Cardiac form | • *Elevation of CK-MB* isoenzyme occurs within 4 hours, maximum in 24 hrs, then falls rapidly.<br>• A ratio of *$CKMB_1 : CKMB_2$ above 1.5 is highly sensitive for the diagnosis of acute MI after 4-6 hours of onset of myocardial ischaemia.* |

## Serine Protease

- These are *protein digesting enzymes.* They contain ***serine residue at the active center***[Q]
- They form *charge relay network* with histidine and asparate. This charge relay network functions as *proton shuttle.* This proton shuttle *donate a proton* to serine & activate it. The activated serine *breaks down peptide.* Serine proteases include - ***Trypsin***[Q], ***Elastase***[Q], **Thrombin**, ***Chymotrypsin***[Q]

## 6 – Classes of enzymes (International Union of Biochemistry = IUB) Mn – "TO HILL"

| Class | Feature | Example |
|---|---|---|
| **Transferase** | ***Catalyze transfer of C – N-, or P- containing group from one substrate to another***[Q], such as<br>$\text{Serine} \underset{\text{SHT}}{\rightleftharpoons} \text{Glycine}$ | - Aspartate & alanine transminase (AST/ALT)<br>- ***Hexokinase***[Q], Hexose 1- phosphate uridyl transferase<br>- Phosphoglucomutase<br>- Ornithine carbamoyl transferase<br>- Serine hydroxy methyl transferase (SHT) |
| **Oxidoreductase** | Catalyze oxidation reduction reactions, such as<br>$\text{Lactate} \overset{\text{Lactate dehydrogenase}}{\rightleftharpoons} \text{Pyruvate}$ | - Alcohol dehydrogenase, lactate dehydrogenase, glucose – 6 – phosphate dehydrogenase<br>- Glutathione reductase<br>- Xanthine oxidase, ***Tyrosinase***[Q] |
| **Hydrolases** | ***Catalyze hydrolysis i.e., cleavage of bonds by addition of water***[Q], such as<br>$Urea + H_2O \xrightarrow[Urease]{} CO_2 + 2NH_3$ | - Pepsin, trypsin, esterases<br>- Glucose 6 phosphatase, glycoside hydrolases<br>- ***Urease***[Q] |
| **Isomerases** | Involved in isomerization of substrate i.e., catalyze racemization of optical or geometric isomers, such as<br>$\text{Methyl Malonyl CoA} \underset{MMCoAM}{\rightleftharpoons} \text{Succinyl CoA}$ | - Triose phosphate isomerase, retinal isomerase<br>- UDP- glucose epimerase, racemase<br>- Methyl malonyl CoA mutase (MMCM) |
| **Lysases** | Catalyze cleavage of C – C , C – S, & certain C – N bonds and facilitate removal of small molecules from a large substrate<br>$Pyruvate \xrightarrow[decarboxylase]{Pyruvate} Acetaldehyde$ | - ***Fumarase***[Q], Argino- succinase<br>- Histidine decarboxylase<br>- Pyruvate decarboxylase |
| **Ligases** | Catalyze *formation of bonds between carbon and O, S, N* coupled *to hydrolysis of high energy phosphates* and involved in joining together two substrates.<br>$Pyruvate + CO_2 \xrightarrow[ATP \rightarrow ADP]{PC} Oxalo\ acetate$ | - DNA ligase, Pyruvate carboxylase (PC)<br>- Alanyl t-RNA synthetase<br>- Glutamine synthetase |

## Oxido- Reductase Enzymes

Oxidation involves *removal of electron /hydrogen or hydride* ion from a (reduced) substrate or *incorporation of* $O_2$ into a (reduced) substrate. After which the reduced substrate becomes oxidized. *Oxygen, flavin nucleotides (FMN, FAD) and nicotinamide coenzymes (NAD+ or NADP+)* are used as hydrogen acceptor. $H_2O_2$ canbe used as e- acceptor & donor both. Thus *oxidation is always accompanied by reduction* of an electron (hydrogen) acceptor.

### Oxidase

- Catalyze removal of hydrogen from substrate using *$O_2$ as hydrogen acceptor* and forming $H_2O$ or $H_2O_2$ as product
- ***Cytochrome oxidase (aa$_3$) contain copper***[Q]
- Flavoprotein containing oxidases are *L amino oxidase (FMN linked), Xanthine oxidase (Mo containing) and aldehyde dehydrogenase* (FAD linked molybdenum & non heme iron containing)

### Dehydrogenase

- Dehydrogenaese **cannot use oxygen as hydrogen acceptor**. So these transfer hydrogen from one substrate to another in a coupled oxidation – reduction reaction
- Cytochromes are iron containing hemoproteins in which iron atoms oscillates between Fe+2 & Fe+3 during oxidation & reduction. All cytochromes (except aa3) i.e. *cytochrome b, $C_1$, c of respiratory chain and cytochrome p-450 & $b_5$ of endoplasmic reticulum* are regarded dehydrogenase
- They use common coenzyme eg NAD+ as hydrogen carrier. Because these reactions are reversible, these reducing equivalents (NAD+) are freely transferred in within the cell.

### Hydroperoxidase

- These use $H_2O_2$ or organic peroxide as substrate & protect body from harmful peroxides.
- Are of 2 types: **peroxidases & catalase**
- Catalase is a hemoprotein containing 4 heme group. In addition to possessing peroxidase activity it uses $H_2O_2$ as electron donor and acceptor

$$2H_2O_2 \xrightarrow[\text{Catalase}]{} 2H_2O + O_2$$

- Peroxidases are found in milk & in leukocytes, platelets, & tissues involved in eicosanoid metabolism. It reduces peroxides using electron acceptors such as **ascorbate, quinines, & cytochrome C**

$$H_2O_2 + AH_2 \xrightarrow{\text{Peroxidase}} 2H_2O + A$$

### Oxygenase

Catalyze direct transfer & incorporation of $O_2$ into a substrate

Many dehydrogenase employ **(niacin) nicotinamide coenzymes (NAD+ or NADP+)**

- Glucose -6 – phosphate dehydrogenase (NADP+)
- Glutamate dehydrogenase (NADP+ or NAD+)
- NAD+:
  - Isocitrate dehydrogenase
  - α-ketoglutarate dehydrogenase
  - Malate dehydrogenase
  - Lactate dehydrogenase
  - Alcohol dehydrogenase
  - Glyceraldehyde-3-PO4 dehydrogenase

Other depend on **(riboflavin) flavoproteins (FMN or FAD)**

- Glycolate oxidase (FMN)
- NADH dehydrogenase / complex I (FMN)
- FAD:
  - Acyl CoA dehydrogenase
  - Dihydrolipoyl dehydrogenase
  - Succinate dehydrogenase
  - Glycerol-3- phosphate dehydrogenase
  - Thioredoxin reductase
  - Electron transferring Flavoprotein (ETF)

## Oxygenase

It *oxidizes a substrate* by catalyzing incorporation of oxygen into a substrate. It belongs to *oxido- reductase family* and is called direct oxidase. It is divided into 2 sub groups

### Dioxygenase

- ***Cause incorporation of both atoms of $O_2$ into substate***[Q] i.e.

$$A + O_2 \xrightarrow[\text{Dioxygenase}]{} AO_2$$

- Examples include liver enzymes, iron containing *3-hydroxy anthranilate* dioxygenase (oxidase), & *homogentisate* dioxygenase (oxidase), and *L- tryptophan 2, 3 dioxygenase (pyrolase)* that utilize heme.

### Monooxygenase (Mised function oxidase, Hydroxylase)

- ***Cause incorporation of only one atom of molecular oxygen into substrate***[Q]. The 2nd $O_2$ atom is reduced to water.
- An electron donor co substrate is necessary. Since main substrate is hydroxylated, it is also c/a **hydroxylase.**

$$\text{A – H (Main substrate)} + O_2 + ZH_2 \text{ (Cosubstrate)} \xrightarrow[\text{Hydroxylase}]{\text{Monooxygenase}} \text{A – OH (hydroxylated)} + H_2O + Z$$

- They are also called mixed function oxidase/oxigenase to indicate that they oxidize two different substrate simultaneously. Examples include **cytochrome P-450** and **phenylalanine hydroxylase** (responsible for PKU).
- ***Cytochromes $P_{450}$ are (heme containing) monoxygenases***[Q] which take part in ***hydroxylase cycle***[Q] (NADH, NADPH & $Fe_2 S_2$ required), ***detoxify drugs in liver microsomes***[Q] (with cytochrome $b_5$, $Fe_2 S_2$ not required).
- **Mitochondrial cytochrome $P_{450}$** is found in *steroidogenic – adrenal cortex, testis, ovary and placenta* and is concerned with *hydroxylation at $C_{22}$ & $C_{20}$ in side chain* cleavage & at *11B & 18* positions during synthesis of steroid chromones from cholesterol. It catalyzes 1 $\alpha$ & 25 hydroxylation in vit. D metabolism (in kidney) and 7 $\alpha$ hydroxylase & 27 hydroxylase in bile acid synthesis (in liver).

## Holoenzyme

It is active enzyme (protein part) with its non protein component

**Apoenzyme (protein part)**

It is inactive enzyme (protein part) without its non protein component.

**Non protein part**

**Transient association**

**Coenzyme**

- If non-protein part is a **small** thermostable low molecular weight **organic molecule**, it is termed coenzyme
- Coenzyme that only transiently associate with the enzyme are called **cosubstrate** (**second substrate** or **coenzyme – cosubstrate**). Co substrate dissociate from enzyme in an altered state. eg ***$NAD^+$ & coenzyme A***[Q]
- Coenzyme ***serve as recyclable substrate shuttles –or group transfer agents***[Q] that transport many substrates from their point of generation to their point of utilization. It also *stabilizes unstable substrates* such as hydrogen atoms or hydride ions.
- Components of coenzymes are- ***vitamin B***[Q], adenine, ribose & phosphoryl moieties of AMP or ADP

**Cofactor**

- If non protein moiety is **metal ion** such as $Fe^{++}$ or $Zn^{++}$, it is termed cofactor
- Bind reversibly in *transient dissociable manner* either to enzyme or substrate
- Enzymes requiring metal ion as cofactor are k/a **metal activated enzymes**.

**Stable & tight incorporation**

**Prosthetic group**

- These are tightly & stability incorporated into protein (enzyme) by covalent or non covalent forces.
- Metals are most common prosthetic groups. Metalloenzymes contain a tightly bound metal ion, that is not dissociated even after several steps of purification.

| Vitamin B component | Part of / coenzyme | Function |
|---|---|---|
| **Pantothenic acid** | *Coenzyme A*[Q] | Co ASH is acyl group carrier |
| **Cobalamine ($B_{12}$)** | **Cobamide** | ***Coenzyme in transfer of 1 carbon fragment & metabolism of folic acid***[Q] |
| **Folic acid** | **Tetrahydro folate** ($TH_4F$) | ***Coenzyme in transfer of 1 carbon fragment***[Q] |
| **Niacin (nicotinamide / nicotinic acid)** | **NAD & NADP** | Coenzyme in redox (oxidation and reduction) reactions |
| **Riboflavin ($B_2$)** | **FMN & FAD** | |
| **Pyridoxine, pyridoxal, pyridoxamine ($B_6$)** | **Pyridoxal phosphate** | Coenzyme in transmination & decarboxylation of amino acids & glycogen phosphorylase |
| **Thiamine ($B_1$)** | - **Thiamine pyro phosphate (TPP)**<br>- **Thiamine di phosphate (TDP)** | • Coenzyme for **oxidative decarboxylation** by 3 multi enzyme complexes<br>- ***Pyruvate dehydrogenase***[Q] (catalyze pyruvate to acetyl CoA)<br>- ***$\alpha$ -ketoglutarate dehydrogenase***[Q] (in citric acid cycle)<br>- Branched chain ketoacid dehydrogenase for leucine, Isoleucine & valine<br>• Coenzyme for Transketolase ($\alpha$ ketoacid decarboxylation) in pemtose phosphate (PPP) |
| **Biotin** | - | ***Coenzyme in carboxylation***[Q] reactions in gluco neogenesis & fatty acid synthesis |
| **Vitamin C (ascorbic acid)** | ***Coenzyme in hydroxylation of proline & lysine in collagen synthesis***[Q] | |
| **Vitamin K (phylloquinoses, menaquinones)** | - Coenzyme in **carboxylation** of glutamate residue in proteins of blood clotting (factor 2, 7, 9, 10, protein C, S and Z) and bone matrix (osteocalcin) to form ***$\gamma$ -carboxy glutamate residue***[Q]. | |

★ **Coenzyme prosthetic group** are small organic molecules that associate permanently with an enzyme & return to their original form by enzyme. Eg are FMN, FAD, TPP, pyridoxal phosphate, biotin.

## Functions of Zinc

**Role in Enzyme action**

Zinc forms an integral part of several enzymes (metallo enzymes) in the body:

- ***Superoxide dismutase***[Q] in cytosol: Cu-Zn protein complex with two $Zn^{++}$ per molecule of the enzyme.
- ***Carbonic anhydrase***[Q] present in RBC, parietal cells and renal tubular epithelial cells, one $Zn^{++}$ per molecule
- **Leucine- Amino- peptidase** of intestinal juice
- **Carboxyl peptidase A** – of *pancreatic* juice
- **Others:**
  - ***Alcohol dehydrogenase, lactate dehydrogenase***[Q], glutamate dehydrogense, malate dehydrogenase, Carbon monoxide dehydrogenase, D-2 hydroxy acid dehydrogenase, galactitol 1 PO4 5 dehydrogenase
  - ***Alkaline phosphatase***[Q], δ ALA dehydratase
  - Retinine reductase, DNA & RNA polymerase, histone deacetylase
  - β lactamase, lactoylglutathione lyase, insulin degrading enzyme.
  - Glutamae carbboxypeptidase II, glutamyl aminopeptidase
  - ADAM (a disintegrin & metalloprotease domain) of proteinases (eg TACE i.e. TNF α converting enzyme)

**Other functions**

- **Role in Vit A metabolism**
  - Stimulate release of Vit A from liver
  - Participate in the regeneration of Rhodopsin in eye during dark adaptation (as present in *Retinine reductase*)
- Role in *insulin secretion*
- Role in *growth & Reproduction*
- Role in *wound healing*

## Selenium & Selenocysteine

- **Selenium** in form of **selenocysteine** is a component (as a prosthetic groop) of **glutathione peroxidase, thioredoxin**, and **deiodinase** that converts thyroxine to triodothyronine.
- **Selenocysteine**, the **21st aminoacid** is present at the active site of enzymes and participate in catalytic mechanism of these enzymes. So the *replacement of selenocysteine by cysteine can significantly impair catalytic activity*.
- Unlike hydroxy proline & hydroxy lysine, selenocysteine arises by **cotranslational insertion from a previously modified t-RNA (t-RNA$^{sec}$). Serine** provides the carbon skeleton of selenocysteine. Biosynthesis of selenocyteine requires **selenate ($SeO_4^{2-}$), cysteine**, ATP, a specific unusual t RNA$^{sec}$ and enzymes. The **UGA anticodon of t RNA$^{sec}$ signals STOP** and this selenocysteine specific UGA stop codon is identified by **selenocysteine insertion element** (ie a stem loop structure in untranslated m RNA).

| Enzymes | Cofactors |
|---|---|
| KG dehydrogenase | *TPP*[Q] |
| **Carbonic anhydrase** | *Zn*[Q] |
| **Lactate/Alcohol dehydrogenase** | *Zn*[Q] |
| Xanthine oxidase | Mo |
| Tyrosinase } Cytochrome oxidase | Cu |
| Carboxylation | *Biotin*[Q] |
| Transamination | *Pyridoxine*[Q] |
| Kinase & peptidase | *Mg*[Q] |
| Hb & Cytochrome | *Fe* |
| Hydrolase, decarboxylase & transferase | Manganese |

**tRNA$^{sec}$ + Serine** —(Ligase)→ **tRNA $^{ser}$**; Selenium —(Selenophosphate Synthetase)→ Selenophosphate

Cysteyl-t RNA$^{sec}$ → Aminoacrylyl tRNA$^{sec}$ → Selenocystelyl tRNA$^{sec}$

- In presence of specific elongation factors that recognize selenocysteyl – t RNA$^{sec}$, selenocysteine is incorporated into protein.
- In erythrocytes pentose phosphate pathway (PPP) is the only source of NADPH for the reduction of oxidized glutathione catalyzed by glutathione reductase (containing FAD). **Reduced glutathione removes $H_2O_2$** in a reaction catalyzed by **glutathione peroxidase. Glutathione peroxidase** ***contains selenium analog of cysteine (selenocysteine) as a prosthetic group***[Q]. In erythrocytes and other tissues, it *catalyzes the destruction of $H_2O_2$ and lipid peroxidases*, protecting membrane lipid and hemoglobin against oxidation. This reaction is important since accumulation of $H_2O_2$ decreases life span of RBCs by causing oxidative damage to cell membrane proteins, lipids & nucleic acids l/t hemolysis. In other tissues, NADPH can also be generated by reaction catalyzed by malic enzyme. So **PPP & glutathione peroxidase protect RBCs against hemolysis**.

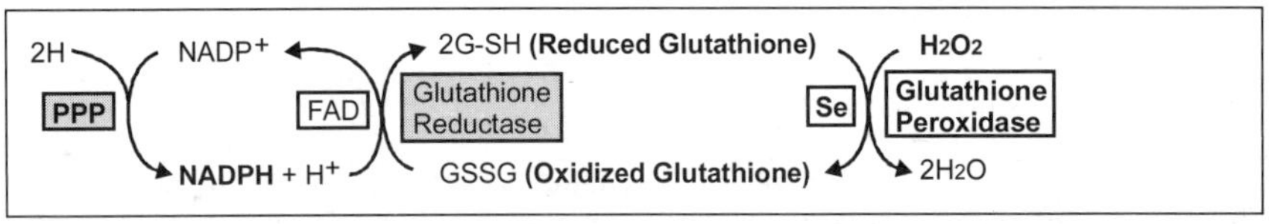


- Selenium has sparing effect on vitamin E reducing its requirements and similarly vitamin E reduces selenium requirement. Selenium & sulphur protect against toxic effects of heavy metals such as cadmium, Hg & Ag (b/o high affinity).
- *Seafood, muscle meat & cereals* are rich dietary sources of selenium, although the Se content of cereals is determined by soil concentration. Scandinavia, China & New Zealand have low soil Se content. Daily requirement's are 0.1 to 0.2 mg/kg (~ 50-100 Hg in 70 kg adult)

### Selenium Deficiency Diseases

1. **Keshan disease**: **Endemic cardiomyopathy** (enlargement, arrhythmia & ECG changes) mainly affecting children & young women with intake < 20μg/d.
2. **Kaschinbeck disease:Endemic degenerative osteoarthritis** (osteopathy) mainly in children between 5 & 13 years with enlarged dysfunctional joints & retarded growth.
3. Liver cell necrosis, exudative diasthesis, pancreatic degeneration, muscular dystrophy, myopathy, infertility, growth failure, and dilatation of heart l/t CCF. (in animals)

### Selenium Toxicity

1. **Selenosis** (chronic exposure) presents with **garlicky breath** (d/t dimethyl selenide), chronic **dermatitis**, skin rash, hair & **nail brittleness and loss**, myopathy, irritability & other abnormalities of nervous system (in humans). Animals develop impaired vision, movement disorder (**blind staggers**), alkali disease (anorexia, alopecia, loss of vitality, myocardial atrophy & liver necrosis), paralysis & death.
2. Acute toxicity in animals present with **diarrhea**, raised PR & temperature, tetanic spasm, laboured breathing, respiratory failure & hemorrhagic necrosis of various tissues.

### Metallothioneins

- Are group of *small proteins (6.5 KDa)*, found in cytosol of cells, particularly of *liver, kidney & intestine*
- They have high content of *cysteine*. The SH group of cysteine binds the metal
- ***Tissue levels of $Cu^{2+}$, $Zn^{2+}$, $Cd^{2+}$ and $Hg^{2+}$ i.e. (Copper, Zinc, Cadmium & mercury)***[Q] are regulated by metallothioneins
- It may function to *store the above metals in nontoxic form* & are involved in their over all metabolism in the body.
- The concentration of metallothionines in tissue is increased by *acute intake of metals or administration of certain hormones or cytokines.*

### Enzymes that contain Copper

- *Amine oxidase*[Q]
- *Superoxide dismutase*[Q]
- *Cytochrome oxidase*[Q]
- *Tyrosinase*[Q]

# Chapter -6 METABOLISM OF PROTEIN & AMINO ACIDS

## QUESTIONS

### Fate of Amino Group

1. **Transfer of an amino group from an amino acid to an alpha keto acid is done by?**
   A. Transaminases ☐
   B. Aminases ☐
   C. Transketolase ☐
   D. Decarboxylase ☐
2. **Transmination of pyruvate with glutamate produces**
   A. Oxaloacetate & aspartate ☐
   B. Alanine & asparate ☐
   C. Oxaloacetate & α-ketoglutarate ☐
   D. Alanine & α-ketoglutarate ☐
3. **Trans-amination of pyruvate and glutamic acid leads to the formation of**
   A. Oxaloacetate ☐
   B. α-ketoglutarate ☐
   C. Aspartate ☐
   D. Malate ☐
4. **All are involved in non toxic transport of ammonia except**
   A. Glutamine synthetase ☐
   B. Glutaminase ☐
   C. Alanine cycle ☐
   D. SGPT ☐
5. **The amino acid which serves as a carrier of ammonia from skeletal muscle to liver is:**
   A. Alanine ☐
   B. Methionine ☐
   C. Arginine ☐
   D. Glutamine ☐
6. **Glutamine in blood acts as:**
   A. $NH_3$ transporter ☐
   B. Toxic element ☐
   C. Stored energy ☐
   D. Abnormal metabolite ☐
7. **Which end product of citric acid cycle is used in detoxification of ammonia in brain**
   A. Oxaloacetate ☐
   B. Alphaketoglutarate ☐
   C. Succinate ☐
   D. Citrate ☐
8. **In Metabolic alkalosis, which is true about excretion in urine:**
   A. More of $NH_3$ ☐
   B. Less of aceto acetic acid ☐
   C. Betahydroxy butyric acid ☐
   D. Less ammonia ☐
9. **Ammonia is detoxified in brain to :**
   A. Urea ☐
   B. Glutamine ☐
   C. GABA ☐
   D. Uric acid ☐
10. **Glutamine synthetase is a -**
   A. Isomerase ☐
   B. Ligase ☐
   C. Lyase ☐
   D. Transferase ☐
11. **Source of ammonia in urine**
   A. Glutaminase ☐
   B. Urease ☐
   C. Glutamate dehydrogenase ☐
   D. Arginase ☐
12. **The amino acid producing (major source of) ammonia in kidney is:**
   A. Glutamine ☐
   B. Alanine, Aspartate ☐
   C. Methionine ☐
   D. Glycine ☐
   E. Glutamate

### Urea Cycle

13. **Which of the following enzyme (s) is/are not involved in urea cycle:**
   A. Glutamate dehydrogenase ☐
   B. Argininosucinate synthetase ☐
   C. α-KG dehydrogenase ☐
   D. Isocitrate dehydrogenase ☐
   E. Fumarase ☐
14. **Urea cycle occurs in :**
   A. Liver ☐
   B. G.I.T. ☐
   C. Spleen ☐
   D. Kidney ☐
15. **Urea cycle enzymes are:**
   A. Glutaminase ☐
   B. Asparginase ☐
   C. Arginosuccinate synthetase ☐
   D. Ornithine transcaroxylase ☐
   E. Glutamate dehydrogenase ☐
16. **Urea is produced by the enzyme-**
   A. Urease ☐
   B. Uricase ☐
   C. Arginase ☐
   D. Glutaminase ☐
17. **Urea is mainly formed in liver and to small extent in-**
   A. Spleen ☐
   B. Heart ☐
   C. Muscle ☐
   D. Brain ☐
18. **Which of the following is true in relation of urea cycle:**
   A. First 2 steps in cytoplasm ☐
   B. First 2 steps in mitochondria ☐
   C. Defect of enzyme of any step can cause deficiency disease ☐
   D. Urea is formed by $NH_3$, glutamic acid and $CO_2$ ☐
   E. Citruline is formed by combination of carbomoyl phosphate and L. Ornithine ☐
19. **Sources of the nitrogen in urea cycle are:**
   A. Aspartate and ammonia ☐
   B. Glutamate and ammonia ☐
   C. Arginine and ammonia ☐
   D. Uric acid ☐
20. **Urea cycle, true is all except**
   A. Aspartate converted to fumarate ☐
   B. Ornithine-citrulline transporter aminoacids ☐
   C. N-acetyl glutamate is allosteric inhibitor ☐
   D. Aspartate-arginino succinate shunt ☐

**21. A child presents with metabolic lactic acidosis along with hyperammonemia and convulsion is due to**
- A. Reye's syndrome ☐
- B. Mitochondrial enzyme disorders (MELAS) ☐
- C. Urea cycle defect ☐
- D. Phenylketonuria ☐

**22. Hyperammonaemia inhibit TCA cycle by depleting:**
- A. Oxaloacetate ☐
- B. α-ketoglutarate ☐
- C. Citrate ☐
- D. Succinyl Co-A ☐
- E. Fumarate ☐

## Amino Acids

**23. A common feature of all serine proteases is:**
- A. Autocatalytic activation of zymogen precursor ☐
- B. Tight binding of pancreatic trypsin inhibitor ☐
- C. Cleavage of protein on the carboxyl site of serine residues ☐
- D. Presence of Ser-His-Asp catalytic triad at the active site ☐

**24. Vitamin $B_{12}$ acts as co-enzyme to which one of the following enzymes?**
- A. Isocitrate dehydrogenase ☐
- B. Homocysteine methyl transferase ☐
- C. Glycogen synthase ☐
- D. G-6-P dehydrogenase ☐

**25. Guanido acitic acid is formed in....from....-**
- A. Kidney; Arginine+Glycine ☐
- B. Liver; Methionine + Glycine ☐
- C. Liver; Cysteine + Arginine ☐
- D. Muscle; Citrulline + Aspartate ☐

**26. Creatinine is synthesised from -**
- A. Glycine, arginine and methionine ☐
- B. Glycine and methionine ☐
- C. Ornithine and glycine ☐
- D. Thymine and ornithine ☐

**27. Creatinine is formed from :**
- A. Arginine ☐
- B. Lysine ☐
- C. Leucine ☐
- D. Histamine ☐

**28. All of the following amino acids are converted to succinyl-CoA, *except*:**
- A. Methionine ☐
- B. Isoleucine ☐
- C. Valine ☐
- D. Histidine ☐

**29. Which one of the following can be a homologous substitution for isoleucine in a protein sequence?**
- A. Methionine ☐
- B. Aspartic acid ☐
- C. Valine ☐
- D. Arginine ☐

**30. At physiological pH, the carboxy-terminal of a peptide is:** *(AIIMS Nov 05)*
- A. Positively charged ☐
- B. Negatively charged ☐
- C. Neural ☐
- D. Infinitely charged ☐

**31. Iso electric pH is :**
- A. Point at which all amino acids are in zwitter ion form. ☐
- B. Point at which pH of ions are same. ☐
- C. Point at which pH of ions does not alter. ☐
- D. Point at which positive and negative charges on the amino acid are equal. ☐

**32. At isoelectric $p^H$ protein:**
- A. Have Net charge 'O' ☐
- B. Are positively charged ☐
- C. Are negatively charged ☐
- D. Don't migrate ☐

**33. The amino acid residue having an iminoside chain is:**
- A. Lysine ☐
- B. Histidine ☐
- C. Tyrosine ☐
- D. Proline ☐

**34. Sulphur containing amino acid is/are:**
- A. Aspartic acid ☐
- B. Glutamine ☐
- C. Methionine ☐
- D. Glycine ☐
- E. Serine ☐

**35. Sulphur containing amino acids are -**
- A. Cysteine ☐
- B. Asparagine ☐
- C. A and B ☐
- D. Methionine ☐
- E. Glycine ☐

**36. Replacing alanine by which amino acid will increase UV absorbance of protein at 280 nm wavelength:**
- A. Leucine ☐
- B. Proline ☐
- C. Arginine ☐
- D. Tryptophan ☐

**37. Property of photochromosity is seen amongst the following amino acids:**
- A. Unsaturated aminoacid ☐
- B. Aromatic aminoacid ☐
- C. Monocarboxylic acid ☐
- D. Dicarboxylic acid ☐

**38. The property of proteins to absorb ultraviolet rays of light is due to :**
- A. Peptide band ☐
- B. Imino group ☐
- C. Di Sulphide bond ☐
- D. Aromatic amino acid ☐

**39. Aromatic amino acids are -**
- A. Tryptophan ☐
- B. Tyrosine ☐
- C. Lysine ☐
- D. Arginine ☐
- E. Phenylalanine ☐

**40. Aromatic ring is present in -**
- A. Arginine ☐
- B. Glycine ☐
- C. Phenylalanine ☐
- D. Phenylalanine Glycine ☐

**41. Hydrophobic aminoacids are:**
- A. Methione ☐
- B. Isoleucine ☐
- C. Tyrosine ☐
- D. Alanine ☐
- E. Asparagine ☐

**42. Polar amino acid (s) is/are:**
- A. Serine ☐
- B. Tryptophan ☐
- C. Tyrosine ☐
- D. Valine ☐
- E. Lysine ☐

43. **Non Polar Amino Acids are:**
   A. Alanine ☐
   B. Tryptophan ☐
   C. Isoleucine ☐
   D. Lysine ☐
   E. Tyrosine ☐
44. **Which of the following side chains is least polar**
   A. Methyl ☐
   B. Carboxyl ☐
   C. Amino ☐
   D. Phosphate ☐
45. **Leucine is a aminoacid with a :**
   A. Nonpolar side chain ☐
   B. Polar side chain ☐
   C. Negatively charged side chain ☐
   D. Positively charged side chain ☐
46. **Most non polar Amino Acid is :**
   A. Leucine ☐
   B. Glycine ☐
   C. Arginine ☐
   D. Lysine ☐
47. **Acidic amino acids are -**
   A. Asparagine ☐
   B. Arginine ☐
   C. Glutamine ☐
   D. Lysine ☐
   E. None ☐
48. **Basic amino acids are :**
   A. Aspartate and glutamate ☐
   B. Serine and glycine ☐
   C. Lysine and arginine ☐
   D. None of the above ☐
49. **Most basic amino acid out of the following is :**
   A. Alanine ☐
   B. Arginine ☐
   C. Histidine ☐
   D. Lysine ☐
50. **Basic amino acid (s) is /are:**
   A. Arginine ☐
   B. Proline ☐
   C. Lysine ☐
   D. Histidine ☐
   E. Methionine ☐
51. **Which of these amino acids will migrate slowest to the anode end at the physiological pH-**
   A. Aspartic acid ☐
   B. Glycine ☐
   C. Lysine ☐
   D. Valine ☐
52. **Non-Essential amino acid is -**
   A. Tyrosine ☐
   B. Phenylalanine ☐
   C. Lysine ☐
   D. Threonine ☐
53. **An essential amino acid in man is -**
   A. L-methionine ☐
   B. L-tyrosine ☐
   C. L-serine ☐
   D. L-proline ☐
54. **Negative nitrogen balance is produced in humans by elimination from the diet of all of the following amino acids except -**
   A. Leucine ☐
   B. Methionine ☐
   C. Lysine ☐
   D. Serine ☐
   E. Threonine ☐
55. **Aminoacid that enters the TCA cycle for gluconeogenesis & Ketogenin in nature -**
   A. Pheylalanine ☐
   B. Alanine ☐
   C. Glycine ☐
   D. Serine ☐
56. **All ar essential amino acid except-**
   A. Phenylalanine ☐
   B. Lysine ☐
   C. Leucine ☐
   D. Glycine ☐
57. **Semiessential amino acids are-**
   A. Arginine ☐
   B. Histidine ☐
   C. Glycine ☐
   D. Phenylalanine ☐
58. **Negative nitrogen balance is produced in humans by elimination from the diet of all of the following amino acids except -**
   A. Leucine ☐
   B. Methionine ☐
   C. Lysine ☐
   D. Serine ☐
   E. Threonine ☐
59. **All of the following are essential aminoacids except:**
   A. Methionine ☐
   B. Lysine ☐
   C. Alanine ☐
   D. Leucine ☐
60. **Substitution of which one of the following amino acids in place of alanine would increase the absorbance of proteins at 280 mm:**
   A. Leucine ☐
   B. Arginine ☐
   C. Tryptophan ☐
   D. Protein ☐
61. **Which one of the following amino acids is most likely to be found in the transmembrane region of a protein**
   A. Lysine ☐
   B. Arginine ☐
   C. Leucine ☐
   D. Aspartate ☐
62. **All biologically active proteins are**
   A. L-forms ☐
   B. D-forms ☐
   C. Mostly D form ☐
   D. D and L form ☐
63. **The conversion of an optically pure isomer (enantiomer) into a mixture of equal amounts of both dextro and levo forms is called as:**
   A. Polymerization ☐
   B. Stereoisomerization ☐
   C. Racemization ☐
   D. Fractionation ☐
64. **Amino acid which lacks chirality is:**
   A. Lysine ☐
   B. Leucine ☐
   C. Histidine ☐
   D. Glycine ☐
65. **Which of these amino acids does not have anomeric carbon atom:**
   A. Valine ☐

B. Alanine ☐
C. Tyrosine ☐
D. Glycine ☐

**66. Optically inactive Amino Acid is**
A. Proline ☐
B. Glycine ☐
C. Lysine ☐
D. Leucine ☐

**67. Flexibility of protein depends on**
A. Glycine ☐
B. Tryptophan ☐
C. Phenylalanine ☐
D. Histidine ☐

**68. Amino acid involved in 1 carbon metabolism:**
A. Folic acid ☐
B. Thiamine ☐
C. Pyridoxine ☐

**69. Which vitamin is related to a co-factor in glycine Metabolism is-**
A. V, E ☐
B. Folic acid ☐
C. Thiamine ☐
D. Pantothenic acid ☐

**70. Conversion of glycine to serine requires:**
A. Folic acid ☐
B. Thiamine ☐
B. Vit. C. ☐
C. $Fe^{2+}$ ☐
D. Pyridoxal phosphate ☐

**71. Amino acid with dissociation constant closest to physiological pH is:**
A. Serine ☐
B. Histidine ☐
C. Threonine ☐
D. Proline ☐

**72. Most stable amino acid at the physiological pH is:**
A. Histidine ☐
B. Lysine ☐
C. Arginine ☐
D. Glycine ☐

**73. Maximum influence of local milieu on ionization is on:**
A. Histidine ☐
B. Protine ☐
C. Glycine ☐
D. Lysine ☐

**74. Which of the following amino acid is active at neutral pH:**
A. Histidine ☐
B. Glycine ☐
C. Arginine ☐
D. *Aspartic acid* ☐

**75. Which amino acid can protonate & deprotonate at neutral pH**
A. Histidine ☐
B. Leucine ☐
C. Glycine ☐
D. Arginine ☐

**76. At physiological pH buffering action in blood is caused by:**
A. Histidine ☐
B. Methionine ☐
C. Hemocysteine ☐
D. Arginine ☐
E. Glycine ☐

**77. Which of the following is true about glutathione**
A. Contain sulfhydral group ☐
B. Forms met Hb from Hb ☐
C. It does not detoxity superoxide radicals ☐
D. Transport aminoacid across cell membrane ☐
E. Part of enzymes ☐

**78. In glutathione which amino acid is reducing agent-**
A. Glutamic acid ☐
B. Glycine ☐
C. Cysteine ☐
D. Alanine ☐

**79. Regarding glutathione which of the following is/are true:**
A. It helps in absorption of certain amino acids ☐
B. It inactivates some enzymes ☐
C. It helps in membrane transport ☐
D. It helps in conjugation reactions ☐

**80. Amino acids secreted in cystinuria are all except:**
A. Ornithine ☐
B. Histidine ☐
C. Arginine ☐
D. Lysine ☐

**81. Cystinuria is associated with excretion of which A.A in urine:**
A. Cystine, lysine, Tyrosine and alanine ☐
B. Cystine, lysine, ornithine and alanine ☐
C. Cystine, ornithine, lysine and arginine ☐
D. Cystine, ornithine, leucine and arginine ☐

**82. Aminoacid containing indole ring is -**
A. Arginine ☐
B. Tryptophan ☐
C. Tyrosine ☐
D. Histidine ☐

**83. The following is false about Tryptophan**
A. Non essential amino acid ☐
B. Involved in serotonin synthsis ☐
C. Involved in niacin synthesis ☐
D. Involved in melatonin synthesis ☐

**84. The amino acid that can be converted into a vitamin**
A. Glycine ☐
B. Tryptophan ☐
C. Phenylalanine ☐
D. Lysine ☐

**85. Which of the following amino acids is involved in the synthesis of thyroxine -**
A. Glycine ☐
B. Methionine ☐
C. Threonine ☐
D. Tyrosine ☐

**86. An amino acid not involved in urea synthesis is -**
A. Ornithine ☐
B. Citrulline ☐
C. Arginine ☐
D. Aspartic acid ☐

**87. Melatonin is synthesised from-**
A. Tryprophan ☐
B. Serotonin ☐
C. Phenylalanine ☐
D. Histidine ☐
E. Leucine ☐

**88. Which of the following is precursor of adrenalin and thyroxine synthesis -**
A. Phenyl alanine ☐
B. Tyrosine ☐
C. Tryptophan ☐
D. None of the above ☐

**89. Which of the following is not synthesised from tyrosine -**
A. Norepinephrine ☐
B. Melatonin ☐
C. Thyroxine ☐
D. Dopamine ☐

90. **The substance from which ammonia is produce by the kidney is-**
   A. Glycine ☐
   B. Alanine ☐
   C. Glutamine ☐
   D. Methionine ☐

91. **Ammonia is detoxified in brain by-**
   A. Uric acid ☐
   B. Glutamine ☐
   C. Creatinine ☐
   D. Urea ☐

92. **The urea in the brain is derived from-**
   A. Glutamine ☐
   B. Glutamine acid ☐
   C. Lactate ☐
   D. Uric acid ☐

93. **Phenylalanine is the precursor of all the following, except** :
   A. Tyrosine ☐
   B. Epinephrine ☐
   C. Thyroxine ☐
   D. Melatonin ☐

94. **Increased risk of Myocardial infarction is associated with which amino acid**
   A. Methionine ☐
   B. Homocystine ☐
   C. Ornithine ☐
   D. Valine ☐

95. **All will predispose to atherosclerosis except**:
   A. Homocystinemia ☐
   B. Fibrinogen ☐
   C. Calcium ☐
   D. Lipoprotein A ☐

96. **In phenylketonuria the main aim for first line therapy is:**
   A. Limiting the substrate for deficient enzyme ☐
   B. Giving the missing amino acids by diet ☐
   C. Replacement of enzyme ☐
   D. To replace deficient product ☐

97. **PKU is a congenital amino acid metabolic disorder. In one of the following rare variants of PKU Dihydro Biopterin synthesis is affected. The enzyme deficient is:**
   A. Histidine decarboxylase ☐
   B. Phenylalanine hydroxylase ☐
   C. Dihydropterin reductase ☐
   D. Tyrosine deficiency ☐

98. **What results due to incomplete oxidation of phenylpyruvic acid**:
   A. Albinism ☐
   B. Alkaptonuria ☐
   C. Phenylketonuria ☐
   D. Tyrosinemia ☐

99. **Ferric chloride test in PKU gives**:
   A. Red ☐
   B. Green ☐
   C. Blue ☐
   D. Yellow ☐

100. **Mousy odour urine is seen in**:
   A. Maple syrup urine ☐
   B. Phenylketonuria ☐
   C. Isovalericaciduria ☐
   D. Cystinuria ☐

101. **Tyrosinemics are more susceptible to develop**:
   A. Adenocarcinoma colon ☐
   B. Melanoma ☐
   C. Retinoblastoma ☐
   D. Hepatic carcinoma ☐

102. **A 40 yr old woman presents with progressive palmoplantar pigmentation. X-ray spine shows calcification of intervertebral discs. On adding Benedict's reagent to urine, it gives greenish brown precipitate and blue-black supernatant fluid. What is the diagnosis?**
   A. Phenylketonuria ☐
   B. Alkaptonuria ☐
   C. Tyrosinemia type-2 ☐
   D. Argininosuccinic aciduria ☐

103. **If urine sample darkens on standing: the most likely condition is** :
   A. Phenylketonuria ☐
   B. Alkaptonuria ☐
   C. Maple syrup disease ☐
   D. Tyrosinemia ☐

104. **Metabolites of tryptophan can give rise to**:
   A. Diarrhoea ☐
   B. Vasoconstriction ☐
   C. Flushing ☐
   D. Can predispose to albinism ☐
   E. Phenylketonuria ☐

105. **In maple syrup urine disease the amino acids. excreted in the urine are -**
   A. Leucine ☐
   B. Isoleucine ☐
   C. Valine ☐
   D. a, b & c ☐
   E. Arginine ☐

106. **Which of the following aminoacid is excreted in urine in maple syrup urine disease** :
   A. Tryptophan ☐
   B. Phenylalanine ☐
   C. Leucine ☐
   D. Arginine ☐

107. **Branched chain ketoacid decarboxylation is defective in**
   A. Maple Syrup urine disease ☐
   B. Hartnup disease ☐
   C. Alkaptonuria ☐
   D. GMI Gangliosidosis ☐

108. **Disease of branched chain amino acid includes:**
   A. Phenylketonuria ☐
   B. Maple syrup disease ☐
   C. Taysach's disease ☐
   D. Isovaleric acidemia ☐
   E. Niemann-pick disease ☐

109. **Sweaty feet odor in body fluids occur d/t deficiency of**
   A. Biotin ☐
   B. FAD linked dehydrogenase ☐
   C. Thiamin linked decarboxylase ☐
   D. Leucine transaminse ☐

110. **Correct combination of urine odour in various metabolic disorders:**
   A. Phenylketonuria-Mousy odour ☐
   B. Tyrosinemia-Rotten cabbage ☐
   C. Hawkinsuria-Potato smell ☐
   D. Maple syrup disease-Rotten tomato ☐
   E. Alkaptonuria-Rotten egg ☐

**111.Phosphorylation of amino acid by:**
- A. Serine ☐
- B. Tyrosine ☐
- C. Leucine ☐
- D. Tryptophan ☐

**112.Succinyl Co-A is formed by:**
- A. Histidine ☐
- B. Leucine ☐
- C. Valine ☐
- D. Lysine ☐

**113.A baby presents with refusal to feed, skin lesions, seizures, ketosis organic acids in urine with normal ammonia; likely diagnosis is:**
- A. Proprionic aciduria ☐
- B. Multiple carboxylase deficiency ☐
- C. Maple syrup urine disease ☐
- D. Urea cycle enzyme deficiency ☐

**114.The comparison of the amino acid sequence of Cytochrome C from different species shows many variations. Most of these variations are found:**
- A. Randomly ☐
- B. Only in helical regions ☐
- C. Only in strand regions ☐
- D. Mainly in loop regions ☐

## Hemoglobin, Bile Pigment & Porphyrin

**115.Hemoproteins are:**
- A. Cytochrome C ☐
- B. Cytochrome 450 ☐
- C. Myoglobin ☐
- D. Hemoglobin ☐
- E. Catalase ☐

**116.Hemoprosthetic group is found in:**
- A. Myoglobin ☐
- B. Cytochrome oxidase ☐
- C. Xanthine oxidase ☐
- D. Tyrosine ☐

**117.Haemoglobin is a buffer because of -**
- A. Histidine residue ☐
- B. Glycoprotein nature ☐
- C. Weak acidic nature ☐
- D. Iron molecule ☐

**118.False statement about hemoglobin structure?**
- A. Hb has 2 polypeptide ☐
- B. Iron is present in ferrous state ☐
- C. Hb structurally similar to myoglobin ☐
- D. Ferrous ions are in porphyrin rings ☐

**119.In hemoglobin, iron is bound to:**
- A. Histidine ☐
- B. Leucine ☐
- C. Isoleucine ☐
- D. Valine ☐

**120.Hemoglobin acts as a buffer because of:**
- A. Glycine ☐
- B. Histidine ☐
- C. Alanine ☐
- D. Valine ☐

**121.In hemoglobin the innate affinity of heme for carbon monoxide is diminished by the presence of :**
- A. His F8 ☐
- B. His E7 ☐
- C. Gly B6 ☐
- D. Thr C4 ☐

**122.Haemoglobin unlike myoglobin shows:**
- A. Parabolic curve of oxygen association ☐
- B. Co-operative effect of combine $O_2$ ☐
- C. Cooperative index of 81 ☐
- D. Hill's coefficient of 1 ☐

**123.Which of the following statement characterize both Hemoglobin and Myoblogin:**
- A. Non-helical ☐
- B. Subunits which are held together by hydrogen bonds. ☐
- C. Binds with 2 Heme ☐
- D. Heme at hydrophobic pockets ☐
- E. Bind with 1 molecule of $O_2$ ☐

**124.Which is an allosteric protein:**
- A. Transferrin ☐
- B. Ceruloplasmin ☐
- C. Phosphofructokinase ☐
- D. Haemoglobin ☐

**125.True regarding conversion of deoxyhemoglobin to oxyhemoglobin is :**
- A. Binding of $O_2$ causes release of $H^+$ ☐
- B. One mole of deoxyhemoglobin binds two moles of 2,3 DPG ☐
- C. pH of blood has no affect on the binding of $O_2$ ☐
- D. Binding of $O_2$ causes increased binding of 2,3,DPG ☐

**126.Decreased glycolytic activity impairs oxygen transport by hemoglobin due to:**
- A. Reduced energy production ☐
- B. Decreased production of 2,3-bisphosphoglycerate ☐
- C. Reduced synthesis of hemoglobin ☐
- D. Low levels of oxygen ☐

**127.Bilirubin is absent in urine because it is :**
- A. Distributed in the body fat ☐
- B. Conjugated with glucoronide ☐
- C. Not filterable ☐
- D. Lipophilic. ☐

**128.Pigment providing colour to stool is:**
- A. Stercobilinogen ☐
- B. Urobilinogen ☐
- C. Mevobilirubin ☐
- D. Bilirubin ☐

**129.The conjugation of bilirubin to glucuronic acid in the liver;**
- A. Converts a hydrophilic compound to a hydrophobic one ☐
- B. Converts a hydrophobic compound to a hydrophilic one ☐
- C. Enables the bilirubin molecule to cross the cell membrane ☐
- D. Is increased during neonatal jaundice ☐

**130.Bilirubin in conjugation with glucoronic acid conjugation has properties:**
- A. Able to cross cell membrane ☐
- B. Hydrophillic to hydrophobic ☐
- C. Hydrophobic to hydrophilic ☐
- D. Lipid soluble ☐

**131.Detergent action of bile salts is due to:**
- A. Hydropathic ☐
- B. Acts as a zwitter ion ☐
- C. Amphipathic ☐
- D. All ☐

**132.Which of the following is luminous :**
- A. Porphyrin ☐
- B. Zymogen ☐
- C. Chromatin ☐
- D. Albumin ☐

**133. Prophobilinogen in urine produces pink colour with:**
A. Fouchet's reagent ☐
B. Benedict's reagent ☐
C. Sodium nitropruside ☐
D. Ehrlich's aldehyde reagent ☐

**134. All of the following types of porphyrias are autosomal dominant except:**
A. Acute intermittent porphyria ☐
B. Porphyria cutanea tarda ☐
C. CEP (Congenital Erythropoietic Porphyria) ☐
D. Hereditary coproporphyria ☐

**135. The enzyme deficient in erythropoietic porphyria is:**
A. PBG deaminase ☐
B. Uroporphyrin II cosynthetase ☐
C. Coprophyrin ☐
D. Ferrochelatase ☐

**136. Hepatomegaly is an essential feature of A/E**
A. Von Gierke's disease ☐
B. Nieman Pick disease ☐
C. Hurler syndrome ☐
D. Hepatic porphyria ☐

**137. Heme synthesis requires**
A. Ferrous iron ☐
B. Glycine ☐
C. Alanine ☐
D. Succhyl CoA ☐
E. Lead ☐

## Answers:

### Fate of Amino Group

1. A i.e. Transaminases *[Ref: Lehninger 5/e p 677-83; Lippincott 5/e p 250-53; Harper 29/e p 274-78; Chatterjea 7/e p 443-50; Vasudevan 6/e p 174-76]*
2. D i.e. Alanine & α- ketoglutarate
3. B i.e. α- ketoglutarate
4. B i.e. Glutaminase
5. A i.e. Alanine
6. A i.e. $NH_3$ transporter
7. B i.e. Alphaketoglutarate
8. D i.e. Less of $NH_3$
9. B i.e. Glutamine

*[Ref: Lippincott's 3/e P-254, 255; Harper's 27/e P-247-250]*

10. B i.e. Ligase
11. A i.e. Glutaminase
12. A i.e. Glutamine

*[Ref: Harper's 28/e p. 242-46; Lippincott's 4/e p. 250-53; Ganong 22/e p. 721; Chatterjea 7/e p. 116]*

### Urea Cycle

13. A, C, D, E i.e. Glutamate dehydrogenase; alpha-KG dehydrogenase; Isocitrate dehydrogemase; Fumarase *[Ref: Harper's 29/e p 267, 274-78; Chattargea 8/e p 476-77]*
14. A i.e. Liver
15. C, D i.e. Arginosuccinate synthetase , Ornithine transcaroxylase
16. C i.e. Arginase
17. D i.e. Brain
18. B i.e. First 2 steps in mitochondria; C i.e Defect of enzyme of any step can cause deficiency disease; E i.e. Citruline is formed by combination of carbomoyl phosphate and L. Ornithine
19. A i.e. Aspartate and ammonia
20. C i.e. N-acetyl glutamate is allosteric inhibitor

*[Ref: Lehninger 5/e p. 683-85; Harper 28/e p. 243-46; Lippincott 5/e p. 253-57; Vasudevan 6/e p. 177-79; Chatterjea 7/e p. 448-50]*

21. A i.e Reye's syndrome *[Ref. Nelson 16/e P-1214, 1246; Harper's 27/e P-100-101]*
22. B i.e. α-ketoglutarate *[Ref: Chatterjea 7/e p. 447-48; Vasudevan 6/e p. 180]*

### Amino Acids

23. D i.e. Presence of Ser-His-Asp catalytic triad at the active site: *[Ref: www.rpc.msoe.edu/lib/sp1.pdf; www.users.rcn.com/jkimball.ma.ultranet/BiologyPages/S/Series/Serine_Proteases.html; www.ebi.ac.uk/interpro/potm/2003_5/Page1.htm]*
24. B i.e. Homoeystine Methyl transferase *[Ref: Lippincott 3rd/373; Chetterjea Shinde 6th/181]*
25. A i.e. Kidney; Arginine + Glycine
26. A i.e. Glycine, arginine and methionine
27. A i.e. Arginine

*[Ref: Harper's 27/e P- 274 – 77 ; Lippincott's 4/e p. 287- 88]*

28. D i.e. Histidine *[Ref: Lippincott's 3/e P-261]*
29. C i.e. Valine *[Ref: Harper's 27/e P-15]*
30. B i.e. Negatively Charged
31. D i.e. Point at which positive and negative charges on the amino acids are equal.
32. A i.e. Have net charge 'O' *[Ref: Lippincott's 3/e P- 1]*
33. D i.e. Proline
34. C i.e. Methionine
35. A i.e. Cysteine; D i.e. Methionine
36. D i.e. Tryptophan
37. B i.e. Aromatic amino acid
38. D i.e. Aromatic amino acid
39. A i.e. Trypthophan; B i.e. Tyrosine; E i.e. phenyl alanine
40. C i.e. Phenyl alanine
41. A, B, C, D i.e. Methione, Isoleucine, Tyrosine, Alanine
42. A, C, E i.e. Serine, Tyrosine, Lysine
43. A, B, C > E i.e. Alanine, Tryptophan, Isoleucine > Tyrosine
44. A i.e. Methyl
45. A i.e. Nonpolar side chain
46. A i.e. Leucine
47. A i.e. Asparagine; C i.e. Glutamine

*Ref: Lehninger 5th/e p.73-76; Lippincott 5th/e p. 2-9; Harper 28th/e p.15-19; Vasudevan 6/e p. 20-23; Chatterjea 7/e p. 74-76]*

48. C i.e. Lysine and arginine
49. B i.e. Arginine
50. A, C, D i.e. Arginine, Lysine, Histidine
51. C i.e. Lysine
52. A i.e. Tyrosine
53. A i.e. L- methionine
54. D i.e. Serine
55. A i.e. Phenyalanine
56. D i.e. Glycine
57. A i.e. Arginine B i.e. Histidine
58. D i.e. Serine
59. C i.e. Alanine

*[Ref: John Baynes 3/e p. 248; Lehinger 5/e p. 686]*

60. C i.e. Tryptophan
61. C i.e. Leucine *[Ref: Lippincott's 3/e P-3- 4]*
62. A i.e. L- forms *[Ref: Harper's 28/e P-14; Chatterjea 6/e P-25]*
63. C i.e. Racemization
64. D i.e. Glycine
65. D i.e. Glycine
66. B i.e. Glycine
67. A i.e. Glycine
68. A i.e. Folic Acid
69. B i.e. Folic Acid
70. A i.e. Folic acid
71. B i.e. Histidine
72. A i.e. Histidine
73. A i.e. Histidine

74. **A i.e. Histidine** 75. **A i.e. Histidine** 76. **A i.e. Histidine**
77. **A i.e. Contain sulfhydral group ; D i.e. Transport aminoacid across cell membrane; E i.e. Part of enzymes**
78. **C i.e. Cysteine** *[Ref: Harper's 27/e P-636; Lippincott's 3/e P-4, 5, 146; Harper's 27/e P-17-18; Lippincott's 3/e P- 4, 5]*
79. **C i.e. It helps in membrane transport, D i.e. It helps in conjugation reaction**
80. **B i.e. Histidine** 81. **D i.e. Cystine, Ornithine, Lysine, Arginine**
82. **B i.e. Tryptophan** 83. **A i.e. Non essential amino acid** 84. **B i.e. Tryptophan**
85. **D i.e. Tyrosine** 86. **C i.e. None** 87. **A i.e. Tryptophan**
88. **B i.e. Tyrosine** 89. **B i.e. Melatonin** 90. **C i.e. Glutamine**
91. **B i.e. Glutamine** 92. **A i.e. Glutamine** 93. **D i.e. Melatonin**
*[Ref: Harper's 27/e P-259-62; 26/e P- 257; Lippincott's 5/e p. 250; Chatterjea 7/e p. 477]*
94. **B i.e. Homocytine** 95. **C i.e. Calcium** *[Ref: Harrison 16/e P. 1430, 1432]*
96. **A i.e. Limiting the substrate for deficient enzyme** 97. **C i.e. Dihydropterin reductase**
98. **C i.e. Phenylketonuria** 99. **B i.e. Green** 100. **B i.e. Phenylketonuria**
*[Ref: Lippincott's 5/e P- 270-71;Lehninger 5/e p. 696-99; Chatterjea 7/e p. 469-70; Harper's 28/e P-254-55, 237; Harrison 17/e p. 2471-70; Nelson 18/e p. 530]*
101. **D i.e. Hepatic carcinoma** *[Ref: Lehninger 5/e p.696-97; Chatterjea: 7/e P- 471; Harper's 28/e P-254; Lippincott 5/e p. 269; Vasudevan 6/e p. 209-10]*
102. **B i.e. Alkaptonuria** 103. **B i.e. Alkaptonuria**
*[Ref: Lehninger 5/e 694-698; Vasudeven 6/e 208-10; Chatterjae 7/e 470-71; Harper 28/e 254; Lippincott 5/e 269, 274; Harrison 17/e 2470-73; Nelson 18/e p 534; Weedon skin pathology 2/e p 440]*
104. **A i.e. Diarrhoea; B i.e. Vasoconstriction; C i.e. Flushing** *[Ref: Chatterjea: 6/e P- 451; Harper's 27/e P-262]*
105. **D i.e. a, b & c** 106. **C i.e. Leucine** 107. **A i.e. Maple Syrup urine disease**
108. **B i.e. Maple syrup disease; D i.e. Isovaleric acidemia**
*[Ref: Harper 29/e p. 284, 293-95; Lippincott 6/e p. 266; Vasudevan 7/e p.230; Chatterjea 7/e p. 493; Satyanarayan 3/e p. 376; Lehninger 5/e p. 694-701]*
109. **B i.e. FAD linked dehydrogenase**
110. **A i.e. Phenylketonuria-Mousy odour; B i.e. Tyrosinemia-Rotten cabbage**
111. **A i.e. Serine, B i.e. Tyrosine** *[Ref: Chatterjea 6/e P-446; Harper's 27/e P-78-79]*
112. **C i.e. Valine**
113. **B i.e. Multiple carboxylase deficiency** *[Ref: Nelson 16/e P-356]*
114. **A i.e. Randomly** (Most probable answer of exclusion)

## Hemoprotein, Hemoglobin, Porphyrins & Bile Pigment

115. **A, B, C, D, E i.e. Cytochrome C; Cytochrome 450; Myoglobin; Hemoglobin; Catalase**
116. **A i.e. Myoglobin B i.e. Cytochrome oxidase** *[Ref: Harper 28/e 271-72; Chattarjae 7/e 82; Lippincott 5/e 25, 34; Lehninger 84-85]*
117. **A i.e. Histidine residue** 118. **A i.e. Hb has 2 polypeptide chain**
119. **A i.e. Histidine** 120. **B i.e. Histidine** *[Ref: Harper's 27/e P- 41-45; 26/e P- 40; Chatterjea 6/e P-133-34]*
121. **B i.e. His E 7** *[Ref: Harper's 27/e P-44; 26/e P- 40]*
122. **B i.e. Co-operative effect of combine $O_2$** 123. **D i.e. Heme at hydrophobic pockets**
*[Ref: Harper's 27/e P- 42-44; Chatterjea 6/e P-134, Lippincott's 3/e P-26]*
124. **D i.e. Hemoglobin** *[Ref: Lehninger 3/e P-214, 278]*
125. **A i.e. Binding of $O_2$ causes of $H^+$** *[Ref: Harper's 27/e P- 42-45]*
126. **B i.e. Decreased production of 2, 3- biphosphoglycerate**
127. **D i.e. Lipophilic**
128. **A i.e. Stercobilinogen** *[Ref: Lippincott's 3/e P- 287, 281; Chatterjea 6/e P- 476, 478; Harper's 27/e P-155]*
129. **B i.e Converts a hydrophobic compound to a hydrophilic one** *[Ref: Lippincott's 3/e P-281; Chatterjea 6/e P-478]*
130. **A i.e., Able to cross cell membrane; C i.e. Hydrophobic to hydrophilic** *[Ref: Lippincott 4/e p. 282; Harper's 27/e p. 289]*
131. **C i.e. Amphipathic** *[Ref: Ganong 21/e P 477, 505]*
132. **A i.e. Porphyrins** *[Ref: Harper's 27/e P-282; 26/e P- 273]*
133. **D i.e. Ehrlich's aldehyde regent** *[Ref: Practical boochemistry, C Raj Gopal and B D Toora 1/e P 47]*
134. **C i.e. CEP** 135. **D i.e. Ferrochelatase**
*[Ref: Harper's 27/e P-283-286; Vasudevan 6/e p. 245-50; Chatterjea 6/e P-472- 73, Lippincott's 3/e P-279]*
136. **D i.e. Hepatic porphyria**
137. **A i.e. Ferrous ion; B i.e. Glycine; D i.e. Succinyl CoA** *[Ref: Harper 26/e Pg 271-275]*

# METABOLISM OF PROTEIN & AMINO ACIDS: REVIEW NOTES

## Biosynthesis of Urea

Biosynthesis of urea has 4 stages (1) **transamination, (2) oxidative deamination of glutamate (3) ammonia transport, and (4) urea cycle.**

### Transamination (Braunstein & Kritzmann Reaction)

- Despite being most abundant in atmosphere, $N_2$ is preciously handled in biological system, because only few micro organism can convert $N_2$ to biologically useful form (as $NH_3$/amino group). Aminoacids derived from dietary protein are the source of amino groups in humans. The presence of this ***α-amino group*** keeps amino acids safely ***locked away from oxidative breakdows***[Q]. So removal of α amino group is essential obligatory step in energy production or catabolism of all aminoacids.
- Transamination is a *reversible* reaction in which α - $NH_2$ group of one aminoacid is transferred to a α - ketoacid resulting in formation of new amino acid a new keto acid. Once they have reached the **liver, transamination** is the first step in catabolism of most amino acids and involves only intermolecular transfer of amino ($NH_2$) group without formation (splitting out) of ammonia ($NH_3$). No net deamination & occurs because α-amino acid is deaminated & α-keto acid (mostly α-keto glutarae) become aminated.

### Aminotransferase (Transaminase) Enzyme

- This transfer of α-amino group from L amino acid to α-ketoacid is enzymed by amino transferase or transaminase enzyme
- Enzyme is found in *mitochondria and cytosol of cells through out the body especially those of liver, kidney, intestine, muscle, heart and brain.*
- Each aminotransferase is specific for one pair of substrate but non specific for other pair. Each is specific for 1 or at most few ***amino group donor on which their names are based. Because the acceptor of aminogroup is almost always α-keto (oxo) glutarate***[Q]***. Other rare recipient ketoacids are oxaloacetate or pyruvate.*** Example are

a. **Alanine (Alanine-Pyruvate) Aminotransferase (ALT)= Serum Glutamate Pyruvate Transaminase and Glutamate (Glutamate α-ketoglutarate) Aminotransferase**

Transfer aminogroup of alanine to α-keto (oxo) glutarate, resulting in formation of pyruvate & glutamate (glutamic acid)

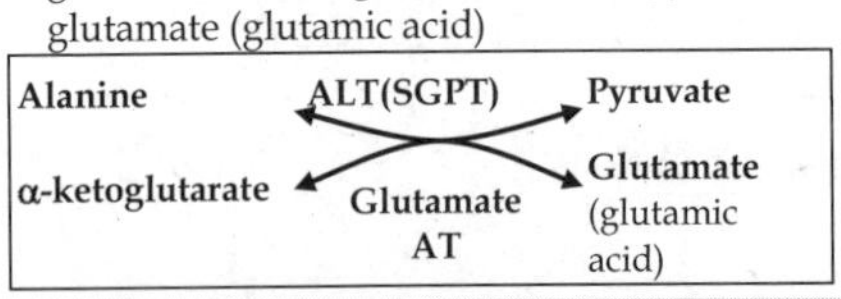


b. **Aspartate Aminotransferase (AST)= Serum Glutamate Oxaloacetate, Transaminase (SGOT)**

Exception to the rule that aminotransferase enzyme funnel amino groups to form glutamate. Because during aa catabolism, it transfer aminogroup of glutamate to oxaloacetate forming **aspartate** (which is used as **source of nitrogen in urea cycle**) & α-ketogluterate.

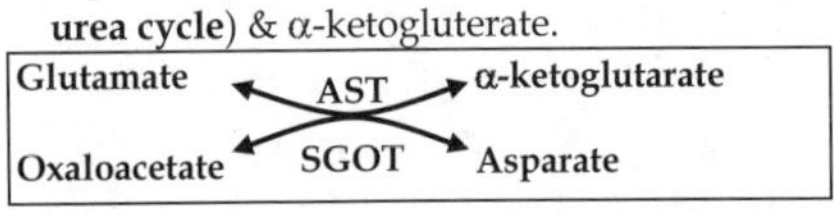


★ However in biosynthesis (when reaction is reversed) the aspartate becomes donor & α-ketoglutarate acceptor.

c. **Formation of alanine by transamination of pyruvate.** Amino donor may be glutamate or aspartate thus forming α-ketoglutarate or oxaloacetate

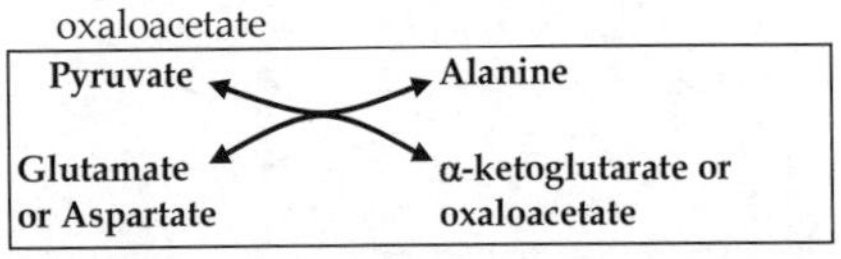


### Salient Features

- **Transamination *interconverts pairs of α-amino acids and α-keto acids, transferring α-amino nitrogen ($NH_2$ group) without splitting out of ammonia ($NH_3$) to α-ketoglutarate forming glutamate*[Q].**
- Alanine pyruvate (or **alanine) aminotransferase** and glutamate – α-ketoglutarate (**or glutamate) aminotransferase** catalyze the transfer of amino (**$NH_2$**) **group to pyruvate (forming alanine) or to α-ketoglutarate (forming glutamate).** Since alanine is also a substrate for glutamate aminotransferase, the α-amino nitrogen from all aminoacids that undergo ***transamination can be concentrated in glutamate. Therefore transamination reaction collects the aminogroup from many different amino acids in form of L-glutamate***[Q]. And then **L-glutamate functions as aminogroup donor for biosynthetic pathways** or **for excretion pathways** that lead to the elimination of nitrogenous waste products.
- **α-ketoglutarate** ***plays a crucial role by accepting amino ($NH_2$) groups from most amino acids and thus becoming glutamate***[Q]. So transamination collects amino groups from many different aminoacids in form of **L-glutamate** (i.e. called *funneling of aminogroups to L-glutamate*). This is important because *L-glutamate is the only amino acid that undergoes oxidative deamination at an appreciable rate* in mammalian tissue. So **formation of ammonia from α-amino group thus occur mainly via α-amino nitrogen of L glutamate**[Q] (by oxidative deamination)
- Transamination occur in almost all amino acids except **threonine, lysine** (loose amino group by deamination), **proline, hydroxyproline**, and *cyclic iminoacids.*
- Transamination is not restricted to α-amino groups. The **δ-amino group** of ornithine (but not ε amino group of lysine) readily undergoes transamination.
- Glutamate produced by transamination can be oxidatively deaminated or used as aminogroup donor in synthesis of non essential amino acids.
- ***Equilibrium constant*** for transamination is ~**1** making it readily reversible and *allowing amino acid biosynthesis* (by addition of amino group to keto acid when supply of amino acid in diet is not adequate) **and amino acid degradation** (by removal of amino group when diet is rich in protein) **both.**

### Deamination

- It is *removal of N of aminoacid as $NH_3$*
- **Oxidative deamination is catalyzed by D & L-aminoacid oxidase.** Despite absence of D aminoacids in tissues, the D-aa-oxidase enzyme is much greater than L-aa-oxidase
- L aminoacid oxidae is *auto oxidizable flavoprotein (FMN),* which is reoxidized, when reduced, at substrate level directly by $O_2$ forming $H_2O_2$ without participation of any electron carrier (like cytochrome or ETS). Toxic $H_2O_2$ is converted to $O_2$ & $H_2O$ by catalase.

| Feature | **L-AA oxidase** | **D-AA oxidase** |
|---|---|---|
| Flavoprotein | FMN | FAD |
| Acts on | L-amino acids | D-amino acids |
| Extracted with water free form | Not; because bound to tissue | Freely |

- **Non oxidative deamination** has a very minor role in $NH_3$ formation and can occur in
  1. **Sulfur containing amino acids** like *cysteine & homocysteine* by **desulfhhydrase** (removing $H_2S$).
  2. **Hydroxy amino acids** like *serine, homoserine & threonine* by **aminoacid dehydrogenases** requiring *pyridoxal (B6)- P as coenzyme.*
  3. **Histidine** by **histidase** forming urocanic acid & $NH_3$.

### Deamination of L-Glutamate = Transdeamination

- L-Glutamate formed as a main product of transamination is not deaminated by L-amino acid oxidase but by hepatic **L-glutamate dehydrogenase (GDH).**
- GDH is a tetramer metalloenzyme containing 1 $Zn^{++}$ in each of 4 polypeptide chain. It can use **NAD+ or NADP+ as coenzymes** and release nitrogen as ammonia. It is **allosterically inhibited by ATP, GTP and NADH** and is **activated by ADP.**
- Reaction is freely reversible and

### Coenzyme Pyridoxal Phosphate (Vitamin $B_6$ derivative)

- ***Pyridoxal phosphate coenzyme (or prosthetic group) is covalently bound to enzyme's active site by an Schiff base (aldimine) linkage***Q to ε amino group of Lys residue and *serves as a carrier of amino group* (and thus generating pyridoxamine phosphate which transfers this amino group to α-keto acid).
- Transamination occurs via **ping pong reaction** which means the 1st substrate reacts & product must leave the active site before 2nd substrate can bind.

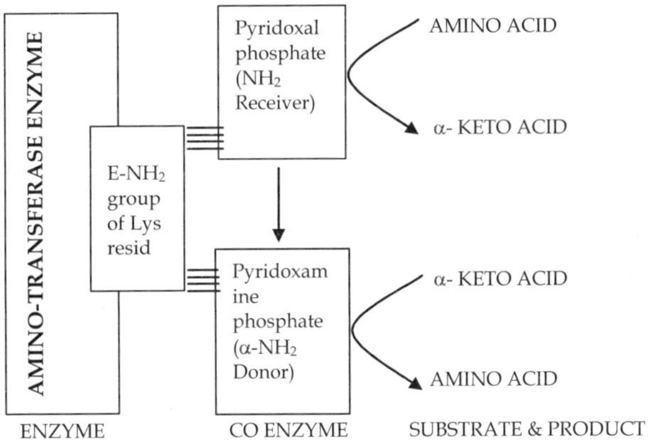


PING-PONG MECHANISM OF TRANSAMINATION

equilibrium constant favours glutamate (amino acid) biosynthesis but quick removal of $NH_3$ to urea cycle & α-ketoglutarate to TCA cycle favours ammonia formation.

$$\text{L-Glutamate} + NAD(P)^+ \underset{\text{L-GDH}}{\rightleftharpoons} \alpha\text{-ketoglutarate} + NH_3 + NAD(P)H + H^+$$

- Conversion of alpha-amino nitrogen to ammonia by **coupled action of glutamate aminotransferase and GDH** is called **transdeamination.**

## Non toxic Transport of Ammonia (& Amino group)

### In Brain & Most other tissue

- In most tissues (especially brain) nucleotide degradation produce free ammonia, which being toxic is immediately trapped by glutamate (glutamic acid) to form **nontoxic glutamine**. This reaction is catabolized by **glutamine synthetase** and require ATP.

$$\underset{\text{Toxic}}{\text{L-Glutamate} + NH_3} \xrightarrow[\text{Glutamine Synthetase}]{ATP \rightarrow ADP} \underset{\textbf{Non toxic}}{\textbf{L- Glutamine}}$$

- Aspartic acid may undergo similar reaction to form **asparagine**, which traps $NH_3$ in brain (minor)
- Glutamine is *non toxic transport form of $NH_3$ and serves as a source of amino group in* biosynthetic reactions. It is normally *present in blood in much higher concentrations* than other amino acids. Excess glutamine (of amount that is required for biosysthesis) is *transported to liver, intestine and kidney*, where enzyme **glutaminase** reverse the reaction and convert glutamine to glutamate (glutamic acid) and $NH_3$ ($NH_4^+$). The toxic $NH_4^+$ from intestine, kidney & other tissues is rapidly removed from blood by liver and converted to urea.
- **In kidney (renal tubular cells)** ***ammonia ($NH_4^+$) production from intra cellular amino acids mainly glutamine increases in metabolic acidosis and decreases in metabolic alkalosis***Q. So in metabolic acidosis not all $NH_4^+$ produced in kidney is released into blood to form urea in liver; *some is excreted directly into the urine thus facilitating cation (positive ion) conservation and regulating acid base balance.*
- **Glutaminase** and **asparaginase** ***deaminate glutamine & asparagines thus releasing toxic $NH_3$***Q

### In Skeletal Muscle

- In tissues that degrade aminoacid for fuel (mainly skeletal muscle), amino group is collected in form of L-glutamate (d/t transamination)
- This **glutamate** (containing toxic α-amino group) can be transported to liver by converting it to glutamine or it can transfer its α-amino group to **pyruvate**, a easily available product of muscle glycolysis by the action of **alanine aminotransferase** (**ALT/SGPT**). The **alanine** so formed passes into blood to liver.
- In liver cell cytosol **alanine aminotransferase** (**ALT/SGPT**) transfers amino group from alanine to α-ketoglutarate forming pyruvate (which enters gluconeogenesis) and glutamate (under go oxidative deamination)
- Vigrously contracting muscles operate anerobically producing pyruvate & lactate (from glycolysis) and $NH_3$ (from aa break down). **Alanine-glucose cycle** in concert with Cori cycle send these products to liver where pyruvate & lactate are incorporated into glucose (by gluconeogenesis and returned back to muscle) and $NH_3$ is converted to urea for excretion. So the **energetic burden of gluconeogenesis is imposed on liver and all available ATP in muscle is devoted to muscle contraction.**

## Transport of Ammonia to Liver

*Ammonia is transported to Liver from peripheral tissue for its ultimate conversion to urea.*

Two mechanisms are available in humans for this transport

- Mechanism found in **Most tissue** → Uses Glutamine
- **Mechanism in Muscle** → Uses Alanine

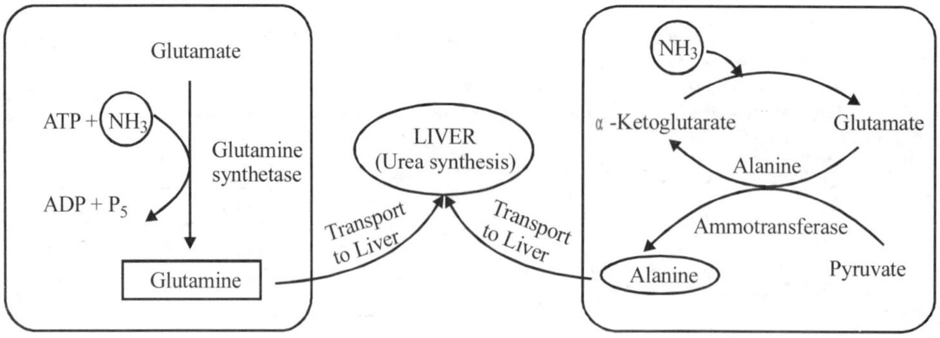


## Ammonia Transport

**Enters Urea Cycle**

- *Most important rout of* disposal
- Formation of urea in liver & then excreted in urine from kidney
- A portion of urea diffuses from blood into intestine & is cleaved to $NH_3$ & $CO_2$ by *bacterial urease*

***As Glutamine***[Q]

- Provide a ***nontoxic storage & transport form of $NH_3$***[Q]
- ***Major mechanism for removal of $NH_3$ in brain***[Q].
- Formation of glutamine from glutamate & NH3 occurs primarily in muscle & Liver
- *Glutamine* is an amide of glutamic acid (glutamate) which is ***formed from α- Ketoglutarate***[Q].

Ammonia production ($NH_4^+$ ion) from renal amino acid (eg glutamine) ***increase in metabolic acidosis and decrease in metabolic alkalosis***[Q]. [To maintain acid- base balance]

**Metabolism of Ammonia**

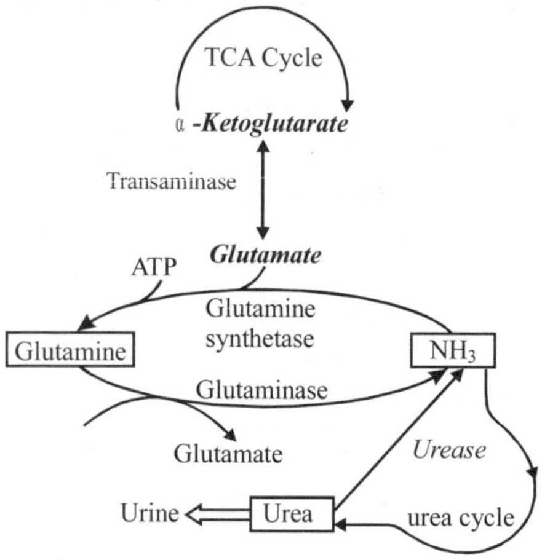


## Hyper-Ammonemia : $NH_3$ Intoxication

- $NH_3$ is produced by protein catabolism and is mainly converted to urea (by urea cycle) in liver. Some $NH_3$ is also used for transamination of α-ketoacid to α-amino acid and in synthesis of glutamine.
- Disorders of urea cycle (i.e. any enzyme of urea cycle) would result in hyper ammonemia, encephalopathy & respiratory alkalosis. Brain is very sensitive to ammonia. Clinical features include mental retardation, lethargy, irritability & vomiting.
- Block in earlier steps of urea cycle results in more symptoms since ammonia itself accumulates, whereas deficiency of later enzymes result in accumulation of less toxic other intermediates and hence symptoms are less. Hyper ammonemia **type I** (d/t **CPS I**- deficiency), hyperammonemia (d/t **OTC** def.), hyperornithinemia (defect in ornithine transporter protein), citrullinemia (def. of argininosuccinate synthetase), argininosuccinicacid uria (def. of argininosuccinate lyase) and *hyperargininemia* (arginase def) are **disorder of urea cycle.** Increase $NH_3$ concentration causes

**Increased tranamination of α-ketoglutrate** (a TCA cycle intermediate) to form glutamate (glutamic acid)

↓

***Decreased mitochondrial poll of α-ketoglutarate inhibiting TCA cycle & cellular respiration***[Q].

**Increased glutamine synthesis** from glutamate (glutamic acid) in brain leading to

- **Decreased** brain cell pool of **glutamic acid**
  ↓
  **Decreased** synthesis of **GABA** (inhibitory neurotransmitter)
- **Increased** brain **glutamine** level and its **outflow**
  
  **Increased tryptophan level** in brain cells because glutamine is carried out by same transporter which allows entery of tryptophan in brain cells
  ↓
  **Increased** synthesis of **serotonin**

## Urea Cycle / Krebs – Henseleit Cycle / Ornithine Cycle

- ***Urea cycle leading to formation of urea takes place in liver***[Q]. Urea is the most important disposal form of $NH_3$ or amino group derived from amino acid catabolism. One mol of urea synthesis requires *1 mol each of NH4+ (ammonium ion) & of α-amino* nitrogen of aspartate and **3 mol of ATP (but 4 high energy phosphate bonds** as 1 ATP of these 3 is converted to AMP thus using 2 $PO_4$ bonds.)
- One nitrogen of urea molecule is supplied by **free ammonia** and other by **aspartate.** However, **glutamate** is the immediate precursor of both ammonia (through oxidative deamination by GDH) and aspartate nitrogen (through trans amination of oxaloacetate by AST). In effect, both nitrogen (N) atoms of urea arise from L-glutamate, which in turn gathers them from aminoacids. The carbon (C) & oxygen (O) atoms of urea are derived from $CO_2$ (or $HCO_3^-$)
- It is a cyclic process with 6 participating aminoacids and 5 enzymes. *There is not net loss or gain of ornithine, citrulline, argininosuccinate, or arginine.* However, **ammonium ion (NH4+), $CO_2$, 3ATP (or 4 high energy phosphate bonds) are consumed and there is net conversion of (oxaloacetate via) aspartate to fumarate.**

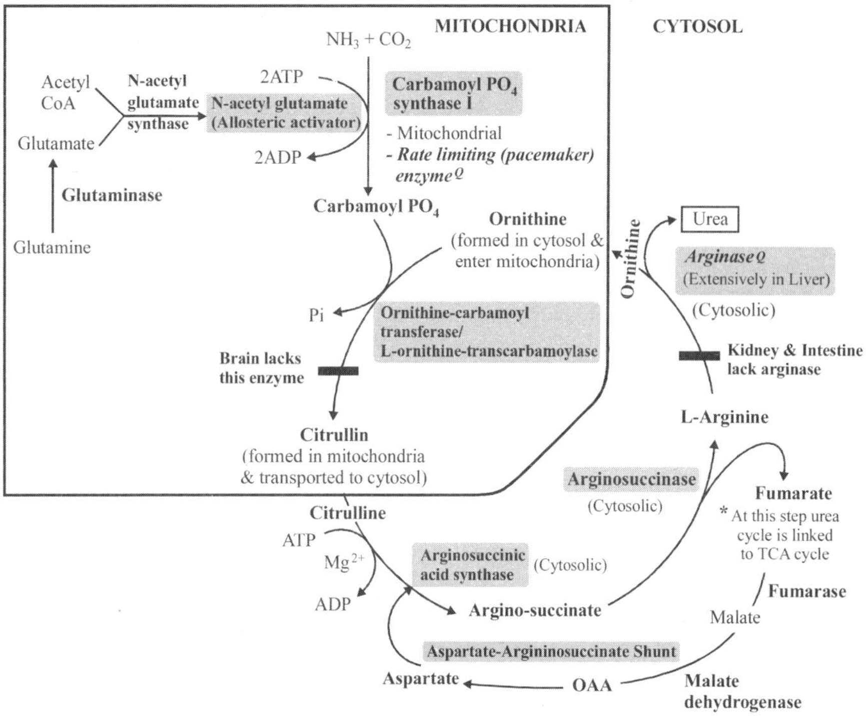


**Sources of Carbon & Nitrogen in Urea ($NH_2CONH_2$)**

Mn: **"OCC-ASA"**

i.e. <u>O</u>rnithine + <u>C</u>arbamoyl

→ <u>C</u>itrullin

→ <u>A</u>rgino-<u>S</u>uccinate

→ <u>A</u>rginine

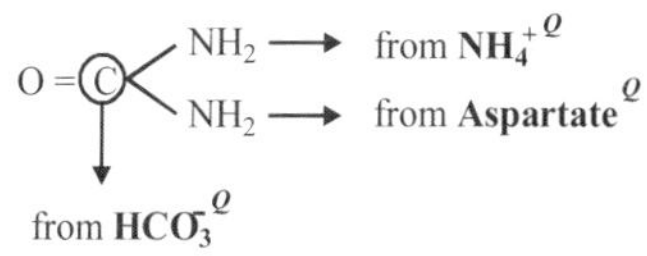


**Aspartate** + $NH_3$ + $CO_2$ + $H_2O$ + **3ATP → Fumarate + Urea** + 2ADP + 2AMP + 2Pi + PPi

However fumarate formed in urea cycle may be converted to malate, which when oxidized to oxaloacetate produce **1 NADPH** equivalent to **2.5 ATP,** so **net energy expenditure** reduces to only **1.5 high energy phosphates**.

- First two reactions i.e. *formation of carbamoyl phosphate* (catabolized by ***carbamoyl phosphate synthetase I enzyme***) and *formation of citrulline* (catabolized by **ornithine transcarbamoylase**) takes place in **mitochondria**. *Citrulline is transported from mitochondria to cytosol* and remaining steps i.e. formation of argininosuccinate (enz. **argininosuccinate synthetase**), its cleavage to arginine & fumarate (enz. **argininosuccinate lyase**), and cleavage of arginine to ornithine and urea (enz **arginase**) takes place in **cytosol**. Ornithine returns to mitochondria to react with another molecule of carbamoyl $PO_4$. Ornithine is regenerated with each turn of urea cycle, much in the same way the oxaloacetate is regenerated in citric acid cycle. **Ornithine & citrulline** are basic aminoacids that are not incorporated **into cellular proteins because there are no codons for these amino acids.**
- 2ATP molecules are required to make carbamoyl $PO_4$ and 1 ATP (2 high energy phosphate bonds) to make argininosuccinate. First step of urea cycle i.e. condensation of $CO_2$, ammonia and 2 ATP l/t **formation of carbomoyl phosphate by carbamoyl $PO_4$ synthetase I is the rate limiting step (& enzyme)**. This enzyme is only active in presence of **N-acetyl glutamate (NAG)** ***an allosteric activator that enhances the affinity of enzyme for ATP***[Q]. NAG is synthesize by N-acety glutamate synthetase from acetyl CoA and glutamate.
- Because fumarate produced in urea cycle is also an intermediate of citric acid cycle, both cycles are inter connected (k/a **Krebs bicycle**) by **aspartate – argininosuccinate shunt**. However each cycle can operate independently. And fumarase & malate dehydrogenase used in urea cycle are cytosolic (not mitochondrial like TCA cycle).
- *Kidney & Intestine* contribute to most of body arginine because they possess all the urea cycle enzyme except arginase.
- Brain can synthesize urea from citrulline, but lacks enzyme for formation of citrulline from ornithine.
- Thus neither brain nor Kidney can form urea in significant amount.

## Serine Proteases

- ***The active site of serine proteases contain three critical amino acids Serine, Histidine and Aspartate. These residues are often referred to as the catalytic triad.*** *Chymotrypsin, Elastase and Trypsin are the three serine proteases that function essentially as enzymes.Each of these enzymes contain the 'catalytic triad' within their active sites but differ with respect to their target cleavage sites.- www.rpc.msue.edu*
- **They are activated by proteolytic activation and not autocatalytic activation.** They are secreted by the pancreas as inactive zymogens into small intestine- and became active through proteolytic cleavage events, either in a subcellular compartment or in an extracellular space where they are required for digestion.
- **Pancreatic trypsin inhibitor** is serine protease inhibitor only for trypsin and not for other serine protease enzymes such as chymotrypsin or elastase. Serine proteases enzymes tightly bind the respective protease inhibitors instead of normal substrates.

| Serine protease | Serine protease inhibitor |
|---|---|
| Trypsin | Pancreatic trypsin inhibitor |
| Chymotrypsin | Alpha-1 antichymotrypsin |
| Elastase | Alpha-1 antitrypsin |

- **Serine proteases attack the carbonyl group of the peptide bond that is to be cleaved (and not essentially the one adjacent to serine residue)**

| Serine protease | Substrate |
|---|---|
| **Chymotrypsin** | Peptide bond next to ***aromatic residues (Phenylalanine, Tyrosine Tryptophan)***[Q] |
| **Trypsin** | Peptide bond next to ***basic residues (Lysine or Arginine)***[Q] |
| **Elastase** | Peptide bonds next to ***Hydrophobic residues (Alanine)***[Q] |

## Metabolic role of vitamin $B_{12}$

Biologically active forms of vitamin $B_{12}$ are called as 'cobamide coenzymes' and act as coenzymes with several enzymes for various metabolic reactions. These include

1. *Isomerization of methyl malonyl co-A to succinyl CoA*[Q]: Methyl malonyl CoA —[Vitamin $B_{12}$ (Deoxyadenosyl cobalamine); Methyl malonyl CoA mutase]→ Succinyl CoA
2. *Methylation of Homocystine to methionine*[Q]: Homocysteine —[Vitamin $B_{12}$ Methyl cobalamine; Homocysteine methyl transferase]→ Methionine (requires methyl tetrahydrofolate As a methyl carrier)
3. *Methylation of pyrimidine ring to form thymine.*
4. *Conversion of ribonucleotides to deoxyribonucleotides in DNA synthesis :* Ribonucleotides —[Vitamin $B_{12}$; Reductase]→ Deoxyribonucleotides
5. *Required for metabolism of diols:* Ethylene glycol —[Vitamin $B_{12}$]→ Acetaldihyde.
6. *In Bacteria for interconversion of glutamate and β methyl aspartate*: Glutamic acid —[Vitamin $B_{12}$]→ β Methyl aspartate.

## Creatinine & Creatinine Biosynthesis

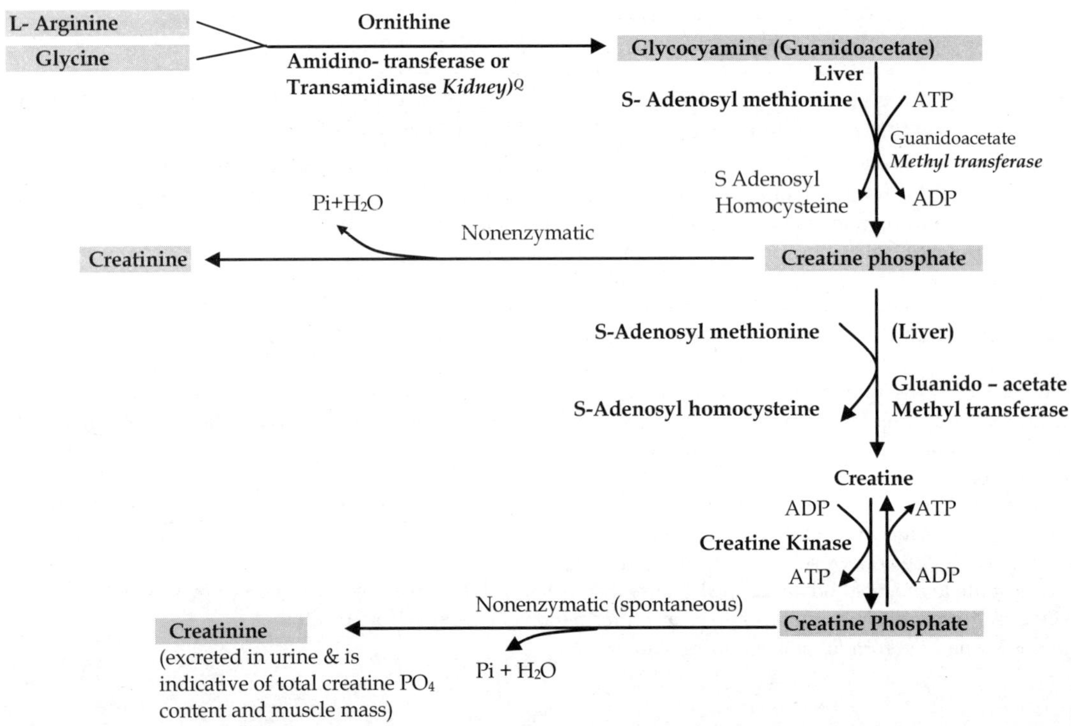

## Catabolism of Carbon Skeletons of Aminoacids

| A.A that form Oxaloacetate |
|---|
| Asparginine (Aspartate) |

| A.A that form Fumarate |
|---|
| - *Phenylalanine* |
| - *Tyrosine* |

| A.A. that form Succinyl CoA | |
|---|---|
| - *Methionine* | - *Isoleucine* |
| - *Valine* | - Threonine |

| A.A That form α-ketoglutarate |
|---|
| - Glutamine |
| - Proline |
| - Arginine |
| - *Histidine* |

| A.A.that form Pyruvate | |
|---|---|
| - Alanine | - Cystine |
| - Serine | - Threonine |
| - Glycine | |

| A.A that form Acetyl CoA/ Acetoacetyl CoA | |
|---|---|
| - Leucine | - Tryptophans |
| - Isoleucine | - Phenyalanine |
| - Lysine | - Tyrosine |

## Classification of Ammino Acids (aa) on the basis of R-Group or Side chains

### Nonpolar (Hydrophobic or Water insoluble) side chains

Nonpolar side chains **does not gain or lose protons or participate in hydrogen or ionic bonds.** Oily or *lipid like* side chains promote *hydrophobic interaction.*

In proteins found in polar environment or aqueous solutions – the side chains of nonpolar aminoacids tend to cluster together in interior of protein (**hydrophobic effect**) and help give it its three dimensional shape. However in hydrophobic environment such as membranes the nonpolar side chains are found on the outside surface of protein interacting with lipid environment

#### Aliphatic (Nonpolar / Hydrophobic) Side chain)

| | |
|---|---|
| Glycine | *Simplest structure*[Q] Very small (H) side chain makes no real contribution to hydrophobic interactions |
| Alanine | *Methyl side chain*[Q] |
| Valine | C3H7 side chain |
| Leucine & Isoleucine | C4H9 side chain |
| **A**lnine, **l**eucine, **I**soleucine & **V**aline (mn "**ALL Is Well**") tend to cluster together within proteins stabilizing protein structure by means of hydrophobic interactions | |
| Methionine | **Sulfur containing** amino acid with **thioether side chain** |
| Proline | Side chain form a distinct **cyclic (ring shaped), rigid 5 membered secondary** (rather than primary **amino group k/a imino group. It reduces structural** flexibility, and contributes in formation of *fibrous structure of collagen* and often **interrupts α-helices** found in globular proteins. |

#### Aromatic (Non polar/ relatively Hydrophobic) Side chain

- All can participate in hydrophobic interactions.
- *Tyrosine & tryptophan* are significantly more polar than **phenyl alanine,** because of tyrosine hydroxyl group& nitrogen of tryptophan indole ring
- Tyrosine hydroxyl (OH) group can form hydrogen bonds
- ***Tryptophan & tyrosine, and to much lesser extent phenylalanine absorb ultraviolet light at a wave length of 280nm.***[Q] **(photochromocity)**
- *Phenylalanine has benzene, tyrosine has phenol and tryptophan has indole groups* respectively.

★ **Hydropathy index is negative** (ΔG< O) for polar or charged aminoacids; and positive (ΔG> O) for nonpolar or more hydrophobic aminoacids. All of aliphatic & aromatic aa have (+) value except **glycine** (- 0.4), **tryptophan** (-0.9), **tyrosine** (- 1.3), and **histidine** (-3.2). Hence histidine is not included & tyrosine is relatively included in non polar group

★ **Histidine** is a positively charged (basic) aa with **$NH_3^+$ side chain.** It also has **aromatic imidazole side** chain. As the only aa. having an imidazole side chain with pKa near neutrality, histadine ***may be positively charged (protonated form) or uncharged at pH 7)***[Q]. It facilitate many reactions by **serving as proton donors / acceptors.**

### Polar (Hydrophillic or Water soluble) side chains

The most hydrophilic (polar) R groups are those that are either positively or negatively charged

#### Polar, Uncharged (Neutral or Non ionic) side chain

- Have **zero (0) net charge at neutral pH,** although cysteine and tyrosine can lose proton at alkali pH
- They contain functional group that form hydrogen bond with water making them hydrophilic & polar

| | |
|---|---|
| **Serine**<br>**Threonine** | Hydroxyl group<br>Hydroxyl group |
| **Cysteine** | Sulfhydryl group (weak acid) |
| **Asparagine**<br>**Glutamine** | Amide group<br>Amide group |
| **Tyrosine** | Hydroxyl group |

- *Asparagine & glutamine* are the amides of 2 other aa, aspartate & glutamate respectively
- Cysteine is oxidized to form a covalently linked dimeric amino acid called **cystine,** in which 2 cysteine molecules are *joined by disulfide bond making it strongly hydrophobic (non polar)*

★ Cysteine & tyrosine may show hydrophobic character when present in interior of protein. Glycine may be included in this group also.

#### Polar ionic, Positively charged (Basic) side chain /aa

| | |
|---|---|
| **Lysine** | Second primary amino at ε position on its aliphatic chain |
| **Arginine** | +ve charged guanidinium group |
| **Histidine** | Aromatic imidazole group |

#### Polar, Ionic, Negatively charged (Acidic) side chains

- 2 aa. with a net negative charge at pH 7 are **aspartate & glutamate** each of which has 2nd carboxyl (COO-) group.
- **Aspartic acid & glutamic acid** contain β carboxyl and γ carboxyl groups respectively.

★ *α- carbon atom of aminoacid is **optically** or **chirally active** as it is attached to 4 different groups. **Glycine** is the exception and is optically inactive b/o 2 hydrogen atoms attached.

★ Aminoacids with asymmetrical α-carbon center can exist in **two 'D' and 'L'** mirror image forms k/a **optical isomers, stereoisomers or enantiomers**. Only 'L' (levorotatory) alpha aminoacids occur in proteins.

★ **Naturally occurring 'D' – aminoacids are free 'D' serine & 'D'-aspartate in brain; 'D' alanine & 'D' glutamate in cell walls of gram (+) bacteria; D aminoacids in some antibiotics & peptides produced by bacteria, fungi etc.**

## (L-α)- Amino acid Classification (Based on Side Chain)

### Polarity and Solubility

#### Hydrophobic (Nonpolar) aa (Lehninger)

| | |
|---|---|
| T | Tryptophan* |
| | Tyrosine** |
| M | Methionine |
| L | Leucine |
| V | Valine |
| I | Isoleucine |
| A | Alanine |
| P | Phenylalanine |
| | Proline |
| G | Glycine* |

**Mn – "Try To Meet Lucy in Valley Is All Phen's problem–G" or "TAMIL VAP-G"**

However in aromatic side chain aa tyrosine > tryptophan are more polar than phenylalanine.

★ = Relative

#### Hydrophollic (Polar) aa

- **Uncharged (Neutral)**
  - *Serine*Q
  - Threonine
  - *Tyrosine*Q
  - Aspargine
  - Cysteine
  - Glutamine
- **Acidic (Negatively charged – Proton donors)**
  Mn: **"Acidic as Glue"**
  - Aspartic acid-Glutamic acid
  - Asparagine★-Glutamine★
- **Basic (Positively charged – Proton acceptor)**
  Mn: **"His basics are loose"**
  - **His**tidine (weakly basic or neutral) ★
  - Hydroxy lysine
  - *Arginine (most basic)*Q
  - *Lysine*Q

### Side Chain Content

#### Aliphatic

- Glycine
- Alanine
- Valine
- Leucine
- Isoleucine
- Proline
- Methionine

Mn: **'GAVLI-PM'**

#### Aromatic

- **Tyr**osine
- **Try**ptophan
- **Phen**ylalanine
- **His**tidine

Mn: **"Try To Pen His Arrow"**

#### Hydroxyl (OH) group

- **Tyrosine**
- **Threonine**
- **Serine**

Mn: **"OH! Try Three sari"**

#### Sulfur atoms

- **Cysteine**
- **Methionine**

Mn: **"Meet Sulphuric Cyst"**

#### Immino acid/ (Secondary amino group)

***Proine*Q**

#### Basic group

- ***Arginine*Q**
- ***Lysine*Q**
- ***Histidine*Q**

#### Acidic Group

- ***Aspartic acid (aspartate)*** Q
- ***Glutamic acid (glutamate)*** Q

#### Amides of acidic group

- Asparagine
- Glutamine

## Polar –Ionic – Charged – Amino acids

### Basic (Positively charged) Monoamino-dicarboxylic acids

- At physiological pH the side chains are *fully ionized (polar) and positively charged* containing an extra positively charged amino group
- These contain one negative charged carboxylic (- COOH / - $COO^-$) group and two positive charged amino ($-NH_2$) groups. Hence called di amino-mono carboxylic acid
- Basic aminoacids accept protons
- Examples include : **Arginine (most basic)**, lysine, hydroxyl-lysine, and ***histidine (weakly basic /neutral)***Q

### Acidic (Negatively charged) Diamino-monocarboxylic acids

- At physiological pH the side chains are fully ionized (polar) and negatively charged *containing an extra negatively charged carboxylic group.*
- Acidic aminoacids contain 1 amino and 2 carboxylic groups. Hence called mono amino dicarboxylic acids
- Acidic aminoacids are *proton donors*
- Examples include **aspartic acid** (or ***aspartate***) and **glutamic acid** (or **glutamate**). These 2 are written in all books but chatterjae also includes ***glutamine & asparagines*** in this group. But these two are included in polar uncharged (neutral) in Lehninger (Go with this)

## Classification of Amino Acids on the Basis of Metabolism

### Essential Amino Acid

| | | | |
|---|---|---|---|
| Lu- | Leucine | Vali- | Valine |
| Ly- | Lysine | Iso- | Isoleucine |
| Thi - | Threonine | Phenyl- | Phenylalanine |
| Her- | Histidine } *Semi-essential*Q | Metho- | Methionine |
| Argi - | Arginine | Trypto- | Tryptophan |

[Mn: **'LuLi Thi His Argi Vali Iso Phenyl Metho Trypto'**] or **"Please Visit To TIM HALL"**

### Conditionally Essential

Required to some degree in young growing animals & during illness

- Arginine – Glutamine – Proline
- Cysteine – Glycine – Tyrosine

### Non essential Amino Acids

- Alanine
- Aspartate
- Serine
- Asparagine
- Glutamine

| Ketogenic A.A | Glucogenic A. A. | Both Glucogenic & Ketogenic A.A. |
|---|---|---|
| Leucine<br>**Lysine** | **V** - Valine<br>**C / see** - Cysteine, Serine<br>**All** - Alanine<br>**His** - Histidine<br>**Three** - Threonine<br>**Asses** - Aspartate<br>**Are** - Arginine<br>**Grass** - Glycine, Glutamate<br>**Prone** - Proline / **Hydroxy proline** | Isoleucine<br>Tyrosine<br>Tryptophan<br>**Phenylalanine** |

★ In Lehninger, **Histidine** is essential and **Arginine** is conditionally essential.

| | Ketogenic | Glucogenic & Ketogenic | Glucogenic |
|---|---|---|---|
| Essential | Leucine<br>Lysine | Isoleucine<br>Phenyl alanine<br>Tryptophan | Methionine<br>Threonine<br>Valine<br>Histidine* |
| Semi Essential | - | - | Histidine<br>Arginine |
| Non - Essential | Hydroxy-lysine | Tyrosine | Arginine*<br>Alanine<br>Asparagine<br>Aspartate<br>Cysteine<br>Glutamate<br>Glutamine<br>Glycine<br>Proline, hydroxyproline<br>Serine |

## Glycine

- **Glycine** does ***not posses asymmetric carbon atom and is therefore optically inactive i.e. lacks chirality (handedness)***[Q].
- The α- Carbon of each a.a is attached to four different chemical groups & is therefore chiral or optically active. *Glycine is an exception because its α- carbon has two Hydrogen atoms* & therefore is optically inactive.

- ***Smallest***[Q] and ***simplest***[Q] amino acid
- Amino acid ***responsible for flexibility of proteins***[Q].
- Is ***optically inactive***[Q], does not exist in isomeric form.
- It ***lacks chirality***[Q].
- **G**lycine with **a**rginine & **m**ethionine (GAM) ***synthesize creatine***[Q].
- Glycine (with succinyl COA) is used for ***Heme synthesis***[Q].

## One Carbon Units

- One carbon units can exist in form of *methane, methanol, formaldehyde, formic acid and carbonic acid*, all of which except methane can be incorporated in various synthetic pathways.
- Sources of one carbon unit are *serine, glycine, choline, histidine, and formate*
- ***Tetrahydrofolate and S-adenosyl methionine are carrier of one carbon units***[Q]. The active form of folic acid, tetra hydrofolic acid (THE) can carry carbon unit bound to nitrogen $N_5$ or $N^{10}$ or to both $N_5$ and $N^{10}$ in form of formyl, formimino, or methyl (attached to $N_5$), methylene, methenyl group (bridging $N_5$ & $N^{10}$) and formyl (attached to $N^{10}$).

★ Biotin functions as coenzyme to transfer $CO_2$ in carboxylation reactions (enzyme carboxylase). But **$CO_2$ is not considered as member of 1 carbon pool**.

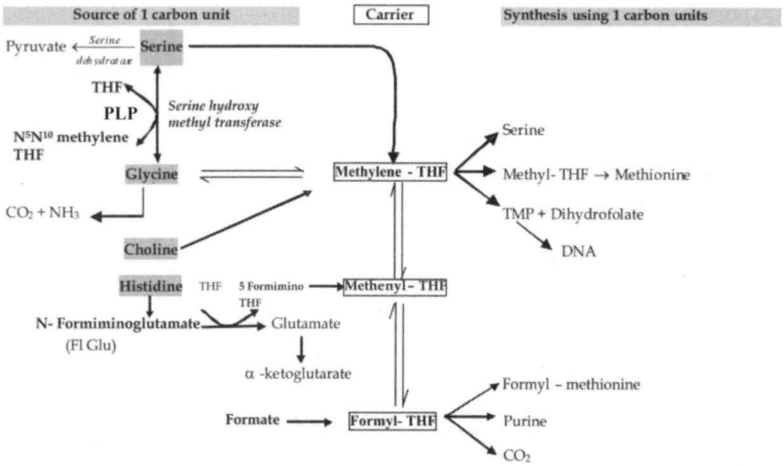


## Histidine

- ***Most stable amino acid at physiological pH***[Q]
- ***Can serve as best buffer at pH 7***[Q]
- Can ***protonate & deprotonate at neutral PH***[Q]

**Histidine** is unique, since pKa of its imidazole group permits it at pH7 (physiological) to function either as a base or as an acid catalyst i.e. it ***has capacity to protonate or deprotonate at neutral pH***[Q].
***Minor change in pH, changes the ionization charge on histidine to buffur pH change***[Q]. Therefore it **can serve as a buffer & is *most stable amino acid at physiological pH***[Q].

## Functions of Glutathione

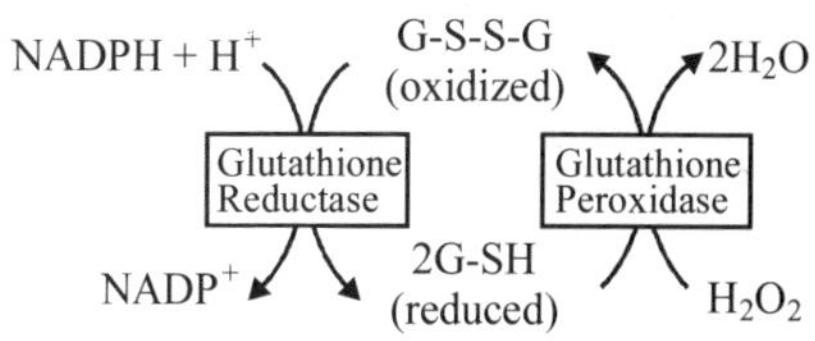


1. **Antioxidant:**
   - Reduced glutathione (GSH) can ***detoxify $H_2O_2$ by glutathione peroxidase***[Q] and itself converted into oxidized form (G-S-S-G).
   - Oxidized glutathione contains two glutathione linked by disulphide bond between its cysteine residue, hence its reducing ***property is because of cysteine sulfhydryl group***[Q].
2. It is important *intracellular reductant*, helping to maintain essential SH gp of enzymes in reduced state.
3. **Membrane transport**: It acts as a ***carrier in transport of certain amino acid across membrane in kidney***[Q].
   Amino acid + GSH → γ - Glutamyl amino acid + Cystein glycine
4. ***Helps in conjugation reaction***[Q]: Toxic xenobiotics are conjugated to nucleophilic GSH (glutathione) to convert to more polar, hydroxylated derivatives.

### Cystinuria [Mn: "COLA"]

- Is a *disorder of proximal tubule's reabsorption of filtered cystine and dibasic amino acid* (Ornithine, Lysine, Arginine). So there is excretion of – **C**ystine, **O**rnithine, **L**ysine & **A**rginine[Q]
- It is *most common* genetic error of amino acid transport affecting aminoacid carrier in small intestine & proximal tubule of kidney (as both share same transport carrier) for COAL amino acids.
- **Complications**: Cystine is relatively insoluble a.a and therefore precipitates in renal tubules, ureter and bladder to form ***cystine calculi***[Q].
- **Diagnosis**: By ***Cyanide- Nitroprusside test***[Q].

### Cysteine

- Cysteine is a ***sulphur containing amino acid***[Q].
- Cystine is formed by two molecules of cysteine, joined together by S- S bond.
- Cysteine can be *synthesized in body from methionine.*
- Prominent a.a in protein of nails, hairs and keratin of skin.

## Amino Acids: Summary

**Glycine**
- *Simplest*[Q] a.a
- ***Optically inactive***[Q]
- ***Lacks chirality***[Q]
- ***Synthesize Creatine***[Q] (with arginine & methionine)
- Used ***in heme synthesis***[Q].

**Histidine**
- ***Most stable a.a at physiological pH***[Q]
- Acts as buffer ***at pH 7***[Q]
- ***Protonate & deprotonate at neutral pH***[Q]
- ***Precursor of histamine***[Q].

**Glutamine**
- ***Storage and transport form of ammonia***[Q].
- Major pathway for removal of $NH_3$ in *brain*
- Precursor of purines and pyrimidines

**Phenylalanine / Tyrosine**
- Phenylalanine is precursor of tyrosine
- Tyrosine is a precursor of:
  - ***Catecholamines***[Q]
  - ***Thyroxine***[Q]
  - ***melanin***[Q]

**Cysteine**
- Sulphur containing amino acid
- Two cysteine joine to form cystine
- Can be *synthesize* in body *from methionine.*
- ***Responsible for reducing action of glulathione***[Q]

**Methionine**
- Sulphur containing a.a
- Methionine form ***S-adenosylmethionine (SAM),*** major ***methyl group donor in body***[Q]
- ***Precursor of homocysteine***[Q]- metabolite ***associated with atherosclerotic vascular disease***[Q].

**Tryptophan**
- Precursor of ***niacin and serotonin***[Q]
- Serotonin form *melatonin*
- ***60mg tryptophan give rise to 1mg Niacin***[Q].
- ***Also kla α - amino β -3 indole propionic acid***[Q]
- **Precursor of Vitamin niacin and serotonin**

**Arginine**
- Member of urea cycle
- ***Precursor of nitric oxide***[Q]

**Alanine**
- ***Most basic amino acid***[Q]
- *Transport form of ammonia from muscle.*

## Risk Factors For Altherosclerosis (Hence MI)

**Major**

Non modifiable
- Increasing age
- Male gender
- Family h/o premature CHD

Potentially modifiable
- Hyperlipidimea
- Hypertension
- Cigarette smoking
- Lifestyle risk factors ***obesity (BMI >30 kg/m²)***[Q].
- Physical inactivity.

**Minor**

Emerging risk factors
- ***Lipoprotein (a)***[Q]
- ***Homocysteine***[Q]
- ***Hyperfibrinogenemia***[Q]
- Proinflammatory factors

## Phenyl Ketonuria (PKU)

- It is ***most common clinically encountered inborn error of aminoacid metabolism. It is biochemically characterized by accumulation of phenylalanine and a deficiency of tyrosine***[Q].
- In this *autosomal recessive* disorder, due to deficiency of ***phenylalanine* hydroxylase** (**PA- 4 monooxygense**, a mixed function oxidase), *phenylalanine can not be converted to tyrosine*, resulting in elevation of phenylalanine in tissue, plasma & urine. **(Type I , Classic PKU)**
- Phenylalanine hydroxylase requires a **cofactor tetra hydrobiopterin**, which carries e- from NADPH to $O_2$ & becomes oxidized to dihydrobiopterin. It is subsequently reduced by **enzyme dihydrobiopterin reductase in a reductase** in a rection that requires NADPH. So **hyper phenylataninemia** may also be caused by deficiency of enzymes synthesizing $BH_4$ or regenerating $BH_4$ from $BH_2$ (i.e. dihydrobiopteridine reductase)

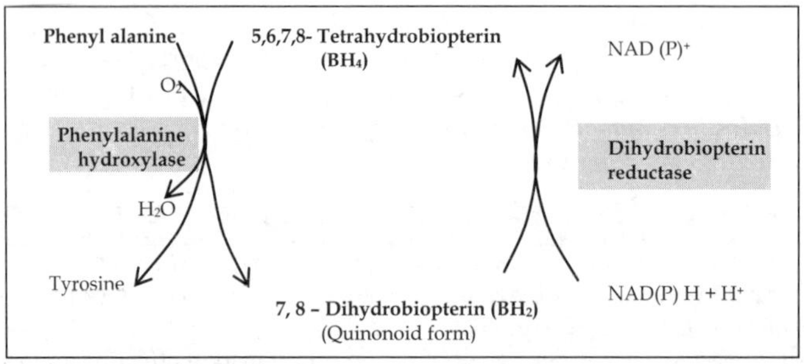

- Hyperphenylalaninemia, d/t **dihydrobiopterine reductase deficiency** (Type II and III), is accompanied with ***$BH_4$ deficiency. BH4 is also required for tyrosine hydroxylase and tryptophan hydroxylase***[Q] leading to synthesis of *neurotransmitters L-DOPA, catecholamines (from tyrosine) and 5-hydroxy tyrptophan & serotonin (from tryptophan)*. So in type II & III PKU simply restricting phenyl alanine and providing tyrosine does not reverse CNS effects d/t deficiencies in neurotransmitters. *Replacement therapy with BH4 or L- DOPA and 5-OH- tryptophan is also needed*. Supplementing the diet with tetrahydro biopterin itself is ineffective as it is unstable and does not cross blood brain barrier.

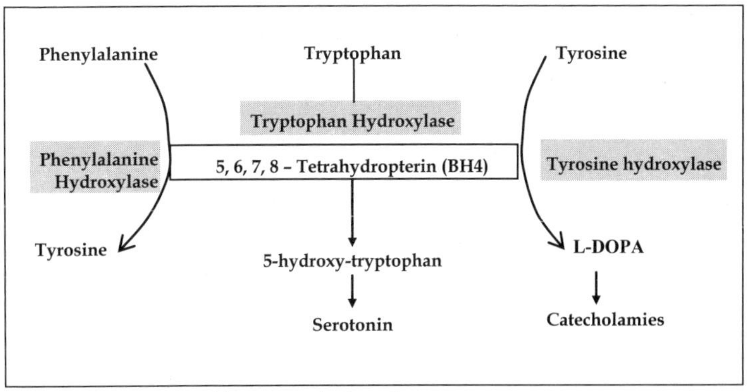


- Elevated phenylalanine undergoes trans amination to form phenyl pyruvate, phenyl lactate and phenyl acetate.

## Pathophysiology

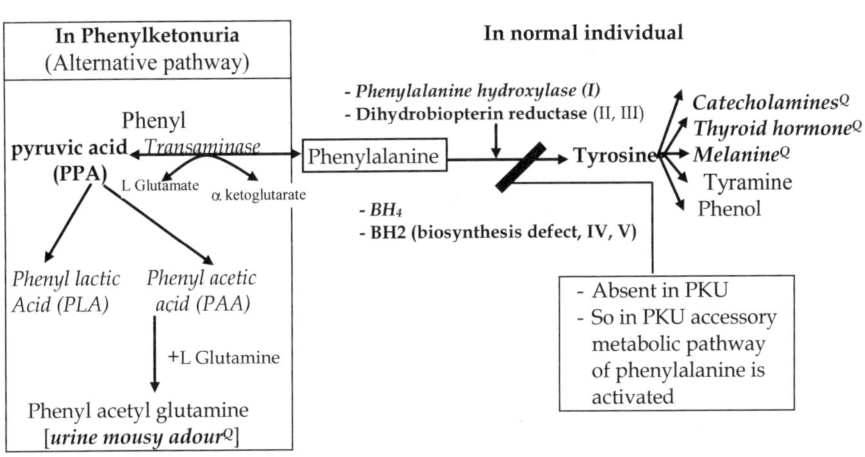


### Types of PKU & other PA metabolism defect

| | |
|---|---|
| I | *Defect in phenylalanine hydroxylase (classic)*[Q] |
| II<br>III | *Defect in dihydrobiopterin ($BH_2$) reductase*[Q]<br>6 Pyruvoyl-tetra hydropterin synthase defect |
| IV<br>V | Defect in dihydrobiopterin (BH2) biosynthesis |
| **Maternal PKU** | When woman with PKU who is not on low phenyl alanine diet become pregnant<br>It causes microcephaly, mental retardation & congenital heart anomalies in fetus) |
| **Transient benign hyper phenylalaninemia** | **Pterin-4 carbinolamine dehydratase deficiency** |
| **GTP Cyclohydrolase I deficiency** | Defect of PA metabolism |

### Treatment

- The **main aim for 1st line therapy** is to ***limit the intake of substrate (i.e. phenyl alanine) for deficient enzyme***[Q].
- In PKU, **blood phenyl alanine is maintained close to the normal range by feeding synthetic amino acid preparations low in PA,** supplemented with some natural food (such as fruits, vegetables & some cereals) selected for their low phenylalanine content.
- Because PA is an essential aminoacid, *overzealous treatment that result in blood PA levels below normal should be avoided* because this can l/t poor growth & neurological symptoms
- In PKU, **tyrosine** cannot be synthesized from PA, and therefore it **becomes an essential aminoacid** that must be supplied in diet.
- Treatment must begin during the first **7-10 days** of life to *prevent mental retardation* (as early as better).
- Discontinuation of PA restricted diet before **8 years of age** is associated with poor performance on IQ test.

### ■ Clinical features:

- ***Hypopigmentation***[Q] d/t impaired melanin synthesis l/t fair hair, light skin, blue eyes
- **CNS symptoms:** Mental retardation, seizures, hyperactivity, tremors, failure to walk, talk & grow and IQ < 50
- Excretion of phenylalanine & its catabolite in urine: PPA, PAA
- ***Mousy (musty) odour urine***[Q]: PAA conjugates with glutamine and excreted as phenyl acetyl glutamine.

### ■ Diagnosis

- **Antenatal prenatal diagnosis** is facilitated by ***DNA probes to detect enzyme defect & tandem mass spectrometry*** (most reliable to estimate blood PA levels).
- ***Neonatal screening and diagnosis* of PKU by elevated blood levels of PA**
- It is important because the *disease is treatable by dietary means* and neonates lack symptoms.
- The *infant with PKU has normal blood levels of phenylalanine (PA) at birth* because the mother clears increased blood PA through placenta.
- Normal PA levels may persist until the new born is exposed to **2-4 days** of protein feeding. Thus screening tests are done after this period to avoid false negatives.
- **False positive** in premature infants may reflect delayed maturation of enzymes of PA catabolism.
- The diagnosis is confirmed through **quantitative determination of PA levels**.
- Plasma phenylalanine level: ↑ed to 15- 65mg% (N- 1- 2mg%)
- **Guthrie** rapid screening **test** uses **Bacillus subtilis** strains which

- **Life long restriction of dietary PA is recommended.** Individuals with PKU are advised to avoid **aspartame**, an artificial sweetner that contains penylalanine.
- Plasma phenylalanine concentrations should be maintained between **2 and 6 mg/dL (120 and 360 µmol/L)** with therapy. And dietary phenylalanine restriction is usually instituted if blood phenylalanine levels are **> 4 mg/dl (250 µmol/L)**
- Some very mild cases of PKU show increased tolerance to dietary proteins & improved metabolic control when treated with **tetra hydro biopterin** (5-20 mg/kg/day) which is an essential cofactor of phenyl hydroxylase
- Pregnancy risks **(Maternal PKU)** can be minimized by assuring strict phenylalanine restrictions 2 ***month prior to conception & through out gestation*** and continuing life long PA restricted diets. Maternal PKU l/t increased risk for congenital defects, microcephaly, congenital heart abnormalities, and severe mental & growth retardation after birth. Phenylalanine is a teratogen.

cannot grow in a medium devoid of phenylalanine and the growth is proportional to its content.

- ***$FeCl_3$ test[Q]: (older less reliable test)***
- Screening test for presence of phenylpyruvate in urine
- $FeCl_3$ gives ***emerald green with urnie in PKU[Q].***
- Phenylalanine load test (iv) detects PKU carriers.

# Hyper Tyrosinemias

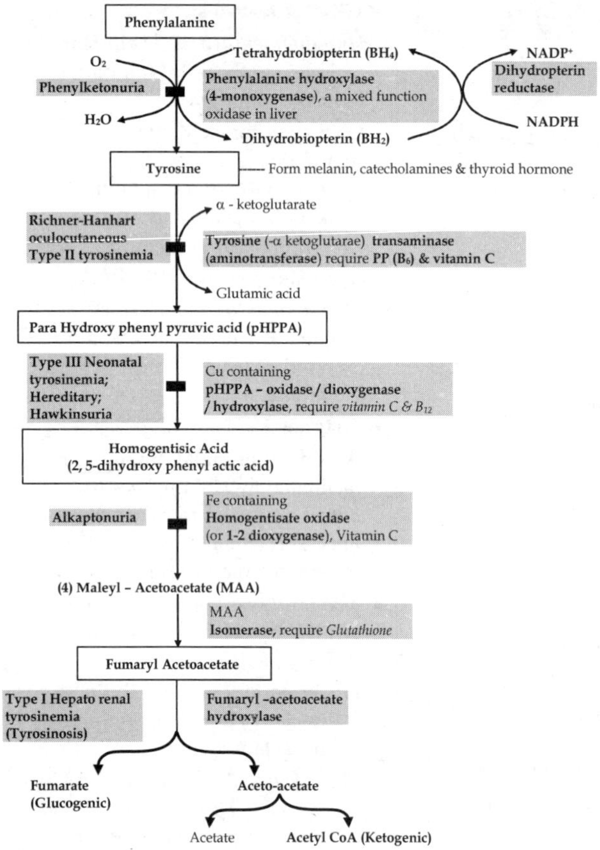


★ - ate & - ic acid are same eg pyruvic acid = pyruvate
★ Tyrosine is converted to DOPA (**dihydroxy phenylalanine**) by **tyrosinase** (or **tyrosine** 3-**monoxygenase**) in melanoblast and **tyrosine hydroxylase** in adrenal medulla. Both are different, so in tyrosinase deficient albinism, epinephrine synthesis is normal. Tyrosine hydroxylase requires NADPH & $BH_4$ (similar to phenylalanine hydroxylase).

| Type / Features | Type I (Tyrosinosis) Hepato renal | Type II (Richner Hanhart syndrome) Oculocutaneous | Neonatal (Type III) | Hereditary | Hawkins-inuria |
|---|---|---|---|---|---|
| **Enzyme defect** | ***Fumaryl acetoacetate hydrolase[Q]*** Malelyl acetoacetate isomerase (+) | ***Tyrosine amino transferase (transaminase)[Q]*** | **pHPPA hydroxylase** | **pHPPA- oxidase** | **PHPPA oxidase** |
| | | | **pHPAA** = para Hydroxy phenyl pyruvic acid = p-OH-phenyl pyruvate = 4-OH-phenyl pyruvate | | |
| **Inheritance** | AR | AR | AR | AR | AD |
| **Clinical Feature** | - Manifest in first 6 months of life (acute form) & cause death rapidly d/t liver failure<br>- **Cabbage like odor,** hypoglycemia, vomiting, diarrhea, failure to thrive, rickets.<br>- Major organs affected are *liver, kidney & peripheral nerves* causing cirrhosis, liver failure, ***hepato cellular carcinoma[Q]*** (in chronic type when children survve beyond 2-10 years); **renal tubular acidosis** and peripheral neuropathy | - Ocular: *painful corneal erosions with photophobia*<br>- Cutaneous: **palmo-plantar keratosis**<br>- Mental retardation (mild to moderate) | - Transient relative deficiency of enzyme d/t delayed maturation or vitamin C deficiency<br>- Transient hypertyrosinemia with normal liver function<br>- Occasional mental delay | Biochemically similar to type III but differs in that it is<br>- More aggressive & severe<br>- Not suppressed by vitamin C<br>- pHP lactic acid excretion is more<br>- Death occurs before 6 months but those who survive later on develop<br>1. Renal tubular absorption defects like aminoacid /protein uria, hyper phosphaturia<br>2. Hypophosphatemic rickets, hypoglycemia<br>3. Nodular cirrhosis, **hepato cellular carcinoma** | - Transient failure to thrive<br>- Metabolic acidosis in infancy<br>- ***Swimming pool odour[Q]*** |
| **Urinarly excretion** | - *Fumaryl acetoacetate* & its metabolite succinyl acetone<br>- pHPPA and pHP lactic acid (PHPLA)<br>- Tyrosine | Tyrosine & its metabolites *N-acetyl tyrosine & tyramine* | - pHPPA and its metabolites pHPLA and pHP acetic acid<br>- Tyrosine, N-acetal tyrosine, tyramine | - Same with more pHPLA | Hawkinsin a derivative of pHPPA |
| **Plasma tyrosine** | 6 -12 mg/dL | 4 -5 mg/dL | - | - | - |
| **Treatment** | - Dietary restriction of protein especially phenylalanine & tyrosine<br>- Substrate restriction using **nitisinone** in tyrosinemia type I<br>- **Vitamin C** (ascorbic acid) in type III neonatal tyrosinemia | | | | |

## Alkaptonuria / Alcaptonuria

### Etio-pathology

- It is *autosomal recessive (AR) inborn error (hereditary defect) in catabolism (degradation ) of phenyl alanine & tyrosine* in which *Garrod's* classic ideas concerning heretable metabolic disorder was proposed. Other disorders of Garrod's tetrad are albinism, cystinuria & pentosuria.
- It occurs d/t **deficiency** of Fe containing liver enzyme **homogentisic (homogentisate) oxidase** also k/a **homogentistate 1, 2-dioxygenase** responsible for *cleavage of aromatic benzene ring* of homogentisic acid resulting in formation of 4-maleyl – acetoacetate.
- With lack of this enzyme, levels of *homogentisic acid increase in blood, and spill over into urine* and tissue. It is oxidized by polyphenol oxidase to *benzoquinone acetate*, which polymerizes and binds to connective tissue l/t pigmentation (ochronosis) & arthritis.
- **Vitamin C deficiency** (in premature infants) and experimental application of α-α'-dipyridyl-chelating agent of Fe may produce alkaptonuria.

**Homogentisic Acid** → (Fe containing liver enzyme **Homogentisic** or **Homogentisate oxidase (or 1-2 dioxygenase)**) → **4- Maleyl Acetoacetate**

**Homogentisic Acid** ↓ *Polyphenol oxidase* | Oxidation → **Benzoquinone acetate**

### Clinical presentation

- *Mild condition compatible with fairly normal life. Patients are usually asymptomatic* until about ***40 years of age***[Q]. However dark staining of diapers may sometimes indicate the disease in infants but usually no symptoms are present until later in life.
- Most striking clinical feature is ***blackening of urine on standing***[Q] which is also the only sign of disorder in children. As other features develop after 30-40 years age.
- Classical triad in includes– "HOA"

### Management

- **Diets low in protein** especially in **phenylalamine** (< 500 mg/day) & **tyrosine** reduce homogentisic acid levels & pigment deposition (Lippincott)
- **Ascorbic acid (vit.C)** may prevent oxidation of homogentisic acid.
- **Nitisinone** [2-(2-Nitro 4-trifluoromethyl benzyl) 1, 3-Cyclo hexanedione], a drug used in tyrosenemia type I reduces excrection of homogentisic acid in urine and *might prevent long term complications* of alkaptonuria, in conjunction with a low protein diet.

### Homogentisic aciduria

- Patient's urinale contain *high levels of homogentisic acid* which is oxidized to dark (black) pigment on standing or exposure to air (sun light and oxygen).
- ***Urine turns black on standing***[Q] or air exposure when it also *becomes alkaline*. (Alkaptonuria meaning to suck up oxygen greedily in alkali)
- When urine is kept in testube *darkening starts from surface* and involves entire sample with in few hours.
- ***Benedict's test is strongly positive***[Q] and so is Ferric chloride ($FeCl_3$) test
- *Urine organic acid analysis* or specific *calorimetric test* detect homogentisic acid in urine.

### Ochronosis

Deposition & accumulation of oxidized homogentisic acid (benzoquinone acetate) pigment in cartilage and collagenous connective tissue l/t **ochronosis**. This results in **black (gray-blue- brown), pigmentation** and (generalized) **darkening** of

- ***Sclera b/w cornea & canthii***[Q]
- **Ear cartilage** (concha, anthelix & fnally helix)
- Nose cartilage
- **Tympanic membrane**, larynx, skin, and heart valves.
- Skin (pigmentation) involving ***palmoplantar area***[Q], dorsum of hand & feet, face & neck
- ***Intervertebral disc & large joints***[Q]
- *Pigmented renal and prostatic calculi (stones)* develop occasionally
- D/t pigmentation, valvulitis & calcification (of mitral & aortic) heart valves, the incidence of degenerative heart disease & MI increases.

### Arthritis

Ochronosis also involves joint cartilage l/t arthritis which may be severely crippling. It

- Starts with pain, stiffness & limitation of movements of **large joints.**
- It involves **large joints of spine (intervertebral disc) followed by hip, knee & shoulder**.
- It resembles rheumatoid arthritis b/o acute excerbations, but **unlike RA small joints of hands & feet are spared**.
- Black pigment deposition at **intervertebral disc** f/b calcification. Radiological findings resemble osteoarthritis with characteristic ***narrowing of joint spaces & calcification of intervertebral disc***[Q].

## Maple Syrup Urine Disease (MSUD) or Branched Chain Ketonuria

### Biochemical Defect

| Reaction | Aminoacids involved | Enzyme |
|---|---|---|
| **Oxidative decarboxylation** | **Leucine** (especially), **isoleucine, valine** | **Branched chain α-ketoacid dehydrogenase** |

- *Autosomal recessive (AR) disorder* in which there is deficiency (partial or complete) in **branched chain α-keto acid dehydrogenase (decarboxylase) enzyme complex.** This enzyme is responsible for ***oxidative decarboxylation of branched chain α- keto acids – leucine, isoleucine and valine***[Q].
- In MSUD, defect or **deficient decarboxylation of leucine, isoleucine & valine d/t deficiency of branched chain α-ketoacid dehydrogenase** enzyme leads to accumulation of these *aminoacids and their corresponding α-keto acids (α-keto isocaproic acid, α-keto- β-methyl valeric acid, α-ketoisovaleric acid) and α-hydroxy acids (reduced α-ketoacids) in blood (plasma or serum), CSF and urine*. Toxic effects interfere with brain functions.
- Unlike other ketoacidosis, **Rothera's test** is positive even in boiled & cooled urine.

### Clinical Features, Types & Management

- Feeding problems, vomiting, dehydration, severe metabolic acidosis and characteristic **sweet maple *syrup or burnt sugar odor of urine***[Q], which gives disease its name. If untreated may l/t mental retardation, physical disability & death
- Variants of MSUD are
  - **Classic type** is most common & most svere, show symptoms with in first few days of life and lethal in first weeks of life. *Leukocytes or cultured skin fibroblasts of patients show little or no enzyme activity.*
  - **Intermediate & intermittent** types have higher (3-15% of normal) enzyme activity. So symptoms are milder & of late onset (from infancy to adulthood)
  - **Thiamin dependent MSUD** achieve increased activity of enzyme if given larger doses of thiamin.
- Early prenatal diagnosis (by enzyme analysis in cell), neonatal screening and life long dietary restriction is essential if the child with MSDU is to develop normal. Treatment entails strict control of diet, *restricting the intake of valine, isoleucine and leucine to the minimum required to permit normal growth.*

★ **Hartnup disease** is d/t defect in membrane transport mechanism of monoamino mono carboxylic (neutral) amino acids such as tryptophan by small intestinal mucosa & proximal renal tubule. Indole derivatives of unabsorbed tryptophan formed by intestinal bacteria are excreted. Large losses d/t intestinal malabsorption and failure of renal reabsorption **limits tryptophan availability for niacin biosynthesis** and accounts for pellagia like features.

★ **GM 1 gangliosidosis** is d/t defect in activity of lysosomal enzyme galactosidase resulting in pathological accumulation of GM1 gangliosides in lysosomes.

## Catabolism of Branched Chain Aminoacids (BCAA)

- BCAA, leucine, isoleucine & valine are **essential aminoacids**. In contrast to most other aminoacis these are metabolized (oxidized) as fuels primarily by peripheral tissues mainy **muscles, adipose, kidney and brain** rather than by liver. Because these tissues contain aminotransferase, **absent in liver**, that acts on BCAA & produce corresponding α-ketoacids.
- **Branched chain α-ketoacid dehydrogenase** enzyme catalyzes **oxidative decarboxylation** of all three α-ketoacids produce their acyl CoA derivatives & release $CO_2$. This reaction is analogus to oxidative decarboxylation caused by pyruvate dehydrogenase complex & α-ketoglutarate dehydrogenase as all 3 enzymes are similar in structure, share same mechanism and cofactors – **TPP, NAD, FAD, Lipoate & CoA.** Defect in this step l/t **maple syrup urine disease.**
- **FAD linked dehydrogenation** (analogous to acyl CoA dehydrogenase of β-oxidation yields α-β-unsaturated acy CoA derivatives. Defective **isovaleryl CoA dehydrogenase** is a/w **seaty feet odor in body fluids**)
- **Methyl malonyl CoA mutase (isomerase)** enzyme and coenzyme **vitamin $B_{12}$ (adenosyl cobalamine)** rearrange MMCoA to succinyl CoA. Deficiency of MMCoA mutase or $B_{12}$ result in **methyl malonic academia & aciduria**, in which both propionate & methyl malonate are excreted in urine. Patient presents with metabolic acidosis, developmental retardation, symptoms resembling **ethylene glycol poisoning and death.**
- Leucine is ketogenic (yields acetyl CoA & acetoacetate); isoleucine is both ketogenic & glucogenic (yields acetyl CoA & succinyl CoA) and valine is glucogenic (yield succinyl CoA).

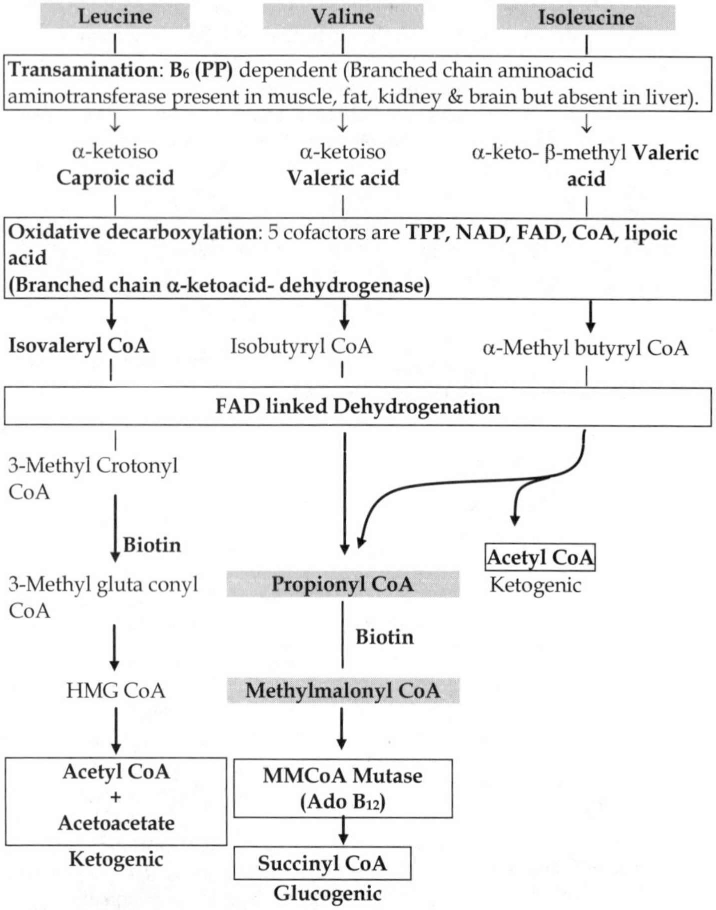


| BCAA Disease | Defective Enzyme |
|---|---|
| **MSUD (BC Ketonuria)** | BCKA Dehydrogenase |
| **Intermittent** branched chain ketonuria | BCKAD (less severe) |
| **Isovaleric acidemia** | Isovaleryl CoA dehydrogenase |
| Hypervalinemia | Valine transaminase |

## Amphibolic Intermediates formed from the Carbon Skeletons of Amio Acid

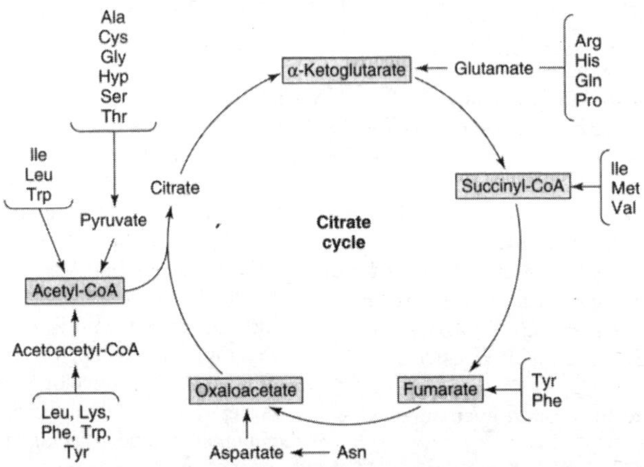

## Heamoglobin

### Heme *(Prosthetic group)*[Q]

It is a Fe- porphyrin compound

#### Iron

- Iron is ***in ferrous state ($Fe^{2+}$)***[Q] in functional Hb
- 4 gm of $Fe^{2+}$ per mole of Hb
- Iron can form six co- ***ordinated bonds***[Q]
  - Linked to four ***pyrrole rings through their nitrogen atom***[Q].
  - ***5th linkage to nitrogen of imidazole ring of histidine of polypeptide***[Q].
  - On other side co-ordinated position of Fe2+ is available to bind to $O_2$

#### Porphyrins

- Is a *tetra pyrrole structure*
- Four pyrrole (I to IV) → joined by ***methylene or Methylodene bridge***[Q]
- *Vinyl* is attached to ***I and II rings***[Q].
- Propionic acid at 6th & 7th position of heme of III & IV Pyrroles

- Within the pH range of 7.0 to 7.8, most of the ***physiological buffering action of Hb is due to imidazole group of amino acid histidine***[Q].
- *Imidazole $H^+$ group* can give up $H^+$ (Proton) and accept H+ depending on pH of medium.
- Other dissociable buffering group responsible for buffering capacity of Hb
  a) Acidic-COOH group
  b) Basic-NH2 group
  c) Guanidino group

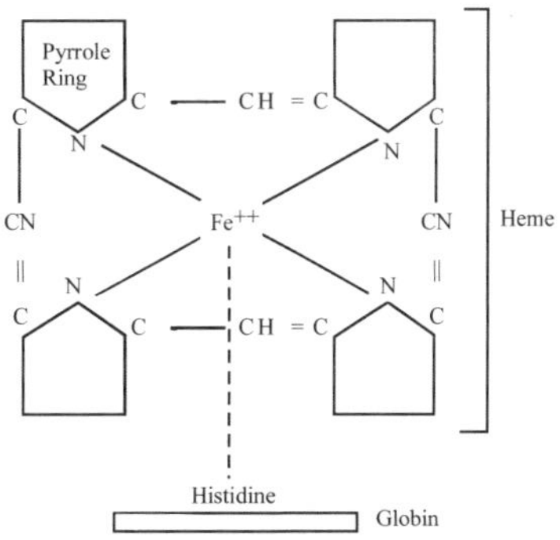


### Globin (Protein part)

- Composed of ***4 polypeptide chains (2α+2β subunits)***[Q]
- The Hb tetramer is arranged a two dimmers $(\alpha\ \beta)_1$ & $(\alpha\ \beta)_2$
- The two polypeptide chains within each dimmer are held together primarily by ***hydrophobic interaction***[Q].
- Each polypeptide chain ***contains a 'heme' in heme Pocket***[Q]. Thus 1 Hb contains 4 heme units
- Hb contains mostly *hydrophobic* amino acids internally ***(forming 'heme pockets')***[Q] & hydrophilic a.a on their surfaces.
- The 'Heme pocket' of α- subunit are adequate for entry of $O_2$ while *β-subunits* heme pockets *blocks entry $O_2$ by valine residue.*

## Comparison between Hb & Myoglobin

### Similarities

- Single polypeptide chain of myoglobin is structurally similar to individual polypeptide chains of Hb.
- Polypeptide chain of Hb & Mb has stretches of ***α-helical structure & a heme binding pockets***[Q].
- Polypetides contain mostly *nonpolar amino acids internally*, these non- polar a.a forming a structure *stabilized by hydrophobic interaction*
- The heme group sits in a cervice, lined with non-polar a.a with exception of two histidine residue (Proximal & distal). Thus ***heme lies in the hydrophobic pocket in both Hb & Mb***[Q].

### Differences

| Hemoglobin | Myoglobin |
|---|---|
| - ***Tetrameric structure***[Q], consists of 4 *polypeptide chains*<br>- Can ***bind 4 $O_2$ molecule***[Q]<br>- Hb-$O_2$ dissociation curve is ***sigmoid shaped***[Q].<br>- ***Positive Co- operativity (or Co-operative binding kinetics***[Q]: binding of heme with $O_2$ facilitates binding of other $O_2$ molecule, a property that permits it to bind a maximal quantity of $O_2$ at the respiratory organ & to deliver a maximal quantity of $O_2$ at peripheral tissue. | - Monomeric structure with *one polypeptide chain*<br>- Combines with ***one mole of $O_2$.***[Q]<br>- Myoglobin -$O_2$ dissociation curve is → ***Rectangular hyperbola.***[Q] |

Carbon monoxide (CO) binds to isolated heme about 25000 times more strongly than does oxygen but to myoglobine only 200 times. CO binds to

#### Hemoglobin

CO binds to isolated heme in its *preferred orientation*, i.e, with all three atoms (Fe, C, O) perpendicular to the plane of heme

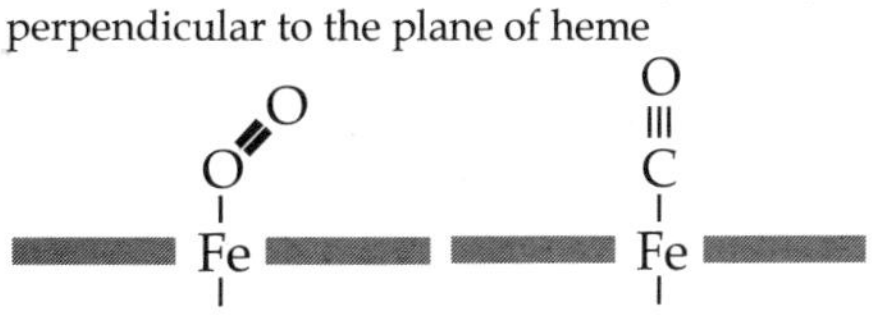


**Preferred angle for bonding of $O_2$ & CO**

#### Myoglobin

Presence of ***distal E-7 histidine***[Q]. Hinders binding or CO at 180° angle (Preferred angle) & forces it to bind in a less favoured configuration and reduce the strength of heme - CO bond.

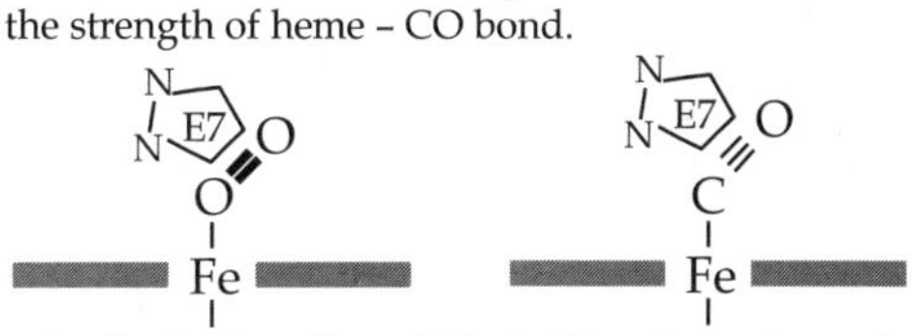


**Angles for bonding of $O_2$ & CO to heme iron of myoglobin**

**Hemoglobin performs two major transport functions**

1. *Transport of $O_2$ from lungs* to peripheral tissues.
2. *Transport of $CO_2$ and protons ($H^+$)* from the peripheral to the lungs.

**In Lungs**

Binding of $O_2$ to deoxyhemoglobin cause release of protons ($H^+$). & this is responsible for the *Bohr effect*

Released $H^+$ combine with $HCO_3^-$, forming carbonic acid. Which is broken down into $CO_2$ & $H_2O$ and $CO_2$ is exhaled out.

**In Tissues**

Binding of protons to Hb causes release of $O_2$.

In tissue ***increase in $H^+$ conc (i.e. ↓pH), decreases the affinity of hemoglobin for $O_2$***Q.

## 2, 3- Di/Bi-Phosphoglycerate (2, 3- DPG)

**Binding with Hb**

- One molecule of BPG is bound per Hb tetramer in the central cavity formed by all four subunits. This cavity is sufficient for BPG, *only when the Hb is in the T form* (deoxy genated form)
- BPG forms salt bridges with the terminal aminogroups of both β- chains via **Val NA1** and **Lys EF6** and **His H21**.
- BPG stabilizes the deoxygenated form (T) of Hb that must be broken prior to conversion to R state.

**Feature**

- ***One mole of deoxyhemoglobin binds one mole of 2, 3 DPG***Q.
- 2,3- DPG binds to deoxygenated (T) form of Hb & binding of $O_2$ to Hb decreases the binding of 2,3- DPG
- 2,3- DPG decreases the affinity of Hb molecule for $O_2$ thus increase in DPG conc. *shifts $O_2$- Hb dissociation curve to right.*
- **Factors that affects conc. of 2,3 DPG in RBC**

| ↑ed 2,3- DPG | ↓ed 2,3- DPG |
|---|---|
| - Hypoxia<br>- GH<br>- Exercise<br>- T3, T4<br>- Anemia<br>- Altitude high | - ***Fetal Hb***Q<br>- In bank blood that is stored→ less $O_2$ is released to the tissues. |

# Porphyria

**Porophyrias**: Are group of disorders *due to abnormalities in the pathway of biosynthesis of heme*, resulting in accumulation & increased excretion of porphyrins or its precursors. Depending on whether enzyme deficiency occurs in Liver or bone marrow.

### Hepatic Porphyria

**Acute Intermittent Porphyria**

- D/t deficiency of ***uroporphyrinogen I synthase (Hydroxymethyl bilane synthase)***Q
- Porphobilinogen & ALA accumulates in urine.
- Urine darkens on exposure to light and air
- Patient are ***not photosensitive*** Q
- Abdominal pain & neuropsychiatric symptoms

**Varigate Porphyria**

- An acute disease caused by deficiency in ***proto porphyrinogen oxidase*** Q
- Protoporphyrinogen III & other intermediates prior to the block accumulate in the urine
- Patients are photosensitive

**Hereditary Coproporphyria**

- An acute disease caused by deficiency in ***coproporphyrino gen oxidase*** Q
- Coproporphyrin ogen III accumulate in the urine
- Patients are photosensitive

### Erythropoietic porphyria

**Erythropoietic Protoporphyria**

- D/t deficiency in ***ferrochelatase***Q
- Protoporphyrins accumulates in erythrocytes, bone marrow and plasma
- Patients are photosensitive

**Congenital Erythropoietic Porphyria**

- D/t deficiency of ***uroporphyrinogen III synthase***Q
- Uroporphyrinogen I & coproporphyrinogen I accumulates in urine
- Patients are photosensitive

### Both

**Porphyrea Cutanea Tarda**

- *Affects both liver and erythropoietic cells.*
- ***Most common type***Q.
- *Chronic* disease caused by deficiency in ***uroporphyrinogen decarboxylase.*** Q
- Uroporphyrin accumulates in urine
- Patients are photosensitive

**Treatment**

- Medical support for pain & vomiting during acute attack
- *I.V hemin*: decreases synthesis of ALA synthase
- Avoidance of sunlight
- Ingestion of β- carotene (free radical scavanger)

★ *All porphyries are AD* disorder *except* congenital erythropoietic porphyria which is AR

★ **Photosensitivity:** patients skin itches & burns (pruritis) when exposed to visible light (result of porphyrin mediated formation of superoxide radicles from $O_2$)

## Heme Synthesis

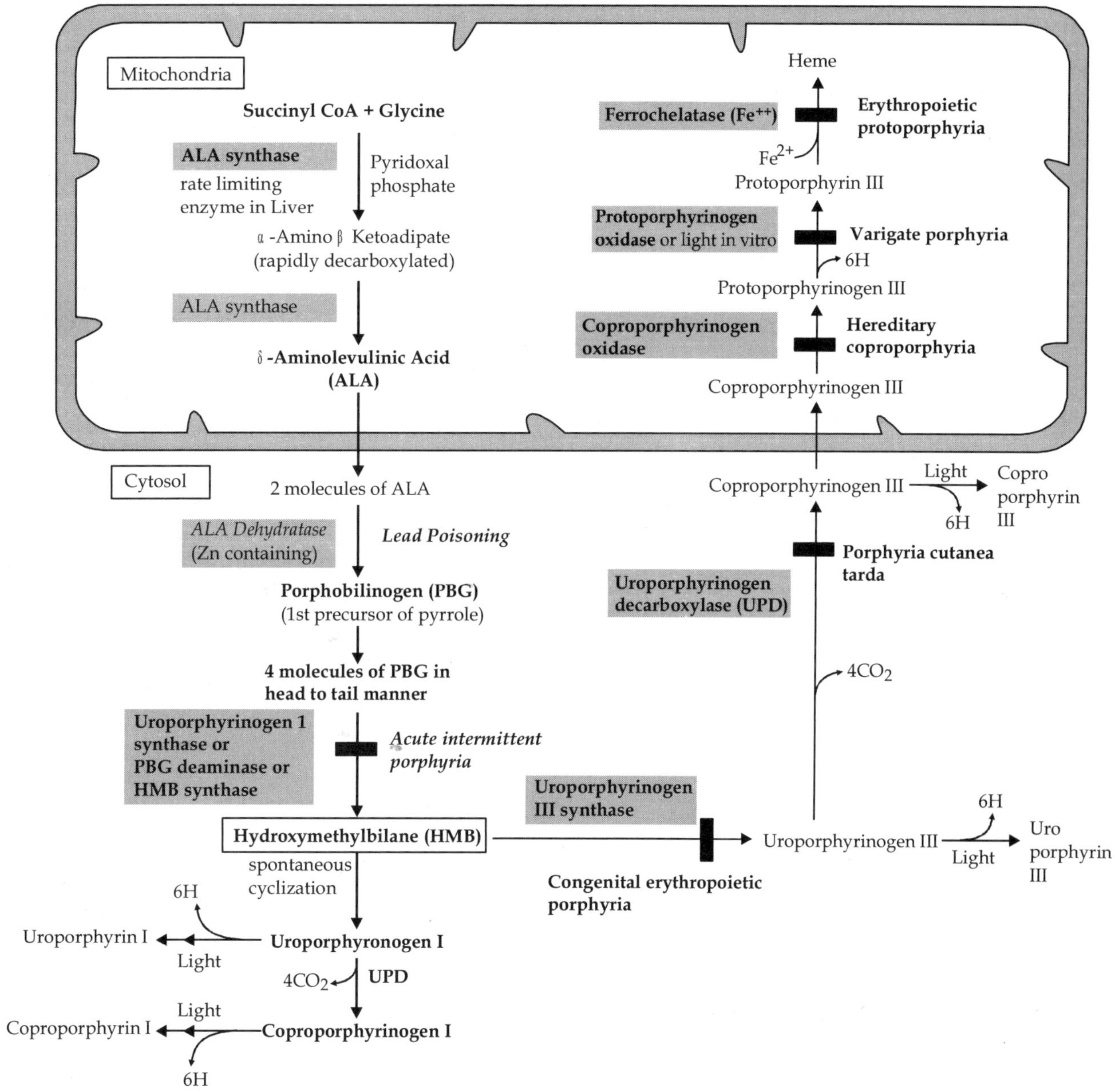


Site of heme biosynthesis are ***Liver & Bone marrow (erythropoietic cells)***[Q]

# *Chapter -7* GENERAL BIOCHEMISTRY

## QUESTIONS

### Water, pH, Buffers & Bioenergetics

**1. Monoprotic acid are**
A. Formic acid ☐
B. Carbonic acid ☐
C. Acetic acid ☐
D. Citric acid ☐
E. Nitric acid ☐

**2. In a solution the concentration of hydrogen ion $[H^+]$ is $1 \times 10^{-6}$ moles/litre. The pH of the solution will be:**
A. Three ☐
B. Six ☐
C. Nine ☐
D. Twelve ☐

**3. The buffering capacity of a buffer is maximum at pH equal to**
A. 0.5 pKa ☐
B. pKa ☐
C. pKa+1 ☐
D. 2pKa ☐

**4. A buffer that is most effective at a pH of about 4.5 is;**
A. Acetate buffer. ☐
B. Bicarbonate buffer ☐
C. Phosphate buffer ☐
D. Tris buffer ☐

**5. The presence of 2 extra pairs of electrons on the oxygen in water molecule results in :**
A. Makes water a non-polar solvent ☐
B. Forms covalent bonds in the ice. ☐
C. Electro negative charge on water molecule ☐
D. Electro positive charge on water molecule ☐

**6. Strongest bond out of the following is :**
A. Electrostatic ☐
B. Hydrogen ☐
C. Hydrophobic ☐
D. Vanderwall's ☐

**7. True statement regarding covalent bonds is :**
A. Electrons have same spin ☐
B. Electrons have opposite spin ☐
C. They are weak bonds ☐
D. None of the above ☐

**8. Strongest bond amongst the following is**
A. Hydrophobic ☐
B. Electrostatic ☐
C. Hydrogen bond ☐
D. Wander wall's ☐

**9. Weakest bond is :**
A. Covalent ☐
B. Hydrogen ☐
C. Electrostatic ☐
D. Vander wall ☐

**10. Energy required for maintenance of bodily functions of a person weighing 40 kgs is:**
A. 1000 kilocalories ☐
B. 15000 kilocalories ☐
C. 2000 kilocalories ☐
D. 2500 kilocalories ☐
E. 3500 kilocalories ☐

**11. Difference between reversible and irreversible reaction is**
A. Entropy ☐
B. Temperature ☐
C. Work done ☐
D. Amount of heat production ☐

**12. Regarding a crystal, the true statement is :**
A. Molecules are arranged in same orientation with different confirmation ☐
B. Molecules are arranged in different oreintation with different confirmation ☐
C. Molecules are arranged in same orientation and same confirmation ☐
D. Molecules are arranged in different oreintation but with same confirmation ☐

### Xenobiotics

**13. All are true about glutathione except:**
A. It is a tripeptide ☐
B. It converts hemoglobin to methemoglobin ☐
C. It conjugates xenobiotics ☐
D. It is co-factor of various enzymes ☐

**14. All are true about glutathione except:**
A. It is a tripeptide ☐
B. It converts hemoglobin to methemoglobin ☐
C. It conjugates xenobiotics ☐
D. It scavenges free radicals and superoxide ions ☐

**15. All are true about glutathione:**
A. It converts Hemoglobin to Methemoglobin ☐
B. It scavenges free radicals & superoxide enzymes ☐
C. It acts as a cofactor for some enzyme ☐
D. Causes sulfate conjugation ☐

**16. Which of the following elements is known to influence the body's ability to handle oxidative stress?**
A. Calcium ☐
B. Iron ☐
C. Potassium ☐
D. Selenium ☐

**17. Which of the following enzyme are associated with break down of $H_2O_2$.**
A. Catalase ☐
B. Perioxidase ☐
C. Oxidase ☐
D. Oxygenase ☐
E. Hydrolase ☐

**18. $H_2O_2$ is breaked or formed by which of the following enzyme:**
A. Oxidase ☐
B. Oxygenase ☐
C. Hydrolase ☐
D. Peroxidase ☐
E. Catalase ☐

**19. Which of the following is not a phase I Reaction:**
A. Oxidation ☐
B. Reduction ☐
C. Hydrolysis ☐
D. Conjugation ☐

**20. The main enzyme responsible for activation of xenobiotics is**
A. Cytochrome P-450 ☐
B. Glutathione S-transferase ☐
C. NADPH cytochrome P-450-reductase ☐
D. Glucuronyl transferase ☐

**21. The conjugation of bilirubin to glucuronic acid in the liver;**
- A. Converts a hydrophilic compound to a hydrophobic one ☐
- B. Converts a hydrophobic compound to a hydrophilic one ☐
- C. Enables the bilirubin molecule to cross the cell membrane ☐
- D. Is increased during neonatal jaundice ☐

**22. What is metabolised like xenobiotics**
- A. Myoglobin ☐
- B. Bilirubin ☐
- C. Biliverdin ☐
- D. Haemoglobin ☐

**23. Bile salts undergo xenobiotics:**
- A. After conjugation with taurine and glycine ☐
- B. After conjugation with lysine ☐
- C. After conjugation with betaglucuronic acid ☐
- D. After conjugation with derived proteins ☐

## Free Radicals

**24. Which of the following reduces oxidative stress except:**
- A. Superoxide dismutase ☐
- B. Catalase ☐
- C. Glutathione peroxidase ☐
- D. Xanthine oxidase ☐
- E. Ceruloplasmin ☐

**25. Which of the following act as antioxidants:**
- A. Vit. D ☐
- B. Vit. C ☐
- C. Selenium ☐
- D. Glutathione peroxidase ☐
- E. Vit. E ☐

**26. Reperfusion injury is caused by:**
- A. Vitamin E ☐
- B. Superoxide ion ☐
- C. Calcium ion ☐
- D. Magnesium ion ☐

**27. Which of these have antioxidant properties:**
- A. Tocopherol ☐
- B. Reduced Glutathione (GSH) ☐
- C. Citrulline ☐
- D. Lycopene ☐

**28. True about Glutathione reductase:**
- A. Sulphur containing enzyme ☐
- B. Important in methemoglobinemia ☐
- C. Free radical scavenger ☐
- D. All ☐

**29. Enzyme responsible for respiratory burst reaction**
- A. Dehydrogenase ☐
- B. Peroxidase ☐
- C. Hydroxylase ☐
- D. NADPH – oxidase ☐

**30. Reactive oxygen intermediates are released by:**
- A. Catalase ☐
- B. NADPH oxidase ☐
- C. Glutathione peroxidase ☐
- D. Superoxide dismutase ☐

## Minerals

**31. Which is non essential mineral:**
- A. Sodium ☐
- B. Manganese ☐
- C. Iron ☐
- D. Lead ☐

## Vitamins

**32. Which of the following is a Water Soluble Vitamin?**
- A. Folic Acid ☐
- B. Vitamin A ☐
- C. Vitamin K ☐
- D. Linolenic Acid ☐

**33. NAD acts as a cofactor for**
- A. Citrate Synthetase ☐
- B. Isocitrate dehydrogenase ☐
- C. α-ketoglutarate dehydrogenase ☐
- D. Malate dehydrogenase ☐
- E. Succinyl thiokinase ☐

**34. Gene for folic acid absorption is present on**
- A. Chromosome X ☐
- B. Chromosome XXI ☐
- C. Chromosome V ☐
- D. Chromosome Xi ☐

**35. The gene for folic acid transporter is located on which chromosome:**
- A. 5 ☐
- B. 15 ☐
- C. 21 ☐
- D. X ☐

**36. Which of the following statement about thiamin is true?**
- A. It is a co-enzyme of lactate deydrogenase ☐
- B. Its deficiency is associated with scurvy ☐
- C. Its co enzyme function is done by thiamine monophosphate ☐
- D. Its co-enzyme for pyruvate dehydrogenase and α-ketoglutarate dehydrogenase ☐

**37. Thiamine requirement increases in excessive intake of:**
- A. Carbohydrate ☐
- B. Amino acid ☐
- C. Fat ☐
- D. Lecithine ☐

**38. Thiamine level is best monitored by :**
- A. Transketolase level in blood ☐
- B. Thiamine level in blood ☐
- C. G6PD activity ☐
- D. Reticulocytosis ☐

**39. Enzyme activity measured in beri beri is:**
- A. Transketolase ☐
- B. Transaminase ☐
- C. Decarboxylase ☐
- D. Deaminases ☐

**40. Thiamine acts as a cofactor in :**
- A. Conversion of pyruvate to acetyl-CoA ☐
- B. Transamination reactions ☐
- C. Oxidation in respiratory chain ☐
- D. Conversion of pyridoxal to pyridoxal phosphate ☐

**41. Thiamine is essential for**
- A. Isocitrate dehydrogenase ☐
- B. Succinate dehydrogenase ☐
- C. Pyruvate dehydrogenase ☐
- D. Acetyl CoA synthetase ☐

**42. Thiamine is not used in which of the following reactions**
- A. Lactate to pyruvate ☐
- B. Alphaketoglutarate to succinyl CoA ☐
- C. Glucose to pentose ☐
- D. Oxidative decarboxylation of α-keto amino acids ☐

**43. Which of the vitamin deficiency lead to lactic acidosis**
- A. Riboflavin ☐
- B. Thiamine ☐
- C. Niacin ☐
- D. Pantothenic acid ☐

**44. The activity of the following enzyme is affected by biotin deficiency:**
- A. Transketolase, ☐
- B. Dehydrogenase. ☐
- C. Oxidase. ☐
- D. Carboxylase. ☐

**45. Active moiety of CoA is**
- A. Acetyl group ☐
- B. Pantoic acid ☐
- C. Thiol of β-alanine ☐
- D. Thiol of pantetheine ☐

**46. Which vitamin is necessary for coenzyme A synthesis**
- A. Pantothenic acid ☐
- B. Ascorbic acid ☐
- C. Biotin ☐
- D. Pyridoxine ☐

**47. Panthothenic acid is coenzyme of which of the following reaction (s):**
- A. Dehydrogenation ☐
- B. Oxidation ☐
- C. Decarboxylation ☐
- D. Reduction ☐
- E. Acetylation ☐

**48. Patient presenting with pellagra, parkinsonism, convulsions, anemia and kidney stones has deficiency of**
- A. Coenzyme A ☐
- B. FADH ☐
- C. Niacin ☐
- D. Pyridoxal phosphate ☐

**49. Which is not pyridoxine dependant:**
- A. Homocystinuria ☐
- B. Maple syrup urine disease ☐
- C. Oxaluria ☐
- D. Xanthinuria. ☐

**50. Cause(s) of homocystinuria:**
- A. Deficiency of vit B6 ☐
- B. Deficiency of vit B 12 ☐
- C. Deficiency of folic acid ☐
- D. Deficiency of pantothenic acid ☐

**51. Co-enzyme used in transamination**
- A. NAD ☐
- B. Biotin ☐
- C. Pyridoxal phosphate ☐
- D. Riboflavin ☐

**52. Intrinsic factor of Castle is secreted by**
- A. Chief cells ☐
- B. Parietal cells ☐
- C. Mucous cells ☐
- D. β cells ☐

**53. Vitamin $B_{12}$ deficiency has A/E**
- A. Folate trap ☐
- B. Decreased methyl malonyl CoA ☐
- C. SACD ☐
- D. Megaloblastic anemia ☐

**54. Vitamin $B_{12}$ is absorbed in the**
- A. Stomach ☐
- B. Duodenum ☐
- C. Ileum ☐
- D. Colon ☐

**55. Cobalt forms a component of which vitamin**
- A. Biotin ☐
- B. Vitamin B12 ☐
- C. Vitamin A ☐
- D. Tocopherol ☐

**56. Not a dietary source of vit. B12-**
- A. Fish ☐
- B. Meat ☐
- C. Soyabean ☐
- D. Liver ☐

**57. Vitamin $B_{12}$ and folic acid supplementation in megaloblastic anemia leads to the improvement of anemia due to :**
- A. Increased DNA synthesis in bone marrow ☐
- B. Increased Hemoglobin production ☐
- C. Erythroid hyperplasia ☐
- D. Increased iron absorption ☐

**58. Vitamin which is excreted in urine is :**
- A. Vitamin A ☐
- B. Vitamin C ☐
- C. Vitamin D ☐
- D. Vitamin K ☐

**59. All of the following are required for hydroxylation of proline in collagen synthesis except :**
- A. $O_2$ ☐
- B. Vitamin C ☐
- C. Dioxygenases ☐
- D. Pyridoxal phosphate ☐

**60. Vitamin required for hydroxyproline to proline conversion:**
- A. Vitamin C ☐
- B. Vitamin E ☐
- C. Pyrodoxal $PO_4$ ☐
- D. Biotin ☐

**61. During the formation of hydroxyproline and hydroxylsine, the essential factors required is/are:**
- A. Pyridoxal phosphate ☐
- B. Ascorbic acid ☐
- C. Thiamine pyrophosphate ☐
- D. Methylcobalamine ☐
- E. Biotin ☐

**62. Aminoacyl t-RNA is required for all except :**
- A. Hydroxyproline ☐
- B. Methionine ☐
- C. Cystine ☐
- D. Lysine ☐

**63. Gamma carboxylation of glutamic acid in clotting factor II, VII and protein C is dependent on**
- A. Vitamin K ☐
- B. Vitamin C ☐
- C. Vitamin A ☐
- D. Vitamin E ☐

**64. Both Vitamin K and C are involved in:**
- A. The synthesis of clotting factors. ☐
- B. Post translational modifications. ☐
- C. Antioxidant mechanisms. ☐
- D. The microsomal hydroxylation reactions. ☐

**65. The Similarity between Vit C & Vit K is :**
- A. Both help in conversion of proline to hydroxy-proline ☐
- B. Both help in post-translational modification ☐
- C. Both have anti infective activity ☐
- D. Both are involved in coagulation cascade ☐

**66. In vitamin C deficiency, post translational modification of which amino acid is defective:**
- A. Lysine ☐
- B. Alanine ☐
- C. Glycine ☐
- D. Arginine ☐

**67. Vitamin K is ivolved in the posttranslational modification?**
- A. Glutamate ☐
- B. Aspartate ☐
- C. Leucine ☐
- D. Lysine ☐

**68. Carboxylation of clotting factors by vitamin K is required to be biologically active. Which of the following amino acid is carboxylated?**
- A. Histidine ☐
- B. Histamine ☐
- C. Glutamate ☐
- D. Aspartate ☐

**69. HDN is seen due to deficiency of vitamin:**

A. A ☐
B. C ☐
C. K ☐
D. E ☐

**70. Vitamin required for post translational modification of coagulants is :**

A. Vitamin A ☐
B. Vitamin C ☐
C. Vitamin B6 ☐
D. Vitamin K ☐

**71. Vit K is needed for which of these post transational modification processes-**

A. Methylation ☐
B. Carboxylation ☐
C. Hydroxylation ☐
D. Transketolation ☐

**72. The vitamin used for post-translational modification of glutamic acid to γ-Carboxy-glutamate is**

A. Vitamin D ☐
B. Vitamin E ☐
C. Vitamin A ☐
D. Vitamin K ☐

**73. Vitamin K dependent coagulation factors include:**

A. II and III ☐
B. IX and X ☐
C. III and V ☐
D. VIII and XII ☐

**74. Vitamin K dependent clotting factor is:**

A. Factor VII ☐
B. Factor I ☐
C. Factor XI ☐
D. Factor XII ☐

**75. Which of the following is a component of the visual pigment rhodopsin:**

A. β-Carotene ☐
B. Retinal ☐
C. Retinol ☐
D. Retinoic acid ☐

**76. Vitamin A is stored mainly as retinol esters in:**

A. Kidney ☐
B. Muscle ☐
C. Liver ☐
D. Retina ☐

**77. Which of the following combinations of biologically active molecules does vitamin A consists of**

A. Retinol, retinal and retinoic acid ☐
B. Retinol, retinal and tetrahydrofolate ☐
C. Retinal, conjugase and retinoic acid ☐
D. PABA, retinal and retinaldehyde ☐

**78. Vitamin A intoxication causes injury to**

A. Lysosomes ☐
B. Mitochondria ☐
C. Endoplasmic reticulum ☐
D. Microtubules ☐

**79. Metabolic bone disease is caused by excess intake of which vitamin:**

A. A ☐
B. B ☐
C. C ☐
D. D ☐
E. E ☐

**80. Which of the following does not contain keratin**

A. Potato ☐
B. Tomato ☐
C. Carrot ☐
D. Spinach ☐

## Answers:

### Water, pH, Buffers & Bioenergenetics

1. **A, C, E i.e. Formic acid, Acetic acid, Nitric acid**
2. **B i.e. Six** *[Ref: Harper's 26/e P-13-8]*
3. **B i.e. pKa** *[Ref: Harper's 27/e P-11-13]*
4. **A i.e. Acetate Buffer** *[Ref. Guyton, 10/e P- 349]*
5. **C ie Electronegative charge on water molecule**
6. **A i.e. Electrostatic**
7. **B i.e. Electrons have opposite Spin**
8. **B i.e. Electrostatic**
9. **D i.e. Vander wall**
*[Ref: Harper's 27/e P- 5-7; Lehninger 2/e P- 39- 45; Chatterjea 6/e P- 84]*
10. **A i.e. 1000 Kcal** *[Ref: CMDT 1263; Park's SPM 424]*
11. **C i.e. Work done** *[Ref: Lehninger 2/e P 390-92; Essentials of Physical Chemistry Bahl,Tuli,Bahl 24/e P-270-74; 200 ]*
12. **C i.e. Same conformation & molecules are arranged in same orientation** *[Ref: Chemistry by Mishra, Bhushan, Sharma/105]*

### Xenobiotics

13. **B i.e. It converts hemoglobin to methemoglobin**
14. **B i.e. It converts hemoglobin to methemoglobin**
15. **A i.e. It converts hemoglobin to methemoglobin**
16. **D i.e. Selenium**
*[Ref: Lippincott's 4/e p. 148; Harper's 27/e p. 620, 636-37, 180- 81, 96; Chattergea 7/e p. 478-79]*
17. **A i.e. Catalase; B i.e. Perioxidase**
18. **A i.e. Oxidase; D i.e. Peroxidase; E i.e. Catalase** *[Ref: Harper's 27/e P-96, 204]*
19. **D i.e. Conjugation** *[Ref: Harper 29/e p 6767-682; Vasudevan 6/e p 447-50]*
20. **A i.e. Cytochrome P-450**
21. **B i.e. Converts a hydrophobic compound to a hydrophilic one**
22. **B i.e. Bilirubin**
23. **C i.e. Conjugation with β glucoronic acid**

### Free Radicles

24. **D i.e. Xanthine oxidase**
25. **B, C, D, E i.e. Vit.C, Selenium, Glutathione peroxidase, Vit E**
26. **B i.e. Superoxide ion** *[Ref: Harper 28/e 482-85; Chattarjae 7/e 198; Lippincott 5/e 148; Vassudevan 6/e 241-388-409-429]*
27. **A i.e. Tocopherol; B i.e. Reduced Glutathione(GSH); D i.e. Lycopene**
28. **C i.e. Free radical scavanger** *[Ref: Harper 29/e p. 200-201]*
29. **D i.e. NADPH – oxidase**
30. **B i.e. NADPH oxidase**
*[Ref: Harper 28/e p. 482-85; Robbins 7/e p. 16-17, 60-61; Guyton 11/e p.16; Ganong 22/e p. 518]*

### Minerals

31. **D i.e. Lead** *[Ref: Vasudevan 6/e p 411; Styanarayan 3/e p 403; Chatterjea 7/e p 707-570]*

### Vitamin

32. **A i.e. Folic Acid** *[Ref:; Lippincott's 4/e p- 373; Ganong 22/e p. 313- 16; Devlin 5/e p- 1154, Harper's 28/e P- 468]*
33. **B, C, D i.e. Isocitrate dehydrogenase, α-ketoglutarate dehydrogenase, Malate dehydrogenase** *[Ref:Chatterjea 7/e p 171;Lehninger 5/e p 518]*
34. **B i.e. Chromosome XXI**
35. **C i.e. 21**
36. **D i.e. Its co-enzyme for pyruvate dehydrogenase and α-ketoglutarate dehydrogenase**
37. **A i.e. Carbohydrate**
38. **A i.e. Transketolase level in blood**
39. **A i.e. Transketolase**
40. **A i.e. Conversion of Pyruvate to acetyl COA**
41. **C i.e. Pyruvate dehydrogenase**
42. **A i.e. Lactate to Pyruvate**
43. **B i.e. Thiamine**
*[Ref: Harper 28/e p. 154, 273-74; Lippincott 5/e p 111, 266, 145-46, 378-79; Vasudevan 6/e p 391-92; Lehninger 5/e p 549-51; Chatterjea 7/e p. 166-67]*
44. **D i.e. Carboxylase** *[Ref: Lippincott 5/e p. 381, 266; Harper 28/e p. 479; Vasudevan 6/e p. 400; Chatterjea 7/e p. 179-80]*
45. **D i.e. Thiol of pantetheine**
46. **A i.e. Pantothenic acid**
47. **E i.e. Acetylation** *[Ref: Harper 28/e p. 479; Chatterjea 7th/ed pg 177-76; Lippincott 5th/ed pg-381; Vasudevan 6/e p. 398-99]*
48. **D i.e. Pyridoxal phosphate**
49. **B i.e. Maple syrup urine disease**
50. **A i.e. Deficiency of vit $B_6$; B i.e. Deficiency of vit $B_{12}$; C i.e. Deficiency of folic acid**
51. **C i.e. Pyridoxal phosphate**
*[Ref: Harper 28/e p. 252-58, 475-76; Lippincott 5/e p. 378; Vasudevan 6/e p. 396-97; Chatterjea 7/e p. 172-73; Lehninger 5/e p. 864-65, 878-83]*

**52.** **B i.e. Parietal cells** **53.** **B i.e. Decreased methylmalonyl CoA**

**54.** **C i.e. Ileum** **55.** **B i.e. Vitamin $B_{12}$** **56.** **C i.e. Soyabean** **57.** **A i.e. Increased DNA synthesis in bone marrow**

*[Ref: Harper's 28/e P-500-02, 476-77; Lippincott 5/e p. 374-76; Vasudevan 6/e p. 403-5; Chatterjea 5/e p. 185-89]*

**58.** **B i.e. Vitamin C** *[Ref: Harrison 16/e p- 406-07, 2469]*

**59.** **D i.e. Pyridoxal phosphate** **60.** **A i.e. Vitamin C** **61.** **B i.e. Ascorbic acid** **62.** **A i.e. Hydroxyproline**

**63.** **A i.e. Vitamin K** **64.** **B i.e. Post translational modification**

**65.** **B i.e. Both help in post translational modification** **66.** **A i.e. Lysine**

*[Ref: Harper's 28/e P-472-473, 479-80; Lippincott's 5/e p. 377-78, 389-90; Vasudevan 6/e p. 407-10; Devlin 5/e p. 1146]*

**67.** **A i.e. Glutamate** **68.** **C i.e. Glutamate**

**69.** **C i.e. K** **70.** **D i.e. Vitamin K** **71.** **B i.e. Carboxylation** **72.** **D i.e. Vitamin K**

**73.** **B i.e. IX and X** *[Ref: Ganong 23/e 535]* **74.** **A i.e. Factor VII**

**75.** **B i.e. Retinal** **76.** **C i.e. Liver** **77.** **A i.e. Retinol, Retinal, and Retinoic acid**

*[Ref: Lippincott's Biochemistry 3/e P-380- 81, Harper's 27/e P-490-92]*

**78.** **A i.e. Lysosome** *[Ref: O.P. Ghai 6/e p. 121; Harrison 16/e p. 408]*

**79.** **A i.e. A; D i.e. D** *[Ref: Harper's 27/e P-492-94]*

**80.** **A i.e. Potato** *[Ref: Chatterjea 6/e P-145]*

# GENERAL BIOCHEMISTRY: REVIEW NOTES

## Acids

### Monoprotic Acids (HA)

These donate *1 proton ($H^+$) per molecule*

Example include

- Mineral acids – ***HCl (hydrochloric acid) & $HNO_3$ (Nitric acid)***[Q]
- Monocarboxylic organic acids like ***formic acid (HCOOH), acetic acid ($CH_3COOH$) and benzoic acid***[Q].

| Monoprotic Acids | | |
|---|---|---|
| Formic | pK | 3.75 |
| Lactic | pK | 3.86 |
| Acetic | pK | 4.76 |
| Ammonium ion | pK | 9.25 |

### Polyprotic Acids

#### Diprotic Acids ($H_2A$)

- Can donate upto **2 protons** per molecule during process of ionization
- Can undero 2 dissociations (ionizations) & have 2 dissociation constants, first typically greater than second **(K1 > K2)**
- Examples include
  - Sulfuric acid ($H_2SO_4$)
  - ***Carbonic acid***[Q] ($H_2CO_3$)

| Diprotic Acids | | |
|---|---|---|
| Carbonic | $pK_1$ | 6.37 |
| | $pK_2$ | 10.25 |
| Succinic | $pK_1$ | 4.21 |
| | $pK_2$ | 5.64 |
| Glutaric | $pK_1$ | 4.34 |
| | $pK_2$ | 5.41 |

#### Triprotic Acids ($H_3A$)

- Can donate upto **3 protons** per molecule during process of ionization
- Can undergo 3 ionization & have 3 dissociation constants (K1>K2>K3)
- Examples include
  - Phosphoric acid ($H_3PO_4$)
  - ***Citric acid***[Q]

| Triprotic Acids | | |
|---|---|---|
| Phosphoric | $pK_1$ | 2.15 |
| | $pK_2$ | 6.82 |
| | $pK_3$ | 12.38 |
| Citric | $pK_1$ | 3.08 |
| | $pK_2$ | 4.74 |
| | $pK_3$ | 5.40 |

## Buffers

- Buffering is the tendency of a solution to resist a change in pH more effectively after addition of a **strong acid or base** than does an equal volume of water.
- Solutions of weak acids & their conjugate bases (& vice versa) exhibit buffering.
- Strong acid/bases do not have buffering quality as great as the weak acid/bases.
- **pKa** refers to the ***pH at which the concentration of the acid equals that of the base***[Q].

### At pH = pKa

the solution would contain acid and base in equal amounts, and therefore would resist a change most effectively in either direction.

### At pH < pK

i.e. more acidic environment much of the acid buffering capacity of the solution has already been neutralized so adding even minute quantities of acid would decrease the pH, i.e. it no more has buffering capacity to acids, but it would still have buffering capacity towards bases.

| Buffer | Pka |
|---|---|
| Phosphate | 6.8 |
| Bicarbonate | 6.1 |
| Acetate | 4.76 |
| Tris [hydroxymethyl aminomethane] | 8.3 |

### At pH > pK

i.e. more alkaline environment, much of the alkaline buffering capacity has been neutralized after all that's the reason why the pH rose above pK in the first place so adding even minute quantities of alkali would increase the pH.

**Note:** The effective range of a buffer is one pH unit higher or lower than pKa.

# Water

**Water is polar solvent and forms dipoles**

A water molecule is an irregular, slightly skewed tetrahedron with oxygen at its center. The two hydrogens and the unshared electrons of the remaining two sp3-hybridized orbitals occupy the corners of the tetrahedron. The 105-degree angle between the hydrogens differs slightly from the ideal tetrahedral angle, 109.5°. Ammonia is also tetrahedral, with 107° angle between its hydrogen. Water is a dipole, a molecule with electrical charge distributed asymmetrically about its structure. The strongly electronegative oxygen atom pulls electrons away from the hydrogen nuclei, leaving them with a partial positive charge, while its two unshared electron pairs constitute a region of local negative charge.

Water, a strong dipole, has a high dielectric constant. As described quantitatively by Coulomb's law, the strength of interaction F between oppositely charged particles is inversely proportionate to the dielectric constant e of the surrounding medium. The dielectric constant for a vaccum is unity; for hexane it is 1.9; for ethanol it is 24.3; and for water it is 78.5. Water therefore greatly decreases the force of attraction between charged and polar species relative to water-free environments with lower dielectric constants. Its strong dipole and high dielectric constant enable water to dissolve large quantities of charged compounds such as salts.

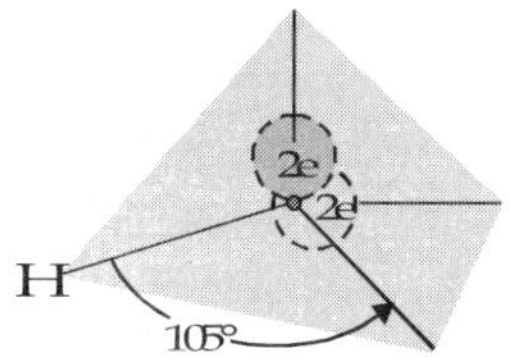


The water molecule has tetrahedral geometry

**Water is an excellent Nucleophile**

Metabolic reactions often involve the attack by lone pairs of electrons on electron-rich molecules termed ***nucleophiles*** on electron-poor atoms called ***electrophiles***. Nucleophiles and electrophiles do not necessarily possess a formal negative or positive charge. Water, whose two lone pairs of $sp^3$ electrons bear a partial negative charge, is an excellent nucleophile. Other nucleophiles of biologic importance include oxygen atoms of phosphates, alcohols and carboxylic acids; the sulfur of thioles; the nitrogen of amines; and the imidazole ring of histidine. Common electrophiles include the carbonyl carbons in amides, esters, aldehydes, and ketones and the phosphorous atoms of phosphoesters.

Nucleophilic attack by water generally results in the cleavage of the amide, glycoside, or ester bonds that hold biopolymers together. This process is termed ***hydrolysis.***

**Forms Hydrogen bond in ice**

Hydrogen bonding favors the self-association of water molecules into ordered arrays. Hydrogen bonding profoundly influences the physical properties of water and accounts for its exceptionally high viscosity, surface tension, and boiling point. On average, each molecule in liquid water associates through hydrogen bond with 3.5 others. These bonds are both relatively weak and transient, with a half-life of about one microsecond. Rupture of a hydrogen bond in liquid water requires only about 4.5 kcal/mol, less than 5% of the energy required to rupture a covalent O-H bond.

Hydrogen bonding enables water to dissolve many organic biomolecules that contain functional groups which can participate in hydrogen bonding. The oxygen atoms of aldehydes, ketones, and amides provide pairs of electrons that can serve as hydrogen acceptors. Alcohols and amines can serve both hydrogen acceptors and donors of unshielded hydrogen atoms for formation of hydrogen bonds.

# Different Types of Bonds

## Covalent Bond

- *Strongest force* that holds molecules together
- ***Electron have opposite spin***[Q]
- *Each individual DNA strand is held together* by covalent bonds; but the two strands of helix are held together by noncovalent interactions (eg. Hydrogen bonds between nucleotide bases (Watson-Crick base pairing) & vandarwall forces.

## Non covalent Interactions

While of lesser magnitude make significant contribution to the structure, stability and functional competence of macro molecules of living cells.

### Electrostatic Bonds / Salt Bridges

- Occurs between oppositely charged groups with in or between molecules
- Comparable in strength to hydrogen bond but *act over larger distances*
- Facilitate the binding of charged molecules & ions to proteins and nucleic acids.

### Hydrogen Bond

- It is the electrostatic interaction between the hydrogen nucleus of one water molecule and unshared electron pair of another
- Compared to covalent bonds, these are quite weak & requires ~ *4.5 k cal / mole* energy to break it (about *4% of energy)* required to rupture the O-H bond ( 110 k cal/mol)
- *Influences the physical properties of water and accounts for its exceptionally high viscosity, surface tension and boiling point.*
- In *solid state* each water molecule is associated with *4 other water molecules* and ~ *3.5 in liquid state*
- Responsible for *ice formation*
- Show phenomenon of *co-operativity*

### Hydrophobic Interactions

- A tendency of nonpolar compounds to self associate in an aqueous environment. This self association is neither attraction nor bond (so hydrophobic bond is misnomer).
- It arises from the need to minimize energetically unfavourable interactions between nonpolar groups and water
- Contribute stability to the interiors of proteins.

### Vandar Wall Forces

- Arise from attraction between transient dipoles *generated by rapid movements of electron* on all neutral atoms
- Significantly weaker than hydrogen bonds but potentially extremely numerous.
- Act over a very short distances (2- 4Å)

## Law of Thermodynamic

**First (Principle of energy Conservation)**

In any process the total energy of the system plus surroundings remains constant. Although energy is neither created nor destroyed it can be transformed from one form to another form.

**Second**

- In all process the entropy of the system + the surroundings i.e. the entropy of universe always increases until equilibrium is attained, at which point the entropy is the maximum possible under the prevailing conditions of temperature & pressure.
- **Entropy** is regarded as *randomness or disorder*. Put in another way 2nd law states that ultimate driving force of all chemical & physical processes is the tendency for the entropy of the universe to be maximized.

However the entropy changes are of limited value in predicting the direction and equilibrium position of chemical reactions. For one thing entropy can not always be directly measured or calculated in chemical processes. More over we must have information about the entropy changes not only in system under study, but also in its surrounding. ***A more useful criterion than the entropy change has been derived for predicting the direction and equilibrium position of chemical reactions, namely the change in free energy***Q, *that form of energy capable of doing work under conditions of constant temperature & pressure.*

### Types of Thermodynamic Systems

| Isolated System | Closed System | Open System | Adiabatic System |
|---|---|---|---|
| When the boundary is both sealed & insulated; no interaction is possible with the surrounding i.e. *neither energy nor matter is transferred* | The boundary is sealed but not insulated i.e. system which *cannot transfer matter but can transfer energy* in form of heat, work & radiation to and from its surroundings | The boundary is open & un-insulted therefore can *transfer both energy & matter* to & from its surroundings | In which no thermal energy passes into or out of system |

### Differences Between

| Irreversible (Spontaneous) Process | | Reversible Process |
|---|---|---|
| It is in equilibrium state only at the initial and final stages of the operation | | It is in equilibrium at all stages of operation |
| After this type of reaction has occurred all changes donot return to the initial state by themselves | | All changes are reversed when the process is carried out in reversible direction |
| It proceeds at measurable speed | | It is extremely slow |
| Work done is ***smaller***Q | **Work done** | Work done is ***greater***Q |
| Decreases (< 0) | **Free Energy Change** | Unchanged (0) |
| Decreases (< 0) | **Enthalpy Change** | Unchanged (0) |
| Increases (> 0) | **Entropy change** | Unchanged (0) |

**Enthalpy/Heat of Reaction**

The heat of a reaction is simply the amount of heat absorbed (endothermic) or evolved (exothermic) in a reaction. At constant temperature & pressure it is called enthalpy.

**Entropy/Internal Energy**

For many years scientists believed that only exothermic changes resulting in lowering of internal energy or enthalpy could occur spontaneously. But melting of ice & evaporation of water are spontaneous endothermic processes.

In other words we can say that the randomness of the water molecule increases as ice melts into water, or water evaporates into space. So increase in randomness favours spontaneous change

Entropy is a thermodynamic state quantity that is a measure of the randomness or disorder of the molecules of the system.

**Free Energy / Work Done**

Change in free energy is of great importance in thermodynamics because it measures net work done, which may be electrical chemical or surface work.

## Glutathione

- Reduced glutathione is ***tripeptide thiol (γ- gluatamyl cystein glycine) consisting of 3 amino acids – glutamic acid, cysteine and glycine***Q. The glutamate is linked to cysteine through γ– carboxyl linkage. And ***sulfhydryl (SH) or thiol group of cysteine, which accounts for its strong electron donating (nucleophilic) character of glutathione***Q, is the business part of molecule.
- Reduced glutathione is important reducing agent in the tissue, and can chemically detoxify hydrogen peroxide. The reaction ***is catabolized by selenium (Se) requiring glutathione peroxidase***Q enzyme and form *oxidized glutathione (glutathione di sulfide GSSG)* which no longer has protective properties. The cell ***regenerates reduced glutathione (GSH) in a reaction catabolized by glutathione reductase, which contains FAD as prosthetic group and uses NADPH as a source of reducing electron***Q.

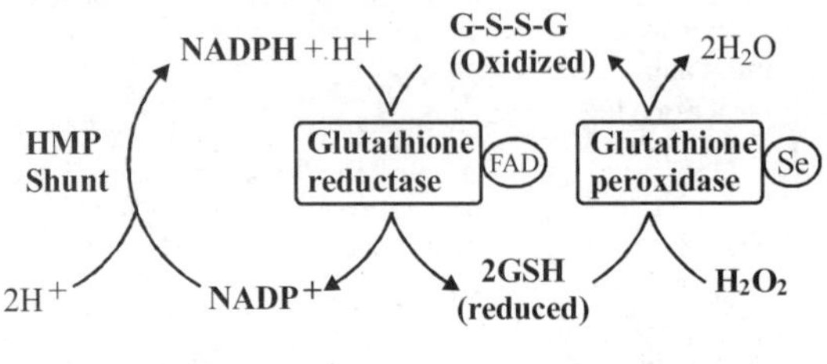


- *Liver is the largest GSH reservoir* and because of its reducing property it has potent ***antioxidant action, protects from oxidative stress conjugates Xenobiotics, acts as carrier and coenzymes & cofactor***Q.

| Xenobiotic metabolic conjugation | Antioxidant: protect from oxidative stress | As a carrier: γ-glutamyl cycle | As intracellular reductant |
|---|---|---|---|
| - Nucleophilic GSH conjugate with toxic electrophilic xenobiotics such as *carcinogens*<br>- **Glutathione S transferase** present in liver cytosol catalyze the reaction.<br>- These conjugates are ultimately excreted in urine as mercpturic acid which is formed by removing glutamyl & glycinyl group and addind acetyl group. | - Accumulation of $H_2O_2$ may decrease life span of RBC by causing oxidative damage of cell membrane l/t hemolysis.<br>- ***Reduced glutathione removes $H_2O_2$ in a reaction catalyzed by glutathione peroxidase***Q an enzyme that contains the ***selenium analogue of cysteine (selenocysteine)***Q<br>- *In RBC, HMP shunt is the only pathway that produces NADPH for reduction of oxidized glutathion* (catalyzed by glutathione reductase)<br>- ***So G6PD deficiency impairs generation of NADPH, and l/t hemolytic anemia***Q when subjected to antimalarial ***primaquin, aspirin, sulfonamides or fava beans (vicia fava – favism)***Q | - It transport certain *amino acids* across membranes in kidney<br>*Aminoacid + GSH → γ- Glutamyl amino acid+ cyteinyl- glycine*<br>- The above reaction I catalyzed by **γ-glutamyl tranferase (GGT)** present in plasma membrane of renal tubular & bile ductular cells and in ER of hepatocytes. | - Prevents oxidation of SH group containing enzymes eg glyceraldehyde-3-P-dehydrogenase<br>- GSH & glutathione trans hydrogenase cause reductive cleavage of S-S linkage of thyroglobulin glycoprotein<br>**Acts as coenzyme / co factor**<br>GSH acts as coenzyme with glutathione transhydrogenase, formaldehyde dehydrogenase, glyoxylase, maleyl acetoacetate isomerase, cyclo- oxygenase (PG synthatase system) and for liver enzyme for activation of methionine to form SAM. |

★ ***Measurement*** of erythrocyte transketolase and its activation by thiamine diphosphate is used to ***assess thiamine nutritional status***Q.

## Oxido-Redutase

In biological systems, oxidation (loss of electron) is always accompanied by reduction of electron acceptor. Enzymes involved in oxidation & reduction are called **Oxidoredutase** and are classified into four groups.

| Oxidase | Dehydrogenase | Hydroperoxidase | Oxygenase |
|---|---|---|---|
| • Catalyze the removal of hydrogen from a substrate *using oxygen as a hydrogen acceptor*, forming $H_2O_2$ or $H_2O$<br>• Some oxidase contain Cu and others are flavoproteins<br>- **Cytochrome oxidase/aa3** is a hemoprotein containing 2 atoms of *Fe atom* (that oscillates between *$Fe^{2+}$ and $Fe^{3+}$*) and 2 *atoms of Cu*.<br>- **Xanthine oxidase** contain ***molybdenum***Q; aldehyde dehydrogenase contain FAD, molebdenum & non heme iron; L-amino acid oxidase contain FMN<br>• Poisoned by ***CO cyanides and $H_2S$***Q. | • *Cannot use oxygen as a hydrogen acceptor*. They transfer H+ from one substrate to another, thus causing one substrate to be oxidized at the expense of another<br>• Useful in enabling *oxidative process* to occur in the *absence of $O_2$* such as during anaerobic phase of glycolysis and *as components of respiratory chain*<br>• These depend on nicotinamide coenzyme (NAD+ or NADP+) or riboflavin (FMN) or FAD<br>• Except for cytochrome oxidase, other cytochromes are classified as dehydrogenase. | Hydroperoxidase ***protect the body against harmful peroxidases***Q (which can generate free radicals). These are of 2 types<br>**1. Catalase**<br>- ***use $H_2O_2$ as electron donor & electron acceptor***Q & its function is assumed to be the destruction of ***$H_2O_2$***Q formed by the action of oxidase<br>- It is found in *blood, bone marrow, mucous membrane, kidney & liver.*<br>**2. Peroxidase**<br>- reduces $H_2O_2$ using various electron acceptors such as ascorbate, quinones & cytochrome C<br>- found in milk, leucocytes, platelets and other tissues involved in eicosanoid metabolism<br>- In erythrocytes ***glutathione peroxidase containing selenium***Q destroy $H_2O_2$. | Catalyze the direct transfer & incorporation of O2 into a substrate molecule<br>- Dioxygenase incorporate both atoms of molecular $O_2$ into the substrate<br>- Monooxygenases (mixed function oxidase hydroxylase) incorporates only one atom of molecular $O_2$ into substrate<br>- Cytochrome p450 are monooxygenase important for detoxification of many drugs & for hydroxylation of steroids. |

★ ***Superoxide dismutase protects aerobic organisms against oxygen toxicity (superoxide anion free radicals $O_2$-)***Q

$$O_2^- + O_2^- + 2H^+ \xrightarrow[\text{Superoxide dismutase}]{} H_2O_2 + O_2$$

## Biotransformation Reactions: Metabolism of Xenobiotics

- Biotransformation is a process of chemical alteration of one compound to another *to change its functions & effects or to achieve detoxification, elimination (excretion) or activation.*
- A **Xenobiotic** is a compound that is foreign to the body eg. *drug, pollutant, chemical carcinogen,* etc. Most of these compounds are subjected to metabolism in human body with in liver ***to increase their water solubility (polarity) and thus excretion from the body***Q in bile or urine. This metabolism occurs in two phases.

### Phase I - Hydroxylation Reaction

- Lipophilic xenobiotics are converted to *more polar hydrophilic* derivative by enzyme ***monooxygenases or cytochrome P-450***[Q].
- Cytochrome P 450 is *most versatile bio-catalyst* known. Almost it metabolize 50% of drugs ingested by humans.
- Types of phase I reactions include

| Hydrolysis | Oxidation (most common) | Reduction |
|---|---|---|
| 1. **Amide hydrolases (amidases)** break amide bonds<br>2. **Ester hydrolases (esterases)** break esters<br>3. **Epoxide hydrolases** break epoxide bonds | 1. **Hydroxylation**<br>2. Oxidation<br>3. Oxidative deamination<br>4. **Dealkylation**<br>5. **Epoxidation** | 1. Azoreduction<br>2. Ketoreduction<br>3. Nitroreduction |

Mn: **High DORE** = Hydrolysis, Hydroxylation, Deamination, Dealkylation, Oxidation, Reduction & Epoxidation.

### Properties of Cytochrome P-450

- Involved in phase I of the metabolism of innumerable xenobiotics, including perhaps 50% of the *drugs* administered to humans.
- Involved in the metabolism of many endogenous compounds (eg *steroids*)
- All are *hemoprotein*
- Often exhibit broad substrate specificity, thus acting on many compounds; consequently, different p450s may catalyze formation of the same product.
- Extremely versatile catalyst, perhaps catalyzing about 60 types of reactions.
- However, basically they catalyze reactions involving introduction of one atom of oxygen into the substrate and one into water.
- Their hydroxylated products are more water-soluble than their generally lipophilic substrate, facilitating excretion.
- *Liver contains highest amounts*, but found in most if not all tissues, including small intestine, brain and lung.
- Located in the *smooth endoplasmic reticulum or in mitochondria* (steroidogenic hormones)
- In some cases, their products are mutagenic or carcinogenic
- May have molecular mass of about 55kDa
- Many are inducible, resulting in one cause of drug interactions
- Many are inhibited by various drugs or their metabolic products, providing another cause of drug interactions
- Some exhibit genetic polymorphisms, which can result in atypical drug metabolism
- Their activities may be altered in diseased tissues (eg cirrhosis), affecting drug metabolism.
- Genotyping the P450 profile of patients (eg to detect polymorphisms) may in the future permit individualization of drug therapy.

### Phase II – Synthetic (Conjugation) Reaction

- Conjugated with glucronic acid, sulfate or glutathione. This renders them even more water soluble & they are eventually excreted in urine or bile. Phase II reaction **may either follow phase I reaction** (in xenobiotics who do not have suitable chemical group for conjugation) or some chemicals **may undergo a phase II reaction directly** (in drugs like morphine who already have polar chemical group suitable for conjugation directly).
- 5types of phase II reactions include **glucronidation, sulfation, conjugation, acetylation & methylation**. Mn "**5G SCAM**"

**1. Glucronidation**

- **Hepatocytes conver non polar bilirubin to polar form which is readily excreted in the bile,** by ***adding glucronic acid molecule***[Q] to it.
- The reaction is catalyzed by UDP-*glucuronosyl transferase* (also called *Bilirubin-UGT*) uses *UDP glucuronic acid as a glucuronosyl donor*
- Most of the bilirubin is excreted in form of *bilirubin diglucronide* whereas in obstructive jaundice they are predominantly monoglucuronide.

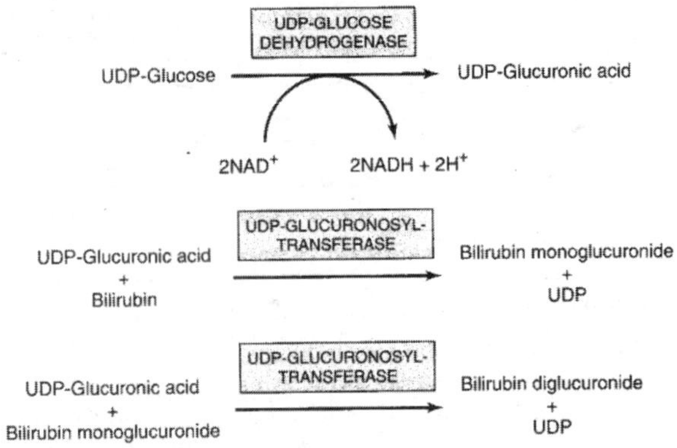


- 2 acetyl aminofluorene (carcinogen), aniline, benzoic acid, meprobamate, phenol and many *steroids* are excreted as glucuronides
- ***Most common conjugation reaction***[Q]

**2. Sulfation**

- Sulfate donor is adenosine ***3′-phosphate-5′-phosphosulphate (PAPS)***[Q] called *active sulfate*.

**3. Conjugation with Glutathione (γ-glutamyl cysteinglycine)**

- Glutathione is a tripeptide consisting of *glutamic acid, cysteine and glycine*, abbreviated as GSH (*Sulfhydryl group* of cysteine is the business part of molecule)
- Nucleophilic GSH conjugate with toxic electrophilic xenobiotics such as *carcinogens*
- **Glutathione S transferase** present in liver cytosol catalyze the reaction.
- These conjugates are ultimately excreted in urine as mercepturic acid which is formed by removing glutamyl & glycinyl group and adding acetyl group.

**4. Other Reactions:**

**A. Acetylation**

- ***Acetyl CoA is a acetyl donor***[Q], acetyl transferase catalyze the reaction
- ***Isoniazid***[Q] is subjected to it

**B. Methylation**

- S-adenosyl methionine (SAM) is the methyl donor and methyl transferase catalyze the reaction

## Oxidative Stress

It is *accumulation of oxygen derived free radicals* due to inappropriate prooxidant - antioxidant balance.

### Pro-oxidant

- These are chemical compounds or reactions capable of generating potentially toxic **reactive oxygen species (ROS)** or **free radicals**, which contain single unpaired electron in an outer orbit. These are produced by/in
- Absorption of radiant energy (UV ray, X-ray, ionizing radiation)
- ***Ischemic - reperfusion injury***[Q] induced by restoration of blood flow in ischemic tissue.
- *Microbial killing by phagocytes* and cellular aging.
- Enzymatic *metabolism of exogenous chemicals* or drugs (eg. $CCl_4$ generate $CCl_3$)
- *Reduction - oxidation reactions* of normal metabolism.
- Transition metals such as **iron (Fe) and copper (Cu)** donate or accept free electrons during intracellular reaction and catalyze free radical formation as in *Fenton reaction* (ferrous form is used)
- **Nitric oxide (NO)**, can act as free radical and can be converted to highly reactive **peroxynitrite anion ($ONOO^-$)** as well as **$NO_2$** and **$NO_3^-$**.

### Antioxidants (AO)

These are compound and reactions that *either block free radical formation or inactivate (scavenge) their action*. These include antioxidants

#### Naturally occurring AO

- Vitamins : **Beta carotene** (a type of vitamin A), **C** (ascorbic acid), **E *(alpha tocopherol)***[Q].
- Zinc (trace element), ***selenium***[Q]
- Caffeine, epigallocatectin gallate = ECGg (in green tea leaves); *clorogenic & melanic acids* (coffee beans); curcuminoids (turmeric); proanthocyanidines (grape seeds); polyphenols (apple); flavonoid querectin (apple & onions); ***lycopene (red tomato)***[Q]; α-lipoic acid (yeast & liver); and lutein & zeaxanthin (egg yolk)

#### Synzyme (M-40403)

A *synthetic enzyme* that works like body's own scavenger anti oxidants (ex SOD) to mop up free radicals. This *manganese based* experimental product (for *treating stroke*) is *more powerful* than traditional antioxidants like vitamin E & C.

#### According to action

- **Preventive AO**: They inhibit chain initiation and initial production of free radicals
  - Catalases
  - Glutathione peroxidase
  - Chelators of metal ions like
    1. ***Transferrin, ferritin, lectoferrin and ceruloplasmin*** are storage and transport proteins that minimize levels of reactive Fe and Cu by binding them (and so OH- formation)
    2. EDTA (ethylene diamine tetra acetate)
    3. DTPA (diethylene triamine penta acetate)
- **Chain Breaking AO**: They interfere with chain propogation
  - Superoxide dismutase both cytosolic & mitochondrial
  - ***Vitamin E (alpha tocopherol)***[Q] is most effective
  - ***Beta carotene***[Q] (a type of vitamin A)
  - Uric acid (urate)
  - ***Selenium containing glutathione peroxidase***[Q]
  - Phenols or aromatic amines
- **Scavanger** of free radicals
  - **Superoxide dismutase** (SOD), scavange superoxide anion ($O_2^{\bullet}$) and produce $H_2O_2$.
  - **Catalse** scavange $H_2O_2$
  - **Glutathione peroxidase *and reduced glutathione (GSH)***[Q] (Se dependent scavenge $H_2O_2$)
  - NADPH dependent Glutathione reductase
  - **Vitamin C, uric acid** and **polyphenols** obtained form plant food act as water soluble free radical trapping AO.
  - **Ubiquinone** & **Beta-carotenes** are lipid soluble radical trapping antioxidants in membranes & plasma lipoproteins.

#### Commercial and therapeutic use

- Used commercially (in vitro) as **food preservatives** to prevent lipid peroxidation (esp PUFA) & increase shelf life
  - Propyl gallate (PG)
  - Butylated hydroxy anisole (BHA)
  - Butylated hydroxy toluene (BHT)
  - Vitamin E
- Used as **therapeutic agents**
  - Dimethyl thio urea
  - Dimethyl sulfoxide
  - Allopurinol
  - Vitamin C
  - Vitamin E

## Free Radicals or Reactive Oxygen Species (ROS)

**Free radicals** or **reactive oxygen species (ROS)** are atoms or groups of atoms that have an unpaired electron and are powerful oxidants. These include **superoxide anion ($O_2^{\cdot-}$), hydrogen peroxide ($H_2O_2$), peroxyl radicals ($ROO^{\cdot}$), hypochlorite (HOCl) and very reactive hydroxyl radicals ($OH^{\cdot}$)** that react with proteins, nucleic acid, lipid etc.

**Reaction & enzyme generating free radicals (and causing damage)**

- *NADPH oxidase (produce superoxide anion)*[Q]
- *Myeloperoxidase (produce hypohalous acids)*[Q]
- *Fenton and Haber – Weiss reaction (produce hydroxyl radicals)*[Q]
- Xanthine oxidase

- **Fenton reaction**:

$Fe^{2+}$ + $H_2O_2$ ⟶ $OH^{\circ}$+ $OH^-$ + $Fe^{3+}$

- **Heber – weiss reaction (iron catalysed)**:

$O_2^{\cdot-}$ + $H_2O_2$ ⟶ $OH^{\circ}$+ $OH^-$ + $O_2$

**Reactions & enaymes scavenging free radicals (protective)**

- **Superoxide dismutase** (SOD), scavange superoxide anion ($O_2^{\bullet}$) and produce $H_2O_2$.
- **Catalse** scavange $H_2O_2$
- **Glutathione peroxidase** (Se dependent scavenge $H_2O_2$)
- NADPH dependent Glutathione reductase

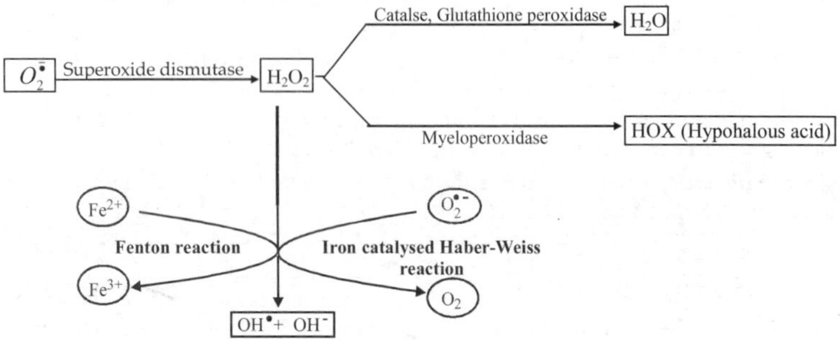


## $H_2O_2$ – Myeloperoxidase (MPO) – Halide System

**$H_2O_2$ - Myeloperoxidase (MPO) - Halide System** is the ***most efficienct bactericidal system in neutrophils***[Q]. It has 3 components.

**NADPH - oxidase**

- Its activation (when phagocytic cell, engulf bacteria) is associated with *a rapid increase in $O_2$ consumption and metabolism* (the ***respiratoryu burst***) and *generation of superoxide ($O_2^{\cdot-}$) anion* by following reaction.

$NADPH + 2O_2 \rightarrow NADP + H^+ + O_2^{\cdot-}$

- There is only a lag of 15-60 seconds in phenomenon of respiratory burst. NADPH is mainly generated by **pentose phosphate pathway**, whose activity increases markedly during phagocytosis. Electron transport chain system – NADPH oxidase is composed of a hetrodimer polypeptide (of 91 KDa + 22KDa) **cytochrome b558**, located in plasma membrane along with two cytoplasmic polypeptides of 47 and 67 KDa
- Two molecules of superoxide anion spontaneously produce hydrogen peroxide ($H_2O_2$) by a process of spontaneous dismutation.

$O_2^{\bullet} + O_2^{\bullet} + 2H+ \rightarrow H_2O_2 + O_2$

**Halide & Myeloperoxidase (MPO)**

- $H_2O_2$ generated by NADPH oxidase system (after spontaneous dismutation) is not able to efficiently kill microbes by itself. This is compensated by *enzyme myeloperoxidase present in azurophilic granules of meutriophils.*
- MPO is responsible for *green colour of pus* and act on $H_2O_2$ in presence of halide to produce **hypophaloius acids**.
- Cl- is the halide usually employed as it is present in high concentration in plasma & body fluids. And hypochlorite (HOCl or bleech) which is a powerful oxidant and is highly microbicidal is usually produced.

$H_2O_2 + H^+ + X^- \xrightarrow{\text{Myeloperoxidase}} HOX + H_2O$

(X- = Cl-, Br-, I- or SCN-; HOX = HOCl etc.)

- In normal tissue, HOCl combines with amine and form *chloramines*, which are less powerful oxidants and act as *microbicidal agents without causing tissue damage.*

- **Superoxide dismutases** tremenduously speed up the above reaction. This group includes both **copper-zinc superoxide dismutase** found in cytosol and **manganese superoxide dismutase** localized in *mitochindria*.

★ **Superoxide dismutase=SOD** (present in cytosol & mitochondria), **catalse** (present in peroxisome) and **glutathione peroxidase** (present in cytosol & mitochondria) protects cells from oxidative stress and damage in following way.

2 Superoxide anion ($O_2^{\cdot-}$) + $2H^+$ $\xrightarrow{\text{SOD}}$ $H_2O_2 + O_2$

$2H_2O + O_2 \xleftarrow{\text{Catalase}} H_2O_2$

$H_2O_2 + 2GSH \xrightarrow{\text{Glutathione peroxidase (GPO)}} GSSG + H_2O$

or

$2OH + 2GSH \xrightarrow{\text{(GPO)}} GSSG + H_2O$

So intracellular **ratio of oxidized glutathione (GSSG) to reduced glutathione (GSH)** is a reflection of oxidative state of cell & its ability to detoxify reactive oxygen species.

# Element /Mineral Requirement

**Group 1:** Components of **organic macro molecules** (carbohydrate, lipid, protein) which form 90% of solid matter
- Carbon (C)
- Hydrogen (H)
- Oxygen (O)
- Nitrogen (N)

**Group 2: Major (Principal or Macro) Elements / Minerals**
Are nutrilionally important and requirement **> 100 mg/day** The deficiency can prove fatal. The 7 macrominerals constitute **60-80% of body's inorganic** matter.
- Calcium (Ca)
- Magnesium (Mg)
- Phosphorus (P)
- ***Sodium (Na)***[Q]
- Potassium (K)
- Chloride (Cl)
- Sulfur (S)

**Group 3: Trace or (Minor or Micro) Elements / Minerals**
These are essential and required in **<100 mg/day** amount. Dificiency can l/t serious disorders
- ***Iron (Fe)***[Q]
- Iodine (I)
- Copper (Cu)
- Cobalt (Co)
- Chromium (Cr)
- ***Manganese (Mn)***[Q]
- Molybdenum (Mo)
- Fluoride (F)
- Selenium (Se)
- Zinc (Zn)

★ Cr & Cd are included in different groups in different books.

**Group 4: Additional Trace Elements**
Are possibly essential (necessary) but exact function is unknown
- Barium (Ba)
- Bromine (B)
- Cadmium (Cd)
- Nickel (Ni)
- Lithium (Li)
- Silicon (Si)
- Sn
- Vanadium (Vn)
- Chromium (Cr)

**Group 5: Non-essential or Toxic Element**
No known role and enter body through pollution or contaminants.

**Non-essential elements**
- Silver (Ag)
- Gold (Au)
- Bismuth (Bi)
- Rubidium (Ru)

**Toxic Elements**
- ***Lead (Pb)***[Q]
- Mercury (Hg)
- Aluminium (Al)
- Cyanide ($CN^-$)
- Arsenic (As)
- Boron (Bo)
- Cadmium (Cd)

# Vitamin

## Water- Soluble Vitamins

Differs from fat soluble vitamins in following ways
- Readily excreted once their concentration surpasses the threshold, so toxicities are rare
- Deficiency is quick on an inadequate diet as their metabolic stores are labile & depletion occurs in few weeks or months
- Are coenzymes so status can be assayed by measuring enzyme activities

### Vitamin B complex[Q]

*Energy releasing*
- Vitamin **B$_1$** (thiamine)
- Vitamin **B$_2$** (riboflavin)
- Vitamin **B$_3$** (niacin)
- Biotin
- Pantothenic acid

**Haemopoietic**
- ***Folic acid***[Q]
- Vitamin **B$_{12}$** (Cobalamine)

**Other**
- Vitamin **B$_6$** (pyridoxine)
- Pyridoxal
- Pyridoxamine

### Vitamin C (ascorbic acid[Q])

## Fat -Soluble Vitamins

- Vitamin **A** (retinol, β carotenes)
- Vitamin **D** (cholecalciferol)
- Vitamin K i.e.
  - **K$_1$ = Phylloquinone** (in green vegetables)
  - **K$_2$ = Menaquinone** (synthesized by intestinal bacteria)
  - **K$_3$ = Menodione** (synthetic compounds that can be metabolized to phylloquinones)
- **Vitamin E** (tocopherols)

| Vitamin | Vit B$_2$ (Riboflavin) | Vit B$_3$ (Niacin) | Folic acid |
|---|---|---|---|
| Coenzyme | FMN & FAD | NAD & NADP | **Tetrahydro folate** ($TH_4F$) |
| Function | • *FMN* and *FAD are 2 coenzymes* of this vit, and are ***electron carriers***[Q] in *oxidoreduction reaction*<br>• Consituent of:<br>- Cytochrome C- reductase<br>- Warburg yellow enzyme<br>- Fumarate dehydrogenase | • *NAD* and *NADP* are its active forms which operate as *hydrogen & electron transfer agent*<br>• **Deficiency seen in:**<br>- ***Maize eater***[Q]<br>- ***Carcinoid syndrome***[Q]<br>- ***Heartnup disease***[Q] | Its active form, Tetrahydrofolate is a **carrier of one carbon unit**; synthesis of methionine, thymine and purine |
| Deficiency | - Seborrhic dermatitis<br>- Angular stomatitis<br>- Cheilosis | ***Pellagra***[Q] c/b "3Ds"<br>- Diarrhoea<br>- Dermatitis<br>- Dementia | - ***Megaloblastic anemia***[Q]<br>- ***Neural tube defect***[Q]. |
| Features | - *Heat & acid resistant*<br>- Destroyed by light & alkali<br>- Used as food additive because of its *yellow color*<br>- Deficiency detected by measurement of ***RBC glutathione reductase***[Q] | - In body ***synthesized from tryptophan***[Q]<br>- 60mg tryptophan= 1mg niacin<br>- High doses used to ***treat hyperlipidemia***[Q]<br>- In *overdose causes cholestatic jaundice* | - ***Folic acid reduces risk of Neural tube defect &***<br>- ***Hyperhomocystinemia***[Q] |

## Vitamin $B_3$ (Niacin)

**NADP⁺ - Cofactor**

- **Glu**cose-6-phosphate dehydrogenase (G-6-PD (glucose-6-$PO_4$ to 6-phosphogluconate)
- **Glu**tathione **reductase**

**Either NADP⁺ or NAD⁺ - Cofactor**

- **Glu**tamate dehydrogenase (glutamate → α-ketoglutarate + $NH_3$)
- **Is**ocitrate dehydrogenase (isocitrate → oxalosuccinate)

Mn- **"Glu³ Is MAL Gly Kit/Pit-PDC"**

All are **dehydrogenase** except glutathione reductase sounds like *"Glue in small gly pit/Kit"*

**NAD⁺ - Cofactor**

- **Mal**ate dehydrogenase (malate → oxaloacetate)
- **Al**cohol dehydrogenase (ethanol → acetaldehyde
- **La**ctate dehydrogenase (pyruvic acid → lactic acid)
- **Gly**ceraldehyde-3-phosphate dehydrogenase (glyceraldehyde 3P → 1, 3 diphosphoglycerate)
- α-**Gly**cero-P-dehydrogenase
- α-**Keto**glutarate dehydrogenase (α-**keto**glutarate → succinyl CoA)
- Pyruvate dehydrogenase complex (**PDC**) (pyruvate → acetyl CoA)

## Vitamin $B_1$ (Thiamin) or Aneurine (i.e. relieves neuritis)

### Chemistry and Mechanism

- Thiamin is a *basic substance* that has a *thiazole ring, pyrimidine & sulphur (S).*
- **Thiamin pyrophosphate (TPP)** also k/a **thiamin diphosphate (TDP)** is **biologically active & storage form** of vitamin B1 and is formed by transfer of pyrophosphate group from ATP

Thiamin —(*ATP* → *AMP*; *TPP Transferase*)→ TPP (TDP)

- **Thiazolium ring**, the functional part of TPP, has a relatively *acidic proton at C-2*. Loss of this acidic ($C_2$) proton produces a **carbanion**, which is the active species in TPP dependent reactions. In other words, *$C_2$ in thiazolium ring of TPP ionizes rapidly, thus producing active species carbanion.* Carbanion readily adds to carbonyl groups (eg pyruvate) and thiazolium ring of TPP stabilizes carbanion intermediate by providing an electron deficient (electrophilic) structure into which the carbanion electrons can be delocalized by **resonance**. This "**electron-sink**" action of thiazolium ring facilitate *carbon-carbon bond cleavage adjacent to carbonyl group in reactions like decarboxylation of α-ketoacids (eliminating $CO_2$) and in chemical rearrangements in which an activated acetaldehyde group is transferred* from one carbon atom to another.

### Physiological Role

- Thiamin has a **central role in energy yielding metabolism** and especially of carbohydrates. ***So thiamin requirements increase in excess intake of carbohydrates and its deficiency leads to decreased energy production***[Q]
- TDP (TPP) is coenzyme for **oxidative decarboxylation and transketolation reactions** such as

**I. Oxidative Decarboxylation of α-Ketoacids**

3 Multienzyme complexes that catalyze oxidative decarboxylation are **pyruvate dehydrogenase/PDH** (in carbohydrate metabolism synthesizing Acetyl CoA from pyruvate); **α-ketoglutarate dehydrogenase** (forming succinyl CoA from α-KG, in citric acid cycle); and ***branched chain ketoacid dehydrogenase*** **/BCKD** (in metabolism of **leucine, isoleucine & valine**).

**Pyruvate** —(**Pyruvate Dehydrogenase (PDH)**; **TPP, FAD, Lipoate, CoA, NAD⁺** → NADH)→ **Acetyl CoA** + $CO_2$

**α-Ketoglutarate** —(**α-KG Dehydrogenase ($Ca^{++}$ activator)**; **TPP, FAD, Lipoate, CoA, NAD⁺** → NADH)→ **Succinyl CoA** + $CO_2$

**Branched chain α-ketoacid dehydrogenase** enzyme (Coenzymes: **TPP, FAD, NAD, Lipoate (Lipoic acid), CoA**):

- **α-Ketoisocaproic acid (Leucine)** → Iso valeryl CoA
- **α-Ketoisovaleric acid (valine)** → Iso butyryl CoA
- **α-Keto β-methyl valeric acid (Isoleucine)** → α-Methyl butyryl CoA

+ $CO_2$ + NADH

### Deficiency

- Thiamin deficiency can l/t 3 distinct syndromes

1. **Chronic peripheral neuritis**
2. **Beriberi** (Singhalese word meaning weakness) occurs in areas where polished rice (lacking aleurone layer) is major diet. It is characterized by dry skin, irritability, disordered thinking, progressive paralysis d/t peripheral neuritis in adults
   - **Acute pernicious (fulminating) beri beri (or shoshin beri beri)** is c/b *high out put cardiac failure, edema and metabolic abnormalities without peripheral neuritis.* **(Wet beri beri)**
   - **Dry beri beri :** Peripheral neuritis & CNS manifestations predominate
   - **Infantile beriberi** occurs in infants born to thiamin deficient mothers and show tachycardia, vomiting, convulsions, death.
3. **Wernicke encephalopathy with Korsakoff psychosis** (W-K syndrome) is a/w thiamin deficiency in ***chronic alcoholism***[Q] & narcotic abuse. It is c/b ***apathy, ataxia, ammesia, nystagmus & opthalmoplegia***[Q]

- **Lactic and pyruvic acidosis**
  High carbohydrate diet in thiamin deficient subjects result in increased level of pyruvic acid **or pyruvate** (d/t **PDH dysfunction**) which is then converted to lactic acid thus causing life threatening **lactic acidosis**. Abnormal blood LA/PA ratio is a specific indicator
- **Decreased energy production** because acetyl CoA is not formed (d/t **PDH dysfunction**) and citric acid cycle is hampered (d/t **α-KGD dysfunction**)
- **Accumulation of pentose (5C) sugar in RBC** d/t retardation of transketolase
- ***Branched chain ketonuria (Maple syrup urine disease)***[Q] variant (d/t retardation of BCKD enzyme)
- Bracken disease, chastek paralysis, opisthotonus, **catatorulin effect** (i.e. decreased $O_2$ uptake by B1 deficient brain) and saturation effect (i.e. low urinary excretion after test dose in thiamin deficient) in animals.

**II. Formation and degradation of α-ketols by transketolase (transferring 2 carbons in PPP/HMP shunt)**

**Ribose-5-PO$_4$**(5C) —(**Transketolase TPP**)→ **Glyceraldehyde-3-PO$_4$** (3C)

**Xylulose-5PO$_4$**(5C) **Sedoheptulose 7-PO$_4$** (7C)

III. Reduction of pyruvate to ethanol (in yeast but not in humans): **Fermentation /Non oxidative decarboxylation**

**Pyruvate** —(**Pyruvate decarboxylase**, **TPP**)→ **Ethanol (alcohol)** + $CO_2$

**Diagnosis**

Thiamin (B1) deficiency is **best diagnosed by** observing an **increase in RBC** ***transketolase activity***[Q] on ***addition of thiamin pyrophosphate (TPP)***[Q]

## Biotin (Vitamin B$_7$)

- *Biotin, carboxybiotin & biocytin (ε-aminobiotinyllysine* which require proteolysis to release biotin) is widely distributed in many foods and *synthesized by intestinal flora in excess of requirement. So dietary deficiency is unknown* except among people
  - Maintained on *total parenteral nutrition* for many months
  - Eat abnormally large amount of (>20) raw eggs per day. Uncooked egg white contains glycoprotein **avidin** that tightly binds biotin and prevents its absorption from intestine.
  - *Multiple carboxylase deficiency*, results from *defect in ability to link or remove biotin from* carboxylases
  - *Congenital holocarboxylase synthetase* deficiency
- Deficiency of biotin l/t anorexia, nausea, glossitis, dermatitis, **spectacle eyed appearance** (d/t circumocular alopecia), and **Leiner's disease** (i.e. exfoliative dermatitis or erythroderma desquamativum in young infants)

**Coenzyme in Carboxylation reaction (by Carboxylase enzyme)**

- Coenzyme biotin serves as a *carrier of activated carbon dioxide in biotin dependent carboxylation* reactions. Biotin *covalently binds to ε-amino groups of lysine residues* of biotin dependent carboxylase (apo) enzymes to form *biocytin residue of holoenzyme*. This conversion is catalyzed by *holocarboxylase synthetase*. **1-N-carboxybiocytin** formed from $CO_2$ in ATP dependent reaction is the *reactive enzyme-biotin-$CO_2$ intermediate*, which transfers carboxy group to substrate.
- **Biotin dependent 4 carboxylase enzymes are**
  - ***Acetyl CoA carboxylase***[Q] : catalyzes Acetyl CoA → Malonyl CoA
  - ***Pyruvate carboxylase***[Q] : Pyruvic acid → Oxaloaceticacid.
  - ***Propionyl CoA Carboxylase***[Q] : Propionyl CoA → Methyl malonyl CoA
  - **3 Methyl-crotonyl CoA carboxylase:** 3 methyl crotonyl CoA → 3 Methyl glutaconyl CoA
- *Carbamoyl phosphate synthetase* (of urea & pyrimidine synthesis), *malic enzyme* (converting pyruvate to malate) and addition of $CO_2$ to form $C_6$ in purine ring are some biotin independent carboxylation reactions.

## Pantothenic Acid (Vitamin B$_5$)

**Biochemistry**

- Pantothenic acid consist of peptide linked β-alanine & pantoic acid (dihydroxy-dimethyl butyric acid).
- Peptide linkage of *pantothenic acid to* ***β-merceptoethanol amine*** (which is obtained from **aminoacid cysteine**) forms **(4-phospho)-pantetheine**. This process requires 2 ATP (or 1 A TP & 1 CTP)
- Terminal **thiol** or **sulfhydryl (-SH)** group of *betamercaptoethanolamine in pantetheine functional moiety is the* **active site** where ***acyl groups are carried***[Q].
- Coenzyme (Co) A is formed when pantoic acid moiety (of pantetheine) is linked to *adenosine 3′ phosphate* by pyrophosphate bridge (a process requiring *2ATP*)
- So CoA is a nucleotide and requires expenditure of 4 high energy bonds (ATP) in synthesis. It can be denoted as *CoA-SH to denote the active thiol site.*

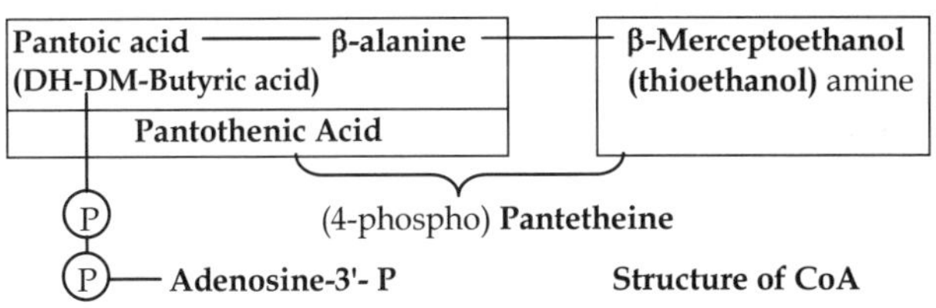


**Structure of CoA**

- It is a *part of coenzyme A (such as acetyl CoA, succinyl CoA, fatty acyl CoA, HMG CoA) and acyl carrier protein (ACP) of fatty acid synthase*[Q]
- It has a central role as a **carrier of acyl group** in metabolism. Active thiol (sulfhydryl-SH) group of betamerceptoethanol amine in *pantetheine functional moiety of CoA or ACP* carries & transfer acyl groups as activated thiol esters.
- Its deficiency is extremely rare as vitamin is widely distributed (Pantos means every where). **Burning foot syndrome**, sleep disturbance & spectacle alopecia may (±) occur
- Its metabolic roles are

| **Formation of acetyl CoA** which is utilized in | **Formation of Succinyl CoA** which is utilized in | |
|---|---|---|
| - ***Acetylation reactions***[Q]<br>- Acetyl choline formation<br>- ***Cholesterol (→steroids), ketone body & fatty acid synthesis***[Q]<br>- Elongation of FA<br>- Synthesis of ether lipids eg plasmalogen & PAF<br>- TCA cycle, Detoxification | - Heme (porphyrin) synthesis<br>- Ketolysis (ketone body degradation) by extrahepatic tissue<br>- TCA cycle, detoxification<br>- Gluconeogenesis, activation of acetoacetate | • Lipid metabolism<br>- β oxidation of FA<br>- Synthesis of FA<br>• Activation of branched chain amino acid such as valine & leucine involve CoA<br>• Formation of adreno cortical hormones. |

# Vitamin $B_6$ / Pyridoxine

- *Six derivatives of pyridine* have vitamin $B_6$ activity: pyridoxine (occurs primarily in plants); *pyridoxal, pyridoxamine* (in animal foods mainly) and their 5′ phosphates.
- ***Biologically active coenzyme is pyridoxal 5′-phosphate***[Q] which can be obtained for from all 3 precursors i.e. pyridoxine (alcohol), pyridoxal (aldehyde) & pyridoxamine (amine).
- *80% of body's total vitamin $B_6$ is pyridoxal (5′) phosphate* (PP) in **muscles** mostly a/w **glycogen phosphorylase**. *This is not available in deficiency, but is released* to become available in starvation, when glycogen reserves become depleted. Then it is mainly available in liver & kidney, to meet increased requirements for gluconeogenesis from aminoacids
- PP *terminates the action of steroid hormone* by removing the hormone receptor complex from DNA binding. So there ***is increased sensitivity to actions of low concentrations of cortisol, androgen, estrogen and vitamin D, which may l/t development of hormone dependent cancers of breast, uterus, & prostate and vitamin $B_6$ status may affect the prognosis***[Q]
- *Isoniazid, OCP, cycloserine and alcohol* may induce B6 deficiency.
- Vit B6 status is assessed by assaying
  - **Activation coefficient** i.e. *activation of RBC transaminase by pyridoxal phosphate added* in vitro.
  - **Xanthurenic acid index (tryptophan loading test)** i.e. *excretion of Xanthurenate (or Xandhurenic acid) in urine after a feeding test dose of tryptophan* is diagnostic of $B_6$ deficiency
- $B_6$ is the only water soluble vitamin with significant toxicity. **Sensory neuropathy** occur at > 200 mg / day doses (used to treat *premenstrual syndrome). Substantial improvement with some residual damage (i.e. recovery is not complete) occurs on discontinuation of vitamin.*

## Physiological role

- $B_6$ is important in ***aminoacid metabolism for transamination, deamination, decarboxylation and condensation***[Q].

| Substrate | Pyridoxal Phosphate ($B_6$) Dependent Decarboxylation | Product |
|---|---|---|
| **Histidine** | | **Histamine** |
| **Tyrosine** | | **Dopamine, NE, Epinephrine** |
| **Glutamate** | | **GABA** |
| **Tryptophan** | | **Serotonin** |
| **Ornithine & Methioine** | | **Spermidine, Spermine** (involved in DNA packaging) |

- So defective allergic response & gastric acid secretion (d/t histamine); deterioration of **parkinson's disease** (d/t dopamine); epileptic seizures (d/t GABA, an inhibitory neurotransmitter) can result from $B_6$ deficiency.

Glycine + Succinyl CoA — **PLP** dependent condensation by rate limiting **ALA synthase** in heme synthesis → δ-ALA (amino levulinic acid)

**Tryptophan** --→ Kynurenine — 3′-OH-Kynurenine — **PLP dependent kynureninase** → 3-OH-Anthranilic acid → **Niacin**

Kynurenine ↓ **Xanthurenic Acid**

- $B_6$ deficiency results in (**sideroblastic** / **sidero achrestic** i.e. microcytic hypochromic) **anemia** (d/t defective ALA synthase in heme /porphyrin synthesis), **xanthurenicaciduria** and **pellagra** (d/t defective kynureninase). One vitamin ($B_6$) is necessary for synthesis of other vitamin (niacin). So niacin is not strictly a vitamin as it can be synthesized from tryptophan (essential aa) in body.

Methionine ---→ **Homocysteine** — (↑ **Serine**) **PLP dependent Transsulfuration** by *Cystathionine β-synthase & γ-cystathionase* → Cystathionine & then cysteine

Homocysteine + **$N^5$ methyl THF** → **Methyl-$B_{12}$ dependent** re methylation by *methionine synthase* ↓ Methionine

- $B_6$ deficiency cases **hyperhomomo cystinemia & homocystinuria** l/t cardiovascular diseases and **oxaluria** l/t **kidney stones.**
- $B_6$ is required in glycogen metabolism as *a cofactor (& constituent of) glycogen phosphorylase* (4 molecule of PLP per enzyme molecule)
- $B_6$ is required in *CoA synthesis, sphingomyelin synthesis (so def.causes peripheral neuritis d/t defective myelination), arachidonic acid* synthesis (from linoleic acid), intramitochondrial FA synthesis and $K^+$ transport (from out to inside).

**$N^5$, $N^{10}$, Methyl THF** ⇄ **THF**

**Glycine** ⇄ **Serine** (PLP dependent serine hydroxyl methyl transferase)

**Glycine** ↓ **Glyoxylate** ↓ Oxalate (Primary **oxaluria type 1**)

## Vitamin $B_{12}$ (Cobalamine, Extrinsic Factor of Castle, Animal protein/Anti Pernicious Anemia-Factor)

### Structure

- Vitamin $B_{12}$ or **cobalamins** are *those* **corrinoids** (i.e. **cobalt containing** compounds possessing **corrin ring**) which show vitamin activity. (some corrinoid growth factors have no vitamin activity & even are antimetabolite)
- Central portion of $B_{12}$, consists of **4 pyrrole rings** (reduced & extensively substituted) surrounding a **single cobalt (Co)** atom and is k/a **Corrin ring system**. This differs from porphyrins only in that 2 of pyrrole rings *(i.e. ring 1 & 4) are linked directly* rather than through a methene bond.
- **1 cobalt (Co) atom** (with 6 valency) is joined to **4 pyrrole rings, 1 DBI** (i.e. 5, 6 Dimethyl Benzimidazole riboside) **ring**. The 6th valency is satisfied by any of the following group **cyanide** (added to get stable crystals in oral preparations CN has no physiological function, k/a cyano- cobalamine); **hydroxyl** (k/a hydroxyl cobalamine or $B_{12}a$ is superior more active form that is retained longer in body; can be injectible), $SO_4$, $Cl^-$ or $NO_2$ (i.e. nitro-cobalamine or $B_{12}c$)
- **Coenzyme forms of cobalamine** are methyl and adenosyl cobalamine. These are formed in body when 6th valency (like CN-) is replaced by methyl or 5' – deoxyadenosine group respectively. **Methyl-cobalamine** is major form seen in cytoplasm of cells & blood circulation, whereas **Ado (adenosine) B12** is the major *storage form seen in liver*

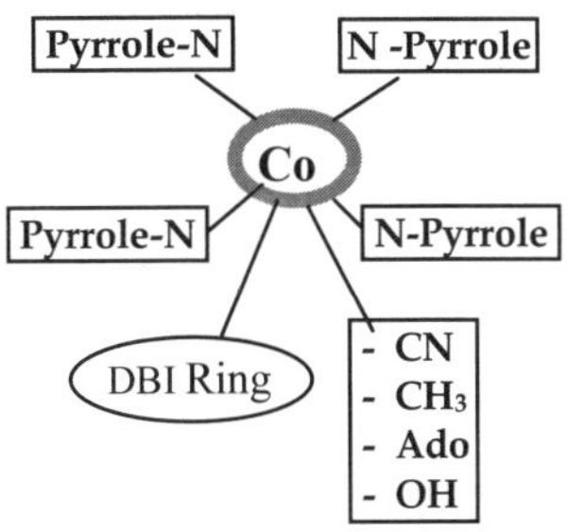


### Source & Absorption

- It is synthesized exclusively by **microorganisms** & (for all practical purposes) ***found only in foods of animal origin***Q. Vit $B_{12}$ has ***no plant sources***Q which means that strict vegetarians (vegans) are at risk of developing $B_{12}$ deficiency.
- Small amounts of $B_{12}$ formed by bacteria on surface of fruits may be adequate to meet the requirements
- 2 factors required for absorption of $B_{12}$ are
  - **Cobalophilin** secreted in *saliva* bind to $B_{12}$ when *gastric acid & pepsin* release the vitamin from protein in food.
  - ***Intrinsic factor (IF) of castle***Q, a small ***glycoprotein secreted by parietal cells of gastric mucosa***Q (in cardiac end & fundus but not in pylorus) **binds only to active vitamin $B_{12}$ vitamers** (and not other corrinoids) **in duodenum**, where cardiophilin is detached (hydrolyzed) from $B_{12}$ by trypsin of pancreatic juice. That's why pancreatic insufficiency result in excretion of cobalophilin bound vitamin $B_{12}$ causing its deficiency. 1 molecule of IF can combine with 2 molecules of $B_{12}$
- ***Vit $B_{12}$ is absorbed from distal third of ileum***Q by receptors that internalize whole IF-$B_{12}$ complex but not free IF or $B_{12}$. $B_{12}$ seperates from IF by **releasing factor (RF)** secreted by duodenum, and $Ca^{++}$
- Vitamin $B_{12}$ is transported in blood as methyl $B_{12}$ with *trans cobalamin glycoprotein;* and stored in liver as ado-$B_{12}$ with transcorrin in amounts sufficient for 2-3 years (an exception as B complex is not stored in body)

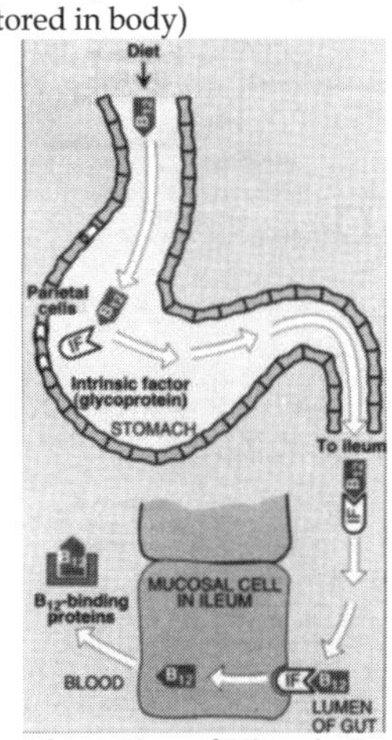


**Absorption of Vitamin $B_{12}$**

### Deficiency

- 3 enzymes **methyl malonyl CoA mutase (or isomerase), leucine amino mutase, and methionine synthase** are $B_{12}$ dependent
- **Methyl malonic acid uria**
  - Methyl malonyl CoA is formed as an intermediate in catabolism of valine, threonine, isoleucine & methenine aminoacids and (by carboxylation of propionyl CoA arising in catabolism of) cholesterol side chains, isoleucine & fatty acids with odd numbers of carbon atoms or directly from proprionate

| - **FA (odd numbers)**<br>- **Cholesterol side chain**<br>- **AA (Valine, Threonine, isoleucine, Methionine)**<br>- **Propionate** | ·····▶ | **L Methyl Malonyl CoA** —($B_{12}$; **MM Isomerase** (mutase))→ **Succinyl CoA** |
|---|---|---|

  - In $B_{12}$ deficiency methyl malonyl accumulates and its *urinary excretion provides a means of assessing $B_{12}$ nutritional status.*
  - Accumulation of unusual fatty acids and their incorporation in cell membrane of nervous system may account for neurological manifestations.
  - ***Hyper homocysteinemia, homo cystinuria l/t cardiovascular diseases, like atherosclerosis, thrombosis, hypertension and MI***Q
- **Folate Trap and Pernicious Anemia**

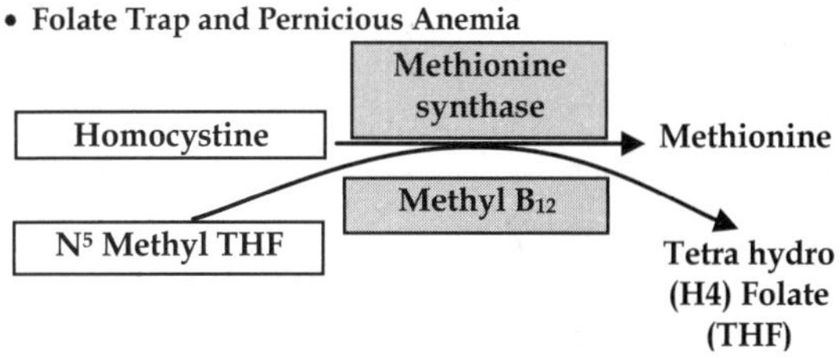


  - Effect of $B_{12}$ def. is most pronounced in rapidly dividing cells of *bone marrow erythropoietic tissue & intestinal mucosa* as these need both the $N_5$ $N_{10}$ methylene & $N_{10}$ formyl forms of THF for ***synthesis of nucleotides required for DNA replication***Q
  - In $B_{12}$ deficiency, d/t dysfunction of methionine synthase methylation of homocysteine by $N_5$ methyl THF is hampered l/t accumulation of both.
  - Because methylated form cannot be directly converted to other forms of tetrahydro folate (THF), the **folate is trapped in $N_5$ methyl form**, which accumulates. The level of other form decreases l/t **functional folate deficiency** (*needed for purine & TMP synthesis*). Decreased DNA synthesis disturbs erythropoiesis, causing immature precursor of RBC to be released in circulation l/t **megaloblastic / pernicious anemia.**
- **Subacute combined degeneration (SACD) & Demyelination**
  - D/t methionine deficiency in CNS, there is irreversible degeneration of spinal cord, as a result of failure of methylation of one arginine residue on myelin basic protein. Therefore inadequate methylation of phosphotidyl ethanolamine to phosphatidyl choline l/t deficient formation of myelin sheath of nerves and demyelination.
  - **Nieweg's hypothesis** explain why only $B_{12}$ def. is a/w neurological lesions whereas, both B12 and folic acid deficiency cause megaloblastic anemia. This occurs because folate is only concerned with DNA synthesis, whereas $B_{12}$ is required for both DNA & RNA synthesis.

Precursor —($B_{12}$)→ Uracil —(**Folic Acid**)→ Thiamine → **DNA** (Bone, marrow mucosa of GI tract)

$B_{12}$ ——→ **RNA** (Nervous system)

- ***Both $B_{12}$ & folate correct megaloblastic anemia by increasing DNA synthesis***Q. Only folate supplements may put some people at risk as this would rectify (correct) megaloblastic anemia but may hasten development of irreversible nerve damage.
- Schilling **(radioactive lebelled Cobalt-60)** test **is done to assess B12 deficiency.**

## Functions of Vit K

### Synthesis & activation of clotting factors

- Vitamin K is required in **hepatic synthesis** and **post translational modification** (by **$\gamma$ carboxylation of glutamate residues**) of **calcium binding clotting factors** (proteins) **prothrombin**, ***2, 7, 9, 10***[Q], ***protein C & protein S***[Q].
- Vitamin K dependent clotting factors are ***2, 7, 9, 10 and protein C & protein S***[Q]
- Carboxylation is inhibited by ***dicumarol (natural analog of vitamin K) and warfarin***[Q] (synthetic analog of vitamin K)
- Vitamin K ***deficiency l/t hemorrhagic disease of newborn (HDN)***[Q]

★ In presence of warfarin, *Vitamin K epoxide* can not be reduced to quinone (by warfarin sensitive reductase), but accumulates & excreted. ***A high dose of vitamin K is an antidote to warfarin overdose***[Q], which is reduced to active hydroquinone by warfarin insensitive enzyme.

### Oxidative phosphorylation

- Being associated with mitochondiral lipid, vitamin K is a necessary cofactor in oxiative phosphorylation.
- ***Dicumarol (vitamin K antagonist)***[Q] is uncoupler of oxidative phosphorylation

### Synthesis of calcium binding bone proteins

- Vit K is required in synthesis of two bone proteins. ***Osteocalcin and bone matrix Gla protein***[Q] that contain $\gamma$- carboxy glutamate.
- **Osteocalcin** also contains **hydroxyproline**, so its synthesis is also dependent *on both vitamin K and C*; and also its synthesis is induced by *vitamin D*. The release of osteocalcin into circulation *provides an index of vitamin D status.*
- Warfarin treatment in pregnancy l/t fetal bone abnormalities (fetal Warfarin syndrome) d/t defective synthesis of bone calcium binding proteins caused by vit K deficiency.

## Functions of Vit C (Acorbic acid)

- Main function of ascorbate is as **reducing agent** in different reactions because it can reversibly chang b/w ascorbic acid & dehydro ascorbic acid (reversible oxidation & reduction)
- Co-enzyme for **copper containing hydroxylases** eg
  - **Dopamine β hydroxylase** involved in synthesis of catecholamines (epinephrine & norepinephrine) from tyrosine in CNS and adrenal medulla.
  - Peptidylglycine hydroxylase, hydroxylating terminal glycine residue
- Co enzyme for **α-ketoglutarate linked iron containing hydroxylases**, in which hydroxylation of substrate is linked to decarboxylation of α-ketoglutarate examples are
  - **Proline & lysine hydroxylases** are required for hydroxylation of ***prolyl (proline) & lysyl (lysine) residues of collagen, in postsynthetic modification of procollagen to colagen***[Q].
  - Proline hydroxylase is also required in synthesis of **osteocalcin & C1q** component of **complement**.
  - **Trimethyllysine & γ-butyrobetaine hydroxylases** are required for **carnitine** synthesis.
  - **Aspartate β-hydroxylase** is required for post translational modification of precursor of protein C (a vitamin K dependent protease that hydrolyse activated factor V in blood clotting cascade)
  - *Vitamin C* is **antioxidant** (just like *vitamin E & β carotene*) and can decrease incidence of common cold; and some chronic diseases like cataract, *coronary heart disease & cancer*. Its deficiency l/t **scurvy**, Barlow's disease (infantile scurvy), hemorrhagic tendency & poor wound healing
  - Help in deposition of **c**ollagen in bone
  - Maintenance of <u>C</u>apillary integrity
  - Help in <u>**A**</u>bsorption of Fe
  - Prevent formation of <u>**A**</u>*theromatous plaque*
  - Involved in Electron <u>**T**</u>ransport chain: contribute to *microsomal hydroxylation reaction.* **[Mn : "C A T"]**

## Vitamin A

### Structure

- Active form
  - ***Retinol***[Q]
  - ***Retinal***[Q]
  - ***Retinoic acid***[Q]
- Retinal is a ***component of visual pigment rhodopsin***[Q].
- **β Carotenes** are found in certain plants, cleaved to yield 2 mol. Of retinal

### Transport & Storage

- Dietary retinal is transported as retinyl esters *in chylomicrons*
- Stored form is ***retinyl esters***[Q] mainly in liver & adipose tissue

↓ Zn

Mobilized form

### Functions

- ***Vision***[Q]
- Maintenance of reproduction
- ***Antinfective***[Q]
- ***Antioxidant***[Q]
- ***Anticarcinogenic***[Q]

### Visual cycle in Retina

All trans retinol
↓
All trans retinal
↓
***11- Cis retinal***[Q]
↓ ← Opsin
**Rhodopsin**
Light ↓ → Opsin
All trans retinal (↺ back to 11-Cis retinal)

### Deficiency

- Night blindness
- Xeropthelmia
- Impotence
- Growth retardation

### Prevalence criteria for determining the xeroplathalamia problem

| Criteria | **Prevalence in population at risk (6 month – 6yr)** |
|---|---|
| Bitol's spot | >0.5% |
| Corneal ulcer | >0.05% |
| Serum retinal | >5% |
| Corneal xerosis | >0.01% |
| Nightblind-ness | >1% |

## Vitamin A Intoxication

### Acute

- Seen after administration of >100 mg in children or > 150 mg in adult
- 1st noticed in arctic explores who ate polar bear liver.
- P manifests as ***increased intracranial pressure, bulging fontanels (in children), seizure, vertigo, diplopia, exfoliative dermatitis***[Q] *and death.*

### Chronic

- Seen after chronic ingestion (for several months) of > *6mg/day in children or >15 mg/day in adults.*
- It manifests as
  - ***Pseudotumor cerebri***[Q] with increased TCP & papilledema
  - Vomiting
  - Alopecia
  - Dryskin
  - Cheliosis
  - Glossitis
  - Bone demineralization
  - Bone pain
  - Hypercalcemia
  - Hyperlipidemia
  - Lymphadenopathy
  - Liver fibrosis
  - Portal hypertension
  - Hyper lipidemia
  - **Teratogenic effects**
    - Amenorrhea
    - Spontaneous abortion
    - Craniofacial abnormality
    - Valvular heart disease

## Vitamin D

$D_2D_3$ (Diet) + 7-OH-cholecalciferol (Skin) ← UV light

→ Vit $D_3$

↓ ***25(OH)*** — ***Liver***[Q]

25(OH) Vit $D_3$

↓ ***1 ∝ (OH)*** — ***Kidney***[Q]

1.25 $(OH)_2$ Vit $D_3$ [Active form]

- ↑absorption of $Ca^{2+}$ from gut
- ↑mineralization of bone

- It behaves like a *steroid hormone,* binding to a nuclear receptor protein.
- **Deficiency:**
  - Rickets (In children)
  - Osteomalacia (In adults)
- **Toxicity:** Vitamin D is most toxic of all vitamins
  - ↑ serum $Ca^{2+}$
    - ↑BP
    - Vaso constriction
    - Calcinosis [soft tissue calcification]
  - Nausea
  - Stupor